Handbook of Experimental Pharmacology

Volume 270

The *Handbook of Experimental Pharmacology* is one of the most authoritative and influential book series in pharmacology. It provides critical and comprehensive discussions of the most significant areas of pharmacological research, written by leading international authorities. Each volume in the series represents the most informative and contemporary account of its subject available, making it an unrivalled reference source.

HEP is indexed in PubMed and Scopus.

More information about this series at https://link.springer.com/bookseries/164

Arnold von Eckardstein • Christoph J. Binder
Editors

Prevention and Treatment of Atherosclerosis

Improving State-of-the-Art
Management and Search for
Novel Targets

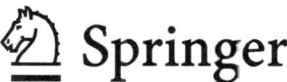 Springer

Editors
Arnold von Eckardstein
Institute of Clinical Chemistry
University Hospital Zurich
Zurich, Switzerland

Christoph J. Binder
Department of Laboratory Medicine
Medical University of Vienna
Vienna, Austria

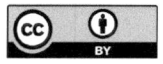

ISSN 0171-2004   ISSN 1865-0325   (electronic)
Handbook of Experimental Pharmacology
ISBN 978-3-030-86075-2   ISBN 978-3-030-86076-9   (eBook)
https://doi.org/10.1007/978-3-030-86076-9

This Springer imprint is published by the registered company Springer Nature Switzerland AG.
The registered company address is: Gewerbestrasse 11, 6330 Cham, Switzerland

Preface

We are proud editors of this follow-up edition of the well-received *Handbook of Experimental Pharmacology* Volume 170 "Atherosclerosis: Diet and Drugs," which was published more than 15 years ago. Since then, major progress has been made in the primary and secondary prevention of atherosclerotic cardiovascular diseases (ASCVDs), thanks to improved control of the classical risk factors with well-established causality in the pathogenesis of ASCVDs, namely, LDL-cholesterol, blood pressure, diabetes, and prothrombotic states. The five chapters in the first part of this book summarize the progress in this evidence-based state-of-the-art management of ASCVDs as well as the perspectives of ongoing drug developments towards better control of these risk factors. The five subsequent chapters of Part II address the state of research and development towards the control of risk factors which are well established by epidemiology but still equivocal due to negative, contradictory, or missing outcomes of randomized controlled trials [triglycerides, HDL-cholesterol, Lipoprotein(a), obesity, nutraceuticals]. Vascular and immune cells, adipose tissue as well as microbiota are important in the pathogenesis of atherosclerosis and intensely investigated. The validation of some anti-inflammatory drugs (e.g., colchicine or methotrexate) or targets (interleukin 1 beta) by clinical trials has been started and generated promising results in first trials. The six chapters of Part III describe the ongoing translational efforts directed to unravel and validate novel target molecules for drug development. Hypothesis-free systems biology approaches have become an important strategy also in atherosclerosis research, which are covered by the four chapters of Part IV. Genomics, transcriptomics, proteomics, and metabolomics have successfully helped to identify novel players in the pathogenesis of atherosclerosis or validate the causality of candidate molecules or processes in the development or clinical manifestation of ASCVDs.

This *Handbook of Experimental Pharmacology* on atherosclerosis is part of the educational activities of the European Atherosclerosis Society (https://www.eas-society.org). EAS finances the open access publication of this handbook, to foster the training and promotion of early career scientists and the dissemination of old and new knowledge on ASCVD and their risk factors to the scientific and medical community as well as the lay public. As the editors of this Handbook of Experimental Pharmacology, we gratefully acknowledge not only this financial but also the moral and intellectual support by the Executive Committee of EAS. We applaud the authors of the 19 chapters for their engagement and reliable cooperation. Finally, we thank Prof. Martin Michel for his sustained interest and guidance as well as Susanne Dathe, Alamelu Damodharan, and Anand Ventakachalam from Springer Nature who supported us with patience and enthusiasm in the production of this book.

Zurich, Switzerland   Arnold von Eckardstein
Vienna, Austria   Christoph J. Binder
August 2021

Acknowledgement

This publication is supported by the European Atherosclerosis Society (EAS; https://www.eas-society.org), which also covered the costs of its Open Access dissemination

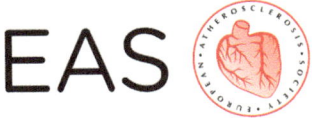

For more than 50 years, the Society's expertise has been used to teach clinicians how to manage lipid disorders and how to prevent atherosclerosis. Through its publications, EAS creates a framework for discussion of new developments in the field. Activities cover the prevention and care of atherosclerosis and its clinical manifestations, and also basic science in the atherosclerosis field. With live and online educational activities including Advanced Courses, Rare Lipid Disorder Courses, and its Annual Congress, EAS supports exchange of knowledge between scientists and clinicians. Many lectures from these events are recorded and available on the Society's educational platform, EAS Academy. By reaching out to involve young scientists and researchers also from related disciplines, EAS strengthens and expands development of the field now and in the future. These activities will ultimately lead to improved healthcare for persons with cardiovascular disease and lipid disorders.

Contents

Part I   Improving the Treatment of Established Targets

Diet, Lifestyle, Smoking   3
Lale Tokgozoglu, Vedat Hekimsoy, Giuseppina Costabile, Ilaria Calabrese,
and Gabriele Riccardi

Blood Pressure-Lowering Therapy   25
Isabella Sudano, Elena Osto, and Frank Ruschitzka

Glycaemic Control in Diabetes   47
D. Müller-Wieland, J. Brandts, M. Verket, N. Marx, and K. Schütt

LDL-Cholesterol-Lowering Therapy   73
Angela Pirillo, Giuseppe D. Norata, and Alberico L. Catapano

**Antithrombotic Therapy: Prevention and Treatment of Atherosclerosis
and Atherothrombosis** 103
R. H. Olie, P. E. J. van der Meijden, H. M. H. Spronk, and H. ten Cate

Part II   Novel Drug Developments Addressing Predefined Targets

Metabolism of Triglyceride-Rich Lipoproteins 133
Jan Borén and Marja-Riitta Taskinen

**High Density Lipoproteins: Is There a Comeback as a Therapeutic
Target?** 157
Arnold von Eckardstein

Lipoprotein(a) 201
Florian Kronenberg

Nonalcoholic Fatty Liver Disease 233
Lingling Ding, Yvonne Oligschlaeger, Ronit Shiri-Sverdlov,
and Tom Houben

**Prevention and Treatment of Atherosclerosis: The Use
of Nutraceuticals and Functional Foods** 271
Francesco Visioli and Andrea Poli

Part III   Hypothesis Based Approaches to Unravel Novel Targets

Novel Adipose Tissue Targets to Prevent and Treat Atherosclerosis   289
Ludger Scheja and Joerg Heeren

Microbiome and Cardiovascular Disease   311
Hilde Herrema, Max Nieuwdorp, and Albert K. Groen

**Smooth Muscle Cell-Proteoglycan-Lipoprotein Interactions as Drivers
of Atherosclerosis**   335
Sima Allahverdian, Carleena Ortega, and Gordon A. Francis

**Anti-inflammatory and Immunomodulatory Therapies
in Atherosclerosis**   359
Justine Deroissart, Florentina Porsch, Thomas Koller,
and Christoph J. Binder

**Neutrophil Extracellular Traps in Atherosclerosis
and Thrombosis**   405
Thomas M. Hofbauer, Anna S. Ondracek, and Irene M. Lang

Part IV   Hypothesis-free Approaches to Unravel Novel Targets

**Genomic Strategies Toward Identification of Novel Therapeutic
Targets**   429
Thorsten Kessler and Heribert Schunkert

Regulatory Non-coding RNAs in Atherosclerosis   463
Andreas Schober, Saffiyeh Saboor Maleki, and Maliheh Nazari-Jahantigh

Lipidomics in Biomarker Research   493
Thorsten Hornemann

The Epigenome in Atherosclerosis   511
Sarah Costantino and Francesco Paneni

Correction to: Blood Pressure-Lowering Therapy   537
Isabella Sudano, Elena Osto, and Frank Ruschitzka

Part I

Improving the Treatment of Established Targets

Diet, Lifestyle, Smoking

Lale Tokgozoglu, Vedat Hekimsoy, Giuseppina Costabile,
Ilaria Calabrese, and Gabriele Riccardi

Contents

1 Diet 5
  1.1 Dietary Fat (Table 1) 6
  1.2 Dietary Carbohydrates (Table 1) 8
  1.3 Salt (Table 1) 10
2 Physical Activity 12
3 Smoking 15
References 17

Abstract

Cardiovascular disease is the leading cause of death globally The past few decades have shown that especially low- and middle-income countries have undergone rapid industrialization, urbanization, economic development and market globalization. Although these developments led to many positive changes in health outcomes and increased life expectancies, they all also caused inappropriate dietary patterns, physical inactivity and obesity. Evidence shows that a large proportion of the cardiovascular disease burden can be explained by behavioural factors such as low physical activity, unhealthy diet and smoking. Controlling these risk factors from early ages is important for maintaining cardiovascular health. Even in patients with genetic susceptibility to cardiovascular disease, risk factor modification is beneficial.

Despite the tremendous advances in the medical treatment of cardiovascular risk factors to reduce overall cardiovascular risk, the modern lifestyle which has led to

L. Tokgozoglu (✉) · V. Hekimsoy
Department of Cardiology, Hacettepe University Faculty of Medicine, Ankara, Turkey

G. Costabile · I. Calabrese · G. Riccardi
Department of Clinical Medicine and Surgery, Federico II University, Naples, Italy
e-mail: riccardi@unina.it

© The Author(s) 2020
A. von Eckardstein, C. J. Binder (eds.), *Prevention and Treatment of Atherosclerosis*,
Handbook of Experimental Pharmacology 270, https://doi.org/10.1007/164_2020_353

3

greater sedentary time, lower participation in active transport and time spent in leisure or purposeful physical activity, unhealthy diets and increased exposure to stress, noise and pollution have diminished the beneficial effects of contemporary medical cardiovascular prevention strategies. Therefore attenuating or eliminating these health risk behaviours and risk factors is imperative in the prevention of cardiovascular diseases.

Keywords

Cardiovascular diseases · Diet · Lifestyle · Prevention

The global burden of disease has dramatically shifted from communicable to non-communicable diseases, making cardiovascular disease (CVD) the leading cause of death in Europe as well as most parts of the world. According to 2017 European Cardiovascular Disease Statistics, there are more than 11 million new cases of cardiovascular disease in Europe, and cardiovascular disease accounts for 45% of all deaths. Europe is in the midst of an epidemiologic, economic, social and nutritional transition. The past few decades have shown that especially low- and middle-income countries have undergone rapid industrialization, urbanization, economic development and market globalization. Although these developments led to many positive changes in health outcomes and increased life expectancies, they all also caused inappropriate dietary patterns, physical inactivity and obesity. Fat and energy consumption is increasing mostly in Eastern Europe, and smoking remains a key public health issue despite decline in some countries.

The causal factors for CVD are well defined today. Genetic susceptibility, environmental factors and lifestyle are the most important determinants of cardiovascular health. Preventable or treatable risk factors such as high blood pressure, high cholesterol, diabetes, smoking and obesity play an important role in the development of cardiovascular disease as well as lifestyle, socioeconomic and environmental conditions. We also know that socioeconomic deprivation increases the dependence on alcohol and tobacco use as well as leading to consumption of unhealthy foods. When we look at the ranking of European countries according to GDP per capita, we see that cardiovascular risk goes hand in hand with low income.

Although genetic susceptibility is extremely important in the development of cardiovascular disease, even the subjects with high genetic risk derive benefit from healthy lifestyles. In a recent study, genetic risk was determined by a polygenic risk score of up to 50 single-nucleotide polymorphisms and adherence to a healthy lifestyle consisting of 4 factors (no current smoking, no obesity, healthy diet and regular physical activity). A favourable lifestyle was associated with a 50% lower relative risk of CAD in all three groups of low, intermediate and high genetic risk (Khera et al. 2016). A healthy lifestyle will modify and decrease traditional risk factors like hypertension, diabetes, dyslipidemia and obesity. In addition lifestyle modification has positive effects beyond attenuation of traditional risk factors. To maintain cardiovascular health, it is important to strive for optimal levels of four health behaviours (non-smoking, body mass index <25 kg/m^2, physical activity and ideal diet) and three health factors (untreated total cholesterol <200 mg/dL, untreated blood pressure $<120/<80$ mmHg and fasting blood glucose <100 mg/dL) (Lloyd-Jones et al. 2010).

Although there have been tremendous advances in the medical treatment of cardiovascular risk factors in the past decades, the same cannot be said for lifestyle. The modern lifestyles have led to greater sedentary time, lower participation in active transport and time spent in leisure or purposeful physical activity, unhealthy diets and increased exposure to stress, noise and pollution.

1   Diet

The evidence that dietary factors influence the development of CVD derives mainly from epidemiological observations and from clinical studies on the impact of dietary changes on traditional risk factors such as plasma lipids, blood pressure or glucose levels.

In fact, epidemiological studies clearly indicate that higher consumption of fruit, non-starchy vegetables, nuts, legumes, fish, vegetable oils, yogurt and whole grains, along with a lower intake of red and processed meats and foods high in refined carbohydrates and salt, is associated with a reduced incidence of cardiovascular events. Moreover, they indicate that the replacement of animal fats, including dairy fats, with PUFAs or other vegetable sources of fats as well as fibre-rich carbohydrate foods can decrease the risk of CVD (Forouhi et al. 2018; Sacks et al. 2017).

Conversely, the evidence from randomized controlled trials (RCTs) is based on few studies that provide, in some cases, conflicting results. In this respect, the difficulties of performing clinical trials that adequately test nutritional interventions for CVD prevention cannot be underestimated since these studies require thousands of participants followed for years or decades. As to the lack of concordance between studies, this is due not only to methodological problems, particularly inadequate sample size or the short duration of many trials, but also to the difficulty of evaluating the impact of a single dietary factor independently of any other change in the diet (Forouhi et al. 2018).

These limitations suggest caution in interpreting the results of RCTs or even meta-analyses of RCTs in relation to the effect of a single dietary change on CVD, particularly where they diverge from the existing global evidence (Catapano et al. 2016). Therefore, in evaluating the role of diet in the prevention of cardiovascular diseases, we will consider not only RCTs on the impact dietary modifications on CVD events but also observational studies and clinical trials on the effects on major CVD risk factors.

Table 1 Summary of the effects of dietary fatty acids, carbohydrates and salt on cardiovascular risk factors and cardiovascular events

	LDL-C	Triglycerides	HDL-C	Plasma glucose	Insulin sensitivity	Blood pressure	CVD
Trans fatty acids	↑↑	–/↑	↓↓	–	↓↓	–	↑↑
SAFA	↑↑	–	–/↑	–	↓↓	↑	↑
MUFA	–	–	–	↓	↑	↓/–	↓
PUFA n-6	–	↓	↓	↓/–	↑	↓/–	↓
PUFA n-3	–	↓↓ (at high dose)	–	–	–	↓ (at high dose)	↓ (at high dose)
Refined starch	–	↑	↓	↑	↓	–	–
Sugars	–	↑↑	↓	↑ (long term)	↓↓	↑/–	↑
Dietary fiber	↓↓	–/↓	–	↓↓	↑	↓	↓
Salt	–	–	–	–	–	↑	↑

↑ increase; ↓ decrease; – no effect

1.1 Dietary Fat (Table 1)

1.1.1 Effects on CVD Risk Factors

The available evidence supports current dietary guidelines recommending that saturated fatty acid (SAFA) intake be reduced and replaced with unsaturated fatty acids. This approach aims at improving blood lipid and lipoprotein profile in order to reduce the risk of coronary heart diseases, since high LDL cholesterol and elevated plasma triglyceride concentrations are established independent CVD risk factors (Catapano et al. 2016; Graham et al. 2012; Reiner 2013; Reiner et al. 2011). A reduction in dietary SAFA intake can be achieved through the isocaloric replacement with unsaturated fatty acids, mainly monounsaturated (MUFA, mostly cis-oleic acid) or polyunsaturated fatty acids (PUFAs) or with dietary carbohydrates. According to the results of meta-analyses of RCTs, replacing 5% of calories from SAFA with MUFA or PUFA (predominantly linoleic acid; C18:2n-6) is able to significantly reduce LDL cholesterol levels by 0.21 mmol/L (8 mg/dL) and 0.28 mmol/L (11 mg/dL), respectively. In addition, this dietary approach is able to significantly improve insulin sensitivity and reduce triglyceride levels, mostly in the postprandial period; notably, the triglyceride-lowering effect is more pronounced with n-6 PUFA than with MUFA. As for HDL cholesterol levels, there is no relevant effect when SAFA is replaced by MUFA, whereas a small decrease occurs when they are substituted by n-6 PUFA (Mensink et al. 2003). Replacing SAFA with refined carbohydrates also reduces LDL cholesterol levels (by 0.16 mmol/L, 6.2 mg/

dL), but has untoward effects on other lipoproteins, namely, HDL cholesterol and plasma triglyceride levels.

Dietary trans-fatty acids (TFAs) are partially hydrogenated fatty acids formed when oils are solidified to produce margarine. Overall, the average intake of trans-fatty acids in western countries is presently low and derives mainly from foods of industrial origin. Quantitatively, dietary trans-fatty acids increase LDL cholesterol levels to the same extent as saturated fat, although, at variance with SAFA, they induce a marked reduction of HDL cholesterol levels (Mensink et al. 2003).

Among the various types of dietary fat, the most relevant effect on plasma triglycerides is achieved with long-chain n-3 polyunsaturated fatty acids; however, in order to reach an intake sufficient to induce a clinically relevant triglyceride-lowering effect (usually 25–30%), it is necessary to rely on foods artificially enriched with n-3 polyunsaturated fat or on pharmacological supplements. Dietary fatty acids may also affect other non-lipid CVD risk factors, particularly, blood pressure (Rasmussen et al. 2006; Zock et al. 2016). In fact, the results from the DIVAS study – a 16-week parallel group RCT on individuals with moderate CVD risk – showed that the isocaloric replacement of 9.5–9.6% of calories from SAFA with MUFA or n-6 PUFA attenuated the increase in night systolic pressure (-4.9 mmHg, $p = 0.019$) and reduced E-selectin. In line with this finding, a multicentre study in which our group was involved demonstrated that in healthy individuals, the consumption of a diet rich in MUFA for 3 months, compared to a SAFA-rich diet, significantly decreased diastolic blood pressure, provided that total fat intake was not exceedingly high (below 35–40% energy intake) (Rasmussen et al. 2006). The beneficial effects of replacing SAFA with unsaturated fat have been summarized in a meta-analysis reporting significantly lower systolic and diastolic blood pressure with high-MUFA diets (Schwingshackl et al. 2011). As to n-3 PUFA, lower blood pressure levels were observed only in hypertensive subjects given >3 g/day as pharmacological supplement (Miller et al. 2014).

Dietary fatty acids are also able to influence insulin sensitivity and, more in general, glucose metabolism; this was suggested by a recent meta-analysis of RCTs indicating that increased PUFA intake is able to improve long-term glycaemic control and reduce insulin resistance (Imamura et al. 2016). In particular, replacing 5% of calories from SAFA partially replacing SAFA or carbohydrates with PUFA or MUFA improved both blood glucose control and insulin sensitivity; moreover, PUFA increased also insulin secretion (Imamura et al. 2016). Other clinical trials have shown that the isocaloric replacement of SAFA with MUFA or PUFA improved insulin sensitivity in healthy subjects (Vessby et al. 2001) and also reduced hepatic fat accumulation (Summers et al. 2002). In line with these findings, Bozzetto and colleagues showed that partially replacing SAFA and carbohydrates with MUFA for an 8-week period induced a clinically relevant reduction of hepatic fat content (29%) in type 2 diabetic patients (Bozzetto et al. 2012).

1.1.2 Effects on CVD Events

TFAs represent one of the few dietary components unanimously considered as deleterious in relation to the cardiovascular risk. Data in the literature are very consistent in showing that TFA intake is associated with a higher risk of CVD and sudden death; this relationship is stronger than with any other nutrient (Mozaffarian et al. 2006). In fact, a meta-analysis of four prospective cohort studies has shown that a 2% increase in energy intake from TFAs is associated with a 23% higher incidence of coronary heart disease (CHD) (Mozaffarian et al. 2006).

In recent years, concern has been expressed regarding the impact of dietary saturated fatty acids (SFAs) on cardiovascular risk. The uncertainty stems from recent meta-analyses failing to find an association between the amount of SFA in the habitual diet and the incidence of CVD (Chowdhury et al. 2014; Siri-Tarino et al. 2010). However, other meta-analyses of prospective studies and RCTs as well as large longitudinal observations clearly indicate that high SFA is linked with a small but potentially important increase in cardiovascular risk (Jakobsen et al. 2009; Li et al. 2015); recently, a Cochrane systematic review has shown that a low-saturated-fat diet induces a 17% reduction in cardiovascular events compared to a control diet (Hooper et al. 2015).

Inconsistencies are due to multiple reasons and, in particular, to the way the data are evaluated; in fact, the meta-analysis by Siri-Tarino overadjusted the outcomes by correcting them for plasma lipid levels, thus eliminating one of the major patho-physiological links between SFA intake and CVD (Siri-Tarino et al. 2010). More in general, in RCTs evaluating the effects of SFAs on CVD, the choice of the foods/nutrients utilized in the control diet to replace SFAs (for instance, unsaturated fat versus refined grains) can influence the effect observed and significantly modify the outcomes of the comparison. The importance of SFA as a risk factor for CVD has been recently underlined by recommendations of scientific societies and public health authorities (Sacks et al. 2017; USDA 2016).

PUFA intake is associated with lower CVD risk, as shown in a meta-analysis of 13 prospective cohort studies (310, 602 subjects) reporting that dietary linoleic acid (LA) intake is inversely associated with the risk of CHD incidence (15%) and mortality (21%) (Farvid et al. 2014).

The available data on the relationship between dietary cholesterol and CVD are inconsistent, probably due to the difficulty to evaluate the impact of dietary choles-terol independently of SAFA that is present in many cholesterol-rich foods. How-ever, a recent meta-analysis from six prospective US cohorts in which many of the possible confounders were properly accounted for showed that each additional 300 mg of dietary cholesterol consumed per day (roughly one egg) was significantly associated with higher risk of CVD incidence (17%) and mortality (18%) (Zhong et al. 2019).

1.2   Dietary Carbohydrates (Table 1)

1.2.1   Effects on CVD Risk Factors

Dietary carbohydrates are the main determinants of postprandial blood glucose levels, which represent an important and independent risk factor for cardiovascular diseases, not only in diabetic patients but also in individuals with normal fasting glucose values (Rivellese et al. 2012). There is a wealth of data indicating that a high intake of refined carbohydrates affects also plasma insulin and triglyceride levels, both at fasting and in the postprandial period, as well as HDL-cholesterol levels (Katan et al. 1997; Riccardi and Rivellese 1991; Sacks and Katan 2002). However, it is worth highlighting that dietary carbohydrates are a heterogeneous class of nutrients that include not only sugars and refined starches but also dietary fibre (i.e. non-starch polysaccharides), with different chemical structures and physical forms and therefore different metabolic effects in relation to their digestion and intestinal activity (Giacco et al. 2016). In line with this concept is the recent evidence supporting the hypothesis that the quality of dietary carbohydrates rather than their amount plays a relevant role in the prevention and development of major cardiovascular risk factors (Reynolds et al. 2019; Riccardi and Costabile 2019). The main indicators of carbohydrate quality refer essentially to the amount of fibre and the glycaemic index of carbohydrate-rich foods as well as the sugar content.

There is consolidated evidence of the beneficial role of consuming low-glycaemic index carbohydrates on blood glucose control, HbA1c levels, fasting and postprandial triglyceride levels and HDL cholesterol levels (Augustin et al. 2015; Riccardi et al. 2008; Thomas and Elliott 2010). However, the best available evidence of the beneficial metabolic impact of low-glycaemic index foods comes from studies in people with type 2 diabetes.

In the last decades, several clinical trials have been conducted to investigate the possible effects of different types of fibre – i.e. fibre from whole grain, legumes, fruit and vegetables and fibre supplements – on body weight changes, blood glucose metabolism, plasma lipids and blood pressure control. The overall evidence shows that soluble fibre, mainly β-glucans from oat and barley but also inulin, guar gum, glucomannan, pectin and psyllium principally found in fruit, vegetables and legumes, are able to significantly reduce plasma LDL-cholesterol levels, improve blood pressure (mainly β-glucan and psyllium) and induce a small reduction in body weight (Bozzetto et al. 2018). Moreover, there is evidence of a triglyceride-lowering effect of dietary fibre and whole grain during the postprandial period (Bozzetto et al. 2014; De Natale et al. 2009; Giacco et al. 2014).

These results support the current nutritional recommendations to replace refined grains with whole grains and increase dietary fibre intake to at least 25–29 g per day to reduce the incidence of the main cardiometabolic risk factors.

Among refined carbohydrates, specific attention should be paid to simple sugars, particularly fructose, whose adverse effects (at amounts higher than 10% of total energy) on human health have been highlighted. According to evidence from observational and intervention studies, the consumption of high fructose-sweetened beverages increases fasting and postprandial triglycerides levels, especially in subjects with obesity and hypertriglyceridemia (Chiavaroli et al. 2015; Stanhope et al. 2009), and also has adverse effects on visceral fat deposition, blood pressure and insulin sensitivity (Stanhope et al. 2009).

1.2.2 Effects on CVD Events

Since dietary carbohydrates are a heterogeneous class of nutrients with different metabolic effects, the evaluation of the relationship between the total amount of carbohydrates in the diet and the incidence of cardiovascular diseases is misleading. In fact, a recent prospective study in 135, 335 individuals from 613 communities in 18 countries has shown, in contrast with the results from meta-analyses of several large cohort studies in North America and Europe, that a high carbohydrate intake is associated with higher risk of total mortality (Dehghan et al. 2017). The reasons for the inconsistency have been highlighted by a recent meta-analysis performed on data from four US communities showing that both very high and very low carbohydrate diets were associated with increased mortality: the lowest mortality was observed in people in whom carbohydrates represented 50–55% of their energy intake (Seidelmann et al. 2018). However, the quality of carbohydrate-rich foods rather than their quantity has the strongest effect on the development of major health outcomes; in this respect, what really matters is the presence of vegetable fibre and/or sugar in the diet.

In fact, a recent meta-analysis reports a 15–30% decrease in all-cause and cardiovascular-related mortality and in the incidence of coronary heart disease between the highest and the lowest dietary fibre intake. The relationship between fibre intake and CVD was linear although the greatest risk reductions were observed for individuals with a fibre intake of 25–29 g/day, mainly provided by cereal fibre; a habitual consumption of 40–50 g/day of whole grains was associated with a risk reduction of 20–30% (Reynolds et al. 2019).

On the other hand, a higher consumption of sugar is associated with an increased risk of coronary events (17% for every serving/day increase in sugar-sweetened beverages consumption) (Xi et al. 2015).

1.3   Salt (Table 1)

1.3.1   Effects on CVD Risk Factors

Extensive scientific evidence shows that reducing dietary salt (sodium chloride) intake significantly decreases systolic and diastolic blood pressure in adults with or without hypertension (He et al. 2013; Stamler et al. 2018). Recent data from the international multicentre population INTERMAP study reported a positive association between salt intake and blood pressure values also within the normal range (Zhou et al. 2019). In addition to sodium reduction, an increase in potassium intake is beneficial to prevent and control blood pressure in people with hypertension, with no adverse effects on plasma lipid concentrations (Aburto et al. 2013a). In line with these findings, current nutritional recommendations include a potassium intake of at least 3.5 g per day in adults. Therefore, a diet that combines low sodium and high potassium intakes is more effective in reducing blood pressure and hypertension risk. An example of this type of approach is the DASH diet, recommended for the non-pharmacological management of hypertension. This diet includes also changes in the quality of fat – promoting unsaturated fat and carbohydrates – favouring unrefined ones. Recent results from a systematic review and meta-analyses of RCTs support the beneficial effect of the DASH diet not only on blood pressure but also on other cardiovascular risk factors, including total and LDL cholesterol concentrations (Siervo et al. 2015).

1.3.2 Effects on CVD Events

Two recent meta-analyses of cohort studies showed a direct relationship between sodium intake and stroke, CVD and CHD mortality; a higher sodium intake was significantly associated with an increased risk of CVD (12%) and CHD (32%) mortality, in addition to a much higher risk of stroke mortality (63%) (Aburto et al. 2013b; Poggio et al. 2015). Consistently, two recent meta-analyses of clinical trials showed that dietary salt reduction induces a significantly lower incidence (−20%) of CVD (Adler et al. 2014; He and MacGregor 2011).

Actually, in many parts of the world, the average sodium consumption (mainly derived from dietary salt intake and food additives, such as sodium glutamate) is above that recommended by guidelines: less than 5 g of salt/day (equivalent to about 2.3 g of sodium daily) (WHO Guidelines Approved by the Guidelines Review Committee 2012).

In the last decades, the science of human nutrition has shifted from a reductionistic approach focused on specific nutrients to a broader view emphasizing the role of food groups/dietary patterns (van Horn et al. 2016). This paradigm change is due to convincing scientific evidence showing that human health is indeed influenced by single nutrients but also by their complex interactions and by their interplay with other bioactive substances present in foods. These are likely to act synergistically, and, therefore, their impact on human health may not be appreciated unless evaluated within the context of the whole diet. Furthermore, characteristics other than nutrient combinations (i.e. physical features of the foods, technological processes, cooking procedures) may influence the absorption and bioavailability of nutrients and in turn modulate their metabolic effects. Therefore, there is growing attention to the identification of dietary patterns associated to the risk of disease or death. The Mediterranean diet is one of dietary patterns for which strong evidence from observational and intervention studies has accumulated on the benefits in the primary and secondary prevention of cardiovascular disease and other major chronic diseases, such as type 2 diabetes, cancer and probably cognitive impairment (de Lorgeril et al. 1999; Estruch et al. 2018; Sofi et al. 2014).

The Mediterranean diet is characterized by a food pattern resembling the healthy food choices outlined above and, in particular, by the regular consumption of plant foods – including vegetables, pulses, nuts, fruits and unrefined cereals – and fish as well as a low intake of red and processed meats and whole fat dairy products; the main source of fat is extra virgin olive oil (Table 1). The optimal nutrient distribution and the balanced food choices of this dietary pattern have supported it as a useful model for the implementation of a healthy diet at the population level. Its strengths are not only the evidence in support of its beneficial impact on cardiovascular disease prevention but also its very deep cultural roots that are the source of the large body of

Table 2 Summary of lifestyle measures and healthy food choices for managing total cardiovascular risk

Dietary recommendations should always take into account local food habits; however, interest in healthy food choices from other cultures should be promoted
A wide variety of foods should be eaten. Energy intake should be adjusted to prevent overweight and obesity
Consumption of fruits, vegetables, legumes, nuts, wholegrain cereal foods and fish (especially oily) should be encouraged
Foods rich in trans-fatty acids should be avoided totally; foods rich in SFAs (tropical oils, fatty or processed meat, sweets, cream, butter, regular cheese) should be replaced with the above foods and with monounsaturated fat (extra virgin olive oil) and polyunsaturated fat (non-tropical vegetable oils) in order to keep SFA intake of <10 En% ($<7\%$ in the presence of high plasma cholesterol values)
Salt intake should be reduced to <5 g/day by avoiding table salt and limiting salt in cooking and by choosing fresh or frozen unsalted foods; many processed and convenience foods, including bread, are high in salt
For those who drink alcoholic beverages, moderation should be advised (<10 g/day for women and <20 g/day for men), and patients with hypertriglyceridaemia should abstain
The intake of beverages and foods with added sugars, particularly soft drinks, should be limited, especially for persons who are overweight, have hypertriglyceridaemia, metabolic syndrome or diabetes
Physical activity should be encouraged, aiming at regular physical exercise for at least 30 min/day every day
Use of and exposure to tobacco products should be avoided

culinary recipes to make a healthy choice a gastronomical adventure (Catapano et al. 2016) (Table 2).

2   Physical Activity

Having a sedentary life is a cardiovascular risk factor in itself. The amount of time spent being sedentary is increasing all over Europe even in young people. Watching TV, being stationary in front of a computer and using vehicles for transportation are the disadvantages of modern living. Especially in middle-aged females, sedentary lifestyle is almost as risky as smoking (Brown et al. 2015). Several studies have shown that sedentary behaviour increases cardiovascular risk. One of the largest prospective registries was the PURE study where physical activity was recorded in 130, 843 participants without existing CVD for 6.9 years. Compared with low physical activity (<600 metabolic equivalents [MET] $\times$ minutes per week or <150 min per week of moderate-intensity physical activity), moderate (600–3,000 MET $\times$ minutes or 150–750 min per week) and high physical activity ($>3,000$ MET $\times$ minutes or >750 min per week) were associated with graded reduction in mortality and major cardiovascular events (Lear et al. 2017).

Experimental studies that mimicked sedentary behaviour have shown greater postprandial glucose and insulin levels during bouts of prolonged sitting compared with individuals taking frequent standing or walking breaks (Pulsford et al. 2017). Compared with prolonged sitting, breaking up sitting time with intermittent, even light-intensity activity, can increase expression of anti-inflammatory and antioxidative pathway modulators (Latouche et al. 2013). A recent meta-analysis investigated the association between sedentary behaviour and incident CVD events using data from nine prospective cohort studies and showed that risk increased with increased sedentary time, with the highest risk being in more than 10 h a day of sedentary time (Pandey et al. 2016). A recent study has shown that sustained physical activity but not weight loss was associated with improved survival in coronary heart disease (Moholdt et al. 2018).

Physical activity has a positive effect on body weight, blood pressure, blood glucose, lipid levels, endothelial function, autonomous regulation and coagulation. The summary of all these effects leads to a decrease in cardiovascular disease incidence and mortality. Physical activity has both acute and chronic effects on blood pressure. With increased physical activity, blood pressure is lowered especially in subjects with prehypertension compared to those with normal blood pressure (Physical Activity Guidelines Advisory Committee 2018). Physical activity combined with calorie restriction can contribute to weight loss and supports the maintenance of weight loss. The risk of type 2 diabetes mellitus is greatly reduced with physical activity, and this benefit is observed irrespective of body weight. Engaging in 150–300 min a week of moderate-intensity physical activity can reduce the risk of developing type 2 diabetes mellitus by 25–35% (Physical Activity Guidelines Advisory Committee 2018). Regular physical activity or exercise can affect serum lipid levels favourably. Men and women who exercise regularly have significantly lower LDL-C and VLDL and higher HDL-C levels compared to age- and gender-matched sedentary controls (Vodak et al. 1980; Wood et al. 1976). Similarly, moderate physical exercise decreases LDL-C and triglycerides and increases HDL in male survivors of myocardial infarction (Ballantyne et al. 1982). The effect of exercise on lipids varies in exercise intervention studies, and there appears to be a minimum exercise volume to increase HDL-C (Kodama et al. 2007). There are additional antiatherogenic effects of physical activity besides those affecting traditional cardiovascular disease risk factors (Green et al. 2017). Exercise intensity improves vascular endothelial function in a dose-dependent manner for aerobic activities (Ashor et al. 2015). Endothelial function is improved with exercise even in the absence of changes in classical risk factors like lipids levels, blood pressure, glucose or BMI (Green et al. 2008). Acute- and moderate-intensity exercises increase shear stress, which stimulates endothelium-dependent vasodilatation through the increased synthesis of nitric oxide (Erkens et al. 2017). Regular exercise training also leads to increased coronary artery size and dilatation capacity (Haskell et al. 1993) and increased luminal diameter of conduit arteries (Green et al. 2008). Exercise training can reduce the wall thickness of conduit arteries and increases the development of coronary collateral blood vessels (Thijssen et al. 2012). Unhealthy gut microbiota has recently been shown to increase the risk of CVD (Fu et al. 2015; Lanter et al. 2014). Regular physical activity or endurance exercise training can positively alter the human gut microbiota by increasing bacterial diversity, increasing faecal concentrations of short-chain fatty acids and increasing the proportion of healthy bacterial species (Allen et al. 2018; Bressa et al. 2017; Estaki et al. 2016). A recent study on endurance training has shown that exercise increases telomerase activity and length, whereas resistance training did not show these effects (Werner et al. 2019). Ideally, a combination of resistance and endurance training should be implemented (Reiner et al. 2019).

Physical activity is any activity that moves the skeletal muscles and consumes energy, whereas systematic physical activity, like swimming and running, is described as exercise. In healthy individuals, regular physical activity decreases all-cause and cardiovascular mortality by 20–30% (Lollgen et al. 2009; Moore et al. 2012; Sattelmair et al. 2011). Regular physical activity increases cardiorespiratory fitness (The American College of Sports Medicine 2014). Cardiorespiratory fitness is associated with reduced prevalence of CVD risk factors and improves prognosis (Harber et al. 2017). A meta-analysis of 33 studies in over 100, 000 individuals observed that every 1 estimated MET increase in CRF was associated with 13 and 15% reductions in all-cause and CVD mortality (Nauman et al. 2017). Cardiorespiratory fitness is important even in the presence of other risk factors and shown to be protective even in men with metabolic syndrome (Katzmarzyk et al. 2004) and obesity (Moholdt et al. 2017).

Although all agree that any level of physical activity is better than none, there is controversy about the optimal dose of physical activity for CVD prevention. The intensity and frequency of exercise should be personalized and adapted to a person's needs as well as lifestyle. We also need to keep in mind that there is a high degree of interindividual variation in cardiorespiratory fitness responses to exercise.

The 2016 ESC prevention guideline recommends (Piepoli et al. 2016) for healthy adults of all ages to perform at least 150 min a week of moderate-intensity or 75 min a week of vigorous-intensity aerobic physical activity (PA) or an equivalent combination. For additional benefits in healthy adults, a gradual increase in aerobic PA to 300 min a week of moderate-intensity or 150 min a week of vigorous-intensity aerobic PA, or an equivalent combination thereof, is recommended. Multiple sessions of PA should be considered, each lasting ≥ 10 min and evenly spread throughout the week. Clinical evaluation, including exercise testing, should be considered for sedentary people with cardiovascular risk factors who intend to engage in vigorous PAs or sports.

Even low-level physical activity, such as low-dose running or commuting to work by bicycle, has been associated with a lower incidence of obesity, arterial hypertension, dyslipidaemia and diabetes mellitus (Grontved et al. 2016). The most recent Physical Activity Guidelines for Americans from the US Department of Health and Human Services has stated that benefits related to physical activity start even earlier and are easier to obtain than was previously thought according to recent evidence (Physical Activity Guidelines Advisory Committee 2018). These guidelines state that although one should try to get to guideline-recommended goals, the threshold at which health benefits begin to start is less than 150 min a week for most outcomes. There is no lower limit to the benefits of physical activity in reducing cardiovascular disease risk. However, getting to goal helps in obtaining benefits for the greatest number of outcomes. Additional physical activity confers additional benefits, and health risk does not seem to increase with high amounts of physical activity, even beyond 3–5 times the 150 min a week recommendation in healthy individuals. Compared with inactive adults, meeting the goals is associated with a 14% reduced risk of developing coronary heart disease (Physical Activity Guidelines Advisory Committee 2018).

2019 ACC/AHA Guideline on the Primary Prevention of Cardiovascular Disease (Arnett et al. 2019) also recommends that adults should engage in at least 150 min per week of accumulated moderate-intensity or 75 min per week of vigorous-intensity aerobic physical activity to reduce atherosclerotic cardiovascular disease. For adults unable to meet the minimum physical activity recommendations, engaging in some moderate- or vigorous-intensity physical activity, even if less than this recommended amount, and decreasing sedentary behaviour can be beneficial to reduce CVD risk.

Although some exercise is beneficial for all, for those with known cardiovascular disease, the dose of exercise needs to be individualised to prevent adverse outcomes. The risk of having an adverse cardiovascular event during exercise is very low, especially during light exercise. However, it is best to do a risk assessment and tailor the exercise program according to the need of the individual. Light- and moderate-intensity exercise can be done with minimal risk, whereas intensive exercise should be preceded by a medical evaluation, especially for middle-aged people. The cardioprotective effects of regular PA, whether performed in low or high volumes, are clear and extend across all ages, gender and race (El Saadany et al. 2017; Nes et al. 2017; O'Donovan et al. 2018). Whether overexercising in healthy individuals can have unfavourable consequences has been questioned. In some studies, long-term strenuous exercise has been shown to increase the risk of atrial fibrillation (Gorenek Chair et al. 2017). It is never too late to start exercising. The Aerobics Center Longitudinal Study has shown that men who were in the lowest percentile of CRF at their first examination but fit at the time of their second examination years later had a 52% reduction in CVD mortality compared with men who remained unfit (Blair et al. 1995). For every one estimated MET increase, all-cause and CVD mortalities were reduced by 15% and 19%, respectively (Lee et al. 2011).

3   Smoking

Smoking is one of the most important modifiable risk factors for CVD. Furthermore, stopping smoking is the most cost-effective prevention intervention. It is well known that smoking and using all forms of tobacco products cause CVD and increase mortality (Mons et al. 2015; Teo et al. 2006). Because tobacco use even in small amounts increases cardiovascular risk, reducing the number of cigarettes or the amount of tobacco consumption is not sufficient. Even smoking one cigarette per day carries a risk (Hackshaw et al. 2018). Therefore there is no safe level of smoking and quitting is mandatory. Passive smoking also increases cardiovascular risk, and studies have shown that second-hand smoke exposure increases CVD and triggers adverse events in non-smokers (Lv et al. 2015).

Cigarette smoke contains more than 4,000 chemicals and toxins like nicotine, carbon monoxide, cadmium and oxidants (Smith and Fischer 2001). Exposure to these chemicals affects all stages of atherosclerotic vascular disease unfavourably. Endothelial dysfunction due to reduced NO bioavailability and activation of NF-kB will lead to functional and eventually physical damage to the endothelium (Collins 1993; Rahman and Laher 2007). Nicotine has been shown to promote MMP expression in smooth muscle cells and decreased collagen synthesis in the arterial wall impairing the stability of the plaque (Carty et al. 1996; Raveendran et al. 2004) Cigarette smoke increases systemic inflammation (Csordas et al. 2008). The catecholamines are increased in the circulation triggering vasospasm (Zhu and Parmley 1995). Smoking also alters the balance between pro- and anticoagulant factors towards procoagulation. Plaque thrombogenicity is increased with increased plasma tissue factor, VWF, thrombin and thrombomodulin and activated platelets (Markuljak et al. 1995; Miller et al. 1998). Upon smoking cessation, several of these prothrombotic changes revert to normal. Blood viscosity is also increased with smoking (Lowe et al. 1980). All of these effects contribute to plaque formation, vulnerability and thrombus development. Interestingly, there is a genetic suscepti-bility to the atherothrombotic effects of smoking. Different variants have been described that alter one's susceptibility to the negative effects of smoking (Wang et al. 1996).

Smoking dependence is a chronic disease that needs to be managed with patience, expertise and time. The ESC prevention guidelines recommend the following strategy for smoking cessation (Piepoli et al. 2016): systematically inquire about smoking status at every opportunity; unequivocally urge all smokers to quit; deter-mine the person's degree of addiction and readiness to quit; agree on a smoking cessation strategy, including setting a quit date, behavioural counselling and phar-macological support; and arrange a schedule of follow-up ("five As" for a smoking cessation strategy for routine practice – ask, advise, assess, assist, and arrange). In case where advice and motivational interventions fail, drug-based interventions can be used to aid quitting smoking. Nicotine replacement therapies, bupropion and varenicline, have been shown to be helpful in increasing quitting (Cahill et al. 2013; Hughes et al. 2014; Stead et al. 2012). Electronic cigarettes emitting an aerosol containing nicotine have been developed to aid quitting; however, they may also emit toxic gases that may increase the risk of cardiovascular and pulmonary diseases, arrhythmias and hypertension (Benowitz and Fraiman 2017). Patients often are concerned about weight gain after smoking cessation. However a recent study from the cohorts of the Nurses' Health Study (NHS), (NHS II) and the Health Professionals Follow-Up Study (HPFS) has shown that even if the smoking cessa-tion was accompanied by substantial weight gain, this did not decrease the benefits of quitting smoking on reducing cardiovascular and all-cause mortality and cardio-vascular mortality decreased in all weight-change groups (Hu et al. 2018).

Modern lifestyles expose us to air pollution and occupational noise which also have a negative impact on cardiovascular diseases. It has been shown that the risk of

STEMI rises within hours of exposure to air pollutants (Sahlen et al. 2019). Furthermore, several investigations support that inhalation of ambient particulate matter triggers pulmonary and systemic inflammation resulting in metabolic syndrome and cardiopulmonary disease (Clementi et al. 2019). Exposure to high occupational noise is also associated with increase in hypertension, cardiovascular disease and cardiovascular mortality (Skogstad et al. 2016; Teixeira et al. 2019).

A healthy lifestyle is critically important to improve cardiovascular health and increase the control of risk factors. Healthy lifestyles should be adapted from birth to childhood and maintained throughout the lifespan. This can be possible only with creating health-promoting environments and improving healthcare policies, the interaction between the patient and the physician and education of the patient and the public about healthy lifestyles.

The WHO has put together a global action plan for the prevention and control of non-communicable diseases (WHO 2013). The goal is to reduce the risk of premature non-communicable disease deaths by 25% by 2025. According to this plan, reductions in tobacco use, salt intake, physical inactivity, harmful use of alcohol, raised blood pressure as well as stopping the diabetes and obesity epidemics are the goals. Early action and aggressive implementation of this plan may decrease the cardiovascular disease epidemic if the individual WHO targets are met and healthcare systems are strengthened. At the individual level, it is important for us to promote healthy lifestyles to everyone, including patients who already have CVD since it is never too late to benefit from a healthy lifestyle.

References

Aburto NJ, Hanson S, Gutierrez H, Hooper L, Elliott P, Cappuccio FP (2013a) Effect of increased potassium intake on cardiovascular risk factors and disease: systematic review and meta-analyses. BMJ (Clin Res Ed) 346:f1378. https://doi.org/10.1136/bmj.f1378

Aburto NJ, Ziolkovska A, Hooper L, Elliott P, Cappuccio FP, Meerpohl JJ (2013b) Effect of lower sodium intake on health: systematic review and meta-analyses. BMJ (Clin Res Ed) 346:f1326. https://doi.org/10.1136/bmj.f1326

The American College of Sports Medicine (2014) ACSM's guidelines for exercise testing and prescription. 9th edn. Wolters Kluwer/Lippincott Williams & Wilkins, Philadelphia, PA

Adler AJ, Taylor F, Martin N, Gottlieb S, Taylor RS, Ebrahim S (2014) Reduced dietary salt for the prevention of cardiovascular disease. Cochrane Database Syst Rev 7:Cd009217. https://doi.org/10.1002/14651858.CD009217.pub3

Allen JM et al (2018) Exercise alters gut microbiota composition and function in lean and obese humans. Med Sci Sports Exerc 50:747–757. https://doi.org/10.1249/mss.0000000000001495

Arnett DK et al (2019) 2019 ACC/AHA guideline on the primary prevention of cardiovascular disease circulation. https://doi.org/10.1161/cir.0000000000000678

Ashor AW, Lara J, Siervo M, Celis-Morales C, Oggioni C, Jakovljevic DG, Mathers JC (2015) Exercise modalities and endothelial function: a systematic review and dose-response meta-analysis of randomized controlled trials sports medicine (Auckland, NZ). Sports Med 45:279–296. https://doi.org/10.1007/s40279-014-0272-9

Augustin LS et al (2015) Glycemic index, glycemic load and glycemic response: An International Scientific Consensus Summit from the International Carbohydrate Quality Consortium (ICQC). Nutr Metab Cardiovasc Dis 25:795–815. https://doi.org/10.1016/j.numecd.2015.05.005

Ballantyne FC, Clark RS, Simpson HS, Ballantyne D (1982) High density and low density lipoprotein subfractions in survivors of myocardial infarction and in control subjects. Metab Clin Exp 31:433–437

Benowitz NL, Fraiman JB (2017) Cardiovascular effects of electronic cigarettes. Nat Rev Cardiol 14:447–456. https://doi.org/10.1038/nrcardio.2017.36

Blair SN, Kohl HW 3rd, Barlow CE, Paffenbarger RS Jr, Gibbons LW, Macera CA (1995) Changes in physical fitness and all-cause mortality. A prospective study of healthy and unhealthy men. JAMA 273:1093–1098

Bozzetto L et al (2012) Liver fat is reduced by an isoenergetic MUFA diet in a controlled randomized study in type 2 diabetic patients. Diabetes Care 35:1429–1435. https://doi.org/10.2337/dc12-0033

Bozzetto L et al (2014) A CHO/fibre diet reduces and a MUFA diet increases postprandial lipaemia in type 2 diabetes: no supplementary effects of low-volume physical training. Acta Diabetol 51:385–393. https://doi.org/10.1007/s00592-013-0522-6

Bozzetto L et al (2018) Dietary fibre as a unifying remedy for the whole spectrum of obesity-associated cardiovascular risk. Nutrients 10. https://doi.org/10.3390/nu10070943

Bressa C et al (2017) Differences in gut microbiota profile between women with active lifestyle and sedentary women. PLoS One 12:e0171352. https://doi.org/10.1371/journal.pone.0171352

Brown WJ, Pavey T, Bauman AE (2015) Comparing population attributable risks for heart disease across the adult lifespan in women. Br J Sports Med 49:1069–1076. https://doi.org/10.1136/bjsports-2013-093090

Cahill K, Stevens S, Perera R, Lancaster T (2013) Pharmacological interventions for smoking cessation: an overview and network meta-analysis. Cochrane Database Syst Rev 5:Cd009329. https://doi.org/10.1002/14651858.CD009329.pub2

Carty CS, Soloway PD, Kayastha S, Bauer J, Marsan B, Ricotta JJ, Dryjski M (1996) Nicotine and cotinine stimulate secretion of basic fibroblast growth factor and affect expression of matrix metalloproteinases in cultured human smooth muscle cells. J Vasc Surg 24:927–934

Catapano AL et al (2016) 2016 ESC/EAS guidelines for the management of dyslipidaemias. Eur Heart J 37:2999–3058. https://doi.org/10.1093/eurheartj/ehw272

Chiavaroli L et al (2015) Effect of fructose on established lipid targets: a systematic review and meta-analysis of controlled feeding trials. J Am Heart Assoc 4:e001700. https://doi.org/10.1161/jaha.114.001700

Chowdhury R et al (2014) Association of dietary, circulating, and supplement fatty acids with coronary risk: a systematic review and meta-analysis. Ann Intern Med 160:398–406. https://doi.org/10.7326/m13-1788

Clementi EA et al (2019) Metabolic syndrome and air pollution: a narrative review of their cardiopulmonary effects. Toxics 7. https://doi.org/10.3390/toxics7010006

Collins T (1993) Endothelial nuclear factor-kappa B and the initiation of the atherosclerotic lesion. Lab Invest 68:499–508

Physical Activity Guidelines Advisory Committee (2018) 2018 Physical Activity Guidelines Advisory Committee Scientific Report. Washington, DC

Csordas A, Wick G, Laufer G, Bernhard D (2008) An evaluation of the clinical evidence on the role of inflammation and oxidative stress in smoking-mediated cardiovascular disease. Biomark Insights 3:127–139

de Lorgeril M, Salen P, Martin JL, Monjaud I, Delaye J, Mamelle N (1999) Mediterranean diet, traditional risk factors, and the rate of cardiovascular complications after myocardial infarction: final report of the Lyon diet heart study. Circulation 99:779–785. https://doi.org/10.1161/01.cir.99.6.779

de Natale C et al (2009) Effects of a plant-based high-carbohydrate/high-fiber diet versus high-monounsaturated fat/low-carbohydrate diet on postprandial lipids in type 2 diabetic patients. Diabetes Care 32:2168–2173. https://doi.org/10.2337/dc09-0266

Dehghan M et al (2017) Associations of fats and carbohydrate intake with cardiovascular disease and mortality in 18 countries from five continents (PURE): a prospective cohort study. Lancet 390:2050–2062. https://doi.org/10.1016/s0140-6736(17)32252-3

el Saadany T, Richard A, Wanner M, Rohrmann S (2017) Sex-specific effects of leisure-time physical activity on cause-specific mortality in NHANES III. Prev Med 101:53–59. https://doi.org/10.1016/j.ypmed.2017.05.029

Erkens R, Suvorava T, Kramer CM, Diederich LD, Kelm M, Cortese-Krott MM (2017) Modulation of local and systemic Heterocellular communication by mechanical forces: a role of endothelial nitric oxide synthase. Antioxid Redox Signal 26:917–935. https://doi.org/10.1089/ars.2016.6904

Estaki M et al (2016) Cardiorespiratory fitness as a predictor of intestinal microbial diversity and distinct metagenomic functions. Microbiome 4:42. https://doi.org/10.1186/s40168-016-0189-7

Estruch R et al (2018) Primary prevention of cardiovascular disease with a Mediterranean diet supplemented with extra-virgin olive oil or nuts. N Engl J Med 378:e34. https://doi.org/10.1056/NEJMoa1800389

Farvid MS et al (2014) Dietary linoleic acid and risk of coronary heart disease: a systematic review and meta-analysis of prospective cohort studies. Circulation 130:1568–1578. https://doi.org/10.1161/circulationaha.114.010236

Forouhi NG, Krauss RM, Taubes G, Willett W (2018) Dietary fat and cardiometabolic health: evidence, controversies, and consensus for guidance. BMJ (Clin Res Ed) 361:k2139. https://doi.org/10.1136/bmj.k2139

Fu J et al (2015) The gut microbiome contributes to a substantial proportion of the variation in blood lipids. Circ Res 117:817–824. https://doi.org/10.1161/circresaha.115.306807

Giacco R et al (2014) A whole-grain cereal-based diet lowers postprandial plasma insulin and triglyceride levels in individuals with metabolic syndrome Nutrition, metabolism, and cardiovascular diseases. Nutr Metab Cardiovasc Dis 24:837–844. https://doi.org/10.1016/j.numecd.2014.01.007

Giacco R, Costabile G, Riccardi G (2016) Metabolic effects of dietary carbohydrates: the importance of food digestion. Food Res Int 88:336–341

Gorenek Chair B et al (2017) European Heart Rhythm Association (EHRA)/European Association of Cardiovascular Prevention and Rehabilitation (EACPR) position paper on how to prevent atrial fibrillation endorsed by the Heart Rhythm Society (HRS) and Asia Pacific Heart Rhythm Society (APHRS). Eur J Prev Cardiol 24:4–40. https://doi.org/10.1177/2047487316676037

Graham I, Cooney MT, Bradley D, Dudina A, Reiner Z (2012) Dyslipidemias in the prevention of cardiovascular disease: risks and causality. Curr Cardiol Rep 14:709–720. https://doi.org/10.1007/s11886-012-0313-7

Green DJ, O'Driscoll G, Joyner MJ, Cable NT (2008) Exercise and cardiovascular risk reduction: time to update the rationale for exercise? J Appl Physiol 105:766–768. https://doi.org/10.1152/japplphysiol.01028.2007

Green DJ, Hopman MT, Padilla J, Laughlin MH, Thijssen DH (2017) Vascular adaptation to exercise in humans: role of hemodynamic stimuli. Physiol Rev 97:495–528. https://doi.org/10.1152/physrev.00014.2016

Grontved A et al (2016) Bicycling to work and primordial prevention of cardiovascular risk: a cohort study among Swedish men and women. J Am Heart Assoc 5. https://doi.org/10.1161/jaha.116.004413

Hackshaw A, Morris JK, Boniface S, Tang JL, Milenkovic D (2018) Low cigarette consumption and risk of coronary heart disease and stroke: meta-analysis of 141 cohort studies in 55 study reports. BMJ (Clin Res Ed) 360:j5855. https://doi.org/10.1136/bmj.j5855

Harber MP, Kaminsky LA, Arena R, Blair SN, Franklin BA, Myers J, Ross R (2017) Impact of cardiorespiratory fitness on all-cause and disease-specific mortality: advances since 2009. Prog Cardiovasc Dis 60:11–20. https://doi.org/10.1016/j.pcad.2017.03.001

Haskell WL, Sims C, Myll J, Bortz WM, St Goar FG, Alderman EL (1993) Coronary artery size and dilating capacity in ultradistance runners. Circulation 87:1076–1082. https://doi.org/10.1161/01.cir.87.4.1076

He FJ, MacGregor GA (2011) Salt reduction lowers cardiovascular risk: meta-analysis of outcome trials. Lancet 378:380–382. https://doi.org/10.1016/s0140-6736(11)61174-4

He FJ, Li J, Macgregor GA (2013) Effect of longer term modest salt reduction on blood pressure: Cochrane systematic review and meta-analysis of randomised trials. BMJ (Clin Res Ed) 346: f1325. https://doi.org/10.1136/bmj.f1325

Hooper L, Martin N, Abdelhamid A, Davey Smith G (2015) Reduction in saturated fat intake for cardiovascular disease. Cochrane Database Syst Rev 6:Cd011737. https://doi.org/10.1002/14651858.Cd011737

Hu Y et al (2018) Smoking cessation, weight change, type 2 diabetes, and mortality. N Engl J Med 379:623–632. https://doi.org/10.1056/NEJMoa1803626

Hughes JR, Stead LF, Hartmann-Boyce J, Cahill K, Lancaster T (2014) Antidepressants for smoking cessation. Cochrane Database of Syst Rev 1:Cd000031. https://doi.org/10.1002/14651858.CD000031.pub4

Imamura F, Micha R, Wu JH, de Oliveira Otto MC, Otite FO, Abioye AI, Mozaffarian D (2016) Effects of saturated fat, polyunsaturated fat, monounsaturated fat, and carbohydrate on glucose-insulin homeostasis: a systematic review and meta-analysis of randomised controlled feeding trials. PLoS Med 13:e1002087. https://doi.org/10.1371/journal.pmed.1002087

Jakobsen MU et al (2009) Major types of dietary fat and risk of coronary heart disease: a pooled analysis of 11 cohort studies. Am J Clin Nutr 89:1425–1432. https://doi.org/10.3945/ajcn.2008.27124

Katan MB, Grundy SM, Willett WC (1997) Should a low-fat, high-carbohydrate diet be recommended for everyone? Beyond low-fat diets. N Engl J Med 337:563–566; discussion 566-567

Katzmarzyk PT, Church TS, Blair SN (2004) Cardiorespiratory fitness attenuates the effects of the metabolic syndrome on all-cause and cardiovascular disease mortality in men. Arch Intern Med 164:1092–1097. https://doi.org/10.1001/archinte.164.10.1092

Khera AV et al (2016) Genetic risk, adherence to a healthy lifestyle, and coronary disease. N Engl J Med 375:2349–2358. https://doi.org/10.1056/NEJMoa1605086

Kodama S et al (2007) Effect of aerobic exercise training on serum levels of high-density lipoprotein cholesterol: a meta-analysis. Arch Intern Med 167:999–1008. https://doi.org/10.1001/archinte.167.10.999

Lanter BB, Sauer K, Davies DG (2014) Bacteria present in carotid arterial plaques are found as biofilm deposits which may contribute to enhanced risk of plaque rupture. mBio 5:e01206–e01214. https://doi.org/10.1128/mBio.01206-14

Latouche C, Jowett JB, Carey AL, Bertovic DA, Owen N, Dunstan DW, Kingwell BA (2013) Effects of breaking up prolonged sitting on skeletal muscle gene expression. J Appl Physiol (Bethesda, MD 1985) 114:453–460. https://doi.org/10.1152/japplphysiol.00978.2012

Lear SA et al (2017) The effect of physical activity on mortality and cardiovascular disease in 130,000 people from 17 high-income, middle-income, and low-income countries: the PURE study. Lancet 390:2643–2654. https://doi.org/10.1016/s0140-6736(17)31634-3

Lee DC et al (2011) Long-term effects of changes in cardiorespiratory fitness and body mass index on all-cause and cardiovascular disease mortality in men: the aerobics center longitudinal study. Circulation 124:2483–2490. https://doi.org/10.1161/circulationaha.111.038422

Li Y et al (2015) Saturated fats compared with unsaturated fats and sources of carbohydrates in relation to risk of coronary heart disease: a prospective cohort study. J Am Coll Cardiol 66:1538–1548. https://doi.org/10.1016/j.jacc.2015.07.055

Lloyd-Jones DM et al (2010) Defining and setting national goals for cardiovascular health promotion and disease reduction: the American Heart Association's strategic impact goal through 2020 and beyond. Circulation 121:586–613. https://doi.org/10.1161/circulationaha.109.192703

Lollgen H, Bockenhoff A Knapp G (2009) Physical activity and all-cause mortality: an updated meta-analysis with different intensity categories. Int J Sports Med 30:213–224. https://doi.org/10.1055/s-0028-1128150

Lowe GD, Drummond MM, Forbes CD, Barbenel JC (1980) The effects of age and cigarette-smoking on blood and plasma viscosity in men. Scott Med J 25:13–17. https://doi.org/10.1177/003693308002500103

Lv X, Sun J, Bi Y, Xu M, Lu J, Zhao L, Xu Y (2015) Risk of all-cause mortality and cardiovascular disease associated with secondhand smoke exposure: a systematic review and meta-analysis. Int J Cardiol 199:106–115. https://doi.org/10.1016/j.ijcard.2015.07.011

Markuljak I, Ivankova J, Kubisz P (1995) Thrombomodulin and von Willebrand factor in smokers and during smoking. Nouv Rev Fr Hematol 37:137–139

Mensink RP, Zock PL, Kester AD, Katan MB (2003) Effects of dietary fatty acids and carbohydrates on the ratio of serum total to HDL cholesterol and on serum lipids and apolipoproteins: a meta-analysis of 60 controlled trials. Am J Clin Nutr 77:1146–1155. https://doi.org/10.1093/ajcn/77.5.1146

Miller GJ, Bauer KA, Cooper JA, Rosenberg RD (1998) Activation of the coagulant pathway in cigarette smokers. Thromb Haemost 79:549–553

Miller PE, van Elswyk M, Alexander DD (2014) Long-chain omega-3 fatty acids eicosapentaenoic acid and docosahexaenoic acid and blood pressure: a meta-analysis of randomized controlled trials. Am J Hypertens 27:885–896. https://doi.org/10.1093/ajh/hpu024

Moholdt T, Lavie CJ, Nauman J (2017) Interaction of physical activity and body mass index on mortality in coronary heart disease: data from the Nord-Trondelag health study. Am J Med 130:949–957. https://doi.org/10.1016/j.amjmed.2017.01.043

Moholdt T, Lavie CJ, Nauman J (2018) Sustained physical activity, not weight loss, associated with improved survival in coronary heart disease. J Am Coll Cardiol 71:1094–1101. https://doi.org/10.1016/j.jacc.2018.01.011

Mons U et al (2015) Impact of smoking and smoking cessation on cardiovascular events and mortality among older adults: meta-analysis of individual participant data from prospective cohort studies of the CHANCES consortium. BMJ (Clin Res Ed) 350:h1551. https://doi.org/10.1136/bmj.h1551

Moore SC et al (2012) Leisure time physical activity of moderate to vigorous intensity and mortality: a large pooled cohort analysis. PLoS Med 9:e1001335. https://doi.org/10.1371/journal.pmed.1001335

Mozaffarian D, Katan MB, Ascherio A, Stampfer MJ, Willett WC (2006) Trans fatty acids and cardiovascular disease. N Engl J Med 354:1601–1613. https://doi.org/10.1056/NEJMra054035

Nauman J, Tauschek LC, Kaminsky LA, Nes BM, Wisloff U (2017) Global fitness levels: findings from a web-based surveillance report. Prog Cardiovasc Dis 60:78–88. https://doi.org/10.1016/j.pcad.2017.01.009

Nes BM, Gutvik CR, Lavie CJ, Nauman J, Wisloff U (2017) Personalized activity intelligence (PAI) for prevention of cardiovascular disease and promotion of physical activity. Am J Med 130:328–336. https://doi.org/10.1016/j.amjmed.2016.09.031

O'Donovan G, Stamatakis E, Stensel DJ, Hamer M (2018) The importance of vigorous-intensity leisure-time physical activity in reducing cardiovascular disease mortality risk in the obese. Mayo Clin Proc 93:1096–1103. https://doi.org/10.1016/j.mayocp.2018.01.016

Pandey A et al (2016) Continuous dose-response association between sedentary time and risk for cardiovascular disease: a meta-analysis. JAMA Cardiol 1:575–583. https://doi.org/10.1001/jamacardio.2016.1567

Piepoli MF et al (2016) 2016 European guidelines on cardiovascular disease prevention in clinical practice: the sixth joint task force of the European Society of Cardiology and Other Societies on cardiovascular disease prevention in clinical practice (constituted by representatives of 10 societies and by invited experts)developed with the special contribution of the European Association for Cardiovascular Prevention & Rehabilitation (EACPR). Eur Heart J 37:2315–2381. https://doi.org/10.1093/eurheartj/ehw106

Poggio R, Gutierrez L, Matta MG, Elorriaga N, Irazola V, Rubinstein A (2015) Daily sodium consumption and CVD mortality in the general population: systematic review and meta-analysis of prospective studies. Public Health Nutr 18:695–704. https://doi.org/10.1017/s1368980014000949

Pulsford RM, Blackwell J, Hillsdon M, Kos K (2017) Intermittent walking, but not standing, improves postprandial insulin and glucose relative to sustained sitting: a randomised cross-over study in inactive middle-aged men. J Sci Med Sport 20:278–283. https://doi.org/10.1016/j.jsams.2016.08.012

Rahman MM, Laher I (2007) Structural and functional alteration of blood vessels caused by cigarette smoking: an overview of molecular mechanisms. Curr Vasc Pharmacol 5:276–292

Rasmussen BM et al (2006) Effects of dietary saturated, monounsaturated, and n-3 fatty acids on blood pressure in healthy subjects. Am J Clin Nutr 83:221–226. https://doi.org/10.1093/ajcn/83.2.221

Raveendran M et al (2004) Cigarette suppresses the expression of P4Hα and vascular collagen production. Biochem Biophys Res Commun 323:592–598. https://doi.org/10.1016/j.bbrc.2004.08.129

Reiner Z (2013) Statins in the primary prevention of cardiovascular disease. Nat Rev Cardiol 10:453–464. https://doi.org/10.1038/nrcardio.2013.80

Reiner Z et al (2011) ESC/EAS guidelines for the management of dyslipidaemias: the task force for the management of dyslipidaemias of the European Society of Cardiology (ESC) and the European Atherosclerosis Society (EAS). Eur Heart J 32:1769–1818. https://doi.org/10.1093/eurheartj/ehr158

Reiner Z, Laufs U, Cosentino F, Landmesser U (2019) The year in cardiology 2018: prevention. Eur Heart J 40:336–344. https://doi.org/10.1093/eurheartj/ehy894

Reynolds A, Mann J, Cummings J, Winter N, Mete E, Te Morenga L (2019) Carbohydrate quality and human health: a series of systematic reviews and meta-analyses. Lancet 393:434–445. https://doi.org/10.1016/s0140-6736(18)31809-9

Riccardi G, Costabile G (2019) Carbohydrate quality is key for a healthy and sustainable diet. Nat Rev Endocrinol 15:257–258. https://doi.org/10.1038/s41574-019-0190-x

Riccardi G, Rivellese AA (1991) Effects of dietary fiber and carbohydrate on glucose and lipoprotein metabolism in diabetic patients. Diabetes Care 14:1115–1125. https://doi.org/10.2337/diacare.14.12.1115

Riccardi G, Rivellese AA, Giacco R (2008) Role of glycemic index and glycemic load in the healthy state, in prediabetes, and in diabetes. Am J Clin Nutr 87:269s–274s. https://doi.org/10.1093/ajcn/87.1.269S

Rivellese AA, Giacco R, Costabile G (2012) Dietary carbohydrates for diabetics. Curr Atheroscler Rep 14:563–569. https://doi.org/10.1007/s11883-012-0278-4

Sacks FM, Katan M (2002) Randomized clinical trials on the effects of dietary fat and carbohydrate on plasma lipoproteins and cardiovascular disease. Am J Med 113(Suppl 9B):13s–24s. https://doi.org/10.1016/s0002-9343(01)00987-1

Sacks FM et al (2017) Dietary fats and cardiovascular disease: a presidential advisory from the American Heart Association. Circulation 136:e1–e23. https://doi.org/10.1161/cir.0000000000000510

Sahlen A et al (2019) Air pollution in relation to very short-term risk of ST-segment elevation myocardial infarction: case-crossover analysis of SWEDEHEART. Int J Cardiol 275:26–30. https://doi.org/10.1016/j.ijcard.2018.10.069

Sattelmair J, Pertman J, Ding EL, Kohl HW 3rd, Haskell W, Lee IM (2011) Dose response between physical activity and risk of coronary heart disease: a meta-analysis. Circulation 124:789–795. https://doi.org/10.1161/circulationaha.110.010710

Schwingshackl L, Strasser B, Hoffmann G (2011) Effects of monounsaturated fatty acids on cardiovascular risk factors: a systematic review and meta-analysis. Ann Nutr Metab 59:176–186. https://doi.org/10.1159/000334071

Seidelmann SB et al (2018) Dietary carbohydrate intake and mortality: a prospective cohort study and meta-analysis. Lancet Public Health 3:e419–e428. https://doi.org/10.1016/s2468-2667(18)30135-x

Siervo M, Lara J, Chowdhury S, Ashor A, Oggioni C, Mathers JC (2015) Effects of the dietary approach to stop hypertension (DASH) diet on cardiovascular risk factors: a systematic review and meta-analysis. Br J Nutr 113:1–15. https://doi.org/10.1017/s0007114514003341

Siri-Tarino PW, Sun Q, Hu FB, Krauss RM (2010) Meta-analysis of prospective cohort studies evaluating the association of saturated fat with cardiovascular disease. Am J Clin Nutr 91:535–546. https://doi.org/10.3945/ajcn.2009.27725

Skogstad M, Johannessen HA, Tynes T, Mehlum IS, Nordby KC, Lie A (2016) Systematic review of the cardiovascular effects of occupational noise. Occup Med 66:10–16. https://doi.org/10.1093/occmed/kqv148

Smith CJ, Fischer TH (2001) Particulate and vapor phase constituents of cigarette mainstream smoke and risk of myocardial infarction. Atherosclerosis 158:257–267

Sofi F, Macchi C, Abbate R, Gensini GF, Casini A (2014) Mediterranean diet and health status: an updated meta-analysis and a proposal for a literature-based adherence score. Public Health Nutr 17:2769–2782. https://doi.org/10.1017/s1368980013003169

Stamler J et al (2018) Relation of dietary sodium (salt) to blood pressure and its possible modulation by other dietary factors: the INTERMAP study. Hypertension 71:631–637. https://doi.org/10.1161/hypertensionaha.117.09928

Stanhope KL et al (2009) Consuming fructose-sweetened, not glucose-sweetened, beverages increases visceral adiposity and lipids and decreases insulin sensitivity in overweight/obese humans. J Clin Invest 119:1322–1334. https://doi.org/10.1172/jci37385

Stead LF, Perera R, Bullen C, Mant D, Hartmann-Boyce J, Cahill K, Lancaster T (2012) Nicotine replacement therapy for smoking cessation. Cochrane Database Syst Rev 11:Cd000146. https://doi.org/10.1002/14651858.CD000146.pub4

Summers LK et al (2002) Substituting dietary saturated fat with polyunsaturated fat changes abdominal fat distribution and improves insulin sensitivity. Diabetologia 45:369–377. https://doi.org/10.1007/s00125-001-0768-3

Teixeira LR et al (2019) WHO/ILO work-related burden of disease and injury: protocol for systematic reviews of exposure to occupational noise and of the effect of exposure to occupational noise on cardiovascular disease. Environ Int 125:567–578. https://doi.org/10.1016/j.envint.2018.09.040

Teo KK et al (2006) Tobacco use and risk of myocardial infarction in 52 countries in the INTERHEART study: a case-control study. Lancet 368:647–658. https://doi.org/10.1016/s0140-6736(06)69249-0

Thijssen DH, Cable NT, Green DJ (2012) Impact of exercise training on arterial wall thickness in humans. Clin Sci 122:311–322. https://doi.org/10.1042/cs20110469

Thomas DE, Elliott EJ (2010) The use of low-glycaemic index diets in diabetes control. Br J Nutr 104:797–802. https://doi.org/10.1017/s0007114510001534

US Department of Agriculture (2016) Agricultural research service, national nutrient database for standard reference. https://ndb.nal.usda.gov/ndb/search/list

van Horn L et al (2016) Recommended dietary pattern to achieve adherence to the American Heart Association/American College of Cardiology (AHA/ACC) guidelines: a scientific statement from the American Heart Association. Circulation 134:e505–e529. https://doi.org/10.1161/cir.0000000000000462

Vessby B et al (2001) Substituting dietary saturated for monounsaturated fat impairs insulin sensitivity in healthy men and women: the KANWU study. Diabetologia 44:312–319

Vodak PA, Wood PD, Haskell WL, Williams PT (1980) HDL-cholesterol and other plasma lipid and lipoprotein concentrations in middle-aged male and female tennis players. Metab Clin Exp 29:745–752

Wang XL, Sim AS, Badenhop RF, McCredie RM, Wilcken DE (1996) A smoking-dependent risk of coronary artery disease associated with a polymorphism of the endothelial nitric oxide synthase gene. Nat Med 2:41–45

Werner CM et al (2019) Differential effects of endurance, interval, and resistance training on telomerase activity and telomere length in a randomized, controlled study. Eur Heart J 40:34–46. https://doi.org/10.1093/eurheartj/ehy585

WHO (2013) Global action plan for the prevention and control of NCDs 2013–2020. WHO, Geneva

WHO Guidelines Approved by the Guidelines Review Committee (2012) Guideline: sodium intake for adults and children. World Health Organization, Geneva

Wood PD, Haskell W, Klein H, Lewis S, Stern MP, Farquhar JW (1976) The distribution of plasma lipoproteins in middle-aged male runners. Metab Clin Exp 25:1249–1257

Xi B et al (2015) Sugar-sweetened beverages and risk of hypertension and CVD: a dose-response meta-analysis. Br J Nutr 113:709–717. https://doi.org/10.1017/s0007114514004383

Zhong VW et al (2019) Associations of dietary cholesterol or egg consumption with incident cardiovascular disease and mortality. JAMA 321:1081–1095. https://doi.org/10.1001/jama.2019.1572

Zhou L et al (2019) Salt intake and prevalence of overweight/obesity in Japan, China, the United Kingdom, and the United States: the INTERMAP study. Am J Clin Nutr 110:34. https://doi.org/10.1093/ajcn/nqz067

Zhu BQ, Parmley WW (1995) Hemodynamic and vascular effects of active and passive smoking. Am Heart J 130:1270–1275. https://doi.org/10.1016/0002-8703(95)90154-x

Zock PL, Blom WA, Nettleton JA, Hornstra G (2016) Progressing insights into the role of dietary fats in the prevention of cardiovascular disease. Curr Cardiol Rep 18:111. https://doi.org/10.1007/s11886-016-0793-y

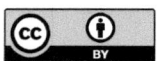

Blood Pressure-Lowering Therapy

Isabella Sudano ⓘ, Elena Osto ⓘ, and Frank Ruschitzka ⓘ

Contents

1 Introduction 26
2 Non-pharmacological Therapy 27
   2.1 Salt Restriction 29
   2.2 Reduce Alcohol Intake 29
   2.3 Weight Loss and Avoidance of Overweight and Obesity 30
   2.4 Regular Physical Activity 31
3 Pharmacological Therapy for the Treatment of Arterial Hypertension 31
   3.1 Who Should Be Treated with Pharmacological Therapy? 32
   3.2 Choice of Initial Antihypertensive Agents 32
   3.3 Combination Therapy 33
   3.4 Direct Effects of Antihypertensive Drugs on Atherosclerosis 34
4 Perspectives of Future Antihypertensive Therapy 36
   4.1 Unresolved Medical Needs 36
   4.2 New Drug Developments 37
   4.3 Device Therapy 37
5 Conclusion 39
References 39

Abstract

Extensive evidence demonstrates that lowering blood pressure can substantially reduce the risk of atherosclerotic cardiovascular disease and death.

The original version of this chapter was revised. A correction to this chapter can be found at https://doi.org/10.1007/164_2020_410

I. Sudano · F. Ruschitzka (✉)
Department of Cardiology, University Heart Center Zurich, Zürich, Switzerland
e-mail: frank.ruschitzka@usz.ch

E. Osto
Department of Cardiology, University Heart Center Zurich, Zürich, Switzerland

Institute of Clinical Chemistry, University of Zurich, University Hospital Zurich, Zürich, Switzerland

© The Author(s) 2020, corrected publication 2020
A. von Eckardstein, C. J. Binder (eds.), *Prevention and Treatment of Atherosclerosis*,
Handbook of Experimental Pharmacology 270, https://doi.org/10.1007/164_2020_372

In light of the latest 2018 European Society of Cardiology/European Society of Hypertension Joint Guidelines, we summarize the current recommendations about lifestyle intervention strategies, pharmacotherapy, and device-based treatments for the management of arterial hypertension. Special attention is given to direct effects exerted by some antihypertensive drugs targeting vascular wall cell components that are involved in the pathogenesis of atherosclerosis.

Keywords

Blood pressure medical treatment · Cardiovascular risk factors · Device therapy · Hypertension · Hypertension-driven atherosclerotic complications · Lifestyle interventions

Abbreviations

ACE	Angiotensin-converting enzyme
Ang II	Angiotensin II
ARBs	Angiotensin II receptor blockers
BP	Blood pressure
CCBs	Calcium channel blockers
CVD	Cardiovascular disease
ESC	European Society of Cardiology
ESH	European Society of Hypertension
MR	Mineralocorticoid receptor
NO	Nitric oxide
ROS	Reactive oxygen species
SHF	Swiss Heart Foundation
SNSF	Swiss National Science Foundation

1   Introduction

Continuous progress in understanding the epidemiology, pathophysiology, and pharmacology of arterial hypertension has consistently improved the possibility of an efficient and safe treatment of elevated blood pressure (BP).

Extensive evidence demonstrates that lowering BP can substantially reduce the risk of cardiovascular disease (CVD) and death with similar proportional reductions across various population subgroups. Every 10 mmHg systolic BP reduction significantly diminished the risk of major CVD events (RR 0.80, 95% CI 0.77–0.83), coronary heart disease (0.83, 0.78–0.88), stroke (0.73, 0.68–0.77), heart failure (0.72, 0.67–0.78), and all-cause mortality (0.87, 0.84–0.91) (Ettehad et al. 2016).

Arterial hypertension is characterized by structural and functional changes in blood vessels, which lead to increased arterial stiffness, vascular inflammation, endothelial dysfunction, fatty streaks, early atherosclerotic plaque, plaque progression, and plaque rapture. Vice versa, arterial stiffness, endothelial dysfunction, and vascular inflammation may also contribute to increased BP. Several lifestyle

Table 1 From ESC/ESH guidelines for hypertension, Eur Heart Journal 2018 (©ESC/ESH 2018)

Table 3. Classification of office blood pressure[a] and definitions of hypertension grade[b]

Category	Systolic (mmHg)		Diastolic (mmHg)
Optimal	<120	and	<80
Normal	120–129	and/or	80–84
High normal	130–139	and/or	85–89
Grade 1 hypertension	140–159	and/or	90–99
Grade 2 hypertension	160–170	and/or	100–109
Grade 3 hypertension	≥180	and/or	≥110
Isolated systolic hypertension[b]	≥140	and	<90

BP blood pressure, *SBP* systolic blood pressure
The same classification is used for all ages from 16 years
[a]BP category is defined according to seated clinic BP and by the highest level of BP, whether systolic or diastolic
[b]Isolated systolic hypertension is graded 1, 2, or 3 according to SBP values in the ranges indicated

interventions and drugs lowering BP were demonstrated to improve endothelial function, decrease arterial stiffness and vascular inflammation, and ultimately prevent the development and/or progression of atherothrombosis.

After exclusion of the main causes of a secondary hypertension, lifestyle modifications should be suggested as BP and cardiovascular risk lowering strategy to every patient with arterial hypertension. However, sooner or later, most patients diagnosed with arterial hypertension will require a pharmacological therapy.

According to the 2018 ESC/ESH Guidelines (Williams et al. 2018), the necessity of a pharmacological therapy will be defined by the grade of arterial hypertension (see Table 1), the cardiovascular risk, and the presence of hypertension-mediated organ damage or concomitant diseases such as a history of cardiovascular events, diabetes mellitus, or chronic kidney disease. The 2018 Guidelines suggest as general rule to reduce office BP below 140/90 mmHg aiming to reach a BP around 130/80 mmHg; see Table 1.

The ultimate goal of antihypertensive therapy is the prevention of cardiovascular events. The higher the absolute cardiovascular risk, the more likely it is that a patient will benefit from a more aggressive BP goal. However, although cardiovascular events generally decrease with more intensive lowering of BP, the risk of adverse effects, cost, and patient inconvenience increase as more medication is added (Ettehad et al. 2016; Williams et al. 2018). See Fig. 1.

This recommendation together with good clinical judgment and shared decision-making between patients and care providers should guide our BP-lowering therapy.

2 Non-pharmacological Therapy

Treatment of hypertension should always include non-pharmacological therapy (Fig. 1) (Williams et al. 2018).

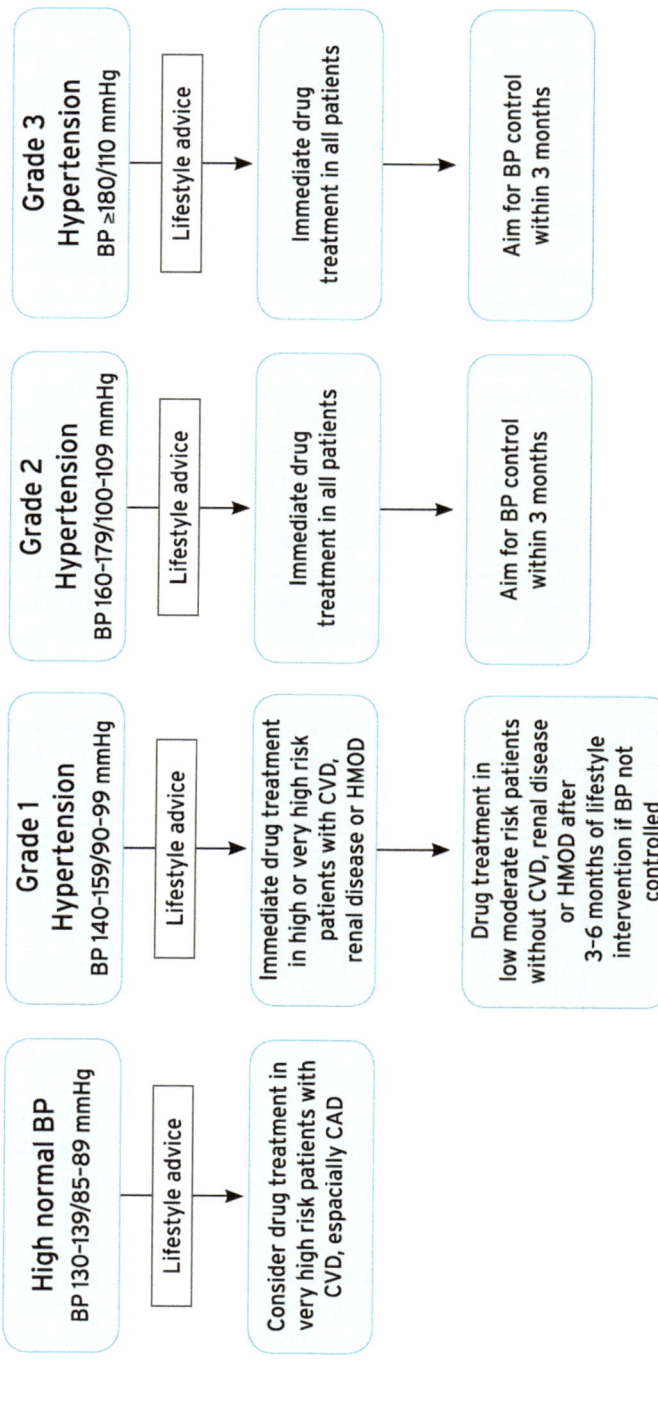

Fig. 1 From ESC/ESH guidelines for hypertension, Eur Heart Journal 2018 (©ESC/ESH 2018)

The ESC/ESH Guidelines (Williams et al. 2018) suggested the following lifestyle changes as contributors for reducing BP and cardiovascular risk to the majority of patients with arterial hypertension: healthy diet including dietary sodium restriction and moderation of alcohol consumption, overweight reduction, regular physical activity, and cessation of consumption of any product containing tobacco or nicotine.

2.1 Salt Restriction

In general, a healthy diet should avoid any excess: moderate sodium reduction is associated with a decrease in BP in hypertensive and normotensive individuals of a maximum of 4.8–2.5 mmHg systolic and 1.9–1.1 mmHg diastolic, respectively (He and MacGregor 2003).

Young patients with hypertension usually are salt-resistant, while older patients as well as obese individuals or patients with diabetes mellitus and chronic kidney disease are characterized by increased salt sensitivity (Weinberger 1996).

Evidence supporting very strong reduction of salt intake is weak. The effect of reduced dietary sodium on cardiovascular event rates remains unclear (Bibbins-Domingo et al. 2010; He et al. 2011; He and MacGregor 2011; Taylor et al. 2011).

Prospective cohort studies have reported an overall increased risk of mortality and cardiovascular events on high sodium intake, but to date, no prospective randomized controlled trial has provided definitive evidence about the optimal sodium intake to minimize cardiovascular events and mortality. However, it was reported that reducing sodium intake below 3 g of sodium per day further reduced BP, but paradoxically was associated with an increased risk of all-cause and cardiovascular mortalities in both the general population and in hypertensive patients, suggesting a J-curve phenomenon (Mente et al. 2016).

Increased potassium intake is associated with BP reduction and may have a protective effect, thereby modifying the association between sodium intake, BP, and CVD. Increasing potassium intake (e.g., including high intake of vegetables and fruits in the diet) could be a problem in patients with diabetes and chronic kidney disease and cannot be applied to all hypertensive patients (Bernabe-Ortiz et al. 2020; Binia et al. 2015; Mente et al. 2016; Miller et al. 2016).

Therefore, every patient with arterial hypertension independently of his/her sodium sensitivity should reduce the sodium consumption and avoid processed and frozen food, which frequently is rich in salt.

2.2 Reduce Alcohol Intake

For a long time, positive linear associations between alcohol consumption, BP, prevalence of hypertension, and cardiovascular risk have been established.

The Prevention and Treatment of Hypertension Study (PATHS) investigated the effects of reduced alcohol consumption on BP; the intervention group had a modest

1.2/0.7 mmHg lower BP than the control group at the end of the 6-month follow-up period. A meta-analysis of 56 epidemiological studies suggested that reduction of alcohol consumption, even for light-moderate drinkers, might be beneficial for cardiovascular health (Holmes et al. 2014). Binge drinking can cause strong increases of BP (Mancia et al. 2013).

Hypertensive men and women, who drink alcohol, should be advised to limit their consumption to 14 units and 8 units per week, respectively (one unit is equal to 125 mL of wine or 250 mL of beer). Alcohol-free days during the week and avoidance of binge drinking are also recommended (Williams et al. 2018).

2.3   Weight Loss and Avoidance of Overweight and Obesity

Weight loss in overweight or obese individuals leads to a significant reduction in BP, independently of exercise and dietary sodium restriction (Appel et al. 2006; Cohen and Gadde 2019), and has multiple beneficial effects against pathologic factors leading to high BP and to end-organ damage in this patient population (Cohen and Gadde 2019).

Weight loss is associated with decreased intra-abdominal pressure exerted on vessels by the excessive visceral fat deposition. Another beneficial effect of weight loss is the amelioration of insulin resistance, which is associated with renal sodium reabsorption and increased sympathetic tone in obesity. Moreover, chronic inflammation associated with overweight/obesity promotes vascular aging, favoring the onset of hypertension. Inflammation also contributes to arterial stiffness and impairs the physiologic anti-contractile effect of perivascular adipocytes on adjacent small arteries (Virdis et al. 2015; Aghamohammadzadeh et al. 2013). Decrease in body weight with lifestyle management, although effective in the short term, is difficult to sustain in the longer-term follow-up. Indeed, the overall efficacy of lifestyle interventions in reducing cardiovascular outcomes has been questioned by the results of the Action for Health in Diabetes (Look AHEAD) Study (Look, Ahead Research Group et al. 2013; Semlitsch et al. 2016). Currently, the most effective pharmacological treatments against obesity include glucagon like peptide-1 (GLP-1) receptor agonists and bariatric surgery. GLP-1 receptor agonists, in particular liraglutide, are cornerstones in antidiabetic therapy, which also have shown positive effects in reducing BP and CVD mortality (Helmstadter et al. 2020; Pi-Sunyer et al. 2015; Mingrone et al. 2015). Liraglutide is currently available also as weight-loss medication in obese patients without diabetes and has promising effects improving hypertension and cardiovascular risk profile over 1-year treatment (Pi-Sunyer et al. 2015; Fonseca et al. 2014; le Roux et al. 2017).

Bariatric surgery has a sustained effect on weight loss, which is superior to pharmacological and lifestyle modifications. Considerable weight loss after bariatric surgery corresponds to high rates of remission of hypertension (Pareek et al. 2019). The GATEWAY trial showed that a reduction of $\geq 30\%$ of the total number of antihypertensive medications while maintaining controlled blood pressure occurred in 83.7% of the patients randomized to receive the Roux-en-Y gastric bypass plus antihypertensive medical therapy compared with only 12.8% patients from the control group with pharmacological therapy alone. Indeed, remission of hypertension was present in almost 50% of patients randomized to gastric bypass, whereas no patient randomized to control therapy was free of antihypertensive drugs at 12-month follow-up (Schiavon et al. 2018).

2.4   Regular Physical Activity

Epidemiological studies suggest that regular aerobic physical activity is beneficial for both reducing BP and decreasing CVD event rates and mortality (Franklin et al. 2020; Williams et al. 2018). As a result and along with the notion that "more exercise is better," more and more normotensive and hypertensive adults have increased their participation in high-intensity interval training or competitive long distance endurance events. However, the quality and intensity of the physical activity is very important. Recent evidence suggests that beyond a safe upper limit, exercise may result in deleterious cardiovascular adaptations. For instance, exercise-induced hypertension and the race distances may contribute to the occurrence of myocardial fibrosis detectable by MRI in asymptomatic triathletes (Tahir et al. 2018).

Aerobic endurance training, dynamic resistance training, and isometric training reduce resting systolic BP and diastolic BP by mean 3.5/2.5, 1.8/3.2, and 10.9/ 6.2 mmHg, respectively, in general populations. Regular physical activity of lower intensity and duration lowers BP less than moderate- or high-intensity training, but is associated with at least a 15% decrease in mortality in cohort studies (Rossi et al. 2012). Thus, the current ESC/EHS Guidelines recommend at least 30 min of moderate dynamic exercise (walking, jogging, cycling, or swimming) on 5–7 days per week (Williams et al. 2018). The impact of isometric exercises on BP and CVD risk is less well-established, although it can be part of a comprehensive treatment regimen (Chrysant 2010).

3   Pharmacological Therapy for the Treatment of Arterial Hypertension

Current evidence suggests that treatment and gradual control of hypertension by the use of the major classes of antihypertensive drugs exert positive effects on atherosclerosis. Randomized controlled trials provided robust evidence that five drug classes lower BP and prevent CVD events. They are therefore recommended by the 2018 ESC/ESH Guidelines (Williams et al. 2018) for the treatment of hypertension: angiotensin-converting enzyme (ACE) inhibitors, angiotensin II receptor blockers (ARBs), beta-blockers, calcium channel blockers (CCBs), and diuretics (thiazides and thiazide-like diuretics such as chlorthalidone and indapamide). ACE-I or ARBs alone or in combination with a calcium antagonist or a diuretic (thiazide-like to be preferred to thiazide) are considered for the first-line treatment. The use of beta-blockers is limited to special indications.

3.1   Who Should Be Treated with Pharmacological Therapy?

The benefits of antihypertensive therapy are clear in the majority of patients with arterial hypertension, but still controversial in subgroups. They include patients with Grade 1 hypertension but without manifest CVD, patients with white coat or masked hypertension and low cardiovascular risk, patients with an estimated 10-year cardiovascular risk <10%, and patients older than 75 years of age who are non-ambulatory or living in nursing homes.

Randomized trials demonstrated that treating hypertension with any antihypertensive therapy reduces cardiovascular morbidity and mortality. According to the ESC/ESH Guidelines, antihypertensive drug therapy should be initiated without any delay in patients with hypertension Grades 2 or 3 or after some time under non-pharmacological therapy in individuals with very high cardiovascular risk and Grade 1 or high-normal BP (Fig. 1). The decision to initiate drug therapy should be individualized and involve shared decision-making between patient and provider.

3.2   Choice of Initial Antihypertensive Agents

Multiple studies and meta-analyses conclude that the degree of BP reduction rather than the kind of antihypertensive medication is the major determinant of reduction in cardiovascular risk in patients with hypertension (Ettehad et al. 2016).

However, not all antihypertensive drugs are equally effective in reducing cardiovascular events and only few reduced mortality (van Vark et al. 2012).

Recommendations for the use of specific classes of antihypertensive medications are based upon clinical trial evidence of decreased cardiovascular risk, BP-lowering efficacy, safety, and tolerability. Most patients with hypertension will require more than one BP medication to reach their BP goal. As the consequence, the new guideline for treatment of hypertension suggests to use combination therapy at early stage and, if possible, a fixed-dose single-pill combination medication to improve adherence (Williams et al. 2018). Having multiple available classes of BP medications, practitioners and clinicians can individualize therapy based upon individual patient characteristics and preferences.

The following drugs are suggested for the start of monotherapy or combination therapy of arterial hypertension:

– ACE inhibitors
– ARBs
– Long-acting CCBs (most often a dihydropyridine such as amlodipine)
– Thiazide-like or thiazide-type diuretics

The previous 2013 Guidelines (Mancia et al. 2013) favored monotherapy for the start of treating hypertension. However, only a minority of patients reach the target blood pressure level under monotherapy, and the combination of two drugs is much more efficient than increasing the dose of a single drug (Williams et al. 2018).

Therefore, the current 2018 Guidelines limit the start of monotherapy to low-risk patients with stage 1 hypertension whose SBP is <150 mmHg, very high-risk patients with high-normal BP, or frail older patients; see Table 1.

3.3 Combination Therapy

Single-agent therapy will not adequately control BP in most patients whose baseline systolic BP is 15 mmHg or more above their goal. Combination therapy with drugs from different classes has a substantially greater BP-lowering effect than doubling the dose of a single agent (Wald et al. 2009).

When more than one agent is needed to control BP, a therapy with a long-acting ACE inhibitor or ARB in combination (fix if this is possible) with a long-acting dihydropyridine CCB or a diuretic is the first choice. Combination of an ACE inhibitor or ARBs with a thiazide diuretic is considered less beneficial, when hydrochlorothiazide instead of thiazide-like diuretic (chlorthalidone or indapamide) is used (Burnier et al. 2019; Williams et al. 2018). ACE inhibitors and ARBs should **not** be used together.

Chlorthalidone and indapamide have been used in several RCTs showing cardiovascular benefits, and these agents are more potent per milligram in lowering BP and have a longer duration of action compared with hydrochlorothiazide without any evidence of more side effects (Williams et al. 2018).

As such, even if head-to-head RCTs are missing, this data suggests that thiazide-like diuretics such as chlorthalidone and indapamide should be preferred over classical thiazide diuretics (e.g., hydrochlorothiazide and bendrofluazide) (Williams et al. 2018; Burnier et al. 2019; Roush et al. 2015).

The Danish Cancer Registry and the Danish Prescription Registry examined the association between the use of hydrochlorothiazide (HCTZ) and the risk of basal cell carcinoma, squamous cell carcinoma, and nodular melanoma (Pedersen et al. 2018a, 2018b, 2019). These two case-control studies showed that high cumulative doses of HCTZ (>50 g) are associated with a dose-dependent increase in the risk of non-melanoma skin cancer, but not of melanoma. The increase of risk was only small for squamous cell carcinoma and negligible for basal cell carcinoma. These studies have several limitations including the investigation of a pale-skinned population and the lack of information on genetic predisposition, sun habits, and ultraviolet exposure. Moreover, the risk reduction of death due to lower BP by HCTZ was much stronger than the small risk increase for squamous cell carcinoma by HCTZ. In general, statistically significant associations from observational studies do not prove any causal relationship.

The next step is the combination of RAAS blocker, Ca antagonists, and thiazide/ thiazide-like diuretics.

If BP is not sufficiently controlled by this triple combination therapy, a mineralocorticoid receptor (MR) antagonist (i.e., spironolactone or eplerenone) may be added (Williams et al. 2015).

In patients with difficult-to-treat/resistant hypertension, a beta-blocker, an alpha-blocker, or a direct arterial vasodilator could be added.

Generally, concomitant use of beta-blockers and non-dihydropyridine CCBs should be avoided, as both drug classes reduce heart rate.

3.4 Direct Effects of Antihypertensive Drugs on Atherosclerosis

Apart from lowering blood pressure and thereby removing an important risk factor, some antihypertensive drugs appear to exert direct effects on vascular cells that are involved in the pathogenesis of atherosclerosis.

3.4.1 ARBs and ACE Inhibitors

ARBs and ACE inhibitors directly affect the renin-angiotensin-aldosterone system (RAAS), by blocking the binding of angiotensin II (Ang II) to the AT1 receptor and decreasing the production of Ang II, respectively. Hypertension promotes and accelerates the atherothrombotic process via inflammatory mechanisms linked to activation of oxidative stress by Ang II, which subsequently leads to endothelial dysfunction and development of atherogenic lesions and plaques. Endothelial dysfunction is observed in the early stages of atherosclerosis. A healthy endothelium induces vasodilatation and has antioxidant and anti-thrombotic effects. The dysfunctional endothelium releases less of nitric oxide (NO) and other protective molecules, has a disrupted redox balance, and acquires pro-constrictive and pro-thrombotic phenotypes (Flammer et al. 2012; Sudano et al. 2011). A dysfunctional endothelium has been associated with cardiovascular risk factors including diabetes mellitus or impaired glucose metabolism, hypertension, cigarette smoking, dyslipidemia, obesity, and/or metabolic syndrome (Flammer et al. 2012; Sudano et al. 2011).

RAAS antagonists, as well as some dihydropyridine CCBs, possess ancillary and synergistic effects that increase NO bioavailability, reduce oxidative stress, and suppress inflammatory responses, thereby improving both endothelial activity and vascular function (Safar and Smulyan 2007; Sudano et al. 2011; Taddei et al. 2002).

3.4.2 Diuretics

Among the diuretics, thiazide-like diuretics such chlorthalidone and indapamide but not hydrochlorothiazide were found to improve endothelial function (Dell'Omo et al. 2005; Vinereanu et al. 2014). Indapamide also reduces arterial stiffness (Agnoletti et al. 2013).

3.4.3 Calcium Antagonists

Dihydropyridine CCBs lower BP mainly through vasodilation and reduction of peripheral resistance. Several clinical studies have demonstrated that they have clinical benefits in patients with CVD. Some studies have indicated that dihydropyridine CCBs have anti-atherogenic effects beyond their BP-lowering effects (Silva et al. 2019; Sudano et al. 2011). In fact, in several animal models, dihydropyridine CCBs were found to suppress the formation of atherosclerotic lesions. It is well-known that the production of reactive oxygen species (ROS) is involved in the progression of atherosclerosis by stimulating the production of inflammatory factors such as chemokines, cytokines, and adhesion molecules (Mason 2002; Ishii et al. 2012). Dihydropyridine CCBs can suppress ROS generation and subsequent inflammatory actions in vascular cells and arterial walls. Furthermore, several reports have revealed that dihydropyridine CCBs suppress the expression of adhesion molecules, thereby inhibiting monocyte adhesion to endothelial cells, which is an early step in the pathogenesis of atherosclerosis. Dihydropyridine CCBs also suppress proliferation and migration of smooth muscle cells both in vitro and in vivo (Mason 2002; Ishii et al. 2012). In macrophages, dihydropyridine CCBs decrease cholesterol accumulation and intracellular cholesterol esterification and increase cholesteryl ester hydrolysis. Moreover, dihydropyridine CCBs suppress the expression of matrix metalloproteinases, which affects the stability of atheromatous plaques. Interestingly, recent studies have revealed that the anti-atherosclerotic effects of dihydropyridine CCBs are mediated, at least in part, via the activation of peroxisome proliferator-activated receptor-γ (Ishii et al. 2012).

3.4.4 Beta-Blockers

In general, beta-blockers usually do not have any effect on endothelial function and atherothrombosis. The only exception is nebivolol, thanks to its high selectivity as beta1-blocker. Nebivolol inhibits the proliferation of human coronary smooth muscle and endothelial cells (Brehm et al. 2001). The specific vasorelaxant properties of nebivolol are mediated by endothelium-dependent NO release and antioxidant activity (do Vale et al. 2018). Unfortunately, nebivolol treatment in patients with non-obstructive coronary artery disease was associated with greater plaque progression and constrictive remodeling as compared to atenolol (Hung et al. 2016). Carvedilol, a nonselective blocker with additional adrenergic receptor antagonist activity, has also been shown to exert beneficial actions against endothelial dysfunction through its antioxidant effects (Bank et al. 2007), although the molecular mechanisms have not yet been fully clarified (Virdis et al. 2011).

3.4.5 Mineralocorticoid Receptor Antagonists

The MR antagonists, spironolactone and eplerenone, have been shown to reduce morbidity and mortality, in part, by blunting the adverse effects of aldosterone on endothelial function and inflammation involved in the development and complications of atherosclerosis. Recent evidence highlight that pharmacological blockade or genetic deletion of endothelial MR blunt vascular inflammation including expression of adhesion molecules, leukocyte-endothelial interactions, and plaque inflammation. Of note, in preclinical studies endothelial MR inhibition is protective only in male, but not in female mice (Moss et al. 2019). Thus, gender- and sex-specific actions of the MR in vascular function and atherosclerosis, so far still poorly investigated, will deserve future attention also in the clinical setting (Shen et al. 2017). Sympathetic hyperactivity with rising catecholamine levels and adrenergic receptors stimulation is a common feature of many CVDs, including hypertension. This is associated with endothelial NO synthase uncoupling and a pro-constrictive vascular phenotype on adjacent small arterial vessel wall components, such as smooth muscle and endothelial cells. Activation of MR signaling in the perivascular adipose tissue surrounding small arteries contributes to β-adrenoceptor overstimulation. Thus, MR antagonists targeting the endothelium and the perivascular adipocytes surrounding small arteries may achieve a dual benefit in hypertension with involvement of sympathetic over-activation, as, for instance, in overweight and obesity (Victorio et al. 2016).

4   Perspectives of Future Antihypertensive Therapy

4.1   Unresolved Medical Needs

Despite large evidence confirming the importance of lowering BP and the availability of many effective and well-tolerated antihypertensive drugs, BP control rate is unfortunately not as high as it should. This is, at least in part, related to poor adherence to lifelong antihypertensive therapy but also, in a minority of patients, due to "difficult to treat" or "resistant" hypertension.

According to the guidelines, resistant or difficult-to-treat hypertension is defined as: *blood pressure that is not controlled to goal despite adherence to an appropriate regimen of three antihypertensive drugs of different classes (including a diuretic) in which all drugs are prescribed at suitable antihypertensive doses* (Williams et al. 2018). Pseudo-resistance as well as secondary causes of hypertension should be excluded before this diagnosis is made.

Pseudo-resistance results from some or all of the following (Williams et al. 2018):

- Inaccurate blood pressure measurement (e.g., use of an inappropriately small blood pressure cuff, not allowing a patient to rest quietly before taking readings)
- Poor adherence to blood pressure medications
- Poor adherence to lifestyle and dietary approaches to lower blood pressure
- Suboptimal antihypertensive therapy, due either to inadequate doses, an inappropriate drug combination, or exclusion of a diuretic from the antihypertensive regimen
- White coat hypertension
- Extracellular volume expansion
- Increased sympathetic activation
- Ingestion of substances that can elevate the blood pressure, such as nonsteroidal anti-inflammatory drugs (NSAIDs) or stimulants
- Secondary or contributing causes of hypertension

4.2   New Drug Developments

Recent research has not yielded major advances in treatment of hypertension: no new targets were identified for development of antihypertensive drugs. In fact, trends show a dramatic slowing of research and development for novel blood pressure-lowering drugs. The reasons are manifold: the field is crowded with relatively effective drugs; there is a lack of major new discoveries and targets; and there are many challenges in developing blockbuster drugs. A short look in clinicaltrial.gov shows that while the development of new classes of antihypertensive drugs is apparently waning, the most current activities by big pharmaceutical companies focused on developing new combination pills, including fixed-dose combination drugs with the exception of a new ARB (fimasartan) and the compound AGSCT101, which is actually tested versus carvedilol. Fimasartan is an Ang II receptor antagonist with selectivity for the AT-1 receptor subtype, developed in 2012 by a Korean company (Boryung Pharmaceutical) as an oral antihypertensive drug (Fimasartan 2011; Chi et al. 2011). Fimasartan reduced BP with a good tolerability profile in a large-scale observational population study – Safe-KanArb (Park et al. 2013). The K-MetS study (Park et al. 2017) included 10,601 patients with metabolic syndrome and evaluated long-term effects of fimasartan on major adverse cardiovascular outcomes.

A recent study evaluated the effects of fimasartan and amlodipine therapy on carotid atherosclerotic plaque inflammation using 18F-fluorodeoxyglucose positron emission tomography imaging. Both drugs similarly decreased carotid atherosclerotic plaque inflammation in patients with acute coronary syndrome (Oh et al. 2019).

Concerning AGSCT101, a new antihypertensive drug developed by Ahn-Gook Pharmaceuticals Co., Ltd., the details are scarce. The Phase III Clinical Trial to Evaluate the Antihypertensive Effect of AGSCT101 Versus Carvedilol in Patient with Stage 1 to 2 Essential Hypertension is described in clinicaltrial.gov. Unfortunately, data about mechanism of action of this drug and status of recruiting of the described study are missing.

4.3   Device Therapy

Various device-based therapies such as renal denervation, carotid baroreceptor stimulation, creation of an arteriovenous fistula, or endovascular carotid body modification have emerged, principally targeted at the treatment of resistant hypertension.

Most data are available for renal denervation. The principle of renal denervation is to destroy some of the sympathetic nerves around the renal artery leading to lower sympathetic nervous activity and lower BP. The first results on renal denervation were obtained with devices using radiofrequency application in the open label SYMPLICITY HTN-1 and SYMPLICITY HTN-2 trials, along with several case series and observational studies. The SYMPLICITY HTN-3 trial proved safety, but was unable to show efficacy of renal denervation using a radiofrequency catheter when compared with sham treatment in patients with severe resistant hypertension on multiple medications (Williams et al. 2018). Post hoc analyses of the SYMPLICITY HTN-3, however, revealed important information concerning patient selection, difference in adherence to antihypertensive medication in the treatment groups, a higher use of antihypertensive drugs in the sham group, as well as technical failure in performing renal denervation, which led to a revision of renal denervation technology and technique. Based on this background, several novel, sham-controlled studies have been conducted and are, in part, published. SPYRAL HTN-OFF MED (Townsend et al. 2017; Bohm et al. 2020), SPYRAL HTN-ON MED (Kandzari et al. 2018), as well as RADIANCE-HTN SOLO (Azizi et al. 2018) showed significant and consistent reductions in BP, both office and ambulatory, in patients with and without concomitant antihypertensive.

The SPYRAL HTN-ON MED was recently published and showed the superiority of catheter-based renal denervation compared with a sham procedure to safely lower BP in the absence of antihypertensive medications (Bohm et al. 2020). Catheter-based renal denervation is superior to a sham procedure to safely lower BP in the absence of antihypertensive medications.

Less data are available about the effect of carotid baroreceptor stimulation and endovascular carotid body modification both techniques aiming to reduce BP through reduction of sympathetic tone and obtained by creation of an arteriovenous fistula. Concerning carotid baroreceptor stimulation, the first-generation device reduced BP in controlled and uncontrolled clinical trials, while controlled clinical trials proving efficacy in BP reduction do not exist for the currently available second-generation carotid sinus stimulator (Jordan et al. 2019; Heusser et al. 2020).

Some, mostly uncontrolled, studies suggest that other techniques such as baroreflex amplification and carotid body modulation may lead to reduction of BP in patients with difficult-to-treat hypertension. However more evidence on safety and efficacy from ongoing large randomized sham-controlled trials is needed before baroreflex amplification and carotid body modulation can be implemented in routine clinical practice (Groenland and Spiering 2020).

Last, but not least, the possibility to safely reduce BP in patients with uncontrolled hypertension by creating a central iliac arteriovenous anastomosis was tested. The ROX CONTROL HTN study (Lobo et al. 2015) tested this hypothesis using the novel arteriovenous ROX Coupler (ROX Medical, San Clemente, CA, USA).

This small study (44 patients treated and 39 patients in the standard of care group) enrolled and showed that creation of an arteriovenous anastomosis was associated with significantly reduced BP.

The actual ESC/ESH Guidelines do not recommend the use of any device-based therapies for the routine treatment of hypertension, unless in the context of clinical studies and RCTs (Williams et al. 2018).

Nevertheless, device-based therapy for hypertension is a fast-moving field, and new data especially data from study evaluating renal denervation are expected in the near future and could change this recommendation.

5 Conclusion

Hypertension represents one of the most important modifiable risk factors for stroke, heart failure, myocardial infarction, and chronic kidney disease, contributing significantly to the global burden of CVD.

The initial assessment of a patient with hypertension is essential for choosing effective therapy. All cardiovascular risk factors as well as hypertension-mediated target organ damage and presence of comorbidities should be taken into account.

The treatment of hypertension should focus on the overall health of the patient, focusing on reducing the risk of future cardiovascular events.

For a long-lasting adherence, it is important that patients are actively involved in the process of choosing the best BP-lowering strategies.

Funding E.O. is supported by the Swiss National Science Foundation (SNSF) (PRIMA: PR00P3_179861/1), the Olga Mayenfisch Foundation, and the Swiss Heart Foundation (SHF), Switzerland. I.S. and F.R received grants from SNSF (Nr 32003B_179519) and the SHF, Switzerland.

Conflict of Interest FR reports grant support for the ESC-HFA Postgraduate Course in Heart Failure from Novartis, Servier, Bayer, Abbott and Astra Zeneca and the VASCEND trial from Novartis (all payments directly to the University of Zurich).

FR has been paid for the time spent as a committee member for clinical trials, advisory boards, other forms of consulting and lectures or presentations. These payments were made directly to the University of Zurich and no personal payments were received in relation to these trials or other activities since January 2018.

Before 2018, FR reports grants and personal fees from SJM/Abbott, Servier, Novartis and Bayer, personal fees from Zoll, Astra Zeneca, Sanofi, Amgen, BMS, Pfizer, Fresenius, Vifor, Roche, Cardiorentis and Boehringer Ingelheim, other from Heartware and grants from Mars, outside the submitted work.

References

Aghamohammadzadeh R, Greenstein AS, Yadav R, Jeziorska M, Hama S, Soltani F, Pemberton PW, Ammori B, Malik RA, Soran H, Heagerty AM (2013) Effects of bariatric surgery on human small artery function: evidence for reduction in perivascular adipocyte inflammation, and the restoration of normal anticontractile activity despite persistent obesity. J Am Coll Cardiol 62:128–135

Agnoletti D, Zhang Y, Borghi C, Blacher J, Safar ME (2013) Effects of antihypertensive drugs on central blood pressure in humans: a preliminary observation. Am J Hypertens 26:1045–1052

Appel LJ, Brands MW, Daniels SR, Karanja N, Elmer PJ, Sacks FM, Association American Heart (2006) Dietary approaches to prevent and treat hypertension: a scientific statement from the American Heart Association. Hypertension 47:296–308

Azizi M, Schmieder RE, Mahfoud F, Weber MA, Daemen J, Davies J, Basile J, Kirtane AJ, Wang Y, Lobo MD, Saxena M, Feyz L, Rader F, Lurz P, Sayer J, Sapoval M, Levy T, Sanghvi K, Abraham J, Sharp ASP, Fisher NDL, Bloch MJ, Reeve-Stoffer H, Coleman L, Mullin C, Mauri L, Radiance-Htn Investigators (2018) Endovascular ultrasound renal denervation to treat hypertension (RADIANCE-HTN SOLO): a multicentre, international, single-blind, randomised, sham-controlled trial. Lancet 391:2335–2345

Bank AJ, Kelly AS, Thelen AM, Kaiser DR, Gonzalez-Campoy JM (2007) Effects of carvedilol versus metoprolol on endothelial function and oxidative stress in patients with type 2 diabetes mellitus. Am J Hypertens 20:777–783

Bernabe-Ortiz A, Rosas Y, Sal VG, Ponce-Lucero V, Cardenas MK, Carrillo-Larco RM, Diez-Canseco F, Pesantes MA, Sacksteder KA, Gilman RH, Miranda JJ (2020) Effect of salt substitution on community-wide blood pressure and hypertension incidence. Nat Med 26:374

Bibbins-Domingo K, Chertow GM, Coxson PG, Moran A, Lightwood JM, Pletcher MJ, Goldman L (2010) Projected effect of dietary salt reductions on future cardiovascular disease. N Engl J Med 362:590–599

Binia A, Jaeger J, Hu Y, Singh A, Zimmermann D (2015) Daily potassium intake and sodium-to-potassium ratio in the reduction of blood pressure: a meta-analysis of randomized controlled trials. J Hypertens 33:1509–1520

Bohm M, Kario K, Kandzari DE, Mahfoud F, Weber MA, Schmieder RE, Tsioufis K, Pocock S, Konstantinidis D, Choi JW, East C, Lee DP, Ma A, Ewen S, Cohen DL, Wilensky R, Devireddy CM, Lea J, Schmid A, Weil J, Agdirlioglu T, Reedus D, Jefferson BK, Reyes D, D'Souza R, Sharp ASP, Sharif F, Fahy M, DeBruin V, Cohen SA, Brar S, Townsend RR, Spyral Htn-Off Med Pivotal Investigators (2020) Efficacy of catheter-based renal denervation in the absence of antihypertensive medications (SPYRAL HTN-OFF MED pivotal): a multicentre, randomised, sham-controlled trial. Lancet

Brehm BR, Wolf SC, Bertsch D, Klaussner M, Wesselborg S, Schuler S, Schulze-Osthoff K (2001) Effects of nebivolol on proliferation and apoptosis of human coronary artery smooth muscle and endothelial cells. Cardiovasc Res 49:430–439

Burnier M, Bakris G, Williams B (2019) Redefining diuretics use in hypertension: why select a thiazide-like diuretic? J Hypertens 37:1574–1586

Chi YH, Lee H, Paik SH, Lee JH, Yoo BW, Kim JH, Tan HK, Kim SL (2011) Safety, tolerability, pharmacokinetics, and pharmacodynamics of fimasartan following single and repeated oral administration in the fasted and fed states in healthy subjects. Am J Cardiovasc Drugs 11:335–346

Chrysant SG (2010) Current evidence on the hemodynamic and blood pressure effects of isometric exercise in normotensive and hypertensive persons. J Clin Hypertens (Greenwich) 12:721–726

Cohen JB, Gadde KM (2019) Weight loss medications in the treatment of Obesity and hypertension. Curr Hypertens Rep 21:16

Dell'Omo G, Penno G, Del Prato S, Pedrinelli R (2005) Chlorthalidone improves endothelial-mediated vascular responses in hypertension complicated by nondiabetic metabolic syndrome. J Cardiovasc Pharmacol Ther 10:265–272

do Vale GT, Simplicio JA, Gonzaga NA, Yokota R, Ribeiro AA, Casarini DE, de Martinis BS, Tirapelli CR (2018) Nebivolol prevents vascular oxidative stress and hypertension in rats chronically treated with ethanol. Atherosclerosis 274:67–76

Ettehad D, Emdin CA, Kiran A, Anderson SG, Callender T, Emberson J, Chalmers J, Rodgers A, Rahimi K (2016) Blood pressure lowering for prevention of cardiovascular disease and death: a systematic review and meta-analysis. Lancet 387:957–967

Fimasartan (2011) Am J Cardiovasc Drugs 11:249–252

Flammer AJ, Anderson T, Celermajer DS, Creager MA, Deanfield J, Ganz P, Hamburg NM, Luscher TF, Shechter M, Taddei S, Vita JA, Lerman A (2012) The assessment of endothelial function: from research into clinical practice. Circulation 126:753–767

Fonseca VA, Devries JH, Henry RR, Donsmark M, Thomsen HF, Plutzky J (2014) Reductions in systolic blood pressure with liraglutide in patients with type 2 diabetes: insights from a patient-level pooled analysis of six randomized clinical trials. J Diabetes Complicat 28:399–405

Franklin BA, Thompson PD, Al-Zaiti SS, Albert CM, Hivert MF, Levine BD, Lobelo F, Madan K, Sharrief AZ, Eijsvogels TMH, Lifestyle American Heart Association Physical Activity Committee of the Council on, Health Cardiometabolic, Cardiovascular Council on, Nursing Stroke, Cardiology Council on Clinical, and Council Stroke (2020) Exercise-related acute cardiovascular events and potential deleterious adaptations following long-term exercise training: placing the risks into perspective-an update: a scientific statement from the American Heart Association. Circulation:CIR0000000000000749

Groenland EH, Spiering W (2020) Baroreflex amplification and carotid body modulation for the treatment of resistant hypertension. Curr Hypertens Rep 22:27

He FJ, MacGregor GA (2003) How far should salt intake be reduced? Hypertension 42:1093–1099

He FJ, MacGregor GA (2011) Salt reduction lowers cardiovascular risk: meta-analysis of outcome trials. Lancet 378:380–382

He FJ, Burnier M, Macgregor GA (2011) Nutrition in cardiovascular disease: salt in hypertension and heart failure. Eur Heart J 32:3073–3080

Helmstadter J, Frenis K, Filippou K, Grill A, Dib M, Kalinovic S, Pawelke F, Kus K, Kroller-Schon S, Oelze M, Chlopicki S, Schuppan D, Wenzel P, Ruf W, Drucker DJ, Munzel T, Daiber A, Steven S (2020) Endothelial GLP-1 (glucagon-like Peptide-1) receptor mediates cardiovascular protection by Liraglutide in mice with experimental arterial hypertension. Arterioscler Thromb Vasc Biol 40:145–158

Heusser K, Thone A, Lipp A, Menne J, Beige J, Reuter H, Hoffmann F, Halbach M, Eckert S, Wallbach M, Koziolek M, Haarmann H, Joyner MJ, Paton JFR, Diedrich A, Haller H, Jordan J, Tank J (2020) Efficacy of electrical Baroreflex activation is independent of peripheral chemoreceptor modulation. Hypertension 75:257–264

Holmes MV, Dale CE, Zuccolo L, Silverwood RJ, Guo Y, Ye Z, Prieto-Merino D, Dehghan A, Trompet S, Wong A, Cavadino A, Drogan D, Padmanabhan S, Li S, Yesupriya A, Leusink M, Sundstrom J, Hubacek JA, Pikhart H, Swerdlow DI, Panayiotou AG, Borinskaya SA, Finan C, Shah S, Kuchenbaecker KB, Shah T, Engmann J, Folkersen L, Eriksson P, Ricceri F, Melander O, Sacerdote C, Gamble DM, Rayaprolu S, Ross OA, McLachlan S, Vikhireva O, Sluijs I, Scott RA, Adamkova V, Flicker L, Bockxmeer FM, Power C, Marques-Vidal P, Meade T, Marmot MG, Ferro JM, Paulos-Pinheiro S, Humphries SE, Talmud PJ, Mateo Leach I, Verweij N, Linneberg A, Skaaby T, Doevendans PA, Cramer MJ, van der Harst P, Klungel OH, Dowling NF, Dominiczak AF, Kumari M, Nicolaides AN, Weikert C, Boeing H, Ebrahim S, Gaunt TR, Price JF, Lannfelt L, Peasey A, Kubinova R, Pajak A, Malyutina S, Voevoda MI, Tamosiunas A, Maitland-van der Zee AH, Norman PE, Hankey GJ, Bergmann MM, Hofman A, Franco OH, Cooper J, Palmen J, Spiering W, de Jong PA, Kuh D, Hardy R, Uitterlinden AG, Ikram MA, Ford I, Hypponen E, Almeida OP, Wareham NJ, Khaw KT, Hamsten A, Husemoen LL, Tjonneland A, Tolstrup JS, Rimm E, Beulens JW, Verschuren WM, Onland-Moret NC, Hofker MH, Wannamethee SG, Whincup PH, Morris R, Vicente AM, Watkins H, Farrall M, Jukema JW, Meschia J, Cupples LA, Sharp SJ, Fornage M, Kooperberg C, LaCroix AZ, Dai JY, Lanktree MB, Siscovick DS, Jorgenson E, Spring B, Coresh J, Li YR, Buxbaum SG, Schreiner PJ, Ellison RC, Tsai MY, Patel SR, Redline S, Johnson AD, Hoogeveen RC, Hakonarson H, Rotter JI, Boerwinkle E, de Bakker PI, Kivimaki M, Asselbergs FW, Sattar N, Lawlor DA, Whittaker J, Davey Smith G, Mukamal K, Psaty BM, Wilson JG, Lange LA, Hamidovic A, Hingorani AD, Nordestgaard BG, Bobak M, Leon DA, Langenberg C, Palmer TM, Reiner AP, Keating BJ, Dudbridge F, Casas JP, Consortium InterAct (2014) Association between alcohol and cardiovascular disease: Mendelian randomisation analysis based on individual participant data. BMJ 349:g4164

Hung OY, Molony D, Corban MT, Rasoul-Arzrumly E, Maynard C, Eshtehardi P, Dhawan S, Timmins LH, Piccinelli M, Ahn SG, Gogas BD, McDaniel MC, Quyyumi AA, Giddens DP, Samady H (2016) Comprehensive assessment of coronary plaque progression with advanced intravascular imaging, physiological measures, and wall shear stress: a pilot double-blinded randomized controlled clinical trial of Nebivolol versus atenolol in nonobstructive coronary artery Disease. J Am Heart Assoc 5

Ishii N, Matsumura T, Shimoda S, Araki E (2012) Anti-atherosclerotic potential of dihydropyridine calcium channel blockers. J Atheroscler Thromb 19:693–704

Jordan J, Tank J, Reuter H (2019) Carotid baroreceptor stimulation. In: Mancia G, Dorobantu M, Grassi G, Voicu V (eds) Hypertension and heart failure. Springer, Cham

Kandzari DE, Bohm M, Mahfoud F, Townsend RR, Weber MA, Pocock S, Tsioufis K, Tousoulis D, Choi JW, East C, Brar S, Cohen SA, Fahy M, Pilcher G, Kario K, Spyral Htn-On Med Trial Investigators (2018) Effect of renal denervation on blood pressure in the presence of antihypertensive drugs: 6-month efficacy and safety results from the SPYRAL HTN-ON MED proof-of-concept randomised trial. Lancet 391:2346–2355

le Roux C, Aroda V, Hemmingsson J, Cancino AP, Christensen R, Pi-Sunyer X (2017) Comparison of efficacy and safety of Liraglutide 3.0 mg in individuals with BMI above and below 35 kg/m (2): a post-hoc analysis. Obes Facts 10:531–544

Lobo MD, Sobotka PA, Stanton A, Cockcroft JR, Sulke N, Dolan E, van der Giet M, Hoyer J, Furniss SS, Foran JP, Witkowski A, Januszewicz A, Schoors D, Tsioufis K, Rensing BJ, Scott B, Ng GA, Ott C, Schmieder RE, Rox Control Htn Investigators (2015) Central arteriovenous anastomosis for the treatment of patients with uncontrolled hypertension (the ROX CON TROL HTN study): a randomised controlled trial. Lancet 385:1634–1641

Look, Ahead Research Group, Wing RR, Bolin P, Brancati FL, Bray GA, Clark JM, Coday M, Crow RS, Curtis JM, Egan CM, Espeland MA, Evans M, Foreyt JP, Ghazarian S, Gregg EW, Harrison B, Hazuda HP, Hill JO, Horton ES, Hubbard VS, Jakicic JM, Jeffery RW, Johnson KC, Kahn SE, Kitabchi AE, Knowler WC, Lewis CE, Maschak-Carey BJ, Montez MG, Murillo A, Nathan DM, Patricio J, Peters A, Pi-Sunyer X, Pownall H, Reboussin D, Regensteiner JG, Rickman AD, Ryan DH, Safford M, Wadden TA, Wagenknecht LE, West DS, Williamson DF, Yanovski SZ (2013) Cardiovascular effects of intensive lifestyle intervention in type 2 diabetes. N Engl J Med 369:145–154

Mancia G, Fagard R, Narkiewicz K, Redon J, Zanchetti A, Bohm M, Christiaens T, Cifkova R, De Backer G, Dominiczak A, Galderisi M, Grobbee DE, Jaarsma T, Kirchhof P, Kjeldsen SE, Laurent S, Manolis AJ, Nilsson PM, Ruilope LM, Schmieder RE, Sirnes PA, Sleight P, Viigimaa M, Waeber B, Zannad F, Redon J, Dominiczak A, Narkiewicz K, Nilsson PM, Burnier M, Viigimaa M, Ambrosioni E, Caufield M, Coca A, Olsen MH, Schmieder RE, Tsioufis C, van de Borne P, Zamorano JL, Achenbach S, Baumgartner H, Bax JJ, Bueno H, Dean V, Deaton C, Erol C, Fagard R, Ferrari R, Hasdai D, Hoes AW, Kirchhof P, Knuuti J, Kolh P, Lancellotti P, Linhart A, Nihoyannopoulos P, Piepoli MF, Ponikowski P, Sirnes PA, Tamargo JL, Tendera M, Torbicki A, Wijns W, Windecker S, Clement DL, Coca A, Gillebert TC, Tendera M, Rosei EA, Ambrosioni E, Anker SD, Bauersachs J, Hitij JB, Caulfield M, De Buyzere M, De Geest S, Derumeaux GA, Erdine S, Farsang C, Funck-Brentano C, Gerc V, Germano G, Gielen S, Haller H, Hoes AW, Jordan J, Kahan T, Komajda M, Lovic D, Mahrholdt H, Olsen MH, Ostergren J, Parati G, Perk J, Polonia J, Popescu BA, Reiner Z, Ryden L, Sirenko Y, Stanton A, Struijker-Boudier H, Tsioufis C, van de Borne P, Vlachopoulos C, Volpe M, Wood DA (2013) 2013 ESH/ESC guidelines for the management of arterial hypertension: the task force for the management of Arterial Hypertension of the European Society of Hypertension (ESH) and of the European Society of Cardiology (ESC). Eur Heart J 34:2159–2219

Mason RP (2002) Mechanisms of plaque stabilization for the dihydropyridine calcium channel blocker amlodipine: review of the evidence. Atherosclerosis 165:191–199

Mente A, O'Donnell M, Rangarajan S, Dagenais G, Lear S, McQueen M, Diaz R, Avezum A, Lopez-Jaramillo P, Lanas F, Li W, Lu Y, Yi S, Rensheng L, Iqbal R, Mony P, Yusuf R, Yusoff K, Szuba A, Oguz A, Rosengren A, Bahonar A, Yusufali A, Schutte AE, Chifamba J, Mann JF, Anand SS, Teo K, Yusuf S, Epidream Pure, and Ontarget Transcend Investigators (2016) Associations of urinary sodium excretion with cardiovascular events in individuals with and without hypertension: a pooled analysis of data from four studies. Lancet 388:465–475

Miller V, Yusuf S, Chow CK, Dehghan M, Corsi DJ, Lock K, Popkin B, Rangarajan S, Khatib R, Lear SA, Mony P, Kaur M, Mohan V, Vijayakumar K, Gupta R, Kruger A, Tsolekile L, Mohammadifard N, Rahman O, Rosengren A, Avezum A, Orlandini A, Ismail N, Lopez-Jaramillo P, Yusufali A, Karsidag K, Iqbal R, Chifamba J, Oakley SM, Ariffin F, Zatonska K, Poirier P, Wei L, Jian B, Hui C, Xu L, Xiulin B, Teo K, Mente A (2016) Availability, affordability, and consumption of fruits and vegetables in 18 countries across income levels:

findings from the prospective urban rural epidemiology (PURE) study. Lancet Glob Health 4: e695–e703

Mingrone G, Panunzi S, de Gaetano A, Guidone C, Iaconelli A, Nanni G, Castagneto M, Bornstein S, Rubino F (2015) Bariatric-metabolic surgery versus conventional medical treatment in obese patients with type 2 diabetes: 5 year follow-up of an open-label, single-centre, randomised controlled trial. Lancet 386:964–973

Moss ME, Lu Q, Iyer SL, Engelbertsen D, Marzolla V, Caprio M, Lichtman AH, Jaffe IZ (2019) Endothelial mineralocorticoid receptors contribute to vascular inflammation in atherosclerosis in a sex-specific manner. Arterioscler Thromb Vasc Biol 39:1588–1601

Oh M, Lee CW, Ahn JM, Park DW, Kang SJ, Lee SW, Kim YH, Moon DH, Park SW, Park SJ (2019) Comparison of fimasartan and amlodipine therapy on carotid atherosclerotic plaque inflammation. Clin Cardiol 42:241–246

Pareek M, Bhatt DL, Schiavon CA, Schauer PR (2019) Metabolic surgery for hypertension in patients with Obesity. Circ Res 124:1009–1024

Park JB, Sung KC, Kang SM, Cho EJ (2013) Safety and efficacy of fimasartan in patients with arterial hypertension (safe-KanArb study): an open-label observational study. Am J Cardiovasc Drugs 13:47–56

Park JB, Kim SA, Sung KC, Kim JY (2017) Gender-specific differences in the incidence of microalbuminuria in metabolic syndrome patients after treatment with fimasartan: the K-MetS study. PLoS One 12:e0189342

Pedersen SA, Gaist D, Schmidt SAJ, Holmich LR, Friis S, Pottegard A (2018a) Hydrochlorothiazide use and risk of nonmelanoma skin cancer: a nationwide case-control study from Denmark. J Am Acad Dermatol 78(673–81):e9

Pedersen SA, Schmidt SA, Klausen S, Pottegard A, Friis S, Holmich LR, Gaist D (2018b) Melanoma of the skin in the Danish Cancer registry and the Danish melanoma database: a validation study. Epidemiology 29:442–447

Pedersen SA, Johannesdottir Schmidt SA, Holmich LR, Friis S, Pottegard A, Gaist D (2019) Hydrochlorothiazide use and risk for Merkel cell carcinoma and malignant adnexal skin tumors: a nationwide case-control study. J Am Acad Dermatol 80(460–65):e9

Pi-Sunyer X, Astrup A, Fujioka K, Greenway F, Halpern A, Krempf M, Lau DC, le Roux CW, Violante Ortiz R, Jensen CB, Wilding JP, Scale Obesity, and N. N. Study Group Prediabetes (2015) A randomized, controlled trial of 3.0 mg of Liraglutide in weight management. N Engl J Med 373:11–22

Rossi A, Dikareva A, Bacon SL, Daskalopoulou SS (2012) The impact of physical activity on mortality in patients with high blood pressure: a systematic review. J Hypertens 30:1277–1288

Roush GC, Ernst ME, Kostis JB, Tandon S, Sica DA (2015) Head-to-head comparisons of hydrochlorothiazide with indapamide and chlorthalidone: antihypertensive and metabolic effects. Hypertension 65:1041–1046

Safar ME, Smulyan H (2007) Atherosclerosis, arterial stiffness and antihypertensive drug therapy. Adv Cardiol 44:331–351

Schiavon CA, Bersch-Ferreira AC, Santucci EV, Oliveira JD, Torreglosa CR, Bueno PT, Frayha JC, Santos RN, Damiani LP, Noujaim PM, Halpern H, Monteiro FLJ, Cohen RV, Uchoa CH, de Souza MG, Amodeo C, Bortolotto L, Ikeoka D, Drager LF, Cavalcanti AB, Berwanger O (2018) Effects of bariatric surgery in obese patients with hypertension: the GATEWAY randomized trial (gastric bypass to treat obese patients with steady hypertension). Circulation 137:1132–1142

Semlitsch T, Jeitler K, Berghold A, Horvath K, Posch N, Poggenburg S, Siebenhofer A (2016) Long-term effects of weight-reducing diets in people with hypertension. Cochrane Database Syst Rev 3:CD008274

Shen ZX, Chen XQ, Sun XN, Sun JY, Zhang WC, Zheng XJ, Zhang YY, Shi HJ, Zhang JW, Li C, Wang J, Liu X, Duan SZ (2017) Mineralocorticoid receptor deficiency in macrophages inhibits atherosclerosis by affecting foam cell formation and Efferocytosis. J Biol Chem 292:925–935

Silva IVG, de Figueiredo RC, Rios DRA (2019) Effect of different classes of antihypertensive drugs on endothelial function and inflammation. Int J Mol Sci 20:3458

Sudano I, Roas S, Noll G (2011) Vascular abnormalities in essential hypertension. Curr Pharm Des 17:3039–3044

Taddei S, Virdis A, Ghiadoni L, Sudano I, Salvetti A (2002) Effects of antihypertensive drugs on endothelial dysfunction: clinical implications. Drugs 62:265–284

Tahir E, Starekova J, Muellerleile K, von Stritzky A, Munch J, Avanesov M, Weinrich JM, Stehning C, Bohnen S, Radunski UK, Freiwald E, Blankenberg S, Adam G, Pressler A, Patten M, Lund GK (2018) Myocardial fibrosis in competitive triathletes detected by contrast-enhanced CMR correlates with exercise-induced hypertension and competition history. JACC Cardiovasc Imaging 11:1260–1270

Taylor RS, Ashton KE, Moxham T, Hooper L, Ebrahim S (2011) Reduced dietary salt for the prevention of cardiovascular disease: a meta-analysis of randomized controlled trials (Cochrane review). Am J Hypertens 24:843–853

Townsend RR, Mahfoud F, Kandzari DE, Kario K, Pocock S, Weber MA, Ewen S, Tsioufis K, Tousoulis D, Sharp ASP, Watkinson AF, Schmieder RE, Schmid A, Choi JW, East C, Walton A, Hopper I, Cohen DL, Wilensky R, Lee DP, Ma A, Devireddy CM, Lea JP, Lurz PC, Fengler K, Davies J, Chapman N, Cohen SA, DeBruin V, Fahy M, Jones DE, Rothman M, Bohm M, Spyral Htn-Off Med trial investigators (2017) Catheter-based renal denervation in patients with uncontrolled hypertension in the absence of antihypertensive medications (SPY RAL HTN-OFF MED): a randomised, sham-controlled, proof-of-concept trial. Lancet 390:2160–2170

van Vark LC, Bertrand M, Akkerhuis KM, Brugts JJ, Fox K, Mourad JJ, Boersma E (2012) Angiotensin-converting enzyme inhibitors reduce mortality in hypertension: a meta-analysis of randomized clinical trials of renin-angiotensin-aldosterone system inhibitors involving 158,998 patients. Eur Heart J 33:2088–2097

Victorio JA, Clerici SP, Palacios R, Alonso MJ, Vassallo DV, Jaffe IZ, Rossoni LV, Davel AP (2016) Spironolactone prevents endothelial nitric oxide synthase uncoupling and vascular dysfunction induced by beta-adrenergic overstimulation: role of perivascular adipose tissue. Hypertension 68:726–735

Vinereanu D, Dulgheru R, Magda S, Dragoi Galrinho R, Florescu M, Cinteza M, Granger C, Ciobanu AO (2014) The effect of indapamide versus hydrochlorothiazide on ventricular and arterial function in patients with hypertension and diabetes: results of a randomized trial. Am Heart J 168:446–456

Virdis A, Ghiadoni L, Taddei S (2011) Effects of antihypertensive treatment on endothelial function. Curr Hypertens Rep 13:276–281

Virdis A, Duranti E, Rossi C, Dell'Agnello U, Santini E, Anselmino M, Chiarugi M, Taddei S, Solini A (2015) Tumour necrosis factor-alpha participates on the endothelin-1/nitric oxide imbalance in small arteries from obese patients: role of perivascular adipose tissue. Eur Heart J 36:784–794

Wald DS, Law M, Morris JK, Bestwick JP, Wald NJ (2009) Combination therapy versus monotherapy in reducing blood pressure: meta-analysis on 11,000 participants from 42 trials. Am J Med 122:290–300

Weinberger MH (1996) Salt sensitivity of blood pressure in humans. Hypertension 27:481–490

Williams B, MacDonald TM, Morant S, Webb DJ, Sever P, McInnes G, Ford I, Cruickshank JK, Caulfield MJ, Salsbury J, Mackenzie I, Padmanabhan S, Brown MJ, Pathway Studies Group British Hypertension Society's (2015) Spironolactone versus placebo, bisoprolol, and doxazosin to determine the optimal treatment for drug-resistant hypertension (PATHWAY-2): a randomised, double-blind, crossover trial. Lancet 386:2059–2068

Williams B, Mancia G, Spiering W, Agabiti Rosei E, Azizi M, Burnier M, Clement DL, Coca A, de Simone G, Dominiczak A, Kahan T, Mahfoud F, Redon J, Ruilope L, Zanchetti A, Kerins M, Kjeldsen SE, Kreutz R, Laurent S, Lip GYH, McManus R, Narkiewicz K, Ruschitzka F, Schmieder RE, Shlyakhto E, Tsioufis C, Aboyans V, Desormais I, E. S. C. Scientific Document Group (2018) 2018 ESC/ESH guidelines for the management of arterial hypertension. Eur Heart J 39:3021–3104

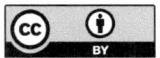

Glycaemic Control in Diabetes

D. Müller-Wieland, J. Brandts, M. Verket, N. Marx, and K. Schütt

Contents

1   Cardiovascular Risk in Diabetes 48
2   Microvascular End-Organ Damage and Cardiovascular Risk 49
3   Role of Hyperglycaemia for Micro- and Macro-vascular Complications 50
4   Role of Hyperglycaemia in Reducing Vascular Risks in Type 1 Diabetes 51
5   Efficacy Trials of Glucose Lowering in Type 2 Diabetes 52
6   Cardiovascular Safety Studies in Type 2 Diabetes 53
7   GLP-1 Receptor Agonists (GLP-1-RA) 54
8   SGLT (Sodium Glucose Transporter) 2 Inhibitors 58
9   Mechanisms of Action for Cardio-Renal Protection Through SGLT-2 Inhibition 62
10 Change in Guidelines and Clinical Recommendations 64
11 Perspectives: Fat Partitioning as a New Target of Diabetes Drugs 65
References 66

Abstract

Reduction of glucose is the hallmark of diabetes therapy proven to reduce micro- and macro-vascular risk in patients with type 1 diabetes. However glucose-lowering efficacy trials in type 2 diabetes didn't show major cardiovascular benefit. Then, a paradigm change in the treatment of patients with type 2 diabetes has emerged due to the introduction of new blood glucose-lowering agents. Cardiovascular endpoint studies have proven HbA1c-independent cardioprotective effects for GLP-1 receptor agonists and SGLT-2 inhibitors. Furthermore, SGLT-2 inhibitors reduce the risk for heart failure and chronic kidney disease. Mechanisms for these blood glucose independent drug target-related effects are still an enigma. Recent research has shown that GLP-1 receptor agonists might have anti-inflammatory and plaque stabilising effects whereas

D. Müller-Wieland (✉) · J. Brandts · M. Verket · N. Marx · K. Schütt
Department of Medicine I, University Hospital RWTH Aachen, Aachen, Germany
e-mail: dirmueller@ukaachen.de

© The Author(s) 2021
A. von Eckardstein, C. J. Binder (eds.), *Prevention and Treatment of Atherosclerosis*,
Handbook of Experimental Pharmacology 270, https://doi.org/10.1007/164_2021_537

SGLT-2 inhibitors primarily reduce pre- and after-load of the heart and increase work load efficiency of the heart. In addition, reduction of intraglomerular pressure, improved energy supply chains and water regulation appear to be major mechanisms for renoprotection by SGLT-2 inhibitors. These studies and observations have led to recent changes in clinical recommendations and treatment guidelines for type 2 diabetes. In patients with high or very high cardio-renal risk, SGLT-2 inhibitors or GLP-1 receptor agonists have a preferred recommendation independent of baseline HbA1c levels due to cardioprotection. In patients with chronic heart failure, chronic kidney disease or at respective risks SGLT-2 inhibitors are the preferred choice. Therefore, the treatment paradigm of glucose control in diabetes has changed towards using diabetes drugs with evidence-based organ protection improving clinical prognosis.

Keywords

GLP-1 receptor agonists · Heart failure · SGLT-2 inhibitors · Type 2 diabetes

Risks for clinical complications of micro- and macro-vascular disease appear to be increased in patients with type 1 and type 2 diabetes. Whereas the relation between elevated glucose levels and microvascular complications seems to be directly correlated and generally specific for diabetes. The relation to macrovascular risk, however, is more complex, multifactorial and not exclusive for diabetes. The link between type 2 diabetes and macrovascular risk is extending beyond glucose levels and may be related to obesity, fat partitioning, and insulin resistance, a concert also called metabolic syndrome.

In the following, we provide epidemiological evidence for increased vascular risk in diabetes, discuss the role of glucose control and introduce the cardiovascular outcome trials (CVOTs) for GLP-1 receptor agonists and SGLT-2-inhibitors. These trials provide direct clinical evidence for cardio-renal protection, independent of baseline HbA1c levels, leading to major changes in treatment algorithms in current guidelines. In conclusion, we will allude to the emerging of efficient obesity treatments, which might ultimately alter pathophysiological features of the metabolic syndrome and potential targets for atherosclerosis.

1 Cardiovascular Risk in Diabetes

The Emerging Risk Factors Collaboration analysed individual data from a total of more than one million people with more than 135,000 deaths (Danesh 2015). The relative risk of mortality was increased approximately twofold in the presence of diabetes or myocardial infarction, almost fourfold for the combination and almost sevenfold for additional stroke.

In the Swedish National Diabetes Registry, 318,083 patients with type 2 diabetes were compared with nearly 1.6 million matched controls over 5–6 years for cardiovascular endpoints and all-cause mortality (Sattar et al. 2019). Patients diagnosed with diabetes before age 40 years had on average a mean twofold increased risk of all-cause mortality, 2.72-fold increased risk of cardiovascular mortality, 4.77-fold increased risk of heart failure and 4.33-fold increased coronary risk. The risk was age-dependent and was no longer increased in a person older than 80 years old. Due to the increased risk of mortality in patients with diabetes, a database of care providers was used to analyse its relative risk in 31,987 newly diagnosed patients with diabetes compared to 162,656 controls over a 9.5-year period (Zucker et al. 2017). During this period, 14% of patients with diabetes died, but only 8% of matched controls without diabetes died. When adjusted for age, sex, socioeconomic status, obesity, smoking and comorbidities incident diabetes was associated with a 38% higher relative risk of all-cause mortality. A systematic review summarised published data over 10 years (2007–2017) on the prevalence of cardiovascular disease in nearly five million people with diabetes (Einarson et al. 2018). 32.2% of patients with type 2 diabetes had clinically manifest cardiovascular disease, 14.9% had clinically manifest heart failure and 10% had myocardial infarction. In 9.9% of cases, cardiovascular disease was the cause of death, which represented 50.3% of the total death rate.

Patients with type 1 diabetes are notably well analysed in the Swedish national registry. In this registry, the patient's mean age between 1998 and 2011 was 35.8 years. Patients were followed for a mean of about 8 years and compared to random control individuals by age, sex and region. Patients with type 1 diabetes had a significantly higher overall mortality of 8.0% compared to 2.9% in subjects without diabetes, corresponding to a relative risk of 3.52 (Lind et al. 2014). Recently, this registry analysed the prognostic significance of 17 risk factors for death, i.e. mortality from all causes, acute myocardial infarction or stroke. Of the 32,611 patients with type 1 diabetes in this Swedish registry cohort, 5.5% died over the course of 10.4 years. The strongest predictors of death and cardiovascular endpoints were HbA1c, albuminuria, diabetes duration, systolic blood pressure and blood LDL cholesterol concentration. An increase of approximately 1.0% in HbA1c was associated with a 22% higher risk. Furthermore, HbA1c levels <7.0% were associated with a significantly lower risk (Rawshani et al. 2019).

2 Microvascular End-Organ Damage and Cardiovascular Risk

Microvascular alterations with increased risk for end-organ damage, such as retino-, nephro- and neuropathy, are increased in diabetes. The duration and intensity of hyperglycaemia appear to play a major role. One clinical relevant question for cardiovascular risk stratification is whether microvascular "end-organ damage" in turn also increases the risk for macrovascular complications. To address this question, a population-based cohort study of 49,027 patients with type 2 diabetes analysed the association between the combined endpoint consisting of cardiovascular death, nonfatal myocardial infarction, stroke and the cumulative presence of retinal, nephro- and peripheral neuropathy over 5.5 years (Brownrigg et al. 2016).

Each microvascular end-organ damage was associated with an increased cardiovascular risk by approximately 35–40%. The accumulation of relative cardiovascular risk in the presence of one, two or three microvascular diseases increased by 32%, 62% and 99%, respectively. Similar trends were seen for cardiovascular death, all-cause mortality and hospitalisation for heart failure.

Therefore, microvascular end-organ damage appears to indicate or even mediate increased cardiovascular risk. In the case of a possible mediating role, common links discussed include damage to the microvascular pathway including endothelial dysfunction. This is clinically relevant because microvascular complications and endothelial dysfunction can be directly influenced by elevated blood glucose concentrations. However, the incidence as well as progression of end-organ damage is also modulated by other factors, such as increased blood pressure, smoking, etc. (Climie et al. 2019; Ziegler et al. 2020).

3 Role of Hyperglycaemia for Micro- and Macro-vascular Complications

Diabetes is not only associated with an increased micro- and macro-vascular risk, but also with a variety of non-vascular changes or syndromes. Since diabetes per se is currently (still) defined by hyperglycaemia, we will briefly discuss the possible roles of hyperglycaemia as an indicator, mediator or modulator of late complications.

Microvascular complications seem to be essentially caused by hyperglycaemia. However, it has to recurrently persist to display clinical consequences or complications. Though, macrovascular complications are more likely to be caused by other factors, such as insulin resistance, altered fat ectopic accumulation (e.g. in the liver, skeletal muscle or heart – see below), dyslipidaemia, hypertension, hypercoagulability, etc. Therefore, these complications are not diabetes-specific and can occur even before diagnosis, e.g. prediabetes or metabolic syndrome (Rask-Madsen and Kahn 2012; Kahn et al. 2019). Numerous non-vascular changes are not specific to diabetes, but are observed more frequently in patients with diabetes, e.g. fatty liver, COPD, certain forms of cancer, depression, cognitive disorders, osteoporosis, disorders of the gastrointestinal tract as well as the genitourinary system, skin changes, increased risk of infection, cheiroarthropathies, etc.

The role of hyperglycaemia in the many facets of vascular and other late complications may vary, i.e. hyperglycaemia may be a mediator, a modulator or just an indicator of increased risk. Moreover, the "damaging thresholds" of hyperglycaemia fluctuate for different micro-, macro- and non-vascular complications. One reason for this may also be that functional loss of the target organ, like retina or glomerular filtration, is not only a direct consequence of microvascular changes, but also involves other non-vascular cells, e.g. pericytes, podocytes, etc. Hitherto, it remains unclear how hyperglycaemia can exactly cause microvascular or organ damage. One common hypothesis is that hyperglycaemia leads to epigenetic and thus long-term changes that are unlikely to be quickly reversible by good blood glucose control. Furthermore, metabolically oriented hypotheses assume that the function, synthesis and degradation of proteins through glycosylation or increased substrate supply for various metabolic pathways can indirectly or directly lead to cell and tissue disorders, e.g. endothelium, nerve cells, proteins in the blood, e.g. of coagulation factors as well as connective tissue proteins. The formation of advanced glycosylation end-products (AGE), increase in sorbitol or hexosamine metabolic pathways, intracellular activation of protein kinase C through an increase in diacylglycerol as well as other signalling cascades and gene regulatory mechanisms play a decisive role. In addition to glycosylation, the formation of reactive oxygen radicals and superoxides in the mitochondria could also have a key biological role in this complex process in a subcellular level. Clinically, it is important to note that glycosylation is usually irreversible, i.e. a near-normal blood glucose control does not acutely lead to a "dissolution" of already manifested alterations, but ensures that no further changes occur and that the cellular metabolism and the pattern of modified proteins reconstitute themselves over (long) time. Therefore, early and long-term control of blood glucose metabolism, especially in younger people who still have a long life expectancy, remains a clinical concept.

In this respect, it is recognised that early and sufficient glucose control may reduce the incidence and possible progression of vascular disease. However, dissolution and cure of already established glucose-related damage, as it occurs in older patients with type 2 diabetes, longer disease duration, or prevalent atherosclerotic cardiovascular disease, appears not feasible. Therefore, it is a milestone that new drug classes like GLP-1 receptor agonists and SGLT-2-inhibitors have HbA1c-independent complication-protective effects even in the short-term.

4   Role of Hyperglycaemia in Reducing Vascular Risks in Type 1 Diabetes

The hypothesis that therapeutic lowering of HbA1c and thus hyperglycaemia is associated with a reduction in late complications has been proven in patients with type 1 diabetes by the DCCT (Diabetes Control and Complications Trial) study. The DCCT study has shown as a proof-of-concept study that early and effective blood glucose lowering can significantly reduce the incidence and progression of microvascular complications in patients with type 1 diabetes; similar associations were found in further follow-up for macrovascular complications. It could be that macrovascular complications or atherosclerosis develops quite differently in type 2 diabetes than in type 1 diabetes, or that the DCCT study examined very young patients in whom the many other modulators of vascular risk (see above) do not yet have the decisive significance as in later adulthood or in most patients with type 2 diabetes. The DCCT study was initiated by the National Institute of Diabetes and Digestive and Kidney Disease (NIDDK) from 1983–1993 with 1,441 patients with type 1 diabetes mellitus and became a milestone for the treatment of patients with type 1 diabetes. This study showed that intensified insulin therapy lasting a mean of 6.5 years halved the incidence and progression of microvascular sequelae compared to conventional therapy. which was associated with a significant difference in

HbA1c (The Diabetes Control and Complication Trial 1993). After a mean follow-up of 17 years in >90% of the initially enrolled patients, the cardiovascular risk was significantly reduced by 42% in the intensified treatment group, and the reduction in HbA1c was significantly associated with this (The Diabetes Control and Complication Trial/Epidemiology of Diabetes Interventions and Complications (DCCT/ EDIC) Study Research Group 2005). In the EDIC (Epidemiology of Diabetes Interventions and Complications) study, patients have now been followed up for over 30 years. In summary, after 30 years the following was concluded (Zinman et al. 2014):

- Hyperglycaemia is the primary modifiable mediator of late complications in type 1 diabetes.
- Near-normal glucose control reduces the incidence and progression of microvascular complications, such as retinopathy, nephropathy and neuropathy.
- Intensive diabetes therapy reduces cardiovascular complications in type 1 diabetes.

Recently, the concept and importance of good glycaemic control has been further explored and discussed in the DCCT/EDIC trial in relation to cardiovascular complications (Riddle and Gerstein 2019). A mediation analysis and multivariable models show (Bebu et al. 2019) that the quality of adjustment of traditional risk factors accounts for only about 50% of the cardioprotective effect of improved metabolic control. HbA1c can be an indicator for changes in other parameters, e.g. lipids, albuminuria, etc., but this explains <10% of the effect. Therefore, about 40% of the cardioprotective effect remains for HbA1c or elevated glucose concentrations per se. Thus, the therapeutic concept is further confirmed that HbA1c lowering in patients with type 1 diabetes is clinically relevant for reducing the incidence and progression of micro- and macro-vascular late complications. The future must show whether the predictability of the clinical prognosis for late complications through other parameters, such as the duration of glucose control in the desired range, so-called time in range (TiR), has a benefit alongside or in addition to HbA1c (Battelino et al. 2019).

5   Efficacy Trials of Glucose Lowering in Type 2 Diabetes

The UKPDS trial randomly assigned 5,102 patients with newly diagnosed type 2 diabetes to intensive glucose control with sulphonylurea or insulin or to management with diet alone. Those who were overweight at study entry also could be randomised in the intensive arm to receive metformin (UKPDS 33 1998; Stratton et al. 2000). In the insulin and sulphonylurea analyses, HbA1c levels of 7.0% vs. 7.9%, respectively, were significantly associated with a relatively decreased risk for a composite endpoint of all diabetes-related complications by 12%, and microvascular disease risk by 25% during an average follow-up of 10 years. Intensive control showed a trend towards decreased risk of myocardial infarction and no effect on stroke. In overweight patients, metformin yielded better glucose control (HbA1c 7.4% vs. 8.0%) and significantly decreased relative risk for myocardial infarction by 39% and for all-cause mortality by 36%. The long-term follow-up of the UKPDS trial cohort suggests a "legacy" of cardiovascular benefit of early and tight glycaemic control. Similarly, this was a finding observed in the long-term follow-up of the Diabetes Control and Complications Trial (DCCT) in patients with type 1 diabetes. However, the results of the following efficacy trials in patients with longer diabetes duration were not so promising.

The ACCORD trial compared intensive vs. standard glucose control in 10,251 patients with type 2 diabetes who had high CVD risk, achieving an HbA1c of 6.4% vs. 7.5% (Gerstein et al. 2008). This trial was halted early due to an excess of all-cause mortality in the intensively treated group (257 vs. 203 events; $p = 0.04$), with no significant difference observed in the primary composite cardiovascular disease endpoint of cardiovascular death, myocardial infarction, and stroke. The ADVANCE trial enrolled 11,140 patients with type 2 diabetes who had cardiovascular disease, microvascular disease, or another vascular risk factor at study entry (Heller 2009). Patients randomly received intensive glucose control with gliclazide plus other drugs in the intensive arm, compared with standard control with other drugs. Similar to the ACCORD trial, the ADVANCE trial did not show statistically significant improvement in the composite outcome of cardiovascular death, myocardial infarction, and stroke with intensive control (achieved HbA1c of 6.4% vs. 7.0%), despite having 1,147 events. In the Veterans Affairs Diabetes Trial (VADT), 1791 US veterans with type 2 diabetes and inadequate glucose control randomly received either intensive or standard glucose control (Duckworth et al. 2009). Despite a wide separation in glucose control levels (HbA1c of 6.9% vs. 8.4%) and ascertainment of 499 primary major adverse cardiovascular events (MACEs), this trial also found no significant improvement in cardiovascular outcomes with intensive control. From post hoc analyses of data for each of these trials and supported by the long-term observations from UKPDS in patients with newly diagnosed diabetes at study entry, the concept has emerged that more intensive glycaemic control may be safer and may have more favourable cardiovascular effects when used earlier in the course of diabetes. In contrast, patients with a longer duration of type 2 diabetes and more intense glucose control has only resulted in modest impact on cardiovascular events over time. In this respect, cardiovascular safety studies are of interest, because they aim to assess the safety of a new drug and possibly a mainly glucose independent superiority effect on predefined endpoints, like cardiovascular or renal complications.

6 Cardiovascular Safety Studies in Type 2 Diabetes

Cardiovascular safety studies are designed in such a way that the substance under investigation is compared with placebo, but that the risk parameter to be influenced, in this case HbA1c or blood glucose, should also be comparably reduced in the placebo arm of the study according to study protocol to achieve glycaemic equipoise. Therefore, this design tests not only the safety of a therapeutic molecule, but also its effect on cardiovascular risk, independent of blood glucose-lowering. Overall, insulin glargine (The ORIGIN Trial Investigators 2012), insulin degludec (Marso et al. 2017) as well as acarbose (Holman et al. 2017b), and sulphonylurea therapy (in directly tested, see Vaccaro et al. 2017, Rosenstock et al. 2019a) are cardiovascular neutral. In this respect it is worthwhile to mention that pioglitazone has been shown to reduce relative risk for myocardial infarction and stroke in a special patient population (subgroup of the PROACTIVE trail), i.e. patients after stroke or transient ischaemic attack (Kernan et al. 2016). Cardiovascular safety studies were conducted for the DPP4 inhibitors alogliptin, linagliptin, saxagliptin and sitagliptin; there is no corresponding prospective endpoint study for vildagliptin. These endpoint studies (Zannad et al. 2015 EXAMINE, Rosenstock et al. 2019b CARMELINA, Scirica et al. 2013 SAVOR-TIMI 53, Green et al. 2015 TECOS) showed safety, but not superiority, in patients with pre-existing cardiovascular disease or multiple risk factors for the primary endpoint, which is in most cases composed of cardiovascular death, myocardial infarction and stroke. In the SAVOR-TIMI (Saxagliptin Assessment of Vascular Outcomes Recorded in Patients with Diabetes Mellitus-Thrombolysis In Myocardial Infarction) 53 trial, 16,492 patients with type 2 diabetes and manifest cardiovascular disease or risk factors were randomised and followed up for a mean of 2.1 years. The primary endpoint, i.e. cardiovascular safety, was proven. However, compared to placebo, a higher hospitalisation due to heart failure was observed in the treatment group with 3.5% vs. 2.8%. For this reason, saxagliptin is not recommended in patients with pre-existing heart failure. Thus, GLP-1-RAs have shown to be cardiovascular protective and SGLT-2 inhibitors provide consistent evidence for cardio- and nephroprotection. Therefore, we will focus on the clinical evidence and potential mechanisms related to these observations.

7   GLP-1 Receptor Agonists (GLP-1-RA)

Therapeutically used GLP (glucagon like peptide)-1 receptor agonists act directly via the GLP-1 receptor, which leads not only to a glucose-dependent metabolically mediated release of insulin from the beta cells, but also to inhibition of glucagon release from the pancreatic alpha cells. Most of them are injected subcutaneously once daily or weekly, depending on the preparation. In addition to effective HbA1c lowering, this therapy also leads to clinically relevant weight loss.

The cardioprotective evidence for GLP1 receptor agonists is based on the results of 7 placebo controlled endpoint trials: LEADER for liraglutide (Marso et al. 2016b); SUSTAIN-6 for subcutaneous semaglutide (Marso et al. 2016a), HARMONY for albiglutide (Hernandez et al. 2018), REWIND for dulaglutide (Gerstein et al. 2019a), and AMPLITUDE-O for efpeglenatide (Gerstein et al. 2021). These trials demonstrated a significant reduction in the 3-point MACE endpoint (cardiovascular death, nonfatal myocardial infarction, or nonfatal stroke). In the PIONEER-6 study with oral semaglutide, the primary endpoint was negative, but cardiovascular death and all-cause mortality were reduced (Husain et al. 2019). In the studies with lixisenatide (Pfeffer et al. 2015) and long acting formulation (LAR) of exenatide (Holman et al. 2017a), the primary endpoint was negative. The clinical results of these trials compared with placebo are summarised in Table 1. The results appear heterogeneous for the individual endpoints, which could be due to the study design and different patient populations. Effects on a reduction in the hospitalisation rate due to heart failure were not observed in any study (Lim et al. 2018). Since the curves between treatment and placebo generally only began to diverge after about 1 year, it is assumed that the cardioprotective effects are rather due to a modulation of atherosclerotic processes (Marx and Libby 2018), see Fig. 1.

In Fig. 1, we have distinguished between direct and indirect mechanisms, which we cannot discuss in detail here and therefore refer to recent reviews (Drucker 2016, Nauck et al. 2017; Müller et al. 2019, Giorgino et al. 2020, Nauck et al. 2020). In case of indirect mechanisms, the reduction of blood pressure and weight are certainly in the foreground, whereby interestingly, ectopic lipid accumulation in the liver (Armstrong et al. 2016; Newsome et al. 2021) and epicardial fat (Iacobellis and Villasante Fricke 2020) is also reduced, see below. In addition, there are first indications that certain intraepithelial T lymphocytes in the intestine modulate metabolism and the risk of atherosclerosis as well as that GLP-1 could play an important role as a mediator (He et al. 2019). In terms of direct mechanisms, it must be emphasised that endothelial function, plaque stabilisation and anti-inflammatory effects are of particular importance for the clinical risk posed by plaque (Libby and Hansson 2019). All these mechanisms can be modified by incretin hormones in experimental studies. Therefore, it is thought that GLP-1 receptor agonists may also directly influence the development and stability of atherosclerotic plaque (Rakipovski et al. 2018; Kahles et al. 2018). For example, GLP-1-receptors in various plaque cells like endothelial cells, vascular smooth muscle cells, monocytes, and macrophages are coupled to responses which might modulate plaque biology (Nauck et al. 2020). Similar to ROS formation, oxLDL activation of inflammatory cells and adhesion molecules are reduced. eNOS formation in endothelial cells is increased. After GLP-1- receptor stimulation, foam cell formation is reduced as well as their caspase-mediated apoptosis and the necrotic core in plaque. Interestingly, GLP-1 receptor agonist treatment of cells reduced MMP expression, potentially leading to less degradation of extracellular matrix and thereby increased plaque stability. It is also interesting that GLP-1 receptor agonists may favourably influence the consequences of an ischaemic event (Giblett et al. 2016; Brott 2015; McCormick et al. 2015).

In addition, reduction in progression of chronic kidney disease and clinical renal endpoints were positive as secondary endpoints in LEADER (Mann et al. 2017) and REWIND (Gerstein et al. 2019b). This effect might relate to GLP-1-RA treatment-associated reduction in the progression of albuminuria and mild natriuresis possibly by some inhibition of NHE-3 in the tubulus system.

Table 1 Overview of the cardiovascular outcome trials for GLP1-RA

	ELIXA	EXSCEL	LEADER	SUSTAIN 6	Harmony outcomes	PIONEER 6	REWIND	AMPLITUDE-O
Study drug	Lixisenatide	Exenatide	Liraglutide	Semaglutide	Albiglutide	Semaglutide	Dulaglutide	Efpeglenatide
Year	2015	2017	2016	2016	2018	2019	2019	2021
Patients (n)	6,068	14,752	9,340	3,297	9,463	3,183	9,901	4,076
Median follow-up (years, IQR)	2.08 (NR)	3.2 (2.2–4.4)	3.8 (NR)	2.1 (NR)	1.5 (NR)	1.3 (0.03–1.6)	5.4 (5.1–5.9)	1.81 (1.69–1.98)
MACE HR (95% CI)	1.02 (0.89–1.17)	0.91 (0.83–1.00)	0.87 (0.78–0.97)	0.74 (0.58–0.95)	0.78 (0.68–0.90)	0.79 (0.57–1.11)	0.88 (0.79–0.99)	0.73 (0.58–0.92)
MACE definition	Death from CV causes, nonfatal stroke, nonfatal MI, or unstable angina	Death from CV causes, nonfatal MI, or nonfatal stroke	Death from CV causes, nonfatal (including silent) MI or nonfatal stroke	Death from CV causes, nonfatal MI, or nonfatal stroke	Death from CV causes, nonfatal MI, nonfatal stroke, or urgent coronary revascularisation for unstable angina	Death from CV causes, nonfatal MI, or nonfatal stroke	Nonfatal MI, nonfatal stroke, and death from CV causes or unknown causes	Nonfatal MI, nonfatal stroke, or death from CV or undetermined causes
Event rate (rate/1,000 patient-year)								
Treatment	64	37	34	32.4	45.7	29	23.5	39
Placebo	63	40	39	44.4	58.7	37	26.6	53
Inclusion criteria								
Age (years)	≥30	≥18	≥50	≥50	≥40	≥50	≥50	≥18

HbA1c (%)	5.5–11.0	6.5–10.0	≥7.0	≥7.0	≥7.0	n/a	≤9.5	≥7.0
BMI (kg/m²)	n/a	n/a	n/a	n/a	n/a	n/a	n/a	n/a
eGFR (mL/min/1.73 m²)	≥30	≥30	n/a	n/a	≥30	≥30	≥15	≥25
ASCVD	Established	Any level of risk	Established	Established or high risk	Established	Established or ≥1 risk factor	Established or ≥2 risk factor	Established or CKD + ≥1 risk factor

ASCVD atherosclerotic cardiovascular disease, *BMI* body mass index, *C cr* creatinine clearance, *CI* confidence interval, *CKD* chronic kidney disease, *CV* cardiovascular, *eGFR* estimated glomerular filtration rate, *HF* heart failure, *HR* hazard ratio, *IQR* interquartile range, *i.v.* intravenous, *MACE* major adverse cardiovascular event, *MI* myocardial infarction

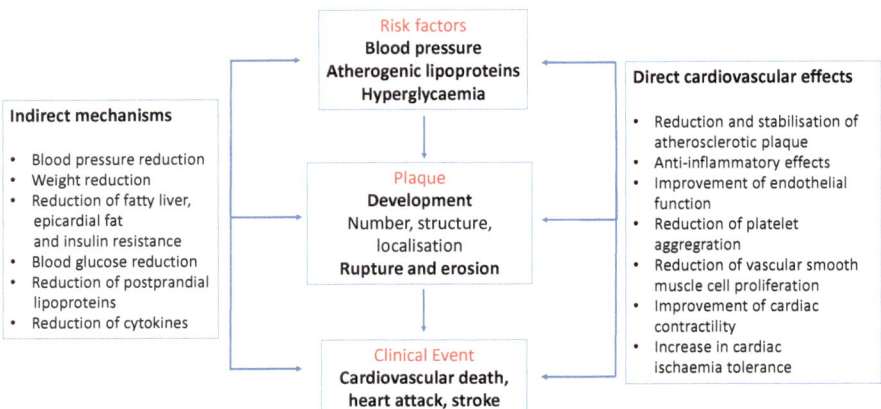

Fig. 1 Potential mechanisms and concepts for modulation of atherosclerotic plaque formation, rupture and erosion and their cardiovascular consequences by GLP-1 receptor agonists. For further explanation see text

8   SGLT (Sodium Glucose Transporter) 2 Inhibitors

SGLT-2 inhibitors are a group of blood glucose-lowering substances that lead to an increased excretion of glucose in the urine by reducing the activity of the transporter selectively in the proximal tubulus of the kidney by approximately 40–60%. CVOTs have been published for canagliflozin, dapagliflozin, empagliflozin, ertugliflozin, and sotagliflozin, mentioned here in alphabetical order and are summarised in Table 2.

The EMPA-REG OUTCOME study (Zinman et al. 2015) enrolled 7,020 patients with pre-existing cardiovascular disease over a mean observation period of 3.1 years and investigated the effect of 10 or 25 mg empagliflozin daily in addition to existing medication. The primary endpoint was a composite of cardiovascular death and nonfatal myocardial infarction and stroke and was significantly reduced with a relative risk reduction (RRR) of 14%; the event rate was 12.1% in the placebo group and 10.5% with empagliflozin treatment. There was no difference between the two doses of empagliflozin. Component analysis showed no effect on nonfatal myocardial infarction or stroke, but cardiovascular mortality was significantly reduced with an RRR of 38%, which also reduced all-cause mortality. In addition, hospitalisation due to heart failure was also significantly lower with an RRR of 35%, an effect that became significant after only a few weeks. The effect on renal function was further analysed. The prespecified secondary renal endpoint was worsening nephropathy (progression to macroalbuminuria, doubling of serum creatinine, initiation of renal replacement therapy or death due to renal causes) and incidence rate of albuminuria. The incidence or relative risk of worsening nephropathy was significantly reduced by 44% with empagliflozin (Wanner et al. 2016). In the primary CANVAS programme (Neal et al. 2017) and in the CREDENCE study (Perkovic

Table 2 Overview of the cardiovascular outcome trials for SLGT2i

	EMPA-REG OUTCOME	CANVAS Programme	DECLARE-TIMI 58	SOLOIST-WHF	VERTIS
Study drug	Empagliflozin	Canagliflozin	Dapagliflozin	Sotagliflozin	Ertugliflozin
Year	2015	2017	2018	2020	2020
Patients (n)	7,020	10,142	17,160	1,222	8,246
Median follow-up (years. IQR)	3.1 (2.2–3.5)	2.4 (NR)	4.2 (3.9–4.4)	0.76	3.5 (NR)
MACE HR (95% CI)	0.86 (0.74–0.99)	0.86 (0.75–0.97)	0.93 (0.84–1.03)	0.67 (0.52–0.85)	0.97 (0.85–1.11)
MACE definition	Death from CV causes, nonfatal MI or nonfatal stroke	Death from CV causes, nonfatal MI or nonfatal stroke	CV death, MI or ischaemic stroke	Deaths from CV causes and hospitalisations and urgent visits for HF	Death from CV causes, nonfatal MI or nonfatal stroke
Event rate (rate/1,000 patient-year)					
Treatment	37.4	26.9	12.2	510	39
Placebo	43.9	31.5	14.7	763	40
Inclusion criteria					
Age (years)	≥18	≥30	≥40	18–85	≥40
HbA1c (%)	7.0–9.0 (with OAD) 7.0–10.0 (without OAD)	7.0–10.5	6.5–12.0	≥ 6.5	7.0–10.5
BMI (kg/m²)	≤45	n/a	n/a	n/a	≥18
eGFR (mL/min/1.73 m²)	≥30	≥30	C cr ≥60 mL/min	≥30	≥30

(continued)

Table 2 (continued)

	EMPA-REG OUTCOME	CANVAS Programme	DECLARE-TIMI 58	SOLOIST-WHF	VERTIS
ASCVD	Established	Established or ≥ 2 risk factors	Established or multiple risk factors	Hospitalised for HF and i.v. diuretic therapy	Established

ASCVD atherosclerotic cardiovascular disease, *BMI* body mass index, *CI* confidence interval, *C cr* creatinine clearance, *CV* cardiovascular, *eGFR* estimated glomerular filtration rate, *HF* heart failure, *HR* hazard ratio, *IQR* interquartile range, *i.v.* intravenous, *MACE* major adverse cardiovascular event, *MI* myocardial infarction, *OAD* oral antidiabetic therapy et al. 2019), the SGLT-2 inhibitor canagliflozin also significantly reduced the risk of the combined cardiovascular endpoint (cardiovascular death, nonfatal myocardial infarction or stroke) by 14% and renal endpoints. This confirmed the concept of cardio-renal risk reduction by a second substance, and the question now arose whether this principle of action could also be observed with a third substance and, above all, also in patients with lower cardio-renal risk. In the DECLARE-TIMI 58 trial, 17,160 patients with type 2 diabetes were studied over a mean of 4.2 years with and without dapagliflozin 10 mg; 10,186 of these patients had no previous atherosclerotic disease (Wiviott et al. 2019). The primary safety analysis confirmed non-inferiority of dapagliflozin for MACE (major cardiovascular events), and the primary efficacy analysis showed a significantly lower event rate for the combined endpoint of cardiovascular death and hospitalisation for heart failure (HHF), although this outcome was substantially driven by HHF. A sub-analysis of 3,586 patients with pre-existing myocardial infarction showed that compared with placebo, dapagliflozin significantly reduced the relative risk of MACE by 16% with an absolute risk reduction of 2.6% (Furtao et al. 2019). The effect of dapagliflozin on nephropathy has been investigated as a renal composite secondary endpoint ($\geq$40% decrease in eGFR in mL/min/1.73 m^2, new manifestation of ESRD, or death due to renal or cardiovascular causes). The relative risk for this renal endpoint was significantly reduced by 24% with dapagliflozin. In the 671 patients with heart failure and impaired left ventricular pump function, dapagliflozin also significantly reduced not only hospitalisation for heart failure but also cardiovascular death with a relative risk reduction of 45% compared to placebo (Kato et al. 2019). Ertugliflozin was investigated in the VERTIS CV trial in 8246 patients with type 2 diabetes and cardiovascular disease over a mean of 3.5 years (Cannon et al. 2020). Ertugliflozin was noninferior to placebo for MACE and clinical renal endpoints. However, results were consistent with other SGLT2-inhibitors in respect of reducing hospitalisation for heart failure in a respective prespecified group and reduction in decline rate of eGFR. Sotagliflozin, an SGLT2 inhibitor with possibly some SGLT-1 blocking potential, was investigated in patients with diabetes and recent worsening of heart failure (SOLOIST-WF) and in patients with diabetes and chronic kidney disease (SCORED) resulting in a significant risk reduction for cardiovascular death and hospitalisation for heart failure in patients with heart failure (Bhatt et al. 2020b) or chronic kidney disease with or without albuminuria (Bhatt et al. 2020a).

In consideration of these very impressive trial results with major impact on risk for heart failure and renal complications to a large extent non-related to baseline HbA1c and glucose-lowering capacity in these trials, the question was emerging, whether SGLT2-inhibitors reduce also clinical risk primarily in patients suffering from chronic heart failure or kidney disease with and also without diabetes. Four studies have been published so far, the DAPA-HF and EMPEROR-Reduced trials for chronic heart failure and CREDENCE for patients with chronic kidney disease (CKD) in patients with diabetes and the DAPA-CKD trial in CKD patients with and also without diabetes.

In the DAPA-HF study (McMurray et al. 2019), 4,744 patients with manifest heart failure and impaired left ventricular function (LVEF $\leq$40%, NT-proBNP

$\geq$600 pg/mL) were enrolled and treated with dapagliflozin 10 mg or placebo in addition to existing standard therapy. The study was event-driven and ran for approximately 3 years. The relative risk for the primary endpoint was significantly reduced by 26% and was composed of cardiovascular death, hospitalisation or urgent medical visit for heart failure. There was no difference between the 42% of patients with or without diabetes. In the EMPEROR-Reduced trial (Packer et al. 2020) 3730 patients with chronic heart failure and reduced left ventricular ejection fraction ($\leq$40%) were investigated over a mean period of 16 months. The relative risk for the primary combined endpoint being cardiovascular death and hospitalisation for heart failure was significantly reduced by 25% regardless of the presence or absence of diabetes. Therefore, both studies show the benefit of SGLT2-inhibition in patients with clinically relevant chronic heart failure independent of diabetes status. These data have an impacted current guidelines for the treatment of patients with chronic heart failure, SGLT2-inhibition being an evidence-based treatment option.

In patients with chronic kidney disease, CREDENCE (Perkovic et al. 2019) was the first study to investigate the effect of an SGLT-2 inhibitor, in this case 100 mg canagliflozin OD, primarily on renal function. The primary renal endpoint was composed of end-stage renal failure (defined by need for dialysis, kidney transplantation or drop in eGFR to <15 mL/ min/1.73 m^2), doubling of serum creatinine levels or death due to renal or cardiovascular causes. 4,401 patients with type 2 diabetes, an eGFR between 30 and 90 mL/min/1.72 m^2 and albuminuria of >300–5,000 mg/g creatinine were included and studied for a mean of 2.62 years. Canagliflozin significantly reduced the relative risk for the primary renal endpoint by 30%, the relative risk for end-stage renal failure by 32% and its combination with creatinine doubling and renal death by 34%. DAPA-CKD (Heerspink et al. 2020) randomly assigned 4,304 patients with an eGFR of 25–75 mL/min/1.73 m^2 and a urinary albumin-to-creatinine ratio of 200–5,000 receiving 10 mg dapagliflozin or placebo over a median time of 2.4 years. The relative risk for the combined endpoint of sustained decline in the eGFR of at least 50%, end-stage kidney disease, or death from renal causes was significantly lower by 44% in the dapagliflozin arm compared to the placebo group. This effect was irrespective of having type 2 diabetes or not. Therefore, SGLT-2 inhibitors are also finding their position in guidelines for the treatment of chronic kidney disease. However, one should be aware that currently there are still differences in specifications of their label in patients with reduced eGFR in different countries and regions of the world.

9   Mechanisms of Action for Cardio-Renal Protection Through SGLT-2 Inhibition

SGLT-2 transports glucose in exchange for sodium in the proximal tubule of the kidney and reabsorbs approximately 90% of the 180 g of glucose normally filtered daily in primary urine, for review see Heerspink et al. (2016); Lytvyn et al. (2017); Verma and McMurray (2018); Marton et al. (2021). SGLT-2 inhibitors selectively

SGLT-2 inhibitors: Potential mechanisms for cardiac protection

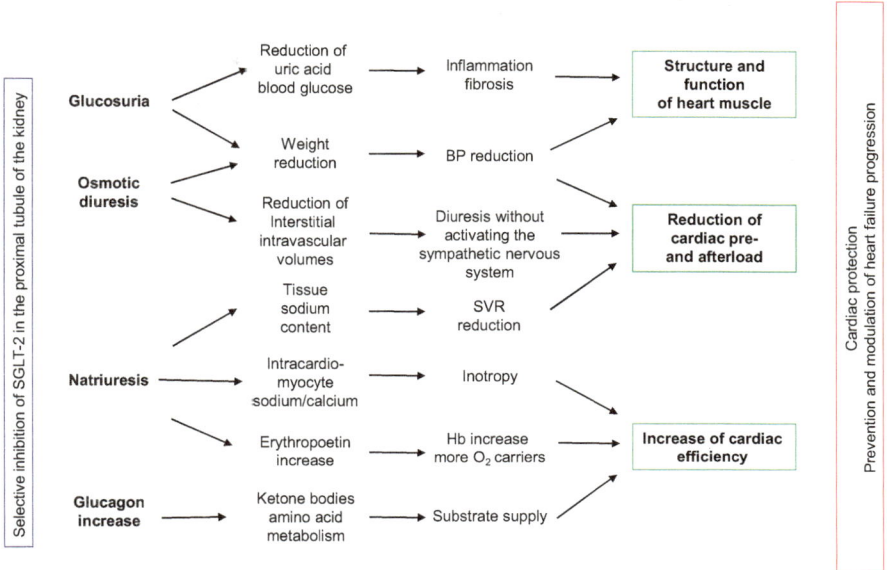

Fig. 2 Potential mechanisms and concepts of cardiac protection by SGLT-2 inhibitors. For further explanation see text

prevent the transporter with high affinity by an average of about 40–60%. This inhibition leads to glucosuria, associated osmotic diuresis, increased natriuresis and an increase in glucagon levels. Figure 2 summarises the principal mechanisms of action and outlines how the cardioprotective effects associated with SGLT-2-inhibitor therapy are currently imagined.

Glucosuria leads to a loss of calories, approx. 70–80 g over 24 h, corresponding to approx. 300 kcal, and weight reduction of approx. 2–3 kg, half of which is due to the reduction of fat mass. The other half is due to the osmotic diuresis of approx. 300 mL/24 h. In contrast to diuretics, this, in combination with natriuresis, leads to an interstitial fluid mobilisation without a significant reduction in intravascular volume, and thus not to an activation of the sympathetic nervous system or an increase in the pulse rate. These effects also cause a reduction in peripheral vascular resistance and, in combination, a reduction in blood pressure of 4–6 mmHg systolic (1–2 mmHg diastolic), which can be even more pronounced at elevated blood pressure levels or in combination with diuretics.

In addition, natriuresis and possibly direct interaction of SGLT-2 inhibitors in the myocardium with sodium proton exchanger-1 (NHE-1) may favourably alter the intracellular ratio of sodium and calcium. The increased natriuresis, also through additional inhibition of tubular NHE-3, probably leads indirectly in the medulla of the kidney to higher consumption of oxygen and thus renally to an increased formation of erythropoietin and an increase in the formation of red blood cells and the oxygen carrier haemoglobin. In a mediation analysis of the cardiovascular endpoint study of empagliflozin, this appears to be clinically relevant for understanding the observed effect in cardioprotection (Inzucchi et al. 2018).

An increase in glucagon levels of about twofold by SGLT-2 inhibitors is associated with an approximately twofold increase in the concentration of ketone bodies during therapy. Ketone bodies in turn can be effective substrates (especially α-hydroxy-butyrate) for cardiac muscle and possibly also lead to altered metabolism of branched-chain amino acids in the cardiac muscle, which can be disturbed in diabetic cardiomyopathy (Wanner and Marx 2018). In summary, therapy with SGLT-2 inhibitors results in a rapid and effective pre- and afterload reduction of the heart as well as possibly a clinically relevant favourable change in metabolism and intracardiomyocyte electrolytes, stabilising the structure and function of the myocardium and increasing work efficiency.

For renoprotection, the key mechanism is probably increased natriuresis in the proximal tubule, leading to activation of the tubuloglomerular feedback (TGF) mechanism. The natriuresis caused by SGLT2 inhibition is sensed by the macula densa in the juxtaglomerular apparatus and leads to a counter-regulation, i.e. specifically a reduction of glomerular filtration by constriction of the vas afferens, probably mediated by adenosine. This lowers the intraglomerular pressure and thus also leads to a reduction in albuminuria and in the long term to a stabilisation and reduced progressive decrease in the glomerular filtration rate. This fascinating observation now also makes the hyperfiltration in the early phase of a renal change in patients with diabetes understandable, because an increased activity of the SGLT-2 transporter in diabetes leads to increased reabsorption of sodium, thus reduction of TGF and vasodilation of the vas afferens and thus hyperfiltration of the glomerulum.

In addition to the aforementioned hypotheses of reduction of cardiac pre-and after-load and intraglomerular pressure reduction by tubuloglomerular feedback mechanisms, a recent hypothesis involves metabolic adaptations. Under SGLT-2-inhibitor treatment, there is an increased caloric loss and an about twofold increase in glucagon levels with a consecutive increase in ketone bodies. These endocrine-metabolic changes provide both a better energy efficient substrate utilisation for the heart and the metabolism switch to a state of chronic hypometabolism and water deprivation. This state is compensated in the long-run by appropriate adaptation of energy homeostasis or metabolic rate and water conservation. This adaptation process, called "aestivation", is evolutionary conserved enabling adaptation to energy and water shortage (Marton et al. 2021). This metabolic switch induced by SGLT-2-inhibition might play a role in improved function and reduced damage progression of different organs, most extensively clinically proven for heart and kidney.

10 Change in Guidelines and Clinical Recommendations

Patient-centred care is the focus of most guidelines and new recommendations (Davies et al. 2018; Consentino et al. 2019; Buse et al. 2020; Landgraf et al. 2020; American Diabetes Association 2021). Based on the clinical evidence provided recently and discussed above, guidelines nowadays don't put HbA1c in focus for decision about treatment strategy in type 2 diabetes, but rather the clinical picture and risk of cardio-renal complications in the foreground. Evidence-based means that the results of large studies, especially cardiovascular endpoint studies, must be translated into practice.

The recent ESC recommendations on "Diabetes, prediabetes and cardiovascular disease" (Consentino et al. 2019), produced in collaboration with the EASD, have incorporated the extensive data from large cardiovascular endpoint studies in recent years with new antidiabetic agents and have led to a new and more specific positioning of metformin and cardioprotective blood glucose-lowering drugs in patients with high and very high cardio-renal risk and diabetes mellitus. The decisive factor for the choice of a glucose-lowering substance for cardiovascular risk reduction is primarily not an HbA1c target anymore, but the risk stratification of patients with diabetes according to the ESC recommendations 2019:

Very high risk patients are those with diabetes and established cardiovascular disease or end organ damage or three or more risk factors or early onset of type 1 diabetes of long duration (>20 years). Patients with diabetes duration ≥ 10 years without end-organ damage but with another risk factor are classified in the high risk category. The moderate-risk category includes young patients (type 1 diabetes under 35 or type 2 diabetes under 50 years) with diabetes duration under 10 years without other risk factors.

The new algorithm for cardiovascular risk reduction with antihyperglycaemic agents in untreated type 2 diabetic patients – regardless of HbA1c level – focuses on the high/very high risk categories. Patients with atherosclerotic cardiovascular disease or high/very high risk should receive an SGLT2 inhibitor or GLP1 receptor agonist monotherapy as a class Ia recommendation, according to the evidence from the studies above. In patients with existing or increased risk for heart failure, SGLT-2 inhibitors are recommended. Similar recommendation belongs to renal protection.

Although the effect of metformin on risk for myocardial infarction was better than expected from degree of glucose lowering in the UKPS trial, it has been questioned whether metformin should continue to be first-line therapy in all patients with type 2 diabetes. The CVOTs described above suggest that in these patient groups GLP-1 RAs and SGLT2-inhibitors should be first choice driven by evidence and not metformin. This is supported by further evaluations of these CVOTs indicating that metformin has no modulating effect on risk protection by GLP-1RA or SGLT2-inhibitors (Marx 2020; Sattar and McGuire 2021).

11 Perspectives: Fat Partitioning as a New Target of Diabetes Drugs

Like treatment of chronic heart failure or chronic kidney disease in patients with and without diabetes by SGLT2-inhibitors initially developed for diabetes, it is also interesting to note that new incretin-based drugs, like "twincretins", reach mean body weight reductions between 8 and 12 kg and absolute reductions in HbA1c of around 2.0% (Rosenstock et al. 2021; Frías et al. 2021). Results of these kind of studies might help decipher new networks between fat tissue, diabetes and atherosclerosis related risks. In this respect, increased and abnormally distributed fat might be a new target. Numerous clinical and pathogenetic studies have changed our understanding of adipose tissue in such a way that the amount of adipose tissue is not the only essential pathophysiological phenomenon, but in particular the abnormal deposition of fat in other cells or organs, called ectopic lipid accumulation or fat partitioning (Blüher 2016; Crewe et al. 2017; Scherer 2016; Stefan et al. 2008; Unger 2002). When the normal storage capacity and plasticity of subcutaneous adipose tissue and its ability to adapt to increased energy balance are exhausted, there is recruitment of inflammatory cells in adipose tissue and increased deposition of fat in other cells, such as visceral fat cells, and in cells of the liver and cardiovascular system. The deposition of fat alters the function of these cells, e.g. resistance to insulin in the liver, release of mediators from visceral fat, or possibly changes in contractility in the case of cardiac muscle cells. A clinically important and classic example of ectopic lipid accumulation is Non-Alcoholic Fatty Liver Disease (NAFLD), which is often associated with insulin resistance, obesity and diabetes (van Heerebeek and Paulus 2016) and diastolic dysfunction of the heart (van Wagner et al. 2015). A growing number of studies show that intracardiomyocyte fat is associated with altered cardiac cell function including heart failure and epicardial fat (EAT) cells may influence cardiac function and cardiovascular risk through release of humoral, inflammatory and metabolic mediators (Unger 2002; McGavock et al. 2007; Fontes-Carvahlo et al. 2014). Recently it has been shown that in patients with diabetes EAT volume was independently associated with coronary calcium score (Cosson et al. 2021) and that extracellular vesicles from EAT facilitate atrial fibrillation and induce proinflammatory and fibrotic responses in cell culture (Shaihov-Teper et al. 2021). Furthermore, considering potential cardiovascular benefit of greater weight reductions, as we have learned from bariatric surgery (Sjöström et al. 2004), CVOTs of these new treatment options are awaited with great curiosity. In addition, these degrees of fat reduction and glucose-lowering open up possibilities to reach "remission" of type 2 diabetes (Lean et al. 2018). Overall perspectives in the treatment of type 2 diabetes are to identify different subgroups with different risk profiles for late complications and to better understand major pathomechanisms that can then be therapeutically targeted therapeutically (Ahlquist et al. 2019; Zaharia et al. 2019).

References

Ahlquist E, Tuomi T, Groop L (2019) Clusters provide a better holistic view of type 2 diabetes than simple clinical features. Lancet Diabetes Endocrinol 7:668–669

American Diabetes Association (2021) Standards in medical care in diabetes – 2021. Pharmacological approaches to glycaemic treatment. Diabetes Care 44(Suppl 1):S111–S125

Armstrong MJ, Gaunt P, Aithal GP et al (2016) Liraglutide safety and efficacy in patients with non-alcoholic steatohepatitis (LEAN): a multicentre, double-blind, randomised, placebo-controlled phase 2 study. Lancet 387:679–690

Battelino T, Danne T, Bergenstal RM et al (2019) Clinical targets for continous glucose monitoring data interpretation: recommendations from the international consensus on time in range. Diabetes Care 42:1593–1603

Bebu I, Braffett BH, Orchard TJ et al (2019) Mediation of the effect of glycemia on the risk of CVD outcomes in type 1 diabetes: the DCCT/EDIC study. Diabetes Care 42:1284–1289

Bhatt DL, Szarek M, Pitt B et al (2020a) Sotagliflozin in patients with diabetes and chronic kidney disease. N Engl J Med. https://doi.org/10.1056/NEJMoa2030186

Bhatt DL, Szarek M, Steg PG et al (2020b) Sotagliflozin in patients with diabetes and recent worsening heart failure. N Engl J Med. https://doi.org/10.1056/NEJMoa2030183

Blüher M (2016) Adipose tissue inflammation: a cause or consequence of obesity-related insulin resistance? Clin Sci 130:1603–1614

Brott BC (2015) Prevention of myocardial stunning during percutaneous coronary interventions: novel insights from pre-treatment with glucagon-like peptide-1. JACC Cardiovasc Interv 8:302–304

Brownrigg JRW, Hughes CO, Burleigh D et al (2016) Microvascular disease and risk of cardiovascular events among individuals with type 2 diabetes: a population-level-cohort study. Lancet Diabetes Endocrinol 4:588–597

Buse JB, Wexler DJ, Tsapas A et al (2020) 2019 update to: Mangement of hyperglycemia in type 2 diabetes, 2018. A consensus report by the American Diabetes Association (ADA) and the European Association for he Study of Diabetes (EASD). Diabetologia 63:221–228 and Diabetes Care 43:487–493

Cannon CP, Pratley R, Dagogo-Jack S et al (2020) Cardiovascular outcomes with ertugliflozin in type 2 diabetes. N Engl J Med 383:1425–1435

Climie RE, Gallo A, Picone DS et al (2019) Measuring the interaction between the macro- and micro-vasculature. Front Cardiovasc Med. https://doi.org/10.3389/fcvm.2019.00169

Consentino F, Grant PJ, Abcyans V et al (2019) 2019 ESC guidelines on diabetes, pre-diabetes, and cardiovascular diseases developed in collaboration with the EASD. Eur Heart J. https://doi.org/10.1093/eurheartj/ehz486

Cosson E, Nguyen MT, Rezgani I et al (2021) Epicardial tissue volume and coronary calcification among people living with diabetes: a cross-sectional study. Cardiovasc Diabetol 20:35. https://doi.org/10.1186/s12933-021-01225-6

Crewe C, An YA, Scherer PE (2017) The omnious triad of adipose tissue dysfunction: inflammation, fibrosis, and impaired angiogenesis. J Clin Invest 127:74–82

Danesh J for The Emerging Risk Factors Collaboration (2015) Association of cardiometabolic multimorbidity with mortality. JAMA 314:52–60

Davies MJ, DÁlessio DA, Fradkin J, Kernan WN, Mathieu C, Mingrone G, Rossing P, Tsapa A, Wexler DJ, Buse JB (2018) Management of hyperglycemia in type 2 diabetes, 2018. A consensus report by the American Diabetes Association (ADA) and the European Association for the Study of Diabetes EASD. Diabetologia 61:2461–2498 and Diabetes Care 41:2669–2701

Drucker DJ (2016) The cardiovascular biology of glucagon-like peptide-1. Cell Metab 24:15–30

Duckworth W, Abraira C, Moritz T et al (2009) for the VADT Investigators. Glucose control and vascular complications in veterans with type 2 diabetes. N Engl J Med 360:129–139

Einarson TR, Acs A, Ludwig C, Panton UH (2018) Prevalence of cardiovascular disease in type 2 diabetes: a systematic literature review of scientific evidence from across the world in 2007-2017. Cardiovasc Diabetol 17:83. https://doi.org/10.1186/s12933-018-0728-6

Fontes-Carvahlo R, Fontes-Oliveira M, Sampaio F et al (2014) Influence of epicardial and visceral fat on left ventricular diastolic and systolic functions in patients after myocardial infarction. Am J Cardiol 114:1663–1669

Frías JP, Davies MJ, Rosenstock J et al (2021) Tirzepatide versus semaglutide once weekly in patients with type 2 diabetes. N Engl J Med. https://doi.org/10.1056/NEJMoa2107519

Furtao RHM, Bonaca MP, Raz I et al (2019) Dapagliflozin and cardiovascular outcomes in patients with type 2 diabetes mellitus and previous myocardial infarction. Subanalysis from DECLARE-TIMI 58 trial. Circulation 139:2516–2527

Gerstein HC, Miller ME, Byington RP et al (2008) for The Action to Control cardiovascular Risk in Diabetes (ACCORD) Study Group. Effects of intensive glucose lowering in type 2 diabetes. N Engl J Med 358:2545–2559

Gerstein HC, Colhoun HM, Dagenais GR et al (2019a) Dulaglutide and cardiovascular outcomes in type 2 diabetes (REWIND): a double-blind, randomised placebo-controlled trial. Lancet 394:121–130

Gerstein HC, Colhoun HM, Dagenais GR et al (2019b) Dulaglutide and renal outcomes in type 2 diabetes: an exploratory analysis oft he REWIND randomised, placebo-controlled trial. Lancet 394:131–138

Gerstein HC, Sattar N, Rosenstock J et al (2021) Cardiovascular and renal outcomes with efpeglenatide in type 2 diabetes. N Engl J Med. https://doi.org/10.1056/NEJMoa2108269

Giblett JP, Clarke SJ, Dutka DP, Hoole SP (2016) Glucagon-like peptide-1: a promising agent for cardioprotection during myocardial ischemia. JACC Basic Transl Sci 1:267–276

Giorgino F, Caruso I, Moellmann J, Lehrke M (2020) Differential indication for SGLT-2 inhibitors versus GLP-1 receptor agonists in patients with established atherosclerotic heart disease or at risk for congestive heart failure. Metabolism 104:154045

Green JB, Bethel MA, Armstrong PW et al (2015) Effect of sitagliptin on cardiovascular outcomes in type 2 diabetes. N Engl J Med 373:232–242

He S, Kahles F, Rattik S et al (2019) Gut intraepithelial T cells calibrate metabolism and accelerate cardiovascular disease. Nature 566:115–119

Heerspink HJL, Perkins BA, Fitchett DH et al (2016) Sodium glucose cotransporter-2 inhibitors in the treatment of diabetes mellitus. Circulation 134:752–772

Heerspink HJL, Stefansson BV, Correa-Rotter R et al (2020) Dapagliflozin in patients with chronic kidney disease. N Engl J Med 383:1436–1446

Heller SR on behalf oft he ADVANCE collabrative group (2009) A summary oft he ADVANCE trial. Diabetes Care 32(Suppl 2):S357–S361

Hernandez AF, Green JB, Janmohamed S et al (2018) Albiglutide and cardiovascular outcomes in patients with type 2 diabetes and cardiovascular disease (Harmony Outcomes): a double-blind, randomised placebo-controlles trial. Lancet 392:1519–1529

Holman RR, Bethel MA, Mentz RJ et al (2017a) Effects of once-weekly exenatide on cardiovascular outcomes in type 2 diabetes. N Engl J Med 377:1228–1239

Holman RR, Coleman RL, Chan JCN et al (2017b) Effects of acarbose on cardiovascular and diabetes outcomes in patients with coronary heart disease and impaired glucose intolerance (ACE): a randomized, double blind, placebo-controlled trial. Lancet Diabetes Endocrinol 5:877–886

Husain M, Birkenfeld AL, Donsmark M et al (2019) Oral semaglutide and cardiovascular outcomes in patients with type 2 diabetes. N Engl J Med 381:841–851

Iacobellis G, Villasante Fricke AC (2020) Effects of semaglutide versus dulaglutide on epicardial fat thickness in subjects with type 2 diabetes and obesity. J Endocr Soc. https://doi.org/10.1210/jendso/bvz042

Inzucchi SE, Zinman B, Fitchett D et al (2018) How does empagliflozin reduce cardiovascular mortality? Insights from a mediation analysis of the EMPA-REG OUTCOME trial. Diabetes Care 41:36–363

Kahles F, Liberman A, Halim C et al (2018) The incretin hormone GIP is upregulated in patients with atherosclerosis and stabilizes plaques in ApoE-/- mice by blocking monocyte/macrophage activation. Mol Metab 14:150–157

Kahn CR, Wang G, Lee KY (2019) Altered adipose tissue and adipocyte function in the pathogenesis of metabolic syndrome. J Clin Invest 129:3990–4000

Kato ET, Silverman MG, Mosenzon O et al (2019) Effect of dapagliflozin on heart failure and mortality in type 2 diabetes mellitus. Circulation 139:2528–2536

Kernan WN, Viscoli CM, Furie KL et al (2016) Pioglitazone after ischemic stroke or transient ischemic attack. N Engl J Med 374:1321–1331

Landgraf R, Aberle J, Birkenfeld AL et al (2020) Therapie des Typ-2-Diabetes. Diabetol Stoffwechs 15(Supplement):S65–S92

Lean ME, Leslie WS, Barnes AC et al (2018) Primary care-led weight management for remission of type 2 diabetes (DiRECT): an open-label, cluster-randomised trial. Lancet 391:541–551. https://doi.org/10.1016/S0140-6736(17)33102-1

Libby P, Hansson GK (2019) From focal lipid storage to systemic inflammation: JACC review topic of the week. J Am Coll Cardiol 74:1594–1607

Lim S, Kim KM, Nauck MA (2018) Glucagon-like peptide-1 receptor agonists and cardiovascular events: class effects versus individual patterns. Trends Endocrinol Metab 29:238–248

Lind M, Svensson A-M, Kosiborod M et al (2014) Glycemic control and excess mortality in type 1 diabetes. N Engl J Med 371:1972–1982

Lytvyn Y, Bjornstad P, Udell JA et al (2017) Sodium glucose cotransporter-2 inhibition in heart failure. Circulation 136:1643–1658

Mann JFE, Orsted DD, Brown-Frandsen K et al (2017) Liraglutide and renal outcomes in diabetes. N Engl J Med 377:839–848

Marso SP, Bain SC, Consoli A et al (2016a) Semaglutide and cardiovascular outcomes in patients with type 2 diabetes. New Engl J Med 375:1834–1844

Marso SP, Daniels GH, Brown-Frandsen K et al (2016b) Liraglutide and cardiovascular outcomes in patients with type 2 diabetes. New Engl J Med 375:311–322

Marso SP, McGuirre DK, Zinman B et al (2017) Efficacy and safety of degludec versus glargine in type 2 diabetes. N Engl J Med 377:723–732

Marton A, Kaneko T, Kovalik J-P et al (2021) Organ protection by SGLT2 inhibitors: role of metabolic energy and water conservation. Nat Rev Nephrol 17:65–77

Marx N (2020) Reduction of cardiovascular risk in patients with T2DM by GLP-1 receptor agonists: a shift in paradigm driven by data from large cardiovascular outcome trials. Eur Heart J 41:3359–3362

Marx N, Libby P (2018) Cardiovascular benefits of GLP-1 receptor agonism. JACC Basic Transl Sci 3:858–860

McCormick LM, Hoole SP, White PA et al (2015) Pre-treatment with glucagon-like Peptide-1 protects against ischemic left ventricular dysfunction and stunning without a detected difference in myocardial substrate utilization. JACC Cardiovasc Interv 8:292–301

McGavock JM, Lingvay I, Zib I et al (2007) Cardiac steatosis in diabetes mellitus: a 1H-magnetic resonance spectroscopy study. Circulation 116:1170–1175

McMurray JJV, Solomon SD, Inzucchi SE et al (2019) Dapagliflozin in patients with heart failure and reduced rejection fraction. N Engl J Med. https://doi.org/10.1056/NEJMoa1911303

Müller TD, Finan B, Bloom SR et al (2019) Glucagon-like peptide 1 (GLP-1). Mol Metab 30:72–130

Nauck MA, Meier JJ, Cavender MA et al (2017) Cardiovascular actions and clinical outcomes with glucagon-like peptide-1 receptor agonists and dipeptidyl peptidase-4 inhibitors. Circulation 136:849–870

Nauck MA, Quast DR, Wefers J, Meier JJ (2020) GLP-1 receptor agonists in the treatment of type 2 diabetes – state-of-the-art. Mol Metab. https://doi.org/10.1016/j.molmet.2020.101102

Neal B, Perkovic V, Mahaffey KW et al (2017) Canagliflozin and cardiovascular and renal events in type 2 diabetes. N Engl J Med 377:644–657

Newsome PN, Buchholtz K, Cusi K et al (2021) A placebo-controlled trial of subcutaneous semaglutide in nonalcoholi steatohepatitis. N Engl J Med 384:1113–1124

Packer M, Anker SD, Butler J et al (2020) Cardiovascular and renal outcomes with empagliflozin in heart failure. N Engl J Med 383:1413–1424

Perkovic V, Jardine MJ, Neal B et al (2019) Canagliflozin and renal outcomes in type 2 diabetes and nephropathy. N Engl J Med 380:2295–2306

Pfeffer MA, Claggett B, Diaz R et al (2015) Lixisenatide in patients with type 2 diabetes and acute coronary syndrome. N Engl J Med 373:2247–2257

Rakipovski G, Rolin B, Nøhr J et al (2018) The GLP-1 analogs liraglutide and semaglutide reduce atherosclerosis in ApoE-/- and LDLr-/- mice by a mechanism that includes inflammatory pathways. JACC Basic Transl Sci 3:844–857

Rask-Madsen C, Kahn CR (2012) Tissue-specific insulin signaling, metabolic syndrome and cardiovascular disease. Arterioscler Thromb Vasc Biol 32:2052–2059

Rawshani A, Rawshani A, Sattar N et al (2019) Relative prognostic importance and optimal levels of risk factors for mortality and cardiovascular outcomes in type 1 diabetes mellitus. Circulation 139:1900–1912

Riddle MC, Gerstein HC (2019) The cardiovascular legacy of good glycemic control: clues about mediators from the DCCT/EDIC study. Diabetes Care 42:1159–1161

Rosenstock J, Kahn SE, Johansen OE et al (2019a) Effect of linagliptin vs glimepiride on major adverse cardiovascular outcomes in patients with type 2 diabetes. The CAROLINA randomized clinical trial. JAMA 322:1155–1166

Rosenstock J, Perkovic V, Johansen OE et al (2019b) Effect of linagliptin vs placebo on major cardiovascular events in adults with type 2 diabetes and high cardiovascular and renal risk: the CARMELINA randomized clinical trial. JAMA 32:69–79

Rosenstock J, Wysham C, Frías JP et al (2021) Efficacy and safety of a novel dual GIP and GLP-1 receptor agonist tirzepatide in patients with type 2 diabetes (SURPASS-1): a double-blind, randomised, phase 3 trial. Lancet 398:143–155. https://doi.org/10.1016/S0140-6736(21)01324-6

Sattar N, McGuire DK (2021) Prevention of CV outcomes in antihyperglycemic drug-naive patients with type 2 diabetes with, or at elevated risk of, ASCVD: to start or not to start with metformin. Eur Heart J 42:2574–2576

Sattar N, Rawshani A, Franzen S et al (2019) Age at diagnosis of type 2 diabetes mellitus and associations with cardiovascular and mortality risks. Circulation 139:2228–2237

Scherer PE (2016) The multifaceted roles of adipose tissue: therapeutic targets for diabetes and beyond: the 2015 banting lecture. Diabetes 65:1452–1461

Scirica BM, Bhatt DL, Braunwald E et al (2013) Saxagliptin and cardiovascular outcomes in patients with type 2 diabetes mellitus. N Engl J Med 369:1317–1326

Shaihov-Teper O, Ram E, Ballan N et al (2021) Extracellular vesicles from epicardial fat facilitate atrial fibrillation. Circulation 143:2475–2493

Sjöström L, Lindroos AK, Peltonen M et al (2004) Swedish Obese Subjects Study Scientific Group. Lifestyle, diabetes, and cardiovascular risk factors 10 years after bariatric surgery. N Engl J Med 351:2683–2693

Stefan N, Kantarzis K, Häring HU (2008) Causes and metabolic consequences of fatty liver. Endocr Rev 29:939–960

Stratton IM, Adler AI, Neil HA et al (2000) Association of glycemia with macrovascular and microvascular complications of type 2 diabetes (UKPDS 35). BMJ 321:405–412

The Diabetes Control and Complication Trial Research Group (1993) The effect of intensive treatment of diabetes on the development and progression of long-term complications in insulin-dependent diabetes mellitus. N Engl J Med 329:977–986

The Diabetes Control and Complication Trial/Epidemiology of Diabetes Interventions and Complications (DCCT/EDIC) Study Research Group (2005) Intensive diabetes treatment and cardiovascular disease in patients with type 1 diabetes. N Engl J Med 353:2643–2653

The ORIGIN Trial Investigators (2012) Basla insulin and cardiovascular and other outcomes in dysglycemia. N Engl J Med 367:319–328

U.K. Prospective Diabetes Study Group (1998) Intensive blood-glucose control with sulfonylureas or insulin compared with conventional treatment and risk of complications in patients with type 2 diabetes (UKPDS 33). Lancet 352:837–853

Unger RH (2002) Lipotoxic diseases. Annu Rev Med 53:19–36

Vaccaro O, Masulli M, Nicolucci A et al (2017) Effects on the incidence of cardiovascular events oft he addition of pioglitazone versus sulfonylureas in patients with type 2 diabetes inadequately controlled with metformin (TOSCA.IT): a randomised, multicentre trial. Lancet Diabetes Endocrinol 5:887–897 van Heerebeek L, Paulus WJ (2016) Understanding heart failure with preserved ejection fraction: where are we today? Neth Heart J 24:227–236

van Wagner LB, Wilcox JE, Colangelo LA et al (2015) Association of nonalcoholic fatty liver disease with subclinical myocardial remodeling and dysfunction: a population-based study. Hepatology 62:773–783

Verma S, McMurray JJV (2018) SGLT2 inhibitors and mechanisms of cardiovascular benefit: a state-of-the-art review. Diabetologia 61(10):2108–2117

Wanner C, Marx N (2018) SGLT-2 inhibitors: the future treatment of type 2 diabetes mellitus and other chronic diseases. Diabetologia 61:2134–2139

Wanner C, Inzucchi SE, Lachin JM, Fitchett D, von Eynatten M, Mattheus M, Johansen OE, Woerle HJ, Broedl UC, Zinman B, EMPA-REG OUTCOME Investigators (2016) Empagliflozin and Progression of Kidney Disease in Type 2 Diabetes. N Engl J Med 375:323–334

Wiviott SD, Raz I, Bonaca MP et al (2019) Dapagliflozin and cardiovascular outcomes in type 2 diabetes. N Engl J Med 380:347–357

Zaharia OP, Strassburger K, Strom A et al (2019) Risk of diabetes-associated diseases in subgroups of patients with recent-onset diabetes: a 5-year follow-up study. Lancet Diabetes Endocrinol 7:684–694

Zannad F, Cannon CP, Cushman WC et al (2015) Heart failure and mortality outcomes in patients with type 2 diabetes taking alogliptin versus placebo in EXAMINE: a multicentre, randomised, double-blind trial. Lancet 385:2067–2076

Ziegler T, Rahmnann FA, Jurisch V, Kupatt C (2020) Atheroclerosis and the capillary network; pathophysiology and potential therapeutic strategies. Cell 50. https://doi.org/10.3390/cells9010050

Zinman B, Genuth S, Nathan DM (2014) The diabetes control and complications trial/epidemiology of diabetes interventions and complications study: 30th anniversary presentations. Diabetes Care 37:8

Zinman B, Wanner C, Lachin JM et al (2015) Empagliflozin, cardiovascular outcomes, and mortality in type 2 diabetes. N Engl J Med 373:2117–2128

Zucker I, Schohat T, Dankner R, Chodick G (2017) New onset diabetes in adulthood is associated with a substantial risk for mortality at all ages: a population based historical cohort study with a decade-long follow-up. Cardiovasc Diabetol 16:105. https://doi.org/10.1186/s12933-017-0583-x

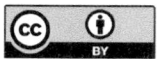

LDL-Cholesterol-Lowering Therapy

Angela Pirillo, Giuseppe D. Norata, and Alberico L. Catapano

Contents

1 Introduction 74
2 Statins in the Prevention of Cardiovascular Disease 75
3 Non-statin Cholesterol-Lowering Drugs 76
   3.1   Ezetimibe 77
   3.2   PCSK9 Inhibitors 78
       3.2.1   Evolocumab 80
       3.2.2   Alirocumab 81
   3.3   Lomitapide 83
   3.4   Mipomersen 84
4 Cholesterol-Lowering Drugs Under Clinical Development 86
   4.1   Inclisiran 86
   4.2   Bempedoic Acid 88
5 The Future of Cholesterol Lowering 90
   5.1   ANGPTL3-L_{Rx} 90
6 Conclusions 91
References 92

A. Pirillo
Center for the Study of Atherosclerosis, E. Bassini Hospital, Milan, Italy

IRCCS MultiMedica, Milan, Italy
e-mail: angela.pirillo@guest.unimi.it

G. D. Norata
Department of Pharmacological and Biomolecular Sciences, Università degli Studi di Milano, Milan, Italy

Center for the Study of Atherosclerosis, E. Bassini Hospital, Milan, Italy
e-mail: danilo.norata@unimi.it

A. L. Catapano (✉)
Department of Pharmacological and Biomolecular Sciences, Università degli Studi di Milano, Milan, Italy

IRCCS MultiMedica, Milan, Italy
e-mail: alberico.catapano@unimi.it

© The Author(s) 2020
A. von Eckardstein, C. J. Binder (eds.), *Prevention and Treatment of Atherosclerosis*,
Handbook of Experimental Pharmacology 270, https://doi.org/10.1007/164_2020_361

Abstract

The causal relation between elevated levels of LDL-C and cardiovascular disease has been largely established by experimental and clinical studies. Thus, the reduction of LDL-C levels is a major target for the prevention of cardiovascular disease. In the last decades, statins have been used as the main therapeutic approach to lower plasma cholesterol levels; however, the presence of residual lipid-related cardiovascular risk despite maximal statin therapy raised the need to develop additional lipid-lowering drugs to be used in combination with or in alternative to statins in patients intolerant to the treatment. Several new drugs have been approved which have mechanisms of action different from statins or impact on different lipoprotein classes.

Keywords

Cardiovascular disease · Dyslipidemias · Ezetimibe · Familial hypercholesterolemia · Hypercholesterolemia · Hypertriglyceridemia · Lipid-lowering drugs · Low-density lipoprotein cholesterol · Low-density lipoprotein receptor · Proprotein convertase subtilisin/kexin type 9 · Statins

1   Introduction

Atherosclerosis is a chronic inflammatory disease affecting arterial wall and characterized by a progressive accumulation of lipids in the subendothelial space. Epidemiological and genetic evidence suggests low-density lipoprotein cholesterol (LDL-C) as a causal factor in cardiovascular disease (Ference et al. 2017), and the results of a large number of randomized clinical trials definitely proved that decreasing LDL-C levels translates in a proportional reduction of the risk of atherosclerotic cardiovascular (CV) events (Baigent et al. 2005, 2010, 2011; Cannon et al. 2015a; Sabatine et al. 2017a; Schwartz et al. 2018).

Populations of modern societies present with LDL-C levels largely exceeding those believed to be physiological. Optimal plasma concentration of LDL-C ranges around 25 mg/dL, since above this value the LDL receptor (LDLR) is saturated (Brown and Goldstein 1986); furthermore, individuals with genetically determined low levels of LDL-C are healthy and exhibit very low incidence of CV events (Glueck et al. 1997; Cohen et al. 2006). These observations, coupled to the results of clinical trials testing the most recent lipid-lowering drugs (i.e., PCSK9 inhibitors), which have shown that LDL-C levels may be lowered well below the values recommended by guidelines without safety concerns (Robinson et al. 2017; Sabatine et al. 2017b), provided the notion that reaching very low LDL-C levels may safely confer additional clinical CV benefits. This concept led to a substantial reduction of the LDL-C goals recommended by the most recent guidelines for the management of dyslipidemias (Mach et al. 2020).

Statins, which represent the cornerstone for the treatment of hypercholesterol-emia, have shown approximately a 20% reduction in the risk of cardiovascular events per each mmol/L LDL-C reduction (Baigent et al. 2005); a more intensive intervention was associated with a greater reduction of the incidence of major vascular events (Baigent et al. 2010), suggesting that the higher the degree of reduction of LDL-C levels, the greater the benefit in terms of reduction of CV events.

Although statin monotherapy could reduce LDL-C levels to a large extent (up to −50% with the highest doses of most potent statins), this might not be enough to reach the desired goals based on the individual CV risk, and therefore additional approaches are needed.

This is even more important in patients with familial hypercholesterolemia (FH) which are considered among those with the highest cardiovascular risk, due to the exposure to high plasma LDL-C levels from birth (Nordestgaard et al. 2013). FH is caused by mutations in genes encoding proteins involved in the LDL catabo-lism, such as LDL receptor (LDLR), apolipoprotein B (apoB), proprotein convertase subtilisin/kexin type 9 (PCSK9), and LDLR adaptor protein (LDLRAP); mutations in LDLR gene account for the vast majority of FH cases (Nordestgaard et al. 2013). Heterozygous FH (HeFH) patients are characterized by two- to threefold elevation in plasma cholesterol levels and development of coronary atherosclerosis at an early age (usually after 30 years); homozygous FH (HoFH) patients, which include either patients with a significantly reduced LDLR activity (2–30% residual activity) or receptor-negative subjects, characterized by a residual LDLR activity <2%, exhibit a more severe cardiovascular condition, due to the exposure to very high LDL-C levels from birth, childhood coronary heart disease, and premature death from myocardial infarction (prior to 20 years of age) if untreated (Cuchel et al. 2014; Sniderman et al. 2014).

These aspects indicate that the choice of the most appropriate therapeutic approach should be done taking into account the LDL-C target and the distance of LDL-C from the target which are dictated by the cardiovascular risk of the patient, and thus the therapy needs to be tailored to each patient. While statins are the first approach, combination therapy is critical when certain LDL-C goals should be achieved (Norata et al. 2013a; Toth et al. 2016; Russell et al. 2018).

2   Statins in the Prevention of Cardiovascular Disease

Statins are competitive inhibitors of 3-hydroxy-3-methylglutaryl coenzyme A (HMG-CoA) reductase, the rate-limiting enzyme of cholesterol synthesis pathway. Following the reduction of intracellular cholesterol synthesis, hepatocytes upregulate surface LDLR expression to increase LDL uptake, resulting in the reduction of circulating LDL-C levels. A large number of clinical trials have established the efficacy of statins in reducing cardiovascular morbidity and mortality in both primary and secondary prevention (Baigent et al. 2010; Chan et al. 2011; Mills et al. 2011a, b; Tonelli et al. 2011; Naci et al. 2013; Taylor et al. 2013). A meta-analysis of 14 randomized clinical trials including >90,000 participants showed a significant reduction in coronary heart disease (CHD) mortality (-19%, $p < 0.0001$), myocardial infarction or coronary death (-23%, $p < 0.0001$), and fatal or nonfatal stroke (-17%, $p < 0.0001$) (Baigent et al. 2005). Overall, there was a significant 21% proportional reduction in the incidence of major vascular events per mmol/L LDL-C reduction (Baigent et al. 2005). A linear relationship between proportional reduction in incidence of major cardiovascular events and mean absolute LDL-C reduction was reported (Baigent et al. 2005). The analysis of more intensive versus less intensive statin regimens showed that treatment with more intensive regimens resulted in an additional 15% ($p < 0.0001$) reduction in major vascular events (Baigent et al. 2010), suggesting that further reducing LDL-C levels safely translates into a further clinical benefit.

Despite the proven efficacy of statin therapy, a relevant percentage of patients still experience cardiovascular events, even in the presence of well-controlled LDL-C levels due to a "residual risk" (Ahn and Choi 2015), likely related to abnormalities in other lipid parameters (such as high triglycerides and low HDL-c) which may account for this effect particularly in specific groups of patients (including obese patients or those with metabolic syndrome or type 2 diabetes) (Fruchart et al. 2014). Moreover, although statin therapy represents the first approach for the treatment of FH, its efficacy is strictly related to the presence of a functional LDLR and thus may be effective in HeFH or in receptor-defective HoFH (Nordestgaard et al. 2013; Cuchel et al. 2014). In HoFH patients carrying null mutations on LDLR gene, statins induce a modest reduction of LDL-C (~20%) likely through pathways LDLR-independent, which however is not sufficient to reduce massively LDL-C levels and reach the goals suggested for their risk category (Hovingh et al. 2013). In addition, although statins are overall well tolerated, statin-associated muscle symptoms may lead to therapy discontinuation and limit clinical benefit (Banach et al. 2015). Muscle-related adverse events occur mainly with high statin doses which are commonly used in high cardiovascular risk patients, but they have been reported also in patients presenting with comorbidities, due to pharmacokinetic interactions with other drugs (Chatzizisis et al. 2010; Taha et al. 2014). Several pharmacological approaches are available for the management of hypercholesterol-emia in patients intolerant to statins, including the possibility to combine a low dose of a statin with another cholesterol-lowering drug which is acting by a complementary mechanism of action (Pirillo and Catapano 2015). Several non-statin drugs approved for the treatment of dyslipidemia, however, failed to further reduce the incidence of cardiovascular events when added to current statin therapy, with the exception of ezetimibe (Ridker 2014; Cannon et al. 2015a) and, more recently, PCSK9 inhibitors (Sabatine et al. 2017a; Schwartz et al. 2018).

3   Non-statin Cholesterol-Lowering Drugs

In recent years several therapeutic approaches have been investigated and developed with the aim of reducing plasma cholesterol levels with a mechanism of action complementary to that of statins. Among them, ezetimibe and, more recently, the monoclonal antibodies targeting PCSK9 have been approved, while other molecules including bempedoic acid and PCSK9 gene silencing are in an advanced phase of clinical development.

3.1   Ezetimibe

Ezetimibe is a lipid-lowering drug acting as an inhibitor of intestinal cholesterol absorption through the inhibition of the sterol transporter Niemann-Pick C1L1 (NPC1L1) protein (Davis and Veltri 2007). This protein, highly expressed at the brushborder membrane of intestinal epithelial cells, plays a central role in the intestinal absorption of cholesterol and the regulation of cholesterol plasma levels (Wang 2007; Wang and Song 2012). The observation that individuals carrying loss-of-function variants in *NPC1L1* have lower LDL-C levels and a 53% relative risk reduction of CHD (Stitziel et al. 2014) has suggested that this protein could represent a potential pharmacological target for the treatment of hypercholesterolemia.

Ezetimibe has a complementary mechanism of action as compared to statins. Statins, by inhibiting cholesterol synthesis pathway, induce the upregulation of hepatic LDLR, thus resulting in increased uptake of LDL particle from the circulation. This effect prompts a feedback mechanism which increases cholesterol absorption in the intestine, thus partially affecting the efficacy of statin therapy. In this context, ezetimibe as monotherapy, by inhibiting intestinal cholesterol absorption, will reduce plasma cholesterol levels, but the effect would be mitigated by the induction of increased cholesterol synthesis in the intestine and the liver (Descamps et al. 2011). Therefore, the combination statin+ezetimibe will reduce both cholesterol synthesis and absorption, thus representing a valuable approach for further reducing plasma LDL-C levels beyond what was observed with statins in monotherapy.

Indeed several clinical trials have shown that adding ezetimibe to statin therapy results in a further 15–20% LDL-C level reduction (Catapano et al. 2005, 2006; Mikhailidis et al. 2007; Norata et al. 2013a). A pooled analysis of over 21,000 subjects from 27 clinical trials showed that co-administration of ezetimibe with a statin produces a greater LDL-C-lowering effect than statin alone in a wide range of patients (Morrone et al. 2012). Furthermore, the reduction in LDL-C levels was more impressive in patients with CHD or CHD risk-equivalents treated with ezetimibe added to current statin dose compared with patients who titrated the statin dose (Foody et al. 2013). This difference has been reported also in diabetic patients treated with ezetimibe+statin, who showed a 24.6% LDL-C reduction compared with a 10.9% reduction observed in those receiving a doubled statin dose; similarly the entire lipid profile was improved more in patients receiving the combination therapy (Sakamoto et al. 2015). A meta-analysis of available randomized clinical trials showed that the addition of ezetimibe to ongoing simvastatin, atorvastatin, or rosuvastatin therapy results in a greater reduction of LDL-C in high CV risk patients compared with doubling the statin dose (Lorenzi et al. 2019).

The combination ezetimibe+statin has been shown to be effective also in FH patients with residual LDLR activity, who achieve lower levels of total cholesterol and LDL-C than patients treated with statin alone (Gagne et al. 2002; Pisciotta et al. 2007; Kastelein et al. 2008).

Adding ezetimibe to statin therapy was also shown to provide a clinical benefit. The SHARP trial showed that ezetimibe+simvastatin administration for 4.9 years in patients with moderate-to-severe kidney disease reduced LDL-C levels by 0.85 mmol/L (33 mg/dL) and decreased the incidence of first major atherosclerotic events (including nonfatal MI, coronary death, non-hemorrhagic stroke, or arterial revascularization) by 17% compared with placebo (Baigent et al. 2011). The *IMPROVE-IT* trial compared the effect of a 6-year administration of ezetimibe +simvastatin or simvastatin alone in patients with a recent acute coronary syndrome (Cannon et al. 2015a). The combination therapy reduced LDL-C level more than simvastatin alone (24% further reduction), resulting in a significant 6.4% lower relative risk reduction of the primary composite endpoint (cardiovascular death, nonfatal myocardial infarction, unstable angina requiring hospitalization, coronary revascularization, nonfatal stroke) (Cannon et al. 2015a). Specific subgroups of patients benefit more from the combination therapy, including women (12% reduction of the relative CV vs 5% in men) (Toda Kato et al. 2015), older patients (<65 years HR 0.98; ≥75 years HR: 0.80), and diabetic patients (15% reduction versus 2% in non-diabetics) (Giugliano et al. 2018). Combined therapy was also superior to simvastatin alone in reducing the incidence of non-hemorrhagic stroke (hazard ratio 0.78, $P = 0.008$) (Wiviott et al. 2015). Adverse event incidence was similar in all subgroups (Wiviott et al. 2015).

3.2   PCSK9 Inhibitors

Proprotein convertase subtilisin kexin 9 (PCSK9) is a serine protease involved in the regulation of hepatic low-density lipoprotein receptor (LDLR) expression and, as a consequence, in the control of plasma LDL-C levels (Fig. 1). In fact, secreted PCSK9 binds to LDLR, and when the complex LDLR/PCSK9 is internalized, the conformational change of LDLR induced by PCSK9 impairs LDLR recycling on cell surface while making it more susceptible to degradation within lysosomes. This leads to a reduced LDLR surface expression, reduced LDL uptake, and therefore increased LDL-C plasma levels (Leren 2014; Norata et al. 2016; Seidah et al. 2019). Individuals carrying loss-of-function mutations in *PCSK9* gene have lower levels of LDL-C and reduced risk of cardiovascular disease (Cohen et al. 2005, 2006; Kathiresan 2008; Benn et al. 2010; Kent et al. 2017), while gain-of-function mutations are associated with an increased risk of premature cardiovascular disease (Naoumova et al. 2005; Hopkins et al. 2015; Qiu et al. 2017). Based on these observations, PCSK9 inhibition has been suggested as a possible approach for the control of hypercholesterolemia (Fig. 1).

Despite the liver is the major organ expressing PCSK9, other tissues express this protein, including the kidney, pancreas, and brain (Norata et al. 2016); this

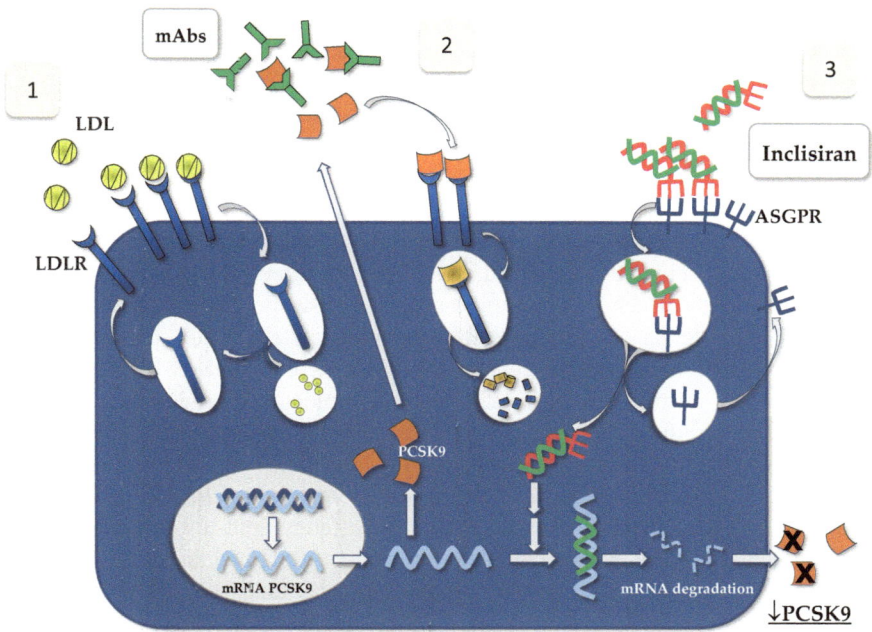

Fig. 1 Mechanism of action of PCSK9 inhibitors. In the absence of PCSK9 (1), LDL binds to LDLR. After internalization, the LDL-LDLR complex dissociates, LDL undergoes lysosomal degradation, and LDLR is recycled to the cell surface. In the presence of PCSK9 (2), LDLR cannot dissociate from LDL and is degraded within the lysosomes, leading to increased levels of circulating LDL-C. Monoclonal antibodies (mAbs) neutralize secreted PCSK9, thus inhibiting its binding to the LDLR and dampening PCSK9-induced LDLR degradation. Inclisiran (3) is a siRNA which is internalized by specific hepatic receptors (ASGPR1) and acts intracellularly by binding to PCSK9 mRNA, thus inducing its degradation and reducing the production of the protein. LDL, low-density lipoprotein; LDLR, LDL receptor; PCSK9, proprotein convertase subtilisin/kexin type 9

observation raises the question of whether the pharmacological inhibition of PCSK9 may also result in extrahepatic effects with a clinical relevance. PCSK9 deficiency in animal models and loss-of-function mutations in humans were associated with increased risk of new-onset diabetes (Ference et al. 2016; Da Dalt et al. 2019), pointing to a role for PCSK9 and LDLR on cholesterol metabolism in pancreatic beta cells (Perego et al. 2019). Available data from clinical trials with anti-PCSK9 monoclonal antibodies excluded this hypothesis (Sabatine et al. 2017a; Schwartz et al. 2018); data from long-term post-marketing surveillance are awaited to clarify this aspect.

Different approaches have been tested or are under evaluation for targeting PCSK9 (Seidah et al. 2019), including two fully human monoclonal antibodies against circulating PCSK9, evolocumab and alirocumab, which inhibit the activity of secreted PCSK9 (approved for the treatment of hypercholesterolemia), and, more recently, a small interfering RNA approach which inhibits PCSK9 synthesis in the liver now under clinical evaluation.

3.2.1 Evolocumab

Several phase 2 trials have shown that evolocumab efficiently reduces LDL-C levels in hypercholesterolemic subjects either as monotherapy or as add-on to background lipid-lowering therapy (LLT) (Giugliano et al. 2012; Koren et al. 2012) and was effective also in FH patients (Raal et al. 2012; Stein et al. 2013) and in statin-intolerant patients (Sullivan et al. 2012).

The PROFICIO (Program to Reduce LDL-C and Cardiovascular Outcomes Following Inhibition of PCSK9 in Different Populations) program of evolocumab included phase 3 clinical trials aimed at assessing the effectiveness of evolocumab in comparison with placebo or ezetimibe across a broad population of patients with hypercholesterolemia. In monotherapy, evolocumab efficiently reduced LDL-C levels compared with either placebo or ezetimibe (Koren et al. 2014); when added to a moderate- or high-intensity statin therapy, evolocumab reduced LDL-C levels more efficiently than adding placebo or ezetimibe, and most patients achieved LDL-C levels <70 mg/dL, compared with the group receiving ezetimibe (Robinson et al. 2014). Similar results were obtained when hypercholesterolemic patients were treated for 52 weeks with evolocumab added to different lipid-lowering therapy with a significant 57% LDL-C level reduction that was maintained throughout the study period, independent of background therapy (Blom et al. 2014). Evolocumab also induced a decrease in percent atheroma volume (PAV) in statin-treated patients (Nicholls et al. 2016).

The efficacy of PCSK9 has been tested also in patients with statin intolerance. In the phase 3 GAUSS-2 study, statin-intolerant patients were treated with evolocumab or ezetimibe for 12 weeks: evolocumab reduced LDL-C levels more efficiently than ezetimibe, and the incidence of myalgia among treated patients was low (Stroes et al. 2014). These findings have been confirmed by the GAUSS-3 trial (Nissen et al. 2016).

Specific studies have evaluated the effect of evolocumab also in FH patients (Raal et al. 2012, 2015b). The RUTHERFORD-2 study showed a significant reduction of LDL-C levels (~60%) in HeFH patients treated with evolocumab (Raal et al. 2015b). The pilot study TESLA part A, performed in six receptor-defective and two receptor-negative HoFH patients, showed that patients with defective LDLR activity had a significant reduction in their LDL-C levels following the treatment with evolocumab (~23%), while, as expected on the basis of the mechanism of action, receptor-negative patients did not respond to the therapy (Stein et al. 2013) further confirming that the mechanism by which evolocumab reduces LDL-C levels is primarily through the upregulation of residual LDLR activity. In the phase 3 TESLA part B trial, a ~31% LDL-C reduction was observed; the analysis of LDL-C reduction according to LDLR mutation status showed that the type of mutation causing FH is the major determinant of evolocumab-induced response (Raal et al. 2015a). An interim analysis of the open-label TAUSSIG trial confirmed that evolocumab reduces LDL-C levels by approximately 20% in HoFH patients (with the exception of receptor-negative patients), a reduction that persisted up to 48 weeks, with a high variability in the percent change of LDL-C from baseline (Raal et al. 2017).

Patients who completed one of the phase 2 or 3 studies have been recruited for the open-label trials OSLER-1 (for phase 2) and OSLER-2 (for phase 3); the analysis of combined data showed that evolocumab reduced LDL-C levels by 61% compared with patients treated with standard therapy; this reduction was sustained through 48 weeks and translated into a lower rate of all CV events (Sabatine et al. 2015). The final report of the OSLER-1 study showed a persistent LDL-C reduction over 5 years with a good safety profile (Koren et al. 2019). The benefit of this massive LDL-C reduction translated also in a clinical benefit. Indeed the FOURIER trial showed that, after a median follow-up of 2.2 years, in statin-treated patients with CVD and LDL-C $\geq$ 70 mg/dL, evolocumab significantly reduced by 15% the risk of the primary endpoint (including cardiovascular death, myocardial infarction, stroke, hospitalization for unstable angina, or coronary revascularization) and by 20% the secondary endpoint (cardiovascular death, myocardial infarction, or stroke) (Sabatine et al. 2017a). The clinical benefit was present in all patient categories, with patients at the highest CV risk showing the greatest absolute risk reduction (Sabatine et al. 2017b, 2018; Bonaca et al. 2018). A prespecified analysis of the FOURIER trial showed a linear relationship between LDL-C levels and CV outcomes down to LDL-C < 0.5 mmol/L (<~20 mg/dL), without safety concerns (Giugliano et al. 2017b). The therapy with evolocumab did not increase the risk of new-onset diabetes and did not worsen glycemia (Sabatine et al. 2017b) nor did affect negatively the cognitive function (Giugliano et al. 2017a). Altogether these results indicate that evolocumab can be used safely used to reduce LDL-C levels and the risk of CV events in patients at high CV risk despite current optimized lipid-lowering therapy.

3.2.2 Alirocumab

Alirocumab is a fully human monoclonal antibody against PCSK9. As for evolocumab, several phase 2 trials have been performed in different patient groups; these trials have reported a significant alirocumab-induced reduction of LDL-C levels in patients taking statins as well as in patients with FH (40% up to 73%) (McKenney et al. 2012; Roth et al. 2012; Stein et al. 2012b; Dufour et al. 2017).

The *ODYSSEY* program included 14 phase 3 trials on alirocumab, aimed at evaluating the efficacy and safety of alirocumab alone or in combination with other lipid-lowering therapies in different groups of hypercholesterolemic patients. As monotherapy, alirocumab reduced LDL-C levels more efficiently than ezetimibe (47.2% vs 15.6%) (Roth and McKenney 2015). Then alirocumab was tested in high CV risk populations as add-on to maximum tolerated statin±other LLT: the COMBO I and II studies showed that alirocumab induced a greater reduction of LDL-C levels compared with either placebo (48.2% vs 2.3%) (Kereiakes et al. 2015) or ezetimibe (50.6% vs 20.7%) (Cannon et al. 2015b). In the ODYSSEY LONG TERM trial, the addition of alirocumab to the maximal tolerated dose of statin produced a 61% reduction of LDL-C levels at week 24, and this reduction persisted up to week 78 (52.4%) (Robinson et al. 2015). Adjudicated major CV events in a post hoc analysis were lower in alirocumab group than in placebo group (1.7% vs 3.3%), with cumulative probability of event curves tending to diverge over time

(Robinson et al. 2015). The ODYSSEY OPTIONS I and II trials compared the effects of adding alirocumab to atorvastatin or rosuvastatin, adding ezetimibe, or doubling the statin dose; these trials reported the greatest LDL-C level reductions in patients treated with alirocumab as add-on (Bays et al. 2015; Farnier et al. 2016).

A specific trial was designed to address the efficacy and safety of alirocumab in statin-intolerant patients, with a statin rechallenge arm. In the ODYSSEY ALTER-NATIVE trial, alirocumab produced greater LDL-C reduction compared with ezetimibe in patients intolerant to statins (45% and 14.6% at week 24, respectively), and a higher percentage of patients reached the recommended LDL-C goal (41.9% vs 4.4%, respectively) (Moriarty et al. 2015). Skeletal muscle-related adverse events were the most common in all treatment groups, but significantly lower with alirocumab vs atorvastatin (HR 0.61, 95% CI, 0.38–0.99, $P = 0.042$) (Moriarty et al. 2015).

The ODYSSEY program included also clinical trials specifically designed to evaluate the effect of alirocumab in HeFH patients. In the ODYSSEY FH I (North America, Europe, South Africa) and FH II (Europe) studies, HeFH patients with an inadequate control of LDL-C levels despite maximally tolerated LLT received alirocumab and showed 57.9% (FH I) and 51.4% (FH II) LDL-C level reductions with alirocumab versus placebo; these reductions were maintained up to week 78 (Kastelein et al. 2015). Similar reductions were observed in HeFH patients presenting with higher LDL-C levels (≥ 4.1 mmol/L; ≥ 160 mg/dL) despite maximally tolerated LLT, in agreement with previous observations (Kastelein et al. 2014; Robinson et al. 2015). The treatment with alirocumab allowed the discontinuation or, at least, prolonged the time to next apheresis treatment in HeFH patients undergoing weekly or biweekly lipoprotein apheresis at baseline (ODYSSEY ESCAPE trial) (Moriarty et al. 2016). The ODYSSEY OLE study, which included HeFH patients who had completed one of the four phase 3 parent studies (FH I, FH II, LONG TERM, HIGH FH), showed a durability of alirocumab-induced LDL-C lowering over time (Farnier et al. 2018).

The ODYSSEY OUTCOMES trial tested the hypothesis that the treatment with alirocumab may reduce the risk of CV events in patients with a recent acute coronary syndrome having LDL-C levels exceeding the recommended goals for this risk category despite high-intensity statin therapy (Schwartz et al. 2018). After a median follow-up of 2.8 years, the risk of composite primary endpoint was significantly reduced by 15% in alirocumab-treated patients, and the greatest absolute reduction was observed in patients with the highest baseline LDL-C levels (≥ 100 mg/dL) (Schwartz et al. 2018). During the study, LDL-C levels were reduced by 62.7% at 4 months and 54.7% at 48 months (Schwartz et al. 2018).

Altogether, the results obtained in these studies have shown a significant efficacy of this pharmacological approach, which, by inducing a remarkable and sustained reduction of LDL-C levels beyond that obtained with statins with/without other LLT, translates into a greater CV benefit.

3.3 Lomitapide

Microsomal triglyceride transfer protein (MTP) localizes in the endoplasmic reticulum (ER) of hepatocytes and enterocytes and acts by transferring triglycerides and cholesteryl esters from the ER membrane to the nascent apoB (Hooper et al. 2015) (Fig. 2). MTP plays an essential role in the assembly and secretion of apolipoprotein B-containing lipoproteins, including very-low-density lipoproteins (VLDL) and chylomicrons (Hooper et al. 2015). Loss-of-function mutations in the gene encoding for MTP (*MTTP*) result in a reduced synthesis of VLDL and chylomicrons, increased apoB degradation, and lower levels of circulating LDL-C; based on these observations, MTP has been proposed as a possible target for the pharmacological control of hypercholesterolemia, particularly for the treatment of HoFH (Sirtori et al. 2014). Lomitapide is an MTP inhibitor which reduces LDL-C levels independent of LDLR (Fig. 2), and preclinical studies in animal models have shown that MTP inhibition resulted in the reduction of atherogenic lipoprotein levels (Wetterau et al. 1998; Shiomi and Ito 2001).

Lomitapide has been approved for the treatment of HoFH (Berberich and Hegele 2017), based on the results of several randomized clinical trials. A phase 2 study showed that the administration of lomitapide for 16 weeks in monotherapy efficiently reduced LDL-C levels in six HoFH patients (5 LDLR-negative and 1 LDLR-defective) (Cuchel et al. 2007); overall the drug was well tolerated, and the most serious adverse events were elevations in liver aminotransferase levels and hepatic fat accumulation (Cuchel et al. 2007). This study highlighted that, although lomitapide was highly effective in reducing LDL-C levels, it also induced liver steatosis in treated patients, casting doubts about long-term safety.

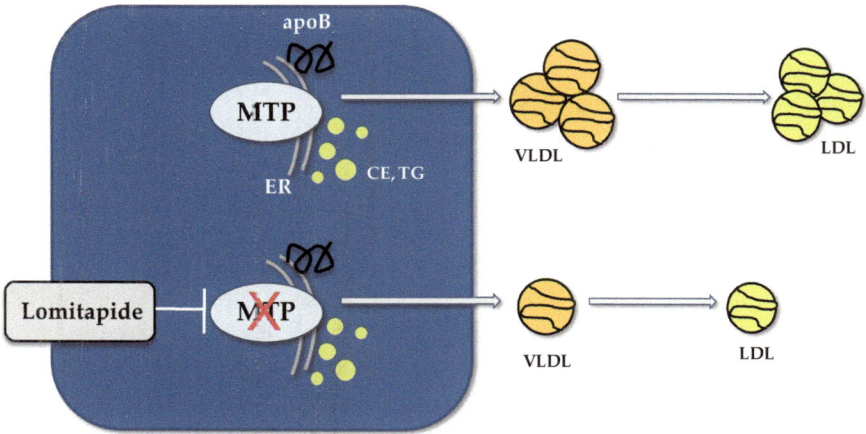

Fig. 2 Mode of action of lomitapide. MTP mediates the transfer of cholesteryl esters (CE) and triglycerides (TG) to apolipoprotein B (apoB) resulting in the synthesis of VLDL and chylomicrons. Lomitapide inhibits the activity of MTP, thus reducing the production of apoB-containing lipoproteins

To address this aspect, lomitapide was administered to 29 HoFH patients in a single-arm, open-label, phase 3 study in addition to conventional lipid-lowering therapy (Cuchel et al. 2013). Mean LDL-C levels were significantly reduced by 50% at the end of efficacy phase (week 26) with some patients able to discontinue or increase the interval between apheresis treatments (Cuchel et al. 2013). At the end of the study (week 78), LDL-C reduction was partially attenuated (−38%); changes in the concomitant lipid-lowering therapies or adjustment of the lomitapide dose in patients experiencing adverse effects can likely explain this result (Cuchel et al. 2013). Many patients reported gastrointestinal adverse reactions, which were controlled by moving patients on a very-low-fat diet. Increased levels of ALT, AST, or both, observed in some patients, were transient, successfully managed by dose reduction or temporary interruption, and were not related to changes of liver function. A modest increase (8.6%) in hepatic fat content was observed (Cuchel et al. 2013); the clinical consequence of this rise in liver fat is still unclear and requires further investigation with longer-term trials in a higher number of patients to assess whether it could have metabolic consequences.

Data from the real-world setting seem to suggest that safety profile of lomitapide is similar to that reported by clinical trials and have confirmed the need of a careful monitoring of transaminase levels and the adherence to a low-fat diet which may minimize gastrointestinal side effects (Roeters van Lennep et al. 2015). A longer follow-up is required to further support safety and establish whether lomitapide therapy may translate into a clinical cardiovascular benefit. To this aim, the LOWER registry for patients treated with lomitapide was created (Blom et al. 2016); it also includes the CAPTURE substudy which is aimed at investigating the effect of lomitapide on the atheroma regression and/or stabilization in the carotid artery and aorta (Blom et al. 2016).

Lomitapide is a weak inhibitor of CYP3A4, thus it might decrease statin metabolism (Tuteja et al. 2014), and therefore careful monitoring for adverse events when these two drugs are administered in combination is required.

3.4   Mipomersen

Elevated levels of apoB, the main apoprotein of all atherogenic lipoproteins, represent an established risk factor in atherosclerosis; mutations in apoB gene causing familial hypobetalipoproteinemia, characterized by very low levels of apoB and LDL-C, have been associated with a reduced risk of coronary disease (Peloso et al. 2019). Furthermore, a Mendelian randomization study showed that genetic variants resulting in reduced apoB levels are associated with comparable lower CHD risk per unit difference in apoB (Ference et al. 2019a), strengthening the concept that the clinical benefit of lipid-lowering therapies may be proportional to the absolute change in apoB levels. Thus, apoB may be a pharmacological target to reduce hypercholesterolemia.

In parallel with the possibility to inhibit MTP activity, it is also possible to target the key structural protein of VLDL and LDL to inhibit lipoprotein biosynthesis

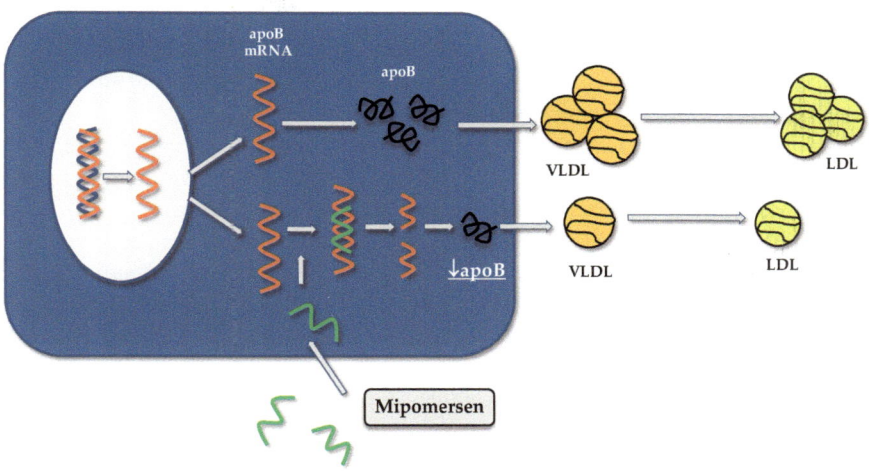

Fig. 3 Mechanism of action of mipomersen. Mipomersen is an antisense oligonucleotide (ASO) that inhibits the synthesis of apolipoprotein B. It binds to the cognate mRNA forming a substrate for a nuclease, thus resulting in mRNA degradation and reduced production of apoB and apoB-containing lipoproteins

(Norata et al. 2013a). Mipomersen is a second-generation antisense oligonucleotide against the coding region of human apolipoprotein B mRNA which, by silencing apoB, results in the reduction of all apoB-containing lipoproteins. The effect of mipomersen is independent of LDLR and thus represents a suitable approach for the treatment of FH with severe LDLR mutations (Crooke and Geary 2013) (Fig. 3). Several trials have shown the lipid-lowering efficacy of mipomersen either as monotherapy or as add-on to current lipid-lowering therapies (Kastelein et al. 2006; Akdim et al. 2010a, b, 2011; Raal et al. 2010; McGowan et al. 2012; Stein et al. 2012a; Visser et al. 2012). A recent meta-analysis on data from 13 randomized clinical trials confirmed that mipomersen significantly reduced LDL-C levels by ~26%, with an overall improvement of all lipid parameters (Fogacci et al. 2019). Nevertheless, mipomersen therapy was associated with several side effects such as injection site reactions, flu-like symptoms, hepatic steatosis, and hepatic enzyme elevations which lead to an elevated number of patients discontinuing the treatment (Fogacci et al. 2019).

The most important side effect expected from the mechanism of action is an increased content of TG in the liver which raised some concerns regarding mipomersen therapy. While short-term studies have in fact reported increased steatosis in mipomersen-treated patients, longer-term trials (up to 104 weeks) showed a return to normal of hepatic triglyceride levels (Sahebkar and Watts 2013; Toth 2013). Further, the analysis of liver biopsies from mipomersen-treated patients revealed a histopathological feature of simple steatosis without signs of inflammation or fibrosis (Hashemi et al. 2014).

In HeFH patients treated with mipomersen, apoB and LDL-C were reduced by ~20% with 200 mg/week dose and by more than 30% with 300 mg/week dose (Akdim et al. 2010b), with the most common adverse effect being injection site erythema (97%). In the same study, four patients treated with mipomersen (three of which in the highest dose group) experienced transaminase elevations >3× ULN with signs of hepatic steatosis (Akdim et al. 2010b). Due to the long half-life of mipomersen, LDL-C levels remain lower than baseline for as long as 2–3 months after the last injection (Akdim et al. 2010b). Similar results have been reported in HeFH patients with CAD (Stein et al. 2012a). Mipomersen is also effective in HoFH patients, with a 24.7% mean LDL-C reduction from baseline observed on top of their maximal tolerated lipid-lowering therapy, associated with an overall improvement of plasma lipid profile (Raal et al. 2010). Also in these patients, the most common adverse event was injection site reactions, followed by ALT elevations ≥3 times ULN which occurred in four mipomersen patients and one patient showing also a significant increase in hepatic fat content (Raal et al. 2010).

A 2-year interim report of a long-term trial showed that mipomersen provides sustained reduction in apoB and LDL-C levels. Of note the median liver fat increased during initial 6–12 months, but returned to baseline with longer treatment, suggesting that a liver metabolic adaptation might occur (Santos et al. 2015). Long-term treatment with mipomersen not only reduces LDL-C and other atherogenic lipoprotein levels but may also reduce the incidence of CV events in patients with FH (Duell et al. 2016).

4 Cholesterol-Lowering Drugs Under Clinical Development

4.1 Inclisiran

Small interfering RNA (siRNA) induces the degradation of a specific mRNA which halts protein synthesis (Norata et al. 2013b). Inclisiran is a specific siRNA which targets PCSK9 mRNA and blocks intracellular PCSK9 synthesis in the liver, as opposed to monoclonal antibodies against PCSK9 which block circulating protein (Fig. 1).

Preclinical studies have shown that a siRNA targeting PCSK9 (ALN-PCS) was effective in reducing plasma PCSK9 and LDL-C levels (Frank-Kamenetsky et al. 2008), and in healthy volunteers, a single intravenous dose of ALN-PCS showed a mean 70% reduction in circulating PCSK9 plasma levels and a 40% reduction in LDL-C levels (Fitzgerald et al. 2014).

Inclisiran (ALN-PCSsc) is a siRNA against PCSK9 conjugated to triantennary N-acetylgalactosamine carbohydrate structure allowing the compound to be recognized by the hepatic asialoglycoprotein receptors, which is selectively expressed in hepatocytes, thus resulting in a specific liver uptake. In healthy volunteers, inclisiran induced a dose-dependent reduction of plasma PCSK9 levels (up to 83.8%) and LDL-C levels (up to 59.7%) (Fitzgerald et al. 2017). The ORION clinical program was started to test the efficacy and safety of inclisiran in people with atherosclerotic CVD and elevated LDL-C levels despite the maximum tolerated dose of LLT, as well as in patients with FH. In the phase 2 trial ORION-1, conducted in patients at high CV risk with elevated LDL-C levels treated with the maximum possible dose of a statin with or without additional LLT, individuals received a single dose or two doses (at days 1 and 90) of inclisiran or placebo (Ray et al. 2017). Inclisiran dose-dependently reduced PCSK9 and LDL-C levels (Ray et al. 2017). At day 240, both PCSK9 and LDL-C were significantly lower than at baseline in all inclisiran regimen groups (Ray et al. 2017). The rate of adverse events was similar in inclisiran and placebo groups, and also injection site reactions were rare and similar to those reported with monoclonal antibodies (Ray et al. 2017; Leiter et al. 2019). The treatment with inclisiran every 6 months resulted in durable LDL-C level reductions over 1 year (Ray et al. 2019b). The *ORION-3 study* is an ongoing open-label extension study of ORION-1 comparing the effect of long-term dosing of inclisiran or evolocumab administration; inclisiran will be administered on day 1 and every 180 days thereafter for up to 4 years (NCT03060577). The interim results showed a favorable safety and tolerability profile for inclisiran, with infrequent, mild, and transient injection site reactions, and no evidence of myalgias or liver or renal adverse events that were related to inclisiran. A robust LDL-C reduction was observed (51% in all patients), and the time-averaged response showed no loss of effect over 3 years (Kastelein 2019).

The phase 3 trials ORION-9, ORION-10, and ORION-11 were designed to assess the efficacy and safety of inclisiran in HeFH, ASCVD, and/or risk equivalent patients with stable LLT. The ORION-9 showed that LDL-C were reduced by 50% at day 210, time-averaged percent change of LDL-C days 90–540 was 45%, and a durable and potent LDL-C-lowering effect was observed over 18 months, independent of the FH genotype; the rate of adverse events was comparable among groups (Raal et al. 2020). Similar effects were reported in the ORION-10 and ORION-11 trials, with prespecified exploratory analysis on CV events showing a lower rate in patients treated with inclisiran compared to placebo (Ray et al. 2020). Inclisiran has been also tested in four HoFH patients in the ORION-2 pilot study, showing a persistent PCSK9-lowering effect independent of the specific mutation and an LDL-C-lowering effect related to the severity of mutation (maximum −43%) (Raal 2019). The ORION-5 trial (NCT03851705) is evaluating the effect of placebo or inclisiran in 45 HoFH patients in a 6-month double-blind period, and then all patients will receive inclisiran during an 18-month open-label follow-up period; the study is expected to end June 2021.

The ongoing ORION-4 aims to assess whether PCSK9 inhibition by inclisiran 300 mg safely lowers the risk of major atherosclerotic cardiovascular events in ≥15,000 patients with pre-existing ASCVD during a median treatment duration of 5 years (NCT03705234). Estimated primary completion date is December 2024.

4.2   Bempedoic Acid

Bempedoic acid is a new drug that inhibits the synthesis of cholesterol by inhibiting the activity of ATP citrate lyase (ACLY), the enzyme catalyzing the transformation of citric acid into oxaloacetate and acetyl-CoA (Fig. 4). The inhibition of ACLY, by blocking cholesterol biosynthesis, results in an increased hepatic expression of the LDL receptor (Pinkosky et al. 2016) and a consequent reduction in the circulating levels of LDL-C. Based on these observations, targeting ACLY activity appears to be a promising approach to lower LDL-C levels. A recent Mendelian randomization study, comparing variants in ACLY gene (mimicking the effect of bempedoic acid) with variants in HMGCR gene (mimicking the effect of statins), seems to suggest that inhibiting ACLY translates into cardiovascular protection (Ference et al. 2019b); in fact, the reduction of the risk of major cardiovascular events for each decrease of 10 mg/dL in LDL-C levels was similar for genetic variants that mimic bempedoic acid or statin activity (Ference et al. 2019b).

Bempedoic acid is a pro-drug, which is converted into its active form by a hepatic enzyme not expressed in skeletal muscle (very-long-chain acyl-CoA sinthetase-1, ACSVL1), which should reduce the potential risk of muscle-related adverse events and may thus represent an important approach in patients intolerant to statins.

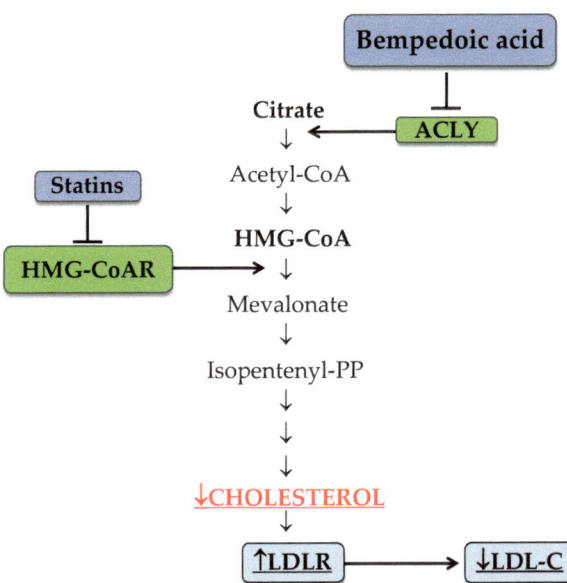

Fig. 4 Mechanism of action of bempedoic acid. Bempedoic acid inhibits cellular cholesterol biosynthesis by blocking the activity of ATP citrate lyase (ACLY), an enzyme upstream of hydroxymethylglutaryl-CoA reductase (the target of statins). Therefore cells upregulate the expression of the LDLR to compensate for reduced cholesterol biosynthesis. A specific enzyme, ACSVL1 (very-long-chain acyl-CoA sinthetase-1), expressed in the liver but not in other peripheral tissues, converts bempedoic acid into the active form thus conferring hepatoselectivity to the drug

Bempedoic acid was also reported to activate the AMP-activated protein kinase (AMPK) subunit beta1 (Pinkosky et al. 2013), however this subunit appears to be less relevant in humans, and therefore whether bempedoic acid positively impact carbohydrate metabolism in humans remains to be demonstrated.

Bempedoic acid dose-dependently lowered LDL-C levels up to 27% in hypercholesterolemic patients, independent on their TG levels (Ballantyne et al. 2013). Non-HDL-C and apoB levels and LDL particle number were also significantly reduced (Ballantyne et al. 2013). Hypercholesterolemic patients with type 2 diabetes showed an even greater LDL-C reduction following the treatment with bempedoic acid (−43%) (Gutierrez et al. 2014). The treatment with bempedoic acid did not result in a worsening of glycemic control, which is another relevant concern associated with statin therapy (Gutierrez et al. 2014). Two studies have specifically evaluated the effect of bempedoic acid in hypercholesterolemic patients intolerant to statins. One study reported a 32% LDL-C level reduction after 8 weeks of treatment (vs a −3.3% with placebo), with an incidence of muscle-related adverse events similar in the two groups (Thompson et al. 2015). In another study, bempedoic acid alone reduced LDL-C levels up to 30%, compared with a 21% reduction observed with ezetimibe; the greatest reduction was observed in patients treated with the combination bempedoic acid+ezetimibe that also improved the levels of other lipids (43–48%) (Thompson et al. 2016). These reductions were similar in statin-tolerant and statin-intolerant patients, and frequencies of muscle-related adverse events were low in all treatment groups (Thompson et al. 2016).

In patients with persistently elevated LDL-C despite a background statin therapy, bempedoic acid induced a significant LDL-C reduction compared with placebo (17%–24% vs 4%), but muscle-related adverse events had similar frequencies in all groups (Ballantyne et al. 2016). Similar results were obtained in patients treated with bempedoic acid added to high-dose atorvastatin background therapy, who showed a 22% LDL-C level reduction compared with placebo and an overall improved lipid profile (Lalwani et al. 2019). In this study, the addition of bempedoic acid to atorvastatin background therapy resulted in an increased exposure (<30%) to atorvastatin, which is suggestive of a weak interaction between the two drugs likely without clinical relevance (Lalwani et al. 2019). The results of these studies suggest that bempedoic acid, alone or in combination with ezetimibe, may represent a valuable approach for the treatment of hypercholesterolemic patients, including those intolerant to statins.

The phase 3 CLEAR program (Cholesterol Lowering via Bempedoic Acid, an ACL-Inhibiting Regimen) includes five studies, four of which have been completed. The CLEAR Harmony and the CLEAR Wisdom studies showed 12.6 and 17.4% LDL-C level reductions in patients with high LDL-C despite receiving maximum tolerated LLT; both studies showed similar incidence of adverse events (Goldberg et al. 2019; Ray et al. 2019a). The CLEAR Serenity study evaluated the effect of bempedoic acid or placebo in patients with a history of intolerance to at least two statins, showing a significant reduction in LDL-C levels (−23.6% vs −1.3% with placebo) and other lipid parameters, with similar incidence of adverse events in the treatment groups (Laufs et al. 2019). Similar results were obtained in the CLEAR

Tranquility trial, which showed that bempedoic acid in combination with ezetimibe further reduced LDL-C levels compared with ezetimibe alone (28.5%) in statin-intolerant patients, with safety profiles comparable between treatment groups (Ballantyne et al. 2018). An ongoing study (CLEAR Cardiovascular Outcomes) is evaluating whether treatment with bempedoic acid treatment reduces the risk of cardiovascular events in patients at high cardiovascular risk with statin intolerance. The results of this study are expected for 2022.

5   The Future of Cholesterol Lowering

5.1   ANGPTL3-L$_{Rx}$

Angiopoietin-like 3 (ANGPTL3) is an endogenous inhibitor of LPL and endothelial lipase (EL), two enzymes playing an important role in lipoprotein metabolism (Tikka and Jauhiainen 2016). Individuals carrying LOF mutations in the *ANGPTL3* gene have lower levels of TG and LDL-C and a significantly reduced CV risk (Dewey et al. 2017; Stitziel et al. 2017; Tarugi et al. 2019). In agreement with this observation, the analysis of plasma levels of ANGPTL3 showed that subjects in the lowest ANGPTL3 level tertile have a significantly reduced risk of myocardial infarction compared to subjects with levels in the highest tertile (Dewey et al. 2017; Stitziel et al. 2017). Based on these observations, ANGPTL3 has been suggested as a possible pharmacological target for the treatment of mixed hyperlipidemias, and for FH patients, due to its cholesterol-lowering effect which is independent of LDLR (Wang et al. 2015). Two different strategies are under investigation to inhibit ANGPTL3: a monoclonal antibody (evinacumab) and an antisense oligonucleotide (ASO, ANGPTL3-L$_{Rx}$) (Fig. 5), both reducing plasma LDL-C and TG levels.

Evinacumab is a fully human monoclonal antibody targeting ANGPTL3 able to reduce LDL-C (up to 23%) and TG (up to 76%) levels in healthy volunteers (Dewey et al. 2017). When tested in HoFH patients, including two null homozygotes and one compound heterozygote with two null alleles, evinacumab added to ongoing LLT further reduced LDL-C levels by 49% (Gaudet et al. 2017). Recently, a phase 3 trial confirmed that evinacumab halves LDL-C levels in HoFH patients independent of the causative mutation, with 47% of patients achieving LDL-C levels <100 mg/dL (http://www.prnewswire.com/news-releases/regeneron-announces-positive-topline-results-from-phase-3-trial-of-evinacumab-in-patients-with-severe-inherited-form-of-high-cholesterol-300901035.html). Ongoing studies are assessing, alongside the lipid-lowering effect, the safety and long-term tolerability (up to 192 weeks) of evinacumab therapy in HoFH patients and the potential development of anti-drug antibodies. Evinacumab is also tested in patients with HeFH or non-FH but with a history of atherosclerotic cardiovascular disease with LDL-C levels persistently elevated despite receiving maximally tolerated LLT.

ANGPTL3-L$_{Rx}$ is an antisense oligonucleotide containing three GalNac residues to promote the specific recognition by hepatic ASGPR1 receptors (Graham et al. 2017). In preclinical studies, the treatment with ANGPTL3-L$_{Rx}$ significantly

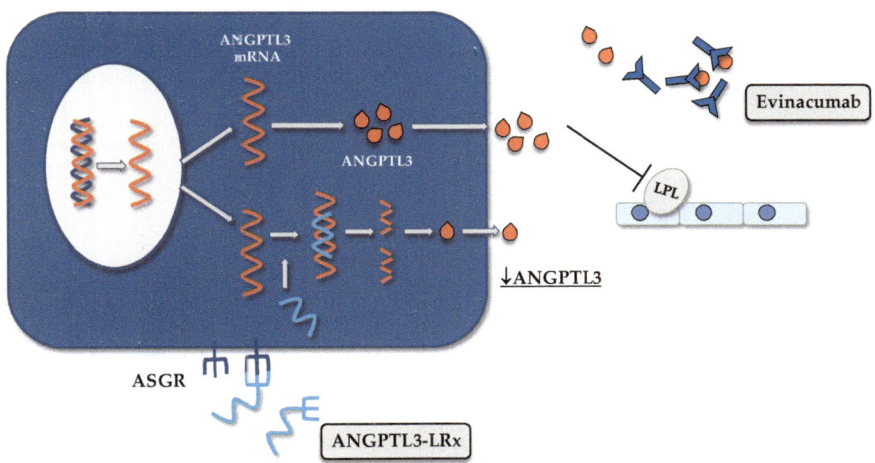

Fig. 5 Mechanism of action of antisense oligonucleotides. ANGPTL3-Lrx and APOA(a)-Lrx are antisense oligonucleotides containing three GalNac residues which promote the specific recognition by hepatic ASGPR receptors. Once internalized, they inhibit protein synthesis of ANGPTL3 or apo (a), respectively, by binding the corresponding mRNAs and inducing their degradation

reduced ANGPTL3 protein levels, which translated into a reduction of plasma TG and LDL-C, hepatic TG content, progression of atherosclerosis, and improvement of insulin sensitivity (Graham et al. 2017). In healthy subjects with elevated TG levels, ANGPTL3-L_{Rx} produced a dose-dependent reduction in circulating levels of ANGPTL3 (47–84%), TG (33–63%), LDL-C (1.3–33%), VLDL-C (28–60%), and apoCIII (19–59%) (Graham et al. 2017). No serious adverse events were reported during treatment, and no evidence of pro-thrombotic effects, bleeding episodes, and reduction of platelet count was reported compared to ASOs of previous generations (Graham et al. 2017).

6   Conclusions

In the last decade, several novel therapeutic approaches have been tested and some approved for reducing plasma lipids and lipoproteins. Some drugs are already available in clinical practice; others are at late stages of development. From a pharmacological perspective, in addition to statins, bempedoic acid was shown to produce an effective inhibition of cholesterol biosynthesis in the liver, while other molecules inhibit cholesterol absorption in the intestine (ezetimibe), inhibit lipoproteins synthesis in the liver and the intestine (lomitapide), or promote lipoprotein catabolism (PCSK9 inhibitors or ANGPTL3 inhibitors). Interest is also emerging on the possibility to target Lp(a).

The new technology of antisense oligonucleotides and small interfering RNAs has clearly opened a fast track for drugs targeting pathways likely to be causal to CVD. The availability of these approaches will definitely improve the management of dyslipidemias, particularly hypercholesterolemias.

References

Ahn CH, Choi SH (2015) New drugs for treating dyslipidemia: beyond statins. Diabetes Metab J 39:87–94. https://doi.org/10.4093/dmj.2015.39.2.87

Akdim F, Stroes ES, Sijbrands EJ et al (2010a) Efficacy and safety of mipomersen, an antisense inhibitor of apolipoprotein B, in hypercholesterolemic subjects receiving stable statin therapy. J Am Coll Cardiol 55:1611–1618. https://doi.org/10.1016/j.jacc.2009.11.069

Akdim F, Visser ME, Tribble DL et al (2010b) Effect of mipomersen, an apolipoprotein B synthesis inhibitor, on low-density lipoprotein cholesterol in patients with familial hypercholesterolemia. Am J Cardiol 105:1413–1419. https://doi.org/10.1016/j.amjcard.2010.01.003

Akdim F, Tribble DL, Flaim JD et al (2011) Efficacy of apolipoprotein B synthesis inhibition in subjects with mild-to-moderate hyperlipidaemia. Eur Heart J 32:2650–2659. https://doi.org/10.1093/eurheartj/ehr148

Baigent C, Keech A, Kearney PM et al (2005) Efficacy and safety of cholesterol-lowering treatment: prospective meta-analysis of data from 90,056 participants in 14 randomised trials of statins. Lancet 366:1267–1278. https://doi.org/10.1016/S0140-6736(05)67394-1

Baigent C, Blackwell L, Emberson J et al (2010) Efficacy and safety of more intensive lowering of LDL cholesterol: a meta-analysis of data from 170,000 participants in 26 randomised trials. Lancet 376:1670–1681. https://doi.org/10.1016/S0140-6736(10)61350-5

Baigent C, Landray MJ, Reith C et al (2011) The effects of lowering LDL cholesterol with simvastatin plus ezetimibe in patients with chronic kidney disease (study of heart and renal protection): a randomised placebo-controlled trial. Lancet 377:2181–2192. https://doi.org/10.1016/S0140-6736(11)60739-3

Ballantyne CM, Davidson MH, Macdougall DE et al (2013) Efficacy and safety of a novel dual modulator of adenosine triphosphate-citrate lyase and adenosine monophosphate-activated protein kinase in patients with hypercholesterolemia: results of a multicenter, randomized, double-blind, placebo-controlled, parallel-group trial. J Am Coll Cardiol 62:1154–1162. https://doi.org/10.1016/j.jacc.2013.05.050

Ballantyne CM, McKenney JM, MacDougall DE, Margulies JR, Robinson PL, Hanselman JC, Lalwani ND (2016) Effect of ETC-1002 on serum low-density lipoprotein cholesterol in hypercholesterolemic patients receiving statin therapy. Am J Cardiol 117:1928–1933. https://doi.org/10.1016/j.amjcard.2016.03.043

Ballantyne CM, Banach M, Mancini GBJ, Lepor NE, Hanselman JC, Zhao X, Leiter LA (2018) Efficacy and safety of bempedoic acid added to ezetimibe in statin-intolerant patients with hypercholesterolemia: a randomized, placebo-controlled study. Atherosclerosis 277:195–203. https://doi.org/10.1016/j.atherosclerosis.2018.06.002

Banach M, Rizzo M, Toth PP et al (2015) Statin intolerance – an attempt at a unified definition. Position paper from an International Lipid Expert Panel. Expert Opin Drug Saf 14:935–955. https://doi.org/10.1517/14740338.2015.1039980

Bays H, Gaudet D, Weiss R et al (2015) Alirocumab as add-on to atorvastatin versus other lipid treatment strategies: ODYSSEY OPTIONS I randomized trial. J Clin Endocrinol Metab 100:3140–3148. https://doi.org/10.1210/jc.2015-1520

Benn M, Nordestgaard BG, Grande P, Schnohr P, Tybjaerg-Hansen A (2010) PCSK9 R46L, low-density lipoprotein cholesterol levels, and risk of ischemic heart disease: 3 independent studies and meta-analyses. J Am Coll Cardiol 55:2833–2842. https://doi.org/10.1016/j.jacc.2010.02.044

Berberich AJ, Hegele RA (2017) Lomitapide for the treatment of hypercholesterolemia. Expert Opin Pharmacother 18:1261–1268. https://doi.org/10.1080/14656566.2017.1340941

Blom DJ, Hala T, Bolognese M et al (2014) A 52-week placebo-controlled trial of evolocumab in hyperlipidemia. N Engl J Med 370:1809–1819. https://doi.org/10.1056/NEJMoa1316222

Blom DJ, Fayad ZA, Kastelein JJ et al (2016) LOWER, a registry of lomitapide-treated patients with homozygous familial hypercholesterolemia: rationale and design. J Clin Lipidol 10:273–282. https://doi.org/10.1016/j.jacl.2015.11.011

Bonaca MP, Nault P, Giugliano RP et al (2018) Low-density lipoprotein cholesterol lowering with evolocumab and outcomes in patients with peripheral artery disease: insights from the FOURIER trial (further cardiovascular outcomes research with PCSK9 inhibition in subjects with elevated risk). Circulation 137:338–350. https://doi.org/10.1161/CIRCULATIONAHA. 117.032235

Brown MS, Goldstein JL (1986) A receptor-mediated pathway for cholesterol homeostasis. Science 232:34–47

Cannon CP, Blazing MA, Giugliano RP et al (2015a) Ezetimibe added to statin therapy after acute coronary syndromes. N Engl J Med 372:2387–2397. https://doi.org/10.1056/NEJMoa1410489

Cannon CP, Cariou B, Blom D et al (2015b) Efficacy and safety of alirocumab in high cardiovascular risk patients with inadequately controlled hypercholesterolaemia on maximally tolerated doses of statins: the ODYSSEY COMBO II randomized controlled trial. Eur Heart J 36:1186–1194. https://doi.org/10.1093/eurheartj/ehv028

Catapano A, Brady WE, King TR, Palmisano J (2005) Lipid altering-efficacy of ezetimibe co-administered with simvastatin compared with rosuvastatin: a meta-analysis of pooled data from 14 clinical trials. Curr Med Res Opin 21:1123–1130. https://doi.org/10.1185/030079905X50642

Catapano AL, Davidson MH, Ballantyne CM, Brady WE, Gazzara RA, Tomassini JE, Tershakovec AM (2006) Lipid-altering efficacy of the ezetimibe/simvastatin single tablet versus rosuvastatin in hypercholesterolemic patients. Curr Med Res Opin 22:2041–2053. https://doi.org/10.1185/030079906X132721

Chan DK, O'Rourke F, Shen Q, Mak JC, Hung WT (2011) Meta-analysis of the cardiovascular benefits of intensive lipid lowering with statins. Acta Neurol Scand 124:188–195. https://doi.org/10.1111/j.1600-0404.2010.01450.x

Chatzizisis YS, Koskinas KC, Misirli G, Vaklavas C, Hatzitolios A, Giannoglou GD (2010) Risk factors and drug interactions predisposing to statin-induced myopathy: implications for risk assessment, prevention and treatment. Drug Saf 33:171–187. https://doi.org/10.2165/11319380-000000000-00000

Cohen I, Pertsemlidis A, Kotowski IK, Graham R, Garcia CK, Hobbs HH (2005) Low LDL cholesterol in individuals of African descent resulting from frequent nonsense mutations in PCSK9. Nat Genet 37:161–165. https://doi.org/10.1038/ng1509

Cohen JC, Boerwinkle E, Mosley TH Jr, Hobbs HH (2006) Sequence variations in PCSK9, low LDL, and protection against coronary heart disease. N Engl J Med 354:1264–1272. https://doi.org/10.1056/NEJMoa054013

Crooke ST, Geary RS (2013) Clinical pharmacological properties of mipomersen (Kynamro), a second generation antisense inhibitor of apolipoprotein B. Br J Clin Pharmacol 76:269–276. https://doi.org/10.1111/j.1365-2125.2012.04469.x

Cuchel M, Bloedon LT, Szapary PO et al (2007) Inhibition of microsomal triglyceride transfer protein in familial hypercholesterolemia. N Engl J Med 356:148–156. https://doi.org/10.1056/NEJMoa061189

Cuchel M, Meagher EA, du Toit TH et al (2013) Efficacy and safety of a microsomal triglyceride transfer protein inhibitor in patients with homozygous familial hypercholesterolaemia: a single-arm, open-label, phase 3 study. Lancet 381:40–46. https://doi.org/10.1016/S0140-6736(12)61731-0

Cuchel M, Bruckert E, Ginsberg HN et al (2014) Homozygous familial hypercholesterolaemia: new insights and guidance for clinicians to improve detection and clinical management. A position paper from the Consensus Panel on Familial Hypercholesterolaemia of the European Athero-sclerosis Society. Eur Heart J 35:2146–2157. https://doi.org/10.1093/eurheartj/ehu274

Da Dalt L, Ruscica M, Bonacina F et al (2019) PCSK9 deficiency reduces insulin secretion and promotes glucose intolerance: the role of the low-density lipoprotein receptor. Eur Heart J 40:357–368. https://doi.org/10.1093/eurheartj/ehy357

Davis HR, Veltri EP (2007) Zetia: inhibition of Niemann-pick C1 like 1 (NPC1L1) to reduce intestinal cholesterol absorption and treat hyperlipidemia. J Atheroscler Thromb 14:99–108. https://doi.org/10.5551/jat.14.99

Descamps OS, De Sutter J, Guillaume M, Missault L (2011) Where does the interplay between cholesterol absorption and synthesis in the context of statin and/or ezetimibe treatment stand today? Atherosclerosis 217:308–321. https://doi.org/10.1016/j.atherosclerosis.2011.06.010

Dewey FE, Gusarova V, Dunbar RL et al (2017) Genetic and pharmacologic inactivation of ANGPTL3 and cardiovascular disease. N Engl J Med 377:211–221. https://doi.org/10.1056/NEJMoa1612790

Duell PB, Santos RD, Kirwan BA, Witztum JL, Tsimikas S, Kastelein JJ (2016) Long-term mipomersen treatment is associated with a reduction in cardiovascular events in patients with familial hypercholesterolemia. J Clin Lipidol 10:1011–1021. https://doi.org/10.1016/j.jacl.2016.04.013

Dufour R, Bergeron J, Gaudet D et al (2017) Open-label therapy with alirocumab in patients with heterozygous familial hypercholesterolemia: results from three years of treatment. Int J Cardiol 228:754–760. https://doi.org/10.1016/j.ijcard.2016.11.046

Farnier M, Jones P, Severance R et al (2016) Efficacy and safety of adding alirocumab to rosuvastatin versus adding ezetimibe or doubling the rosuvastatin dose in high cardiovascular-risk patients: the ODYSSEY OPTIONS II randomized trial. Atherosclerosis 244:138–146. https://doi.org/10.1016/j.atherosclerosis.2015.11.010

Farnier M, Hovingh GK, Langslet G et al (2018) Long-term safety and efficacy of alirocumab in patients with heterozygous familial hypercholesterolemia: an open-label extension of the ODYSSEY program. Atherosclerosis 278:307–314. https://doi.org/10.1016/j.atherosclerosis.2018.08.036

Ference BA, Robinson JG, Brook RD et al (2016) Variation in PCSK9 and HMGCR and risk of cardiovascular disease and diabetes. N Engl J Med 375:2144–2153. https://doi.org/10.1056/NEJMoa1604304

Ference BA, Ginsberg HN, Graham I et al (2017) Low-density lipoproteins cause atherosclerotic cardiovascular disease. 1. Evidence from genetic, epidemiologic, and clinical studies. A con-sensus statement from the European Atherosclerosis Society Consensus Panel. Eur Heart J 38:2459–2472. https://doi.org/10.1093/eurheartj/ehx144

Ference BA, Kastelein JJP, Ray KK et al (2019a) Association of triglyceride-lowering LPL variants and LDL-C-lowering LDLR variants with risk of coronary heart disease. JAMA 321:364–373. https://doi.org/10.1001/jama.2018.20045

Ference BA, Ray KK, Catapano AL et al (2019b) Mendelian randomization study of ACLY and cardiovascular disease. N Engl J Med 380:1033–1042. https://doi.org/10.1056/NEJMoa1806747

Fitzgerald K, Frank-Kamenetsky M, Shulga-Morskaya S et al (2014) Effect of an RNA interference drug on the synthesis of proprotein convertase subtilisin/kexin type 9 (PCSK9) and the concentration of serum LDL cholesterol in healthy volunteers: a randomised, single-blind, placebo-controlled, phase 1 trial. Lancet 383:60–68. https://doi.org/10.1016/S0140-6736(13)61914-5

Fitzgerald K, White S, Borodovsky A et al (2017) A highly durable RNAi therapeutic inhibitor of PCSK9. N Engl J Med 376:41–51. https://doi.org/10.1056/NEJMoa1609243

Fogacci F, Ferri N, Toth PP, Ruscica M, Corsini A, Cicero AFG (2019) Efficacy and safety of mipomersen: a systematic review and meta-analysis of randomized clinical trials. Drugs 79:751–766. https://doi.org/10.1007/s40265-019-01114-z

Foody JM, Toth PP, Tomassini JE et al (2013) Changes in LDL-C levels and goal attainment associated with addition of ezetimibe to simvastatin, atorvastatin, or rosuvastatin compared with titrating statin monotherapy. Vasc Health Risk Manag 9:719–727. https://doi.org/10.2147/VHRM.S49840

Frank-Kamenetsky M, Grefhorst A, Anderson NN et al (2008) Therapeutic RNAi targeting PCSK9 acutely lowers plasma cholesterol in rodents and LDL cholesterol in nonhuman primates. Proc Natl Acad Sci U S A 105:11915–11920. https://doi.org/10.1073/pnas.0805434105

Fruchart JC, Davignon J, Hermans MP et al (2014) Residual macrovascular risk in 2013: what have we learned? Cardiovasc Diabetol 13:26. https://doi.org/10.1186/1475-2840-13-26

Gagne C, Gaudet D, Bruckert E (2002) Efficacy and safety of ezetimibe coadministered with atorvastatin or simvastatin in patients with homozygous familial hypercholesterolemia. Circulation 105:2469–2475

Gaudet D, Gipe DA, Pordy R et al (2017) ANGPTL3 inhibition in homozygous familial hypercholesterolemia. N Engl J Med 377:296–297. https://doi.org/10.1056/NEJMc1705994

Giugliano RP, Desai NR, Kohli P et al (2012) Efficacy, safety, and tolerability of a monoclonal antibody to proprotein convertase subtilisin/kexin type 9 in combination with a statin in patients with hypercholesterolaemia (LAPLACE-TIMI 57): a randomised, placebo-controlled, dose-ranging, phase 2 study. Lancet 380:2007–2017. https://doi.org/10.1016/S0140-6736(12)61770-X

Giugliano RP, Mach F, Zavitz K et al (2017a) Cognitive function in a randomized trial of evolocumab. N Engl J Med 377:633–643. https://doi.org/10.1056/NEJMoa1701131

Giugliano RP, Pedersen TR, Park JG et al (2017b) Clinical efficacy and safety of achieving very low LDL-cholesterol concentrations with the PCSK9 inhibitor evolocumab: a prespecified secondary analysis of the FOURIER trial. Lancet 390:1962–1971. https://doi.org/10.1016/S0140-6736(17)32290-0

Giugliano RP, Cannon CP, Blazing MA et al (2018) Benefit of adding ezetimibe to statin therapy on cardiovascular outcomes and safety in patients with versus without diabetes mellitus: results from IMPROVE-IT (improved reduction of outcomes: vytorin efficacy international trial). Circulation 137:1571–1582. https://doi.org/10.1161/CIRCULATIONAHA.117.030950

Glueck CJ, Kelley W, Gupta A, Fontaine RN, Wang P, Gartside PS (1997) Prospective 10-year evaluation of hypobetalipoproteinemia in a cohort of 772 firefighters and cross-sectional evaluation of hypocholesterolemia in 1,479 men in the National Health and Nutrition Examination Survey I. Metabolism 46:625–633

Goldberg AC, Leiter LA, Stroes ESG et al (2019) Effect of bempedoic acid vs placebo added to maximally tolerated statins on low-density lipoprotein cholesterol in patients at high risk for cardiovascular disease: the CLEAR wisdom randomized clinical trial. JAMA 322:1780–1788. https://doi.org/10.1001/jama.2019.16585

Graham MJ, Lee RG, Brandt TA et al (2017) Cardiovascular and metabolic effects of ANGPTL3 antisense oligonucleotides. N Engl J Med 377:222–232. https://doi.org/10.1056/NEJMoa1701329

Gutierrez MJ, Rosenberg NL, Macdougall DE et al (2014) Efficacy and safety of ETC-1002, a novel investigational low-density lipoprotein-cholesterol-lowering therapy for the treatment of patients with hypercholesterolemia and type 2 diabetes mellitus. Arterioscler Thromb Vasc Biol 34:676–683. https://doi.org/10.1161/ATVBAHA.113.302677

Hashemi N, Odze RD, McGowan MP, Santos RD, Stroes ES, Cohen DE (2014) Liver histology during Mipomersen therapy for severe hypercholesterolemia. J Clin Lipidol 8:606–611. https://doi.org/10.1016/j.jacl.2014.08.002

Hooper AJ, Burnett JR, Watts GF (2015) Contemporary aspects of the biology and therapeutic regulation of the microsomal triglyceride transfer protein. Circ Res 116:193–205. https://doi.org/10.1161/CIRCRESAHA.116.304637

Hopkins PN, Defesche J, Fouchier SW et al (2015) Characterization of autosomal dominant hypercholesterolemia caused by PCSK9 gain of function mutations and its specific treatment

with alirocumab, a PCSK9 monoclonal antibody. Circ Cardiovasc Genet 8:823–831. https://doi.
org/10.1161/CIRCGENETICS.115.001129

Hovingh GK, Davidson MH, Kastelein JJ, O'Connor AM (2013) Diagnosis and treatment of
familial hypercholesterolaemia. Eur Heart J 34:962–971. https://doi.org/10.1093/eurheartj/
eht015

Kastelein JJP (2019) ORION-3. Presented at National Lipid Association (NLA) Scientific Sessions,
Miami, May 2019

Kastelein JJ, Wedel MK, Baker BF et al (2006) Potent reduction of apolipoprotein B and
low-density lipoprotein cholesterol by short-term administration of an antisense inhibitor of
apolipoprotein B. Circulation 114:1729–1735. https://doi.org/10.1161/CIRCULATIONAHA.
105.606442

Kastelein JJ, Akdim F, Stroes ES et al (2008) Simvastatin with or without ezetimibe in familial
hypercholesterolemia. N Engl J Med 358:1431–1443. https://doi.org/10.1056/NEJMoa0800742

Kastelein JJ, Robinson JG, Farnier M et al (2014) Efficacy and safety of alirocumab in patients with
heterozygous familial hypercholesterolemia not adequately controlled with current lipid-
lowering therapy: design and rationale of the ODYSSEY FH studies. Cardiovasc Drugs Ther
28:281–289. https://doi.org/10.1007/s10557-014-6523-z

Kastelein JJ, Ginsberg HN, Langslet G et al (2015) ODYSSEY FH I and FH II: 78 week results with
alirocumab treatment in 735 patients with heterozygous familial hypercholesterolaemia. Eur
Heart J 36:2996–3003. https://doi.org/10.1093/eurheartj/ehv370

Kathiresan S (2008) A PCSK9 missense variant associated with a reduced risk of early-onset
myocardial infarction. N Engl J Med 358:2299–2300. https://doi.org/10.1056/NEJMc0707445

Kent ST, Rosenson RS, Avery CL et al (2017) PCSK9 loss-of-function variants, low-density
lipoprotein cholesterol, and risk of coronary heart disease and stroke: data from 9 studies of
blacks and whites. Circ Cardiovasc Genet 10:e001632. https://doi.org/10.1161/
CIRCGENETICS.116.001632

Kereiakes DJ, Robinson JG, Cannon CP, Lorenzato C, Pordy R, Chaudhari U, Colhoun HM (2015)
Efficacy and safety of the proprotein convertase subtilisin/kexin type 9 inhibitor alirocumab
among high cardiovascular risk patients on maximally tolerated statin therapy: the ODYSSEY
COMBO I study. Am Heart J 169:906–915. https://doi.org/10.1016/j.ahj.2015.03.004

Koren MJ, Scott R, Kim JB et al (2012) Efficacy, safety, and tolerability of a monoclonal antibody
to proprotein convertase subtilisin/kexin type 9 as monotherapy in patients with
hypercholesterolaemia (MENDEL): a randomised, double-blind, placebo-controlled, phase
2 study. Lancet 380:1995–2006. https://doi.org/10.1016/S0140-6736(12)61771-1

Koren MJ, Lundqvist P, Bolognese M et al (2014) Anti-PCSK9 monotherapy for hypercholesterolemia: the MENDEL-2 randomized, controlled phase III clinical trial of evolocumab. J Am Coll
Cardiol 63:2531–2540. https://doi.org/10.1016/j.jacc.2014.03.018

Koren MJ, Sabatine MS, Giugliano RP et al (2019) Long-term efficacy and safety of evolocumab in
patients with hypercholesterolemia. J Am Coll Cardiol 74:2132–2146. https://doi.org/10.1016/j.
jacc.2019.08.1024

Lalwani ND, Hanselman JC, MacDougall DE, Sterling LR, Cramer CT (2019) Complementary
low-density lipoprotein-cholesterol lowering and pharmacokinetics of adding bempedoic acid
(ETC-1002) to high-dose atorvastatin background therapy in hypercholesterolemic patients: a
randomized placebo-controlled trial. J Clin Lipidol 13(4):568–579. https://doi.org/10.1016/j.
jacl.2019.05.003

Laufs U, Banach M, Mancini GBJ et al (2019) Efficacy and safety of bempedoic acid in patients
with hypercholesterolemia and statin intolerance. J Am Heart Assoc 8:e011662. https://doi.org/
10.1161/JAHA.118.011662

Leiter LA, Teoh H, Kallend D et al (2019) Inclisiran lowers LDL-C and PCSK9 irrespective of
diabetes status: the ORION-1 randomized clinical trial. Diabetes Care 42:173–176. https://doi.
org/10.2337/dc18-1491

Leren TP (2014) Sorting an LDL receptor with bound PCSK9 to intracellular degradation. Atherosclerosis 237:76–81. https://doi.org/10.1016/j.atherosclerosis.2014.08.038

Lorenzi M, Ambegaonkar B, Baxter CA, Jansen J, Zoratti MJ, Davies G (2019) Ezetimibe in high-risk, previously treated statin patients: a systematic review and network meta-analysis of lipid efficacy. Clin Res Cardiol 108:487–509. https://doi.org/10.1007/s00392-018-1379-z

Mach F, Baigent C, Catapano AL et al (2020) 2019 ESC/EAS Guidelines for the management of dyslipidaemias: lipid modification to reduce cardiovascular risk. Eur Heart J 41:111–188. https://doi.org/10.1093/eurheartj/ehz455

McGowan MP, Tardif JC, Ceska R et al (2012) Randomized, placebo-controlled trial of mipomersen in patients with severe hypercholesterolemia receiving maximally tolerated lipid-lowering therapy. PLoS One 7:e49006. https://doi.org/10.1371/journal.pone.0049006

McKenney JM, Koren MJ, Kereiakes DJ, Hanotin C, Ferrand AC, Stein EA (2012) Safety and efficacy of a monoclonal antibody to proprotein convertase subtilisin/kexin type 9 serine protease, SAR236553/REGN727, in patients with primary hypercholesterolemia receiving ongoing stable atorvastatin therapy. J Am Coll Cardiol 59:2344–2353. https://doi.org/10.1016/j.jacc.2012.03.007

Mikhailidis DP, Sibbring GC, Ballantyne CM, Davies GM, Catapano AL (2007) Meta-analysis of the cholesterol-lowering effect of ezetimibe added to ongoing statin therapy. Curr Med Res Opin 23:2009–2026. https://doi.org/10.1185/030079907X210507

Mills EJ, O'Regan C, Eyawo O, Wu P, Mills F, Berwanger O, Briel M (2011a) Intensive statin therapy compared with moderate dosing for prevention of cardiovascular events: a meta-analysis of >40 000 patients. Eur Heart J 32:1409–1415. https://doi.org/10.1093/eurheartj/ehr035

Mills EJ, Wu P, Chong G et al (2011b) Efficacy and safety of statin treatment for cardiovascular disease: a network meta-analysis of 170,255 patients from 76 randomized trials. QJM 104:109–124. https://doi.org/10.1093/qjmed/hcq165

Moriarty PM, Thompson PD, Cannon CP et al (2015) Efficacy and safety of alirocumab vs ezetimibe in statin-intolerant patients, with a statin rechallenge arm: the ODYSSEY ALTERNATIVE randomized trial. J Clin Lipidol 9:758–769. https://doi.org/10.1016/j.jacl.2015.08.006

Moriarty PM, Parhofer KG, Babirak SP et al (2016) Alirocumab in patients with heterozygous familial hypercholesterolaemia undergoing lipoprotein apheresis: the ODYSSEY ESCAPE trial. Eur Heart J 37:3588–3595. https://doi.org/10.1093/eurheartj/ehw388

Morrone D, Weintraub WS, Toth PP et al (2012) Lipid-altering efficacy of ezetimibe plus statin and statin monotherapy and identification of factors associated with treatment response: a pooled analysis of over 21,000 subjects from 27 clinical trials. Atherosclerosis 223:251–261. https://doi.org/10.1016/j.atherosclerosis.2012.02.016

Naci H, Brugts JJ, Fleurence R, Tsoi B, Toor H, Ades AE (2013) Comparative benefits of statins in the primary and secondary prevention of major coronary events and all-cause mortality: a network meta-analysis of placebo-controlled and active-comparator trials. Eur J Prev Cardiol 20:641–657. https://doi.org/10.1177/2047487313480435

Naoumova RP, Tosi I, Patel D et al (2005) Severe hypercholesterolemia in four British families with the D374Y mutation in the PCSK9 gene: long-term follow-up and treatment response. Arterioscler Thromb Vasc Biol 25:2654–2660. https://doi.org/10.1161/01.ATV.0000190668.94752.ab

Nicholls SJ, Puri R, Anderson T et al (2016) Effect of evolocumab on progression of coronary disease in statin-treated patients: the GLAGOV randomized clinical trial. JAMA 316:2373–2384. https://doi.org/10.1001/jama.2016.16951

Nissen SE, Stroes E, Dent-Acosta RE et al (2016) Efficacy and tolerability of evolocumab vs ezetimibe in patients with muscle-related statin intolerance: the GAUSS-3 randomized clinical trial. JAMA 315:1580–1590. https://doi.org/10.1001/jama.2016.3608

Norata GD, Ballantyne CM, Catapano AL (2013a) New therapeutic principles in dyslipidaemia: focus on LDL and Lp(a) lowering drugs. Eur Heart J 34:1783–1789. https://doi.org/10.1093/eurheartj/eht088

Norata GD, Tibolla G, Catapano AL (2013b) Gene silencing approaches for the management of dyslipidaemia. Trends Pharmacol Sci 34:198–205. https://doi.org/10.1016/j.tips.2013.01.010

Norata GD, Tavori H, Pirillo A, Fazio S, Catapano AL (2016) Biology of proprotein convertase subtilisin kexin 9: beyond low-density lipoprotein cholesterol lowering. Cardiovasc Res 112:429–442. https://doi.org/10.1093/cvr/cvw194

Nordestgaard BG, Chapman MJ, Humphries SE et al (2013) Familial hypercholesterolaemia is underdiagnosed and undertreated in the general population: guidance for clinicians to prevent coronary heart disease: consensus statement of the European Atherosclerosis Society. Eur Heart J 34:3478–3490a. https://doi.org/10.1093/eurheartj/eht273

Peloso GM, Nomura A, Khera AV et al (2019) Rare protein-truncating variants in APOB, lower low-density lipoprotein cholesterol, and protection against coronary heart disease. Circ Genom Precis Med 12:e002376. https://doi.org/10.1161/CIRCGEN.118.002376

Perego C, Da Dalt L, Pirillo A, Galli A, Catapano AL, Norata GD (2019) Cholesterol metabolism, pancreatic beta-cell function and diabetes. Biochim Biophys Acta Mol Basis Dis 1865:2149–2156. https://doi.org/10.1016/j.bbadis.2019.04.012

Pinkosky SL, Filippov S, Srivastava RA et al (2013) AMP-activated protein kinase and ATP-citrate lyase are two distinct molecular targets for ETC-1002, a novel small molecule regulator of lipid and carbohydrate metabolism. J Lipid Res 54:134–151. https://doi.org/10.1194/jlr.M030528

Pinkosky SL, Newton RS, Day EA et al (2016) Liver-specific ATP-citrate lyase inhibition by bempedoic acid decreases LDL-C and attenuates atherosclerosis. Nat Commun 7:13457. https://doi.org/10.1038/ncomms13457

Pirillo A, Catapano AL (2015) Statin intolerance: diagnosis and remedies. Curr Cardiol Rep 17:27. https://doi.org/10.1007/s11886-015-0582-z

Pisciotta L, Fasano T, Bellocchio A et al (2007) Effect of ezetimibe coadministered with statins in genotype-confirmed heterozygous FH patients. Atherosclerosis 194:e116–e122. https://doi.org/10.1016/j.atherosclerosis.2006.10.036

Qiu C, Zeng P, Li X et al (2017) What is the impact of PCSK9 rs505151 and rs11591147 polymorphisms on serum lipids level and cardiovascular risk: a meta-analysis. Lipids Health Dis 16:111. https://doi.org/10.1186/s12944-017-0506-6

Raal FJ (2019) ORION-2. Presented at EAS, Maastricht, May 2019

Raal FJ, Santos RD, Blom DJ et al (2010) Mipomersen, an apolipoprotein B synthesis inhibitor, for lowering of LDL cholesterol concentrations in patients with homozygous familial hypercholesterolaemia: a randomised, double-blind, placebo-controlled trial. Lancet 375:998–1006. https://doi.org/10.1016/S0140-6736(10)60284-X

Raal F, Scott R, Somaratne R, Bridges I, Li G, Wasserman SM, Stein EA (2012) Low-density lipoprotein cholesterol-lowering effects of AMG 145, a monoclonal antibody to proprotein convertase subtilisin/kexin type 9 serine protease in patients with heterozygous familial hyper-cholesterolemia: the Reduction of LDL-C with PCSK9 Inhibition in Heterozygous Familial Hypercholesterolemia Disorder (RUTHERFORD) randomized trial. Circulation 126:2408–2417. https://doi.org/10.1161/CIRCULATIONAHA.112.144055

Raal FJ, Honarpour N, Blom DJ et al (2015a) Inhibition of PCSK9 with evolocumab in homozygous familial hypercholesterolaemia (TESLA part B): a randomised, double-blind, placebo-controlled trial. Lancet 385:341–350. https://doi.org/10.1016/S0140-6736(14)61374-X

Raal FJ, Stein EA, Dufour R et al (2015b) PCSK9 inhibition with evolocumab (AMG 145) in heterozygous familial hypercholesterolaemia (RUTHERFORD-2): a randomised, double-blind, placebo-controlled trial. Lancet 385:331–340. https://doi.org/10.1016/S0140-6736(14)61399-4

Raal FJ, Hovingh GK, Blom D et al (2017) Long-term treatment with evolocumab added to conventional drug therapy, with or without apheresis, in patients with homozygous familial hypercholesterolaemia: an interim subset analysis of the open-label TAUSSIG study. Lancet Diabetes Endocrinol 5:280–290. https://doi.org/10.1016/S2213-8587(17)30044-X

Raal FJ, Kallend D, Ray KK et al (2020) Inclisiran for the treatment of heterozygous familial hypercholesterolemia. N Engl J Med. https://doi.org/10.1056/NEJMoa1913805

Ray KK, Landmesser U, Leiter LA et al (2017) Inclisiran in patients at high cardiovascular risk with elevated LDL cholesterol. N Engl J Med 376:1430–1440. https://doi.org/10.1056/NEJMoa1615758

Ray KK, Bays HE, Catapano AL et al (2019a) Safety and efficacy of bempedoic acid to reduce LDL cholesterol. N Engl J Med 380:1022–1032. https://doi.org/10.1056/NEJMoa1803917

Ray KK, Stoekenbroek RM, Kallend D et al (2019b) Effect of 1 or 2 doses of inclisiran on low-density lipoprotein cholesterol levels: one-year follow-up of the ORION-1 randomized clinical trial. JAMA Cardiol 4(11):1067–1075. https://doi.org/10.1001/jamacardio.2019.3502

Ray KK, Wright RS, Kallend D et al (2020) Two phase 3 trials of Inclisiran in patients with elevated LDL cholesterol. N Engl J Med. https://doi.org/10.1056/NEJMoa1912387

Ridker PM (2014) LDL cholesterol: controversies and future therapeutic directions. Lancet 384:607–617. https://doi.org/10.1016/S0140-6736(14)61009-6

Robinson JG, Nedergaard BS, Rogers WJ et al (2014) Effect of evolocumab or ezetimibe added to moderate- or high-intensity statin therapy on LDL-C lowering in patients with hypercholesterolemia: the LAPLACE-2 randomized clinical trial. JAMA 311:1870–1882. https://doi.org/10.1001/jama.2014.4030

Robinson JG, Farnier M, Krempf M et al (2015) Efficacy and safety of alirocumab in reducing lipids and cardiovascular events. N Engl J Med 372:1489–1499. https://doi.org/10.1056/NEJMoa1501031

Robinson JG, Rosenson RS, Farnier M et al (2017) Safety of very low low-density lipoprotein cholesterol levels with alirocumab: pooled data from randomized trials. J Am Coll Cardiol 69:471–482. https://doi.org/10.1016/j.jacc.2016.11.037

Roeters van Lennep J, Averna M, Alonso R (2015) Treating homozygous familial hypercholesterolemia in a real-world setting: experiences with lomitapide. J Clin Lipidol 9:607–617. https://doi.org/10.1016/j.jacl.2015.05.001

Roth EM, McKenney JM (2015) ODYSSEY MONO: effect of alirocumab 75 mg subcutaneously every 2 weeks as monotherapy versus ezetimibe over 24 weeks. Futur Cardiol 11:27–37. https://doi.org/10.2217/fca.14.82

Roth EM, McKenney JM, Hanotin C, Asset G, Stein EA (2012) Atorvastatin with or without an antibody to PCSK9 in primary hypercholesterolemia. N Engl J Med 367:1891–1900. https://doi.org/10.1056/NEJMoa1201832

Russell C, Sheth S, Jacoby D (2018) A clinical guide to combination lipid-lowering therapy. Curr Atheroscler Rep 20:19. https://doi.org/10.1007/s11883-018-0721-2

Sabatine MS, Giugliano RP, Wiviott SD et al (2015) Efficacy and safety of evolocumab in reducing lipids and cardiovascular events. N Engl J Med 372:1500–1509. https://doi.org/10.1056/NEJMoa1500858

Sabatine MS, Giugliano RP, Keech AC et al (2017a) Evolocumab and clinical outcomes in patients with cardiovascular disease. N Engl J Med 376:1713–1722. https://doi.org/10.1056/NEJMoa1615664

Sabatine MS, Leiter LA, Wiviott SD et al (2017b) Cardiovascular safety and efficacy of the PCSK9 inhibitor evolocumab in patients with and without diabetes and the effect of evolocumab on glycaemia and risk of new-onset diabetes: a prespecified analysis of the FOURIER randomised controlled trial. Lancet Diabetes Endocrinol 5:941–950. https://doi.org/10.1016/S2213-8587(17)30313-3

Sabatine MS, De Ferrari GM, Giugliano RP et al (2018) Clinical benefit of evolocumab by severity and extent of coronary artery disease. Circulation 138:756–766. https://doi.org/10.1161/CIRCULATIONAHA.118.034309

Sahebkar A, Watts GF (2013) New LDL-cholesterol lowering therapies: pharmacology, clinical trials, and relevance to acute coronary syndromes. Clin Ther 35:1082–1098. https://doi.org/10.1016/j.clinthera.2013.06.019

Sakamoto K, Kawamura M, Kohro T et al (2015) Effect of ezetimibe on LDL-C lowering and atherogenic lipoprotein profiles in type 2 diabetic patients poorly controlled by statins. PLoS One 10:e0138332. https://doi.org/10.1371/journal.pone.0138332

Santos RD, Duell PB, East C, Guyton JR, Moriarty PM, Chin W, Mittleman RS (2015) Long-term efficacy and safety of mipomersen in patients with familial hypercholesterolaemia: 2-year interim results of an open-label extension. Eur Heart J 36:566–575. https://doi.org/10.1093/eurheartj/eht549

Schwartz GG, Steg PG, Szarek M et al (2018) Alirocumab and cardiovascular outcomes after acute coronary syndrome. N Engl J Med 379:2097–2107. https://doi.org/10.1056/NEJMoa1801174

Seidah NG, Prat A, Pirillo A, Catapano AL, Norata GD (2019) Novel strategies to target proprotein convertase subtilisin kexin 9: beyond monoclonal antibodies. Cardiovasc Res 115:510–518. https://doi.org/10.1093/cvr/cvz003

Shiomi M, Ito T (2001) MTP inhibitor decreases plasma cholesterol levels in LDL receptor-deficient WHHL rabbits by lowering the VLDL secretion. Eur J Pharmacol 431:127–131. https://doi.org/10.1016/s0014-2999(01)01419-4

Sirtori CR, Pavanello C, Bertolini S (2014) Microsomal transfer protein (MTP) inhibition-a novel approach to the treatment of homozygous hypercholesterolemia. Ann Med 46:464–474. https://doi.org/10.3109/07853890.2014.931100

Sniderman AD, Tsimikas S, Fazio S (2014) The severe hypercholesterolemia phenotype: clinical diagnosis, management, and emerging therapies. J Am Coll Cardiol 63:1935–1947. https://doi.org/10.1016/j.jacc.2014.01.060

Stein EA, Dufour R, Gagne C et al (2012a) Apolipoprotein B synthesis inhibition with mipomersen in heterozygous familial hypercholesterolemia: results of a randomized, double-blind, placebo-controlled trial to assess efficacy and safety as add-on therapy in patients with coronary artery disease. Circulation 126:2283–2292. https://doi.org/10.1161/CIRCULATIONAHA.112.104125

Stein EA, Gipe D, Bergeron J et al (2012b) Effect of a monoclonal antibody to PCSK9, REGN727/SAR236553, to reduce low-density lipoprotein cholesterol in patients with heterozygous familial hypercholesterolaemia on stable statin dose with or without ezetimibe therapy: a phase 2 randomised controlled trial. Lancet 380:29–36. https://doi.org/10.1016/S0140-6736(12)60771-5

Stein EA, Honarpour N, Wasserman SM, Xu F, Scott R, Raal FJ (2013) Effect of the proprotein convertase subtilisin/kexin 9 monoclonal antibody, AMG 145, in homozygous familial hypercholesterolemia. Circulation 128:2113–2120. https://doi.org/10.1161/CIRCULATIONAHA.113.004678

Stitziel NO, Won HH, Morrison AC et al (2014) Inactivating mutations in NPC1L1 and protection from coronary heart disease. N Engl J Med 371:2072–2082. https://doi.org/10.1056/NEJMoa1405386

Stitziel NO, Khera AV, Wang X et al (2017) ANGPTL3 deficiency and protection against coronary artery disease. J Am Coll Cardiol 69:2054–2063. https://doi.org/10.1016/j.jacc.2017.02.030

Stroes E, Colquhoun D, Sullivan D et al (2014) Anti-PCSK9 antibody effectively lowers cholesterol in patients with statin intolerance: the GAUSS-2 randomized, placebo-controlled phase 3 clinical trial of evolocumab. J Am Coll Cardiol 63:2541–2548. https://doi.org/10.1016/j.jacc.2014.03.019

Sullivan D, Olsson AG, Scott R et al (2012) Effect of a monoclonal antibody to PCSK9 on low-density lipoprotein cholesterol levels in statin-intolerant patients: the GAUSS randomized trial. JAMA 308:2497–2506. https://doi.org/10.1001/jama.2012.25790

Taha DA, De Moor CH, Barrett DA, Gershkovich P (2014) Translational insight into statin-induced muscle toxicity: from cell culture to clinical studies. Transl Res 164:85–109. https://doi.org/10.1016/j.trsl.2014.01.013

Tarugi P, Bertolini S, Calandra S (2019) Angiopoietin-like protein 3 (ANGPTL3) deficiency and familial combined hypolipidemia. J Biomed Res 33:73–81. https://doi.org/10.7555/JBR.32.20170114

Taylor F, Huffman MD, Macedo AF et al (2013) Statins for the primary prevention of cardiovascular disease. Cochrane Database Syst Rev 1:CD004816. https://doi.org/10.1002/14651858.CD004816.pub5

Thompson PD, Rubino J, Janik MJ, MacDougall DE, McBride SJ, Margulies JR, Newton RS (2015) Use of ETC-1002 to treat hypercholesterolemia in patients with statin intolerance. J Clin Lipidol 9:295–304. https://doi.org/10.1016/j.jacl.2015.03.003

Thompson PD, MacDougall DE, Newton RS et al (2016) Treatment with ETC-1002 alone and in combination with ezetimibe lowers LDL cholesterol in hypercholesterolemic patients with or without statin intolerance. J Clin Lipidol 10:556–567. https://doi.org/10.1016/j.jacl.2015.12.025

Tikka A, Jauhiainen M (2016) The role of ANGPTL3 in controlling lipoprotein metabolism. Endocrine 52:187–193. https://doi.org/10.1007/s12020-015-0838-9

Toda Kato E, Giugliano RP, Blazing MA et al (2015) Benefit and safety of adding ezetimibe to statin therapy on cardiovascular outcomes in 4416 women in the IMPROVE-IT trial. Circulation 132:A17862

Tonelli M, Lloyd A, Clement F et al (2011) Efficacy of statins for primary prevention in people at low cardiovascular risk: a meta-analysis. CMAJ 183:E1189–E1202. https://doi.org/10.1503/cmaj.101280

Toth PP (2013) Emerging LDL therapies: mipomersen-antisense oligonucleotide therapy in the management of hypercholesterolemia. J Clin Lipidol 7:S6–S10. https://doi.org/10.1016/j.jacl.2013.02.004

Toth PP, Farnier M, Tomassini JE, Foody JM, Tershakovec AM (2016) Statin combination therapy and cardiovascular risk reduction. Futur Cardiol 12:289–315. https://doi.org/10.2217/fca-2015-0011

Tuteja S, Duffy D, Dunbar RL, Movva R, Gadi R, Bloedon LT, Cuchel M (2014) Pharmacokinetic interactions of the microsomal triglyceride transfer protein inhibitor, lomitapide, with drugs commonly used in the management of hypercholesterolemia. Pharmacotherapy 34:227–239

Visser ME, Wagener G, Baker BF et al (2012) Mipomersen, an apolipoprotein B synthesis inhibitor, lowers low-density lipoprotein cholesterol in high-risk statin-intolerant patients: a randomized, double-blind, placebo-controlled trial. Eur Heart J 33:1142–1149. https://doi.org/10.1093/eurheartj/ehs023

Wang DQ (2007) Regulation of intestinal cholesterol absorption. Annu Rev Physiol 69:221–248. https://doi.org/10.1146/annurev.physiol.69.031905.160725

Wang LJ, Song BL (2012) Niemann-pick C1-like 1 and cholesterol uptake. Biochim Biophys Acta 1821:964–972. https://doi.org/10.1016/j.bbalip.2012.03.004

Wang Y, Gusarova V, Banfi S, Gromada J, Cohen JC, Hobbs HH (2015) Inactivation of ANGPTL3 reduces hepatic VLDL-triglyceride secretion. J Lipid Res 56:1296–1307. https://doi.org/10.1194/jlr.M054882

Wetterau JR, Gregg RE, Harrity TW et al (1998) An MTP inhibitor that normalizes atherogenic lipoprotein levels in WHHL rabbits. Science 282:751–754

Wiviott SD, Giugliano RP, Blazing MA et al (2015) Reduction in non-hemorrhagic stroke with Ezetimibe/simvastatin compared with simvastatin alone in the IMPROVE-IT trial. Circulation 132:A19694

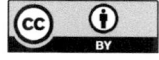

Antithrombotic Therapy: Prevention and Treatment of Atherosclerosis and Atherothrombosis

R. H. Olie, P. E. J. van der Meijden, H. M. H. Spronk, and H. ten Cate

Contents

1   Atherogenesis and the Role of Blood Coagulation Components 104
    1.1   Blood Coagulation: Impact on Vascular Endothelial Cells 105
    1.2   Platelets and Extracellular Vesicles 107
    1.3   Antiplatelet Agents and Atherosclerosis 108
    1.4   Coagulation Proteases 109
2   From Atherosclerosis to Atherothrombosis 111
3   Antithrombotic Therapy Clinical Principles and Applications 112
    3.1   Single Antiplatelet Agents: Mode of Action and Side Effects 112
    3.2   Primary Prevention in the Population; Selecting the Right Subject? 114
    3.3   Primary Prevention in Subjects with Atherosclerosis 114
    3.4   Secondary Prevention of Atherothrombosis in Patients with Arterial Vascular
           Disease 118
4   The Effects of Antithrombotic Therapy on the Vessel Wall and Atherogenesis: Clinical
       Relevance? 120
5   Novel Antiplatelet and Anticoagulant Targets 121
References 122

R. H. Olie
Internal Medicine and CARIM School for Cardiovascular Research, Maastricht University Medical Center, Maastricht, The Netherlands

Thrombosis Expertise Center, Heart+ Cardiovascular Center, and Department of Biochemistry, Maastricht University Medical Center, Maastricht, The Netherlands

P. E. J. van der Meijden · H. M. H. Spronk
Thrombosis Expertise Center, Heart+ Cardiovascular Center, and Department of Biochemistry, Maastricht University Medical Center, Maastricht, The Netherlands

H. ten Cate (✉)
Internal Medicine and CARIM School for Cardiovascular Research, Maastricht University Medical Center, Maastricht, The Netherlands

Thrombosis Expertise Center, Heart+ Cardiovascular Center, and Department of Biochemistry, Maastricht University Medical Center, Maastricht, The Netherlands
e-mail: h.tencate@maastrichtuniversity.nl

© The Author(s) 2020   103
A. von Eckardstein, C. J. Binder (eds.), *Prevention and Treatment of Atherosclerosis*,
Handbook of Experimental Pharmacology 270, https://doi.org/10.1007/164_2020_357

Abstract

Atherosclerosis is a multifactorial vascular disease that develops in the course of a lifetime. Numerous risk factors for atherosclerosis have been identified, mostly inflicting pro-inflammatory effects. Vessel injury, such as occurring during erosion or rupture of atherosclerotic lesions triggers blood coagulation, in attempt to maintain hemostasis (protect against bleeding). However, thrombo-inflammatory mechanisms may drive blood coagulation such that thrombosis develops, the key process underlying myocardial infarction and ischemic stroke (not due to embolization from the heart). In the blood coagulation system, platelets and coagulation proteins are both essential elements. Hyperreactivity of blood coagulation aggravates atherosclerosis in preclinical models. Pharmacologic inhibition of blood coagulation, either with platelet inhibitors, or better documented with anticoagulants, or both, limits the risk of thrombosis and may potentially reverse atherosclerosis burden, although the latter evidence is still based on animal experimentation.

Patients at risk of atherothrombotic complications should receive a single antiplatelet agent (acetylsalicylic acid, ASA, or clopidogrel); those who survived an atherothrombotic event will be prescribed temporary dual antiplatelet therapy (ASA plus a P2Y12 inhibitor) in case of myocardial infarction (6-12 months), or stroke (<6 weeks), followed by a single antiplatelet agent indefinitely. High risk for thrombosis patients (such as those with peripheral artery disease) benefit from a combination of an anticoagulant and ASA. The price of gained efficacy is always increased risk of (major) bleeding; while tailoring therapy to individual needs may limit the risks to some extent, new generations of agents that target less critical elements of hemostasis and coagulation mechanisms are needed to maintain efficacy while reducing bleeding risks.

Keywords

Anticoagulants · Antiplatelet therapy · Aspirin · Atherosclerosis · Atherothrombosis · Clopidogrel · Coagulation · Platelets · Thrombosis

1   Atherogenesis and the Role of Blood Coagulation Components

Atherosclerosis is a multifactorial vascular disease that develops in the course of a lifetime. Numerous risk factors for atherosclerosis have been identified, mostly inflicting pro-inflammatory effects, hence, the term "chronic inflammatory disease" (Ross 1999). The blood coagulation system has a primary role in maintaining hemostasis, preventing fatal bleeding (Spronk et al. 2003a). A second function relates to wound healing in a broader sense. Blood coagulation becomes activated in response to any vascular injury causing contact between the vascular matrix and/or cells with blood. This clotting process likely is meant to seal the wound surface and help to repair the underlying wound bed. Platelets, coagulation, and fibrinolysis factors, as well as fibrin are key elements in this wound healing process, and the administration of some of these components (platelets, fibrinogen) is also studied in clinical trials on wound healing of the skin (Hoffman 2018; Opneja et al. 2019). In the vasculature, pro-atherogenic changes of the vascular endothelium, involving endothelial cell (EC) activation, dysfunction, or damage (exposing subendothelial matrix), trigger the coagulation system in an attempt to vascular wound healing.

1.1   Blood Coagulation: Impact on Vascular Endothelial Cells

The blood coagulation system consists of different pathways that together provide the hemostatic plug or, in pathological situations, the thrombus. Platelets and coagulation proteins act in concert to build the fibrin-platelet clot on top of the damaged vessel wall, while the fibrinolytic system helps to limit clot formation and acts to restore blood flow upon (partial) clot lysis.

In atherogenesis, early inflammatory endothelial perturbation (Gimbrone Jr. and Garcia-Cardena 2016) may trigger activation of platelets that together with leukocyte populations provide a first thrombo-inflammatory response to injury (Fig. 1) (Messner and Bernhard 2014). Activation of platelets (but also other cells) yields extracellular vesicles (EVs) that promote thrombo-inflammatory reactions, amplifying fibrin formation (Badimon et al. 2017). Extracellular vesicles are particles that are naturally released from nearly all kinds of cells; carry a cargo of proteins, RNA, and lipids from the parent cell; and are thus considered to be key components in cell-cell communication. Repeated and/or ongoing inflammatory pressure (endogenous factors like oxidized lipoproteins, glycated end products, homocysteine, etc. and exogenous factors like smoking and other sources of particulate matter) challenges the vascular endothelium to become activated and permeable for inflammatory cells, lipids, and other toxic components (Mozaffarian et al. 2008).

Disruption of the endothelial cell barrier is induced or aggravated by pro-inflammatory cytokines, metalloproteases, and cellular enzymes like elastase and trypsin as well as by the influence of coagulation serine proteases like factor Xa and thrombin, acting on protease-activated receptors (PARs) (Coughlin 2005; Posma et al. 2016; Ruf 2018). Physiologically, PARs are expressed at the endothelial cell surface to mediate endothelial *protective* effects of activated protein C (APC), through activation of PAR1 (Mosnier et al. 2012). Besides activation of protein C, the thrombin-thrombomodulin (TM) complex also converts plasma pro-carboxypeptidase B2 (proCPB2 or thrombin-activatable fibrinolysis inhibitor, TAFI). Activated TAFI (TAFIa) inhibits plasmin formation and hence stabilizes fibrin clots by inhibiting plasmin generation and fibrinolysis (Fujiwara et al. 2012; Mcrser et al. 2010; Myles et al. 2003; Shao et al. 2015). TAFIa also has anti-inflammatory properties including the inactivation of pro-inflammatory mediators like bradykinin, anaphylatoxins C3a and C5a, and thrombin-cleaved OPN (Myles et al. 2003; Naito et al. 2013; Nishimura et al. 2007; Relja et al.

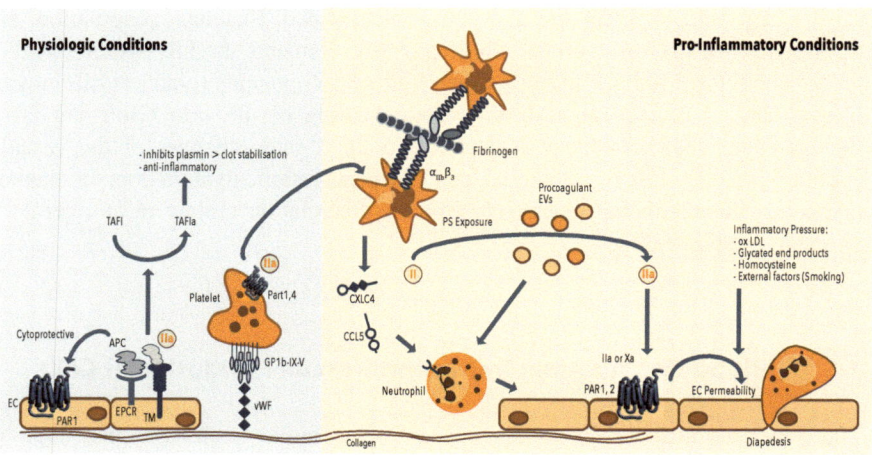

Fig. 1 Interactions of platelets, leucocytes, coagulation factors, and vascular endothelial cells in atherogenesis and atherothrombosis. Under *physiologic conditions*, thrombin (IIa) supports endothelial cell integrity through endothelial cell-mediated APC and TAFIa generation. PARs are expressed at the endothelial cell (EC) surface to mediate cytoprotective effects of APC through activation of PAR1. APC is activated by the thrombin-thrombomodulin (TM) complex, which also converts TAFI into activated TAFI (TAFIa), which has anti-inflammatory properties. Under *pro-inflammatory conditions*, several pro-inflammatory cytokines alter PAR expression patterns and downregulate the protective cellular receptors like TM and EPCR. The result is a shift to prothrombotic and offensive functions of PAR-EC interactions. Thrombin-induced PAR1 activation in combination with endogenous factors like smoking and oxidized lipoproteins challenges the vascular endothelium to become permeable for inflammatory cells. Damage of the endothelial layer results in exposure of highly reactive subendothelial proteins, such as collagen. Under arterial shear stress, vWF bound to collagen enables platelet adhesion via the glycoprotein (GP)Ib-IX-V complex. Activation of platelets yields extracellular vesicles that promote thrombo-inflammatory reactions, including attraction of leukocytes. Activated platelets deposit chemokines, such as CXCL4 and CCL5, on the inflamed endothelium, thereby recruiting leucocytes, which bind to platelets adhering to the (sub)endothelium. Platelets and leukocytes secrete pro-inflammatory and pro-angiogenic factors that further support atherogenesis. Traces of thrombin activate platelets through PAR1 and PAR4. These activated platelets provide a procoagulant phosphatidylserine (PS)-rich surface on which coagulation factors can gather, ultimately leading to the conversion of prothrombin (II) to thrombin (IIa). Thrombin-induced PAR activation induces inflammatory damage to the vascular endothelium. *EC* endothelial cells, *APC* activated protein C, *PAR* protease-activated receptor, *EPCR* endothelial cell protein C receptor, *TM* thrombomodulin, *TAFI* thrombin-activatable fibrinolysis inhibitor, *GP1b-IX-V* glycoprotein Ib-IX-V, *vWF* von Willebrand factor, *CXCL4* chemokine ligand 4, *CCL5* chemokine ligand 5, *PS* phosphatidylserine, *EV* extracellular vesicle

2013). This way, under physiologic conditions thrombin supports endothelial cell integrity through endothelial cell-mediated APC and TAFIa generation.

Under inflammatory pressure, pro-inflammatory cytokines alter PAR expression patterns and downregulate protective cellular receptors like TM and endothelial cell protein C receptor (EPCR) (Esmon 1995, 2014). The result is a shift from anticoagulant (and protective) to prothrombotic (and offensive) functions of serine protease-PAR-EC interactions (Fig. 1). In the case of PAR-1, the shift from protective (APC induced) to inflammatory (thrombin induced) is referred to as "biased" signaling (Griffin et al. 2015).

1.2 Platelets and Extracellular Vesicles

Mouse studies provide mechanistic insight in the pro-atherogenic functions of blood components including platelets, EVs, and coagulation proteins. Platelets and platelet-derived EVs are important messengers of various mediators including microRNAs that modify inflammation and atherogenesis. A range of studies provided evidence for involvement of EVs on various key pathways in atherogenesis, including inflammation, calcification, and cell trafficking (Badimon et al. 2017; Paone et al. 2019; Alique et al. 2018; Bouchareychas and Raffai 2018; Miller et al. 2016). Ongoing research is addressing ways to utilize some of these functions of EVs including transportation of microRNA for potential therapeutic purposes in atherosclerosis (Yin et al. 2015). Majority of EVs are platelet-/megakaryocyte-derived and contain cytokines, RNA species, coagulation factors, etc. EVs can interact with, e.g., leukocytes and regulate activity (Vasina et al. 2013).

Platelets roll and adhere to activated endothelium (Schulz and Massberg 2012). Platelets promote the differentiation and activation of leukocytes (Lievens and von Hundelshausen 2011). Activated platelets deposit chemokines, mainly chemokine ligand 4 (CXCL4) and chemokine ligand 5 (CCL5), on the inflamed endothelium, thereby recruiting leukocytes and exacerbating atherosclerosis (von Hundelshausen et al. 2005; Huo et al. 2003). Also, secreted chemokines attract leukocytes, which bind to platelets adhering to the (sub) endothelium. Platelets and leukocytes secrete pro-inflammatory and pro-angiogenic factors that further support atherogenesis (Semple et al. 2011). Multiple (receptor) interactions between platelets-leukocytes and platelets-vessel wall have been observed in inflammatory conditions such as atherosclerosis (Koupenova et al. 2018; Koenen 2016). Platelet-neutrophil interactions and the release of neutrophil activation products including neutrophil extracellular traps (NETs) may also trigger coagulation.

Cross talk between platelets and coagulation is another important mechanism that operates at different levels. Traces of thrombin activate platelets through PAR1, with PAR4 activation as a delayed, secondary mechanism. Activated platelets provide a phosphatidylserine (PS)-rich surface on which coagulation reactions take place (tenase and prothrombinase complex formation). Upon induction with strong agonists such as a combination of thrombin and collagen, PS exposure allows binding of Gla domain-containing coagulation factors which enhances the activity of coagulation factor complexes. This procoagulant platelet response is supported by the secretion of coagulation factors (prothrombin, Factor V, Factor 8 transcript, Factor XIII, and fibrinogen) and modified by anticoagulation factors (e.g., antithrombin, tissue factor pathway inhibitor (TFPI), protein S).

Platelet-derived factor V may be an important determinant of local prothrombinase formation, driving atherogenesis (Ren et al. 2017). Additional factors that are secreted by platelets are tissue factor (TF) (the origin still somewhat controversial) and protein disulfide-isomerase (PDI) that acts to de-encrypt TF in an active conformation. Polyphospate (PolyP) is secreted that may activate factor XII. Platelet-bound factor XI drives coagulation in an angiotensin-dependent manner (Kossmann et al. 2017). Another mechanism that bridges platelets and coagulation is by binding coagulation factors via the glycoprotein (Gp) complexes GPIb-V-IX, GPIIb/IIIa, and GPVI (Swieringa et al. 2018). Finally, platelets alter fibrin structure (via regulating local thrombin concentration) and mediate clot contraction. This process involves different platelet populations, including procoagulant platelets that primarily stimulate fibrin formation in the periphery of the clot, associated with clot contraction (Nechipurenko et al. 2019). In the course of this process, thrombin-activated platelets become fragmented, a process that limits further dissemination of activated platelets (Kim et al. 2019).

1.3   Antiplatelet Agents and Atherosclerosis

From the described thrombo-inflammatory mechanisms, one may infer that platelet inhibition with antiplatelet medication could potentially attenuate atherogenesis and atherosclerosis. In addition to the inhibition of thromboxane A2 (TXA2) production, aspirin (acetylsalicylic acid (ASA) being the active component) increases platelet nitric oxide (NO) synthesis, protects NO from its inactivation, and improves endothelial dysfunction (Russo et al. 2017). Aspirin also has anti-inflammatory effects, but whether the doses used to prevent platelet aggregation are sufficient to produce meaningful anti-inflammatory effects in humans remains uncertain. In mice, low-dose aspirin improves vascular inflammation and stabilizes plaques (Cyrus et al. 2002) or limits plaque severity, maybe related to reduced fractalkine levels (Liu et al. 2010). In humans, aspirin has been shown to reduce the levels of pro-inflammatory cytokines including interleukin (Il)-6 and monocyte colony-stimulating factor (Ikonomidis et al. 1999) and to protect the endothelium against inflammatory challenge (Kharbanda et al. 2002). In spite of these and other possible protective effects, the net effect on human atherosclerosis remains uncertain (Tousoulis et al. 2016). With regard to thrombosis, literature points to effects of aspirin on fibrin clot formation and stability that may contribute to its antithrombotic action (Gurbel et al. 2019).

Evidence for a role of the P2Y12 receptor in atherogenesis comes from studies in mice with a double apoE and P2Y12 deletion genotype that show reduced lesion area, increased fibrous content at the plaque site, and decreased monocyte/macrophage infiltration of the lesions in the double knockout animals as compared to control apoE$^{-/-}$ mice (Li et al. 2012; West et al. 2014). The P2Y12 inhibitor clopidogrel reduced levels of p-selectin, e-selectin, monocyte chemoattractant protein-1, and platelet-derived growth factor β, reduced macrophage and T-cell infiltration in atherosclerotic lesions, and delayed the development and progression of de novo atherosclerosis (Heim et al. 2016).

In preclinical models clopidogrel attenuated atherosclerosis (Heim et al. 2016; Afek et al. 2009; Takeda et al. 2012), although these protective effects were not evident in other studies (Schulz and Massberg 2012; West et al. 2014). Similarly, ticagrelor reduced the initiation of atherosclerosis in apoE$^{-/-}$ mice (Schirmer et al. 2012) although this effect was not observed by West et al. (West et al. 2014). Discrepancies between the positive and negative studies may be related to drug dose, timing, and duration of treatment (Nylander and Schulz 2016). Furthermore, stabilization and reduced necrotic core were seen in mice with established plaques at 20 weeks of age, for ticagrelor (Buchheiser et al. 2011).

1.4 Coagulation Proteases

Coagulation proteins are for the large part synthesized in the liver and secreted in blood after posttranslational modification. Many of the proteins are zymogens (or proenzymes) that require limited proteolysis to become fully active. It requires one or more triggers like tissue factor (TF) and amplifiers like thrombin, to activate a cascade response yielding fibrin formation at the sites of injury. The liver also makes a series of anticoagulant proteins including antithrombin and protein C that act to dampen the coagulation cascade physiologically. A fairly large number of coagulation proteins are also expressed outside the liver; this can be *constitutive* (like protein S that is for 50% synthesized in vascular EC; tissue factor pathway inhibitor (TFPI) that is partially liver, partially megakaryocyte derived; factor VIII from liver sinusoidal endothelial cells; TF expressed in fibroblasts of the arterial adventitia) or *inducible* under conditions of inflammation: an example is production of TF in blood leukocytes (monocytes/macrophages, neutrophils) and possibly platelets, vascular smooth muscle cells (VSMC), and other cell types (Grover and Mackman 2018). Other proteins like factor VII (Wilcox et al. 2003) and factor X (Sanada et al. 2017) can be expressed by VSMC and fibroblasts. Proteins like factor XI, XII, and prothrombin have been demonstrated in extravascular localizations including atherosclerotic vessels, but whether these are deposited or locally synthesized remains unknown (Borissoff et al. 2010; Wilcox 1994; Soardi et al. 1961). Of interest, coagulation enzymes including thrombin and aPC participate in the control of hematopoiesis in the bone marrow (Nguyen et al. 2018), which may be relevant for the response to stress situations including inflammation.

Within atherosclerotic lesions, coagulation proteins like TF and factors VII and X contribute to form catalytic complexes driving thrombin and fibrin formation (Borissoff et al. 2010). The local formation of fibrin and its split products are modifiers of angiogenesis and cell trafficking within the plaques (Fay 2004; Binder et al. 2017; Badimon and Vilahur 2014; Spronk et al. 2018). The important role of plasminogen activator (receptor)-plasmin and plasminogen activator

1 (PAI-1) system in regulating controlled proteolysis in atherosclerosis, with impact on inflammation (Foley 2017), falls beyond the scope of this chapter.

In general, hypercoagulability and/or thrombophilia has a modest but detectable effect on atherosclerosis, at least coronary artery disease (CAD), peripheral artery disease (PAD), and other manifestations of atherosclerosis (Borissoff et al. 2012; Kleinegris et al. 2013; Lowe and Rumley 2014). This association is not unequivocal, and the lack of protective effect of specific coagulation deficiencies such as in hemophilia, which is not associated with reduced burden of atherosclerosis, argues against very strong influence of coagulation activity in human atherogenesis (Biere-Rafi et al. 2012; Kamphuisen and ten Cate 2014). Nevertheless, evidence from preclinical models is quite striking (Borissoff et al. 2011). Coagulation proteases tend to aggravate atherogenesis toward atherosclerosis in mouse models of atherosclerosis, mostly apoE$^{-/-}$ mice, under pressure of a Western-type diet. In these mice, any hypercoagulable effect introduced by backcrossing apoE$^{-/-}$ mice on a specific mouse with increased procoagulant tendency such as factor V Leiden, or TM$^{Pro/pro}$ mutation, results in worsening atherogenesis. In contrast, mice with a less procoagulant phenotype like FXI$^{-/-}$, FVII$^{+/-}$, or some of the FVIII$^{-/-}$ traits tend to be protected against atherosclerosis progression (Borissoff et al. 2011; Shnerb Ganor et al. 2016; Mackman 2016).

Application of direct oral anticoagulants that inhibit thrombin (dabigatran) or factor Xa (rivaroxaban) slows down atherosclerosis in apoE$^{-/-}$ mice. At least five of such studies document protection against progression of atherosclerosis, including improved plaque stability, while on dabigatran (Lee et al. 2012; Kadoglou et al. 2012; Borissoff et al. 2013; Pingel et al. 2014; Preusch et al. 2015). One protective mechanism may involve the dabigatran-mediated attenuation of pro-inflammatory M1 macrophages in the vessel wall, observed in Lldr$^{-/-}$ mice (Feldmann et al. 2019).

Detrimental effects of dabigatran exposure have also been published; in a diabetic rat model, dabigatran exposure caused increased platelet reactivity, increased coronary lipid deposition, as well as increased PAR4 expression in vessels (Scridon et al. 2019).

Rivaroxaban, the direct factor Xa inhibitor, also attenuates atherosclerosis in apoE$^{-/-}$ mice (Zhou et al. 2011; Hara et al. 2015) or even reverses existing atherosclerosis in apoE$^{-/-}$ mice (Posthuma et al. 2019). Overall, most studies suggest that applying direct oral anticoagulants (DOAC) in atherogenic mice slows down but also stabilizes atherosclerotic lesions and alter the plaque phenotype toward more (Borissoff et al. 2013) or sometimes less stability features (Seehaus et al. 2009), the latter depending on age and sex and probably additional factors like diet. The observed regression on rivaroxaban similarly showed diminished instability markers, but the actual mechanisms explaining diminished plaque volume on anticoagulation remain to be determined (Posthuma et al. 2019).

These proof-of-concept studies support important roles for coagulation proteases FXa and thrombin in driving atherogenesis and altering the phenotype in different directions. Inhibiting factor Xa to actually reverse atherosclerosis in mice raises many new questions regarding the underlying mechanisms of factor Xa-mediated cell signaling and its impact on plaque progression/regression. The protection is thought to involve reducing the impact of FXa and thrombin on PAR1 and 2 activation, respectively. The importance of these PARs in regulating atherosclerosis is emerging; recently, protection against atherosclerosis in PAR2$^{-/-}$ × apoE$^{-/-}$ mice was shown, associated with reduced activity of nuclear factor-κB (NFκB)-regulated inflammation (Hara et al. 2018). However, the importance of coagulation proteases as compared to other possible ligands remains to be demonstrated.

2   From Atherosclerosis to Atherothrombosis

During atherogenesis there are different possible stages of *atherothrombosis* development that could be characterized by combinations of acute or acute on chronic thrombus formation. The occurrence of atherothrombosis is not a single event in time; in series of autopsy studies, it was convincingly demonstrated that coronary thrombi of all stages of development can be found in patients that suddenly died (Kramer et al. 2010). These studies demonstrate that atherothrombosis is part of an ongoing process with temporary, sometimes partial occlusions, subsequent remodeling of thrombus and vessel, gradually changing the vessel wall morphology, and affecting the lumen (Mastenbroek et al. 2015).

Atherogenesis and atherosclerosis may go through several stages of disease. A first and early stage relates to "perturbation" of the vascular endothelium (Nawroth et al. 1984; de Groot et al. 1987), referring to a state of endothelial cell activation associated with a disturbance of the anticoagulant/procoagulant balance, in a pro-inflammatory and thrombotic direction. It could be imagined that this perturbation may in fact be a first trigger in specific types of arterial thrombosis that may form in absence of visible atherosclerosis with sensitive imaging of coronary arteries. A second, more frequent scenario is the formation of a thrombus based on a damaged atherosclerotic plaque. Since long, two fundamentally different scenarios, plaque erosion versus plaque rupture, are recognized (Fuster et al. 1992a, b; Arbab-Zadeh et al. 2012).

While plaque rupture was previously recognized as the dominant pathophysiologic mechanism, recent studies suggest a gradual shift toward less plaque rupture and persistently frequent plaque erosion. One hypothesis for this change in time is declining impact of smoking and increased attention for and management of cardiovascular risk factors (e.g., statins, smoking cessation) that might translate into vascular protective effects and a more stable plaque phenotype (Quillard et al. 2017; Pasterkamp et al. 2017). Currently, about 30% of ST-elevation myocardial infarction (STEMI) is thought to result from eroded plaque lesions (Libby 2013).

Although known for a long time and recognized also as a predilection site for atherothrombosis in the aforementioned autopsy studies, erosion probably triggers fundamentally different mechanisms than rupture of a vulnerable cap (Quillard et al. 2017). Plasma from patients with STEMI showed higher levels of epidermal growth factor and thrombospondin-1 in patients with intact fibrotic cap versus those with ruptured cap lesions, while interferon-inducible T-cell alpha chemoattractant (I-TAC) was lower in coronary blood from intact cap lesion subjects (Chandran et al. 2017). In thrombectomy specimens from these patients, I-TAC mRNA expression levels were markedly increased in patients with eroded lesions. Eroded lesions are characterized by fewer inflammatory cells, abundant extracellular matrix, and the presence of neutrophil extracellular traps (NETs). Eroded plaques contain more myeloperoxidase (MPO)-positive inflammatory cells; MPO is a marker of NETs. Patients with plaque erosion have more MPO in peripheral blood than those with plaque fissure (Ferrante et al. 2010). In addition, components from extracellular matrix including hyaluronan that interact with prohemostatic proteins like fibrinogen, fibrin, and fibronectin are important erosion determinants (Pedicino et al. 2018; Wight 2018). Inflammation and NETs may be complimentary mechanisms to trigger blood coagulation toward thrombus formation. Ruptured lesions typically express inflammatory cells, matrix containing oxidized lipids, and subendothelial proteins from the matrix and on inflammatory cells, including procoagulant tissue factor, factors VII and X, as well as platelets localizing and activating proteins including von Willebrand factor (vWF), collagen, and thrombospondin (Quillard et al. 2017; Pasterkamp et al. 2017). If, indeed, there are fundamental differences in the phenotypes of eroded versus ruptured lesions, it may be anticipated that thrombus formation also follows different pathways. On the other hand, it has been suggested that the main difference between eroded and ruptured plaque is the absence of direct contact between blood components and the necrotic core (Badimon and Vilahur 2014). Better insight into the mechanisms involved in atherothrombosis related to erosion or rupture of plaques is important in order to tailor antithrombotic protection in a more mechanistically founded direction. As will be discussed below, current antithrombotic management does not yet consider such differences.

3 Antithrombotic Therapy: Clinical Principles and Applications

3.1 Single Antiplatelet Agents: Mode of Action and Side Effects

Aspirin is the common name for acetylsalicylic acid, a compound that acts by inhibiting prostaglandin synthesis in different cells; the relevant antithrombotic effect is thought to be mostly based on inhibition of the cyclooxygenase-1 production of thromboxane A2 in platelets (Gresele 2002). It is prescribed at doses between ±75 and 325 mg od, mostly related to regional differences (higher doses more common in the USA than Europe). Its intake results in irreversible inhibition of platelet activation and aggregation. To achieve continued effect, daily intake of aspirin is needed to suppress newly formed platelets, about 10% per day.

Clopidogrel is a prodrug that needs metabolization in the liver (Coukell and Markham 1997). It is ingested as a single dose of 75 mg/day, and the active metabolite shows a large interindividual variation in blood. This variability is partly explained by genetic polymorphisms encoding cytochrome P450 (CYP) 2C19, the hepatic enzyme involved in biotransformation of the prodrug clopidogrel to its active metabolite (Shuldiner et al. 2009). The active metabolite interferes with the binding of ADP to the P2Y12 receptor. This pharmacodynamic variation translates into variation in clopidogrel effectiveness after percutaneous coronary intervention (PCI) (Mega et al. 2010; Sibbing et al. 2009). The interindividual variation in response to clopidogrel, commonly known as clopidogrel "resistance," was first identified in patients with coronary disease, occurring up to 25% of cases in platelet function testing (depending on the test used). Given the association between clopidogrel high on-treatment platelet reactivity (HTPR) and increased incidences of major adverse cardiovascular events (MACE), several studies addressed the question whether dose adjustment based on platelet function testing would correct this problem. Unfortunately, none of the studies demonstrated that test-based adjusted clopidogrel dosing could improve clinical efficacy of such interventions (Price et al. 2011; Collet et al. 2012). In part, the variation in clopidogrel activity is "corrected" for by the development of more potent P2Y12 inhibitors with a more predictable pharmacodynamic profile including prasugrel, ticagrelor, and cangrelor.

The principal side effect of aspirin is bleeding, and the regular use of aspirin increases the risk of particularly gastrointestinal bleeding twofold (Garcia Rodriguez et al. 2016). Risk factors for bleeding should therefore be taken into account, including (recent) GI ulcer (*H. pylori* infection may be additional factor), old age, and use of interacting medication including other antiplatelet therapy (APT), NSAIDs, COX-2 selective inhibitors, oral anticoagulants, and corticosteroids. In individual decision-making, balancing the pros (risk of atherothrombotic complications) and the cons (mostly bleeding) needs to be done, and certain decision support tools like the app "Aspirin Guide" can be helpful in this regard. In general, the risk of GI bleeding with aspirin can be effectively reduced with proton pump inhibitors (PPI), better than with histamine-2 receptor antagonists (Mo et al. 2015; Szabo et al. 2017). Recently, a fixed-dose combination of aspirin and omeprazole (Yosprala) was approved by the FDA, hoping that the simultaneous intake of these agents would improve adherence by reducing gastric side effects (Veltri 2018). Although clopidogrel does not interfere with prostaglandins in gastric mucosal tissue, its use is also associated with an increased risk of bleeding, of which GI bleeds are the most common type. The standard use of PPI in patients on clopidogrel has been disputed; in fact there is evidence that its concomitant use is associated with an increased risk of MACE (Bundhun et al. 2017). Compared to clopidogrel, the newer and more potent P2Y12 inhibitors prasugrel and ticagrelor are associated with an increase in the risk of major bleeding. These agents are generally not prescribed as single APT, although ticagrelor may be used as single agent in selected PAD patients (Hiatt et al. 2017).

3.2   Primary Prevention in the Population; Selecting the Right Subject?

In patients with atherosclerotic vascular disease, antithrombotic medication has been applied since the late 1950s of the past century. Traditionally, platelets were regarded key players in atherothrombosis; hence much focus has been put on antiplatelet agents, initially mostly aspirin. Given the efficacy/safety profile, *primary prevention* with aspirin has been extensively studied. Recent studies and meta-analyses of decades of large trials refute a major role for aspirin in primary prevention. Exceptions may be subjects with diabetes in whom aspirin showed to reduce the incidence of major vascular events including myocardial infarction, at a price of increased major bleeding risk (Group ASC et al. 2018). Otherwise, primary prevention with aspirin in apparently healthy subjects may require additional risk factors like coronary calcification to yield sufficient net clinical benefit. A recent discussion paper on the pros and cons of aspirin for primary prevention in elderly subjects shows the jury is still out (McNeil et al. 2018a, b, c; Fernandes et al. 2019).

3.3   Primary Prevention in Subjects with Atherosclerosis

Primary prevention (of MACE) with aspirin or other APT is warranted in all subjects with *symptomatic* atherosclerotic disease, including angina, or symptomatic PAD. Here, the risk/benefit ratio is clearly in favor of indefinite APT. In patients with any evidence of coronary artery disease, indefinite single APT with aspirin is recommended. This policy is adjusted in case of emerging interventions like PCI; see further.

Remarkably, aspirin was not better than placebo in patients with *asymptomatic* lower extremity artery disease (LEAD), in spite of the fact that their mortality is comparable to patients with symptomatic disease (Fowkes et al. 2010). In symptomatic PAD, there is a certain preference for the P2Y12 inhibitor clopidogrel over aspirin, as the PAD subgroup in the CAPRIE trial that compared aspirin with clopidogrel in subjects at high risk for cardiovascular complications showed better antithrombotic efficacy for clopidogrel at comparable bleeding risk (Table 1) (Committee 1996). However, both aspirin and clopidogrel are still used for this indication. Stronger acting APT like ticagrelor may be used as alternative in patients with PAD in case of failure, allergy, or "resistance" to aspirin or clopidogrel, based on the EUCLID trial showing non-inferiority of ticagrelor versus clopidogrel (Hiatt et al. 2017). Table 1 presents an overview of different therapeutic strategies in symptomatic patients with stable CAD or PAD, referring to the large trials supporting these strategies.

The principle of combining APT was established in the CURE trial, comparing the efficacy and safety of aspirin plus clopidogrel with aspirin alone in the secondary prevention of MACE in patients with coronary disease (Mehta et al. 2001). Since then, dual antiplatelet therapy (DAPT) has become a cornerstone treatment in secondary prevention following PCI (see further). However, the

Table 1 Studies evaluating different antithrombotic strategies in patients with coronary artery disease (CAD) and peripheral artery disease (PAD) (adapted from Olie et al. (2018))

Therapeutic strategy	Stable coronary artery disease (CAD); outcome		Stable peripheral artery disease (PAD); outcome				Bleeding complications in PAD and CAD patients	
	MACE	Ref.	MACE	Ref.	MALE	Ref.	Bleeding	Ref.
Aspirin	↓	[1]	↓/–	[1, 2]	↓	[3, 4]	↑	[1–4]
MONOTHERAPY compared to aspirin								
Clopidogrel	↓	CAPRIE [5]	↓	CAPRIE [5]			↑	CAPRIE [5]
Ticagrelor			↓[a]	EUCLID [6]	–[a]	EUCLID [6]	↑	EUCLID [6]
Rivaroxaban 5 mg B.I.D.	–	COMPASS [7]	–	COMPASS [7]	↓	COMPASS [7]	↑↑	COMPASS [7]
COMBINATION THERAPY compared to aspirin								
Aspirin + clopidogrel	↓	CHARISMA [8, 9]	–	CHARISMA [10]	–	CHARISMA [10]	↑↑	CHARISMA [8–10]
Aspirin + ticagrelor	↓↓	PEGASUS-TIMI 54 [11]	↓↓[b]	PEGASUS-TIMI 54 [12]	↓↓[b]	PEGASUS-TIMI 54 [12]	↑↑	PEGASUS-TIMI 54 [11, 12]
Aspirin / DAPT + vorapaxar	↓↓↓	TRA2°P-TIMI 50 [13]	–	TRA2°P-TIMI 50 [13, 14]	↓	TRA2°P-TIMI 50 [13, 14]	↑↑↑	TRA2°P-TIMI 50 [13, 14]
Aspirin + VKA	↓↓↓	WARIS, ASPECT [15, 16]	–	WAVE [17]	↓	WAVE [17]	↑↑↑	WARIS, ASPECT, WAVE [15–17]
DAPT + rivaroxaban 2.5 mg B.I.D. (*post-ACS*)	↓↓↓↓	ATLAS ACS2-TIMI 51 [18]					↑↑↑	ATLAS ACS2-TIMI 51 [18]
Aspirin + rivaroxaban 2.5 mg B.I.D.	↓↓↓↓	COMPASS [7]	↓↓↓	COMPASS [7]	↓↓↓	COMPASS [7]	↑↑	COMPASS [7]

Study population, control groups, and definition of primary efficacy and safety outcomes are highly variable between different studies. This table is based on the authors' interpretation of clinical trials and meta-analyses and is clearly not based on head-to-head comparisons of the different therapeutic strategies

($\downarrow$) to ($\downarrow\downarrow\downarrow$) indicates modest to strong decrease in MACE/MALE

($\uparrow$) to ($\uparrow\uparrow\uparrow$) indicates modest to strong increase in bleeding complications

(−) indicates no beneficial effect compared to aspirin monotherapy

($\downarrow$/−) indicates contradictory results

Gray boxes indicate that these results are not available and/or not applicable

MACE major adverse cardiovascular events, *MALE* major adverse limb events, *DAPT* dual antiplatelet therapy, *VKA* vitamin K antagonist, *B.I.D.* bis in die, twice a day, *ACS* acute coronary syndrome, ref. reference

Table adapted from Olie et al. (2018)

1. Antithrombotic Trialists C. Collaborative meta-analysis of randomised trials of antiplatelet therapy for prevention of death, myocardial infarction, and stroke in high risk patients. BMJ. 2002;324(7329):71–86

2. Berger JS, Krantz MJ, Kittelson JM, Hiatt WR. Aspirin for the prevention of cardiovascular events in patients with peripheral artery disease: a meta-analysis of randomized trials. JAMA. 2009;301(18):1909–19

3. Critical Leg Ischaemia Prevention Study G, Catalano M, Born G, Peto R. Prevention of serious vascular events by aspirin amongst patients with peripheral arterial disease: randomized, double-blind trial. J Intern Med. 2007;261(3):276–84

4. Collaborative overview of randomised trials of antiplatelet therapy–II: Maintenance of vascular graft or arterial patency by antiplatelet therapy. Antiplatelet Trialists' Collaboration. BMJ. 1994;308(6922):159–68

5. Committee CS. A randomised, blinded, trial of clopidogrel versus aspirin in patients at risk of ischaemic events (CAPRIE). CAPRIE Steering Committee. Lancet. 1996;348(9038):1329–39

6. Hiatt WR, Fowkes FG, Heizer G, Berger JS, Baumgartner I, Held P, et al. Ticagrelor versus Clopidogrel in Symptomatic Peripheral Artery Disease. N Engl J Med. 2017;376(1):32–40

7. Eikelboom JW, Connolly SJ, Bosch J, Dagenais GR, Hart RG, Shestakovska O, et al. Rivaroxaban with or without Aspirin in Stable Cardiovascular Disease. N Engl J Med. 2017

8. Bhatt DL, Fox KA, Hacke W, Berger PB, Black HR, Boden WE, et al. Clopidogrel and aspirin versus aspirin alone for the prevention of atherothrombotic events. N Engl J Med. 2006;354(16):1706–17

9. Helton TJ, Bavry AA, Kumbhani DJ, Duggal S, Roukoz H, Bhatt DL. Incremental effect of clopidogrel on important outcomes in patients with cardiovascular disease: a meta-analysis of randomized trials. Am J Cardiovasc Drugs. 2007;7(4):289–97

10. Cacoub PP, Bhatt DL, Steg PG, Topol EJ, Creager MA, Investigators C. Patients with peripheral arterial disease in the CHARISMA trial. Eur Heart J. 2009;30(2):192–201

11. Bonaca MP, Bhatt DL, Cohen M, Steg PG, Storey RF, Jensen EC, et al. Long-term use of ticagrelor in patients with prior myocardial infarction. N Engl J Med. 2015;372(19):1791–800

(continued)

Table 1 (continued)

12. Bonaca MP, Bhatt DL, Storey RF, Steg PG, Cohen M, Kuder J, et al. Ticagrelor for Prevention of Ischemic Events After Myocardial Infarction in Patients With Peripheral Artery Disease. J Am Coll Cardiol. 2016;67(23):2719–28

13. Morrow DA, Braunwald E, Bonaca MP, Ameriso SF, Dalby AJ, Fish MP, et al. Vorapaxar in the secondary prevention of atherothrombotic events. N Engl J Med. 2012;366(15):1404–13

14. Bonaca MP, Scirica BM, Creager MA, Olin J, Bounameaux H, Dellborg M, et al. Vorapaxar in patients with peripheral artery disease: results from TRA2 {degrees}P-TIMI 50. Circulation. 2013;127(14):1522-9, 9e1–6

15. Effect of long-term oral anticoagulant treatment on mortality and cardiovascular morbidity after myocardial infarction. Anticoagulants in the Secondary Prevention of Events in Coronary Thrombosis (ASPECT) Research Group. Lancet 1994;343(8896):499 503

16. Smith P, Arnesen H, Holme I. The effect of warfarin on mortality and reinfarction after myocardial infarction. N Engl J Med. 1990;323(3):147–52

17. Warfarin Antiplatelet Vascular Evaluation Trial I, Anand S, Yusuf S, Xie C, Pogue J, Eikelboom J, et al. Oral anticoagulant and antiplatelet therapy and peripheral arterial disease. N Engl J Med. 2007;357(3):217–27

18. Mega JL, Braunwald E, Wiviott SD, Murphy SA, Plotnikov A, Gotcheva N, et al. Comparison of the efficacy and safety of two rivaroxaban doses in acute coronary syndrome (from ATLAS ACS 2-TIMI 51). Am J Cardiol. 2013;112(4):472–8

19. Olie RH, van der Meijden PEJ, Ten Cate H. The coagulation system in atherothrombosis: Implications for new therapeutic strategies. Res Pract Thromb Haemost. 2018;2(2):188–98

[a]No direct comparison with aspirin monotherapy but compared to clopidogrel monotherapy

[b]In patients with concomitant PAD and CAD

concept also triggered studies as to the potential benefits DAPT would offer in patients with high-risk cardiovascular disease. Large trials like CHARISMA (Bhatt et al. 2006) tested this concept, the outcome of which was however negative in failing to show improved efficacy while increasing the bleeding risk. Consequently, DAPT is not recommended in any patient for *primary* prevention of MACE, unless there are subject-specific reasons for this more potent combination.

In PAD, in general, *combined* antiplatelet therapy does not add benefit to the patient and increases bleeding risk; for this reason, it is only applied for short-term use, e.g., after endovascular interventions (Hess et al. 2017). The use of oral anticoagulants (mostly vitamin K antagonists) in therapeutic intensity is not indicated in patients with PAD, except for those that underwent venous bypass grafting (Dutch Bypass Oral Anticoagulants or Aspirin (BOA) Study Group 2000). The most recent regimen studied in patients with high-risk vascular disease, including PAD, is the combination of an anticoagulant rivaroxaban 2.5 mg bd plus low-dose aspirin, which reduced cardiovascular mortality as well as major acute limb events in patients with PAD (patients with LEAD or carotid artery disease) (Anand et al. 2018). From a mechanistic perspective, targeting platelets and the plasmatic coagulation system seems rational, given the postulated pathophysiologic mechanisms discussed above. Moreover, targeting FXa, herewith also inhibiting the formation of thrombin, reduces the potential interactions between these proteases and cellular PARs. Thus, vascular protective effects may be an additional consequence of a strategy that includes an anticoagulant (although the clinical evidence is still weak).

3.4   Secondary Prevention of Atherothrombosis in Patients with Arterial Vascular Disease

Secondary prevention with APT, following myocardial infarction or ischemic stroke (not due to cardiac embolism, thus including a spectrum of non-embolic strokes), is straightforward and based on class 1A evidence.

Combined APT (dual (DAPT) antiplatelet therapy) is indicated in all settings of acute coronary syndrome, with or without PCI with stent placement (DAPT for 6–12 months, longer in selected cases) (Roffi et al. 2016; Authors/Task Force et al. 2014; Amsterdam et al. 2014). In acute ischemic stroke, DAPT is only indicated for a very limited duration, up to 6 weeks, due to the observed increased bleeding risk (Wang et al. 2013; Johnston et al. 2018). Following these time windows, single APT will be continued indefinitely, comprising of aspirin in most patients with CAD and aspirin or, more commonly, clopidogrel in patients after atherothrombotic stroke (Hackam and Spence 2019).

In most combined APT regimens, aspirin remains an element; in patients with CAD, DAPT comprises aspirin plus a P2Y12 inhibitor, prasugrel or ticagrelor (unless contraindicated clopidogrel, a weaker P2Y12 inhibitor, is used in combination with aspirin). Although the thienopyridine prasugrel is a prodrug like clopidogrel, it only requires a single oxidation step to form its active metabolite, and it seems to be not affected by genetic variations in CYP enzymes. Compared to clopidogrel its use is associated with an increase in the risk of major bleeding, especially among those with age ≥75 years or body weight <60 kg, and is contraindicated in patients with prior stroke (Wiviott et al. 2007). Ticagrelor, an oral, direct acting, reversible P2Y12 receptor antagonist, provides faster and greater platelet inhibition with less patient-to-patient variation (Wallentin et al. 2009).

Despite intensification of APT in recent years, an approximately 10% risk for recurrent ischemic events at 1 year after coronary events still remains (Wiviott et al. 2007; Wallentin et al. 2009). With blockade of the TXA2 pathway and the P2Y12 receptor, platelets can still be activated by thrombin, via the PAR1 and PAR4 receptor on their surface (Olie et al. 2019). Vorapaxar is an orally administered, competitive PAR1 antagonist that blocks thrombin-mediated platelet activation via PAR1, without inhibiting other modes of thrombin activity, such as fibrin formation, protein C activation, and PAR4 activation. On top of standard antiplatelet therapy (consisting of aspirin in almost all cases and a thienopyridine or dipyridamole in a significant proportion), addition of vorapaxar led to significant reduction in rates of ischemic cardiovascular events in patients with stable CAD or PAD, but at the price of increased major bleeding, limiting its use in clinical practice (Morrow et al. 2012). Non-platelet-mediated effects of PAR inhibition on the vascular endothelium have been speculated on, since PAR1 is also present on endothelial cells and VSMCs, where it mediates mitogenic effects (Posma et al. 2016). Thus, PAR1 inhibition might be effective in reducing vascular remodeling and consecutive progression of atherosclerosis.

In patients with atherosclerotic disease, oral anticoagulants were not routinely applied until recently. One reason for not using anticoagulants was the assumption that atherothrombosis primarily is a platelet-dependent phenomenon, given the efficacy data of all APT trials. A second reason to refrain from anticoagulants was the concern of cholesterol embolization that could follow anticoagulant-associated instability and plaque rupture; however, the evidence for a causal effect of anticoagulants is poor.

Early trials with vitamin K antagonists (van Bergen et al. 1994; Smith et al. 1990) in CAD patients had provided proof of principle that inhibition of coagulation may be of additional benefit in atherothrombotic disease, although in daily practice, their use was practically abandoned due to markedly increased bleeding and more effective protection by DAPT. Nonetheless, after the introduction of direct oral anticoagulants (DOACs), the role of these anticoagulants in secondary prevention of ischemic events was re-evaluated in several trials (Olie et al. 2018). Addition of low-dose rivaroxaban (2.5 mg twice daily) on top of APT reduced major adverse cardiac events both in patients with acute coronary syndrome (in the ATLAS-ACS-2 TIMI 51 trial (Mega et al. 2012)) and in patients with stable CAD or PAD (in the COMPASS trial (Eikelboom et al. 2017)). In COMPASS also cardiovascular mortality was reduced in patients receiving the combination of vascular doses of rivaroxaban (2.5 mg bd) and aspirin as compared to either agent alone, which means a breakthrough in the efficacy of antithrombotic management (Coppens et al. 2019).

4 The Effects of Antithrombotic Therapy on the Vessel Wall and Atherogenesis: Clinical Relevance?

Platelets are pivotal in atherogenesis, but the impact of antiplatelet agents beyond inhibition of platelet activation and aggregation (including the procoagulant role platelets play in catalyzing phospholipid-dependent coagulation reactions) remains controversial. As discussed, low-dose aspirin may have local anti-inflammatory effects in the vessel wall, but evidence for diminished atherosclerosis related to aspirin intake is not present.

Human studies revealed several anti-inflammatory effects and reduction in platelet CD40 ligand and CD62, respectively, associated with clopidogrel (less evident in those with clopidogrel "resistance") and prasugrel, both thienopyridines (summarized in (Nylander and Schulz 2016)). Ticagrelor had anti-inflammatory effects including reduced formation of platelet-neutrophil aggregates in inflammation models and more profound reduction in Il-6 in a human sepsis model as compared to clopidogrel, suggesting that stronger inhibition of the P2Y12 receptor (ticagrelor) may provide greater anti-inflammatory effect (Nylander and Schulz 2016). Off-target effects of ticagrelor on endothelial function and vascular biomarkers have been speculated on, but a recent study comparing ticagrelor to prasugrel and clopidogrel found no evidence for any non-platelet-mediated effects in post-acute coronary syndrome patients (Ariotti et al. 2018).

The previous generation of oral anticoagulants, the vitamin K antagonists (VKA), has defined effects on the vasculature due to inhibition of carboxylation of specific vitamin K-dependent proteins like matrix Gla protein, a protein involved in the inhibition of both medial and intimal calcification. Ample mouse studies support these effects, where VKA rapidly induces calcification that can be partially prevented by additional vitamin K administration (Spronk et al. 2003b). Whether the VKA achieved inhibition of FXa and thrombin generation also in part affects atherosclerosis remains difficult to dissect, because of the overwhelming effect of calcification. Whether VKA affects plaque *stability* in humans is still uncertain. Observational studies suggest more plaque instability in patients on VKA due to intraplaque hemorrhage particularly upon prolonged exposure and higher intensity of anticoagulation (Mujaj et al. 2018; Li et al. 2014). However, in the Rotterdam study, the effects were comparable for anticoagulants (VKA) and aspirin, so the specificity and causal contribution of anticoagulation versus antiplatelet effects remain unproven. More direct evidence for effects of inhibiting coagulation protease needs to come from studies with DOACs. Two studies that either randomized patients to rivaroxaban or warfarin (Lee et al. 2018) or performed propensity score matching yielding three populations that used DOAC, warfarin, or no anticoagulants (Plank et al. 2018) were recently published. Both studies show diminished calcification and less instability features in patients on DOAC versus VKA. These somewhat preliminary data seem to point to a possibly favorable impact of DOAC (hence, FXa/thrombin inhibition) on atherosclerosis and the vessel wall.

5   Novel Antiplatelet and Anticoagulant Targets

In spite of the available array of antithrombotic agents, there is still a need for further improvement. One of the critical downsides of all antithrombotic agents is a risk of bleeding, linked to the potency of the drug. Thus, more effective antiplatelet agents like prasugrel or ticagrelor will generally inflict more bleeding risk than the less potent P2Y12 inhibitor clopidogrel. Combinations of APT like in DAPT or even triple therapy will also show increased bleeding risk as compared to single agents.

Although the current class of DOAC has a better safety profile with regard to intracranial bleeding as compared to VKA, there is still a substantial risk of other clinically relevant bleeding complications, including gastrointestinal bleeds. Combined anticoagulant and APT therapy also has increased bleeding potential, and even the relatively low doses of rivaroxaban in the COMPASS regimen, combined with aspirin, increase the risk of major bleeding (Eikelboom et al. 2017).

With existing antiplatelet drugs, a therapeutic ceiling seems to be reached, whereby increased potency is offset by elevated bleeding risk. Ongoing research on developing new antiplatelet drugs therefore focuses on identifying targets that inhibit thrombosis while maintaining hemostasis. Developing thrombi at sites of endothelial injury are now known to be composed of two distinct regions: the hemostatic plug (composed of highly activated platelets and rich in fibrin) and the propagating platelet thrombus (composed of platelets in a low activation state) (Stalker et al. 2013). The latter region of the propagating thrombus is regulated by phosphatidylinositol 3-kinase-β (PI3Kβ), glycoprotein (GP)IIb/IIIa outside-in signaling, and activation of protein disulfide-isomerase (PDI). Inhibition of these factors that regulate thrombus propagation seems to protect against thrombotic occlusion while preserving hemostasis. Therefore, novel agents include PI3Kβ inhibitors, PDI inhibitors, conformation-specific targeting of activated GPIIb/IIIa, and selective inhibition of GPIIb/IIIa outside-in signaling (McFadyen et al. 2018).

Other candidate drugs include inhibitors of the GPIb-vWF axis, novel PAR1 and PAR4 inhibitors, and blockade of platelet GPVI-mediated adhesion pathways. The GPIb-IX-V receptor binds to vWF during injury and under conditions of high shear stress, allowing early platelet adhesion to the subendothelium. Therefore, various inhibitors of this axis have been developed. Although two antibodies against vWF (ARC1779 and caplacizumab) have demonstrated to have antithrombotic effects, their development has been halted owing to an increased incidence of bleeding (Markus et al. 2011; Muller et al. 2013). However, additional agents, directly targeting GPIb or the vWF binding domain, are under development. As discussed, the use of the currently available PAR-1 antagonist vorapaxar is limited by substantially increased rates of bleeding. Besides orthosteric antagonists like vorapaxar, another class of PAR1 inhibitors, called paramodulins, has been developed. These target the cytoplasmic face of PAR1, contrary to blocking the ligand-binding site like vorapaxar, which inhibits all signaling downstream of the PAR1 receptor. This may allow paramodulins to selectively block platelet and endothelial cell activation mediated by PAR1 while maintaining the cytoprotective signaling pathways in endothelial cells (Aisiku et al. 2015). As thrombin activates platelets via both PAR1 and PAR4, also the PAR4 receptor is currently under investigation as a target for platelet antagonism (McFadyen et al. 2018). Another promising target is the interaction between GPVI and collagen. The observation that GPVI is platelet-specific, in combination with the fact that patients with GPVI deficiency usually suffer from only a mild bleeding phenotype, has led to strategies targeting GPVI. Phase II trials, studying the anti-GPVI agent Revacept in patients with stable CAD and symptomatic carotid stenosis, are currently underway (Majithia and Bhatt 2019).

In recent years, the contribution of the proteins of the contact system (factors VIII, IX, XI, and XII, prekallikrein, and high-molecular-weight kininogen) to the process of atherothrombosis has gained more attention. Factor XII-deficient humans have a normal hemostatic capacity, while animal models have revealed an important role of factor XIIa-driven coagulation in arterial thrombosis (Kuijpers et al. 2014). Furthermore, factor XIIa contributes to inflammation through the activation of the inflammatory bradykinin-producing kallikrein-kinin system (Nickel et al. 2017; Long et al. 2016). Thus, pharmacological inhibition of factor XII(a) may not only be a safer therapeutic strategy (by inhibition of thrombosis while preserving hemostasis) but also has additional beneficial anti-inflammatory and anti-atherogenic effects. Currently, factor XII(a) and its activator polyphosphate are being studied as potential targets for prevention of thrombosis. However, factor XIIa also stimulated the fibrinolytic pathway (Long et al. 2016), and inhibition may thus have potential prothrombotic side effects. Moreover, when thrombosis is initiated by TF exposure, small amounts of thrombin generated by extrinsic tenase have the potential to activate FXI, thereby bypassing FXII inhibition. Therefore, FXI inhibition may be a better target than FXII inhibition. Furthermore, besides attenuation of coagulation, factor XI deprivation has also been shown to slow down atherogenesis in apoE/factor XI double knockout mice (Shnerb Ganor et al. 2016). Several potential strategies to target FXI are currently under investigation, including antisense oligonucleotides (ASOs) that reduce hepatic synthesis of FXI, monoclonal antibodies that suppress FXIa generation and inhibit FXIa activity, and aptamers that block the binding site and small molecules that bind reversibly to the active site of FXIa and inhibits its activity (Weitz and Chan 2019). Clinical phase 2 studies with FXI-directed ASOs, monoclonal antibodies against FXIa, and an oral FXIa inhibitor have been performed (Buller et al. 2015) or are currently underway (Weitz and Chan 2019).

References

Afek A, Kogan E, Maysel-Auslender S, Mor A, Regev E, Rubinstein A et al (2009) Clopidogrel attenuates atheroma formation and induces a stable plaque phenotype in apolipoprotein E knockout mice. Microvasc Res 77(3):364–369

Aisiku O, Peters CG, de Ceunynck K, Ghosh CC, Dilks JR, Fustolo-Gunnink SF et al (2015) Parmodulins inhibit thrombus formation without inducing endothelial injury caused by vorapaxar. Blood 125(12):1976–1985

Alique M, Ramirez-Carracedo R, Bodega G, Carracedo J, Ramirez R (2018) Senescent microvesicles: a novel advance in molecular mechanisms of atherosclerotic calcification. Int J Mol Sci 19(7):2003

Amsterdam EA, Wenger NK, Brindis RG, Casey DE Jr, Ganiats TG, Holmes DR Jr et al (2014) 2014 AHA/ACC guideline for the management of patients with non-ST-elevation acute coronary syndromes: a report of the American College of Cardiology/American Heart Association task force on practice guidelines. J Am Coll Cardiol 64(24):e139–e228

Anand SS, Bosch J, Eikelboom JW, Connolly SJ, Diaz R, Widimsky P et al (2018) Rivaroxaban with or without aspirin in patients with stable peripheral or carotid artery disease: an international, randomised, double-blind, placebo-controlled trial. Lancet 391:219–229

Arbab-Zadeh A, Nakano M, Virmani R, Fuster V (2012) Acute coronary events. Circulation 125(9):1147–1156

Ariotti S, Ortega-Paz L, van Leeuwen M, Brugaletta S, Leonardi S, Akkerhuis KM et al (2018) Effects of ticagrelor, prasugrel, or clopidogrel on endothelial function and other vascular biomarkers: a randomized crossover study. JACC Cardiovasc Interv 11(16):1576–1586

Authors/Task Force M, Windecker S, Kolh P, Alfonso F, Collet JP, Cremer J et al (2014) 2014 ESC/EACTS guidelines on myocardial revascularization: the Task Force on Myocardial Revascularization of the European Society of Cardiology (ESC) and the European Association for Cardio-Thoracic Surgery (EACTS) developed with the special contribution of the European Association of Percutaneous Cardiovascular Interventions (EAPCI). Eur Heart J 35(37):2541–2619

Badimon L, Vilahur G (2014) Thrombosis formation on atherosclerotic lesions and plaque rupture. J Intern Med 276(6):618–632

Badimon L, Suades R, Arderiu G, Pena E, Chiva-Blanch G, Padro T (2017) Microvesicles in atherosclerosis and angiogenesis: from bench to bedside and reverse. Front Cardiovasc Med 4:77

Bhatt DL, Fox KA, Hacke W, Berger PB, Black HR, Boden WE et al (2006) Clopidogrel and aspirin versus aspirin alone for the prevention of atherothrombotic events. N Engl J Med 354(16):1706–1717

Biere-Rafi S, Tuinenburg A, Haak BW, Peters M, Huijgen R, De Groot E et al (2012) Factor VIII deficiency does not protect against atherosclerosis. J Thromb Haemost 10(1):30–37

Binder V, Bergum B, Jaisson S, Gillery P, Scavenius C, Spriet E et al (2017) Impact of fibrinogen carbamylation on fibrin clot formation and stability. Thromb Haemost 117(5):899–910

Borissoff JI, Heeneman S, Kilinc E, Kassak P, van Oerle R, Winckers K et al (2010) Early atherosclerosis exhibits an enhanced procoagulant state. Circulation 122(8):821–830

Borissoff JI, Spronk HM, ten Cate H (2011) The hemostatic system as a modulator of atherosclerosis. N Engl J Med 364(18):1746–1760

Borissoff JI, Joosen IA, Versteylen MO, Spronk HM, ten Cate H, Hofstra L (2012) Accelerated in vivo thrombin formation independently predicts the presence and severity of CT angiographic coronary atherosclerosis. JACC Cardiovasc Imaging 5(12):1201–1210

Borissoff JI, Otten JJ, Heeneman S, Leenders P, van Oerle R, Soehnlein O et al (2013) Genetic and pharmacological modifications of thrombin formation in apolipoprotein e-deficient mice determine atherosclerosis severity and atherothrombosis onset in a neutrophil-dependent manner. PLoS One 8(2):e55784

Bouchareychas L, Raffai RL (2018) Apolipoprotein E and atherosclerosis: from lipoprotein metabolism to MicroRNA control of inflammation. J Cardiovasc Dev Dis 5(2):30

Buchheiser A, Ebner A, Burghoff S, Ding Z, Romio M, Viethen C et al (2011) Inactivation of CD73 promotes atherogenesis in apolipoprotein E-deficient mice. Cardiovasc Res 92(2):338–347

Buller HR, Bethune C, Bhanot S, Gailani D, Monia BP, Raskob GE et al (2015) Factor XI antisense oligonucleotide for prevention of venous thrombosis. N Engl J Med 372(3):232–240

Bundhun PK, Teeluck AR, Bhurtu A, Huang WQ (2017) Is the concomitant use of clopidogrel and proton pump inhibitors still associated with increased adverse cardiovascular outcomes following coronary angioplasty?: a systematic review and meta-analysis of recently published studies (2012–2016). BMC Cardiovasc Disord 17(1):3

Chandran S, Watkins J, Abdul-Aziz A, Shafat M, Calvert PA, Bowles KM et al (2017) Inflammatory differences in plaque erosion and rupture in patients with ST-segment elevation myocardial infarction. J Am Heart Assoc 6(5):e005868

Collet JP, Cuisset T, Range G, Cayla G, Elhadad S, Pouillot C et al (2012) Bedside monitoring to adjust antiplatelet therapy for coronary stenting. N Engl J Med 367(22):2100–2109

Committee CS (1996) A randomised, blinded, trial of clopidogrel versus aspirin in patients at risk of ischaemic events (CAPRIE). CAPRIE steering committee. Lancet 348(9038):1329–1339

Coppens M, Weitz JI, Eikelboom JWA (2019) Synergy of dual pathway inhibition in chronic cardiovascular disease. Circ Res 124(3):416–425

Coughlin SR (2005) Protease-activated receptors in hemostasis, thrombosis and vascular biology. J Thromb Haemost 3(8):1800–1814

Coukell AJ, Markham A (1997) Clopidogrel. Drugs 54(5):745–750; Discussion 51

Cyrus T, Sung S, Zhao L, Funk CD, Tang S, Pratico D (2002) Effect of low-dose aspirin on vascular inflammation, plaque stability, and atherogenesis in low-density lipoprotein receptor-deficient mice. Circulation 106(10):1282–1287

de Groot PG, Reinders JH, Sixma JJ (1987) Perturbation of human endothelial cells by thrombin or PMA changes the reactivity of their extracellular matrix towards platelets. J Cell Biol 104(3):697–704

Dutch Bypass Oral Anticoagulants or Aspirin (BOA) Study Group (2000) Efficacy of Oral anticoagulants compared with aspirin after infrainguinal bypass surgery (The Dutch Bypass Oral Anticoagulants or Aspirin Study): a randomised trial. Lancet 355(9201):346–351

Eikelboom JW, Connolly SJ, Bosch J, Dagenais GR, Hart RG, Shestakovska O et al (2017) Rivaroxaban with or without aspirin in stable cardiovascular disease. N Engl J Med 377:1319–1330

Esmon CT (1995) Inflammation and thrombosis: the impact of inflammation on the protein C anticoagulant pathway. Haematologica 80(2 Suppl):49–56

Esmon CT (2014) Targeting factor Xa and thrombin: impact on coagulation and beyond. Thromb Haemost 111(4):625–633

Fay WP (2004) Plasminogen activator inhibitor 1, fibrin, and the vascular response to injury. Trends Cardiovasc Med 14(5):196–202

Feldmann K, Grandoch M, Kohlmorgen C, Valentin B, Gerfer S, Nagy N et al (2019) Decreased M1 macrophage polarization in dabigatran-treated Ldlr-deficient mice: implications for atherosclerosis and adipose tissue inflammation. Atherosclerosis 287:81–88

Fernandes A, McEvoy JW, Halvorsen S (2019) Doctor, should I keep taking an aspirin a day? N Engl J Med 380(20):1967–1970

Ferrante G, Nakano M, Prati F, Niccoli G, Mallus MT, Ramazzotti V et al (2010) High levels of systemic myeloperoxidase are associated with coronary plaque erosion in patients with acute coronary syndromes: a clinicopathological study. Circulation 122(24):2505–2513

Foley JH (2017) Plasmin(ogen) at the nexus of fibrinolysis, inflammation, and complement. Semin Thromb Hemost 43(2):135–142

Fowkes FG, Price JF, Stewart MC, Butcher I, Leng GC, Pell AC et al (2010) Aspirin for prevention of cardiovascular events in a general population screened for a low ankle brachial index: a randomized controlled trial. JAMA 303(9):841–848

Fujiwara A, Taguchi O, Takagi T, D'Alessandro-Gabazza CN, Boveda-Ruiz D, Toda M et al (2012) Role of thrombin-activatable fibrinolysis inhibitor in allergic bronchial asthma. Lung 190(2):189–198

Fuster V, Badimon L, Badimon JJ, Chesebro JH (1992a) The pathogenesis of coronary artery disease and the acute coronary syndromes (1). N Engl J Med 326(4):242–250

Fuster V, Badimon L, Badimon JJ, Chesebro JH (1992b) The pathogenesis of coronary artery disease and the acute coronary syndromes (2). N Engl J Med 326(5):310–318

Garcia Rodriguez LA, Martin-Perez M, Hennekens CH, Rothwell PM, Lanas A (2016) Bleeding risk with long-term low-dose aspirin: a systematic review of observational studies. PLoS One 11(8):e0160046

Gimbrone MA Jr, Garcia-Cardena G (2016) Endothelial cell dysfunction and the pathobiology of atherosclerosis. Circ Res 118(4):620–636

Gresele P (2002) Platelets in thrombotic and non-thrombotic disorders: pathophysiology, pharmacology, and therapeutics. Cambridge University Press, Cambridge

Griffin JH, Zlokovic BV, Mosnier LO (2015) Activated protein C: biased for translation. Blood 125(19):2898–2907

Group ASC, Bowman L, Mafham M, Wallendszus K, Stevens W, Buck G et al (2018) Effects of aspirin for primary prevention in persons with diabetes mellitus. N Engl J Med 379(16):1529–1539

Grover SP, Mackman N (2018) Tissue factor: an essential mediator of hemostasis and trigger of thrombosis. Arterioscler Thromb Vasc Biol 38(4):709–725

Gurbel PA, Fox KAA, Tantry US, Ten Cate H, Weitz JI (2019) Combination antiplatelet and oral anticoagulant therapy in patients with coronary and peripheral artery disease. Circulation 139(18):2170–2185

Hackam DG, Spence JD (2019) Antiplatelet therapy in ischemic stroke and transient ischemic attack. Stroke 50(3):773–778

Hara T, Fukuda D, Tanaka K, Higashikuni Y, Hirata Y, Nishimoto S et al (2015) Rivaroxaban, a novel oral anticoagulant, attenuates atherosclerotic plaque progression and destabilization in ApoE-deficient mice. Atherosclerosis 242(2):639–646

Hara T, Phuong PT, Fukuda D, Yamaguchi K, Murata C, Nishimoto S et al (2018) Protease-activated receptor-2 plays a critical role in vascular inflammation and atherosclerosis in apolipoprotein E-deficient mice. Circulation 138(16):1706–1719

Heim C, Gebhardt J, Ramsperger-Gleixner M, Jacobi J, Weyand M, Ensminger SM (2016) Clopidogrel significantly lowers the development of atherosclerosis in ApoE-deficient mice in vivo. Heart Vessel 31(5):783–794

Hess CN, Norgren L, Ansel GM, Capell WH, Fletcher JP, Fowkes FGR et al (2017) A structured review of antithrombotic therapy in peripheral artery disease with a focus on revascularization: a TASC (InterSociety Consensus for the Management of Peripheral Artery Disease) initiative. Circulation 135(25):2534–2555

Hiatt WR, Fowkes FG, Heizer G, Berger JS, Baumgartner I, Held P et al (2017) Ticagrelor versus clopidogrel in symptomatic peripheral artery disease. N Engl J Med 376(1):32–40

Hoffman M (2018) The tissue factor pathway and wound healing. Semin Thromb Hemost 44(2):142–150

Huo Y, Schober A, Forlow SB, Smith DF, Hyman MC, Jung S et al (2003) Circulating activated platelets exacerbate atherosclerosis in mice deficient in apolipoprotein E. Nat Med 9(1):61–67

Ikonomidis I, Andreotti F, Economou E, Stefanadis C, Toutouzas P, Nihoyannopoulos P (1999) Increased proinflammatory cytokines in patients with chronic stable angina and their reduction by aspirin. Circulation 100(8):793–798

Johnston SC, Easton JD, Farrant M, Barsan W, Conwit RA, Elm JJ et al (2018) Clopidogrel and aspirin in acute ischemic stroke and high-risk TIA. N Engl J Med 379(3):215–225

Kadoglou NP, Moustardas P, Katsimpoulas M, Kapelouzou A, Kostomitsopoulos N, Schafer K et al (2012) The beneficial effects of a direct thrombin inhibitor, dabigatran etexilate, on the development and stability of atherosclerotic lesions in apolipoprotein E-deficient mice: dabigatran etexilate and atherosclerosis. Cardiovasc Drugs Ther 26(5):367–374

Kamphuisen PW, ten Cate H (2014) Cardiovascular risk in patients with hemophilia. Blood 123(9):1297–1301

Kharbanda RK, Walton B, Allen M, Klein N, Hingorani AD, MacAllister RJ et al (2002) Prevention of inflammation-induced endothelial dysfunction: a novel vasculo-protective action of aspirin. Circulation 105(22):2600–2604

Kim OV, Nevzorova TA, Mordakhanova ER, Ponomareva AA, Andrianova IA, Le Minh G et al (2019) Fatal dysfunction and disintegration of thrombin-stimulated platelets. Haematologica 104(9):1866–1878

Kleinegris MC, ten Cate H, ten Cate-Hoek AJ (2013) D-dimer as a marker for cardiovascular and arterial thrombotic events in patients with peripheral arterial disease. A systematic review. Thromb Haemost 110(2):233–243

Koenen RR (2016) The prowess of platelets in immunity and inflammation. Thromb Haemost 116(4):605–612

Kossmann S, Lagrange J, Jackel S, Jurk K, Ehlken M, Schonfelder T et al (2017) Platelet-localized FXI promotes a vascular coagulation-inflammatory circuit in arterial hypertension. Sci Transl Med 9(375):eaah4923

Koupenova M, Clancy L, Corkrey HA, Freedman JE (2018) Circulating platelets as mediators of immunity, inflammation, and thrombosis. Circ Res 122(2):337–351

Kramer MC, Rittersma SZ, de Winter RJ, Ladich ER, Fowler DR, Liang YH et al (2010) Relationship of thrombus healing to underlying plaque morphology in sudden coronary death. J Am Coll Cardiol 55(2):122–132

Kuijpers MJ, van der Meijden PE, Feijge MA, Mattheij NJ, May F, Govers-Riemslag J et al (2014) Factor XII regulates the pathological process of thrombus formation on ruptured plaques. Arterioscler Thromb Vasc Biol 34(8):1674–1680

Lee IO, Kratz MT, Schirmer SH, Baumhakel M, Bohm M (2012) The effects of direct thrombin inhibition with dabigatran on plaque formation and endothelial function in apolipoprotein E-deficient mice. J Pharmacol Exp Ther 343(2):253–257

Lee J, Nakanishi R, Li D, Shaikh K, Shekar C, Osawa K et al (2018) Randomized trial of rivaroxaban versus warfarin in the evaluation of progression of coronary atherosclerosis. Am Heart J 206:127–130

Li D, Wang Y, Zhang L, Luo X, Li J, Chen X et al (2012) Roles of purinergic receptor P2Y, G protein-coupled 12 in the development of atherosclerosis in apolipoprotein E-deficient mice. Arterioscler Thromb Vasc Biol 32(8):e81–e89

Li X, Vink A, Niessen HW, Kers J, de Boer OJ, Ploegmakers HJ et al (2014) Total burden of intraplaque hemorrhage in coronary arteries relates to the use of coumarin-type anticoagulants but not platelet aggregation inhibitors. Virchows Arch 465(6):723–729

Libby P (2013) Mechanisms of acute coronary syndromes and their implications for therapy. N Engl J Med 368(21):2004–2013

Lievens D, von Hundelshausen P (2011) Platelets in atherosclerosis. Thromb Haemost 106(5):827–838

Liu H, Jiang D, Zhang S, Ou B (2010) Aspirin inhibits fractalkine expression in atherosclerotic plaques and reduces atherosclerosis in ApoE gene knockout mice. Cardiovasc Drugs Ther 24(1):17–24

Long AT, Kenne E, Jung R, Fuchs TA, Renne T (2016) Contact system revisited: an interface between inflammation, coagulation, and innate immunity. J Thromb Haemost 14(3):427–437

Lowe G, Rumley A (2014) The relevance of coagulation in cardiovascular disease: what do the biomarkers tell us? Thromb Haemost 112(5):860–867

Mackman N (2016) The clot thickens in atherosclerosis. Arterioscler Thromb Vasc Biol 36(3):425–426

Majithia A, Bhatt DL (2019) Novel antiplatelet therapies for atherothrombotic diseases. Arterioscler Thromb Vasc Biol 39(4):546–557

Markus HS, McCollum C, Imray C, Goulder MA, Gilbert J, King A (2011) The von Willebrand inhibitor ARC1779 reduces cerebral embolization after carotid endarterectomy: a randomized trial. Stroke 42(8):2149–2153

Mastenbroek TG, van Geffen JP, Heemskerk JW, Cosemans JM (2015) Acute and persistent platelet and coagulant activities in atherothrombosis. J Thromb Haemost 13(Suppl 1):S272–S280

McFadyen JD, Schaff M, Peter K (2018) Current and future antiplatelet therapies: emphasis on preserving haemostasis. Nat Rev Cardiol 15(3):181–191

McNeil JJ, Nelson MR, Woods RL, Lockery JE, Wolfe R, Reid CM et al (2018a) Effect of aspirin on all-cause mortality in the healthy elderly. N Engl J Med 379(16):1519–1528

McNeil JJ, Wolfe R, Woods RL, Tonkin AM, Donnan GA, Nelson MR et al (2018b) Effect of aspirin on cardiovascular events and bleeding in the healthy elderly. N Engl J Med 379(16):1509–1518

McNeil JJ, Woods RL, Nelson MR, Reid CM, Kirpach B, Wolfe R et al (2018c) Effect of aspirin on disability-free survival in the healthy elderly. N Engl J Med 379(16):1499–1508

Mega JL, Simon T, Collet JP, Anderson JL, Antman EM, Bliden K et al (2010) Reduced-function CYP2C19 genotype and risk of adverse clinical outcomes among patients treated with clopidogrel predominantly for PCI: a meta-analysis. JAMA 304(16):1821–1830

Mega JL, Braunwald E, Wiviott SD, Bassand JP, Bhatt DL, Bode C et al (2012) Rivaroxaban in patients with a recent acute coronary syndrome. N Engl J Med 366(1):9–19

Mehta SR, Yusuf S, Peters RJ, Bertrand ME, Lewis BS, Natarajan MK et al (2001) Effects of pretreatment with clopidogrel and aspirin followed by long-term therapy in patients undergoing percutaneous coronary intervention: the PCI-CURE study. Lancet 358(9281):527–533

Messner B, Bernhard D (2014) Smoking and cardiovascular disease: mechanisms of endothelial dysfunction and early atherogenesis. Arterioscler Thromb Vasc Biol 34(3):509–515

Miller VM, Lahr BD, Bailey KR, Hodis HN, Mulvagh SL, Jayachandran M (2016) Specific cell-derived microvesicles: linking endothelial function to carotid artery intima-media thickness in low cardiovascular risk menopausal women. Atherosclerosis 246:21–28

Mo C, Sun G, Lu ML, Zhang L, Wang YZ, Sun X et al (2015) Proton pump inhibitors in prevention of low-dose aspirin-associated upper gastrointestinal injuries. World J Gastroenterol 21(17):5382–5392

Morrow DA, Braunwald E, Bonaca MP, Ameriso SF, Dalby AJ, Fish MP et al (2012) Vorapaxar in the secondary prevention of atherothrombotic events. N Engl J Med 366(15):1404–1413

Morser J, Gabazza EC, Myles T, Leung LL (2010) What has been learnt from the thrombin-activatable fibrinolysis inhibitor-deficient mouse? J Thromb Haemost 8(5):868–876

Mosnier LO, Sinha RK, Burnier L, Bouwens EA, Griffin JH (2012) Biased agonism of protease-activated receptor 1 by activated protein C caused by noncanonical cleavage at Arg46. Blood 120(26):5237–5246

Mozaffarian D, Wilson PW, Kannel WB (2008) Beyond established and novel risk factors: lifestyle risk factors for cardiovascular disease. Circulation 117(23):3031–3038

Mujaj B, Bos D, Muka T, Lugt AV, Ikram MA, Vernooij MW et al (2018) Antithrombotic treatment is associated with intraplaque haemorrhage in the atherosclerotic carotid artery: a cross-sectional analysis of the Rotterdam study. Eur Heart J 39(36):3369–3376

Muller O, Bartunek J, Hamilos M, Berza CT, Mangiacapra F, Ntalianis A et al (2013) von Willebrand factor inhibition improves endothelial function in patients with stable angina. J Cardiovasc Transl Res 6(3):364–370

Myles T, Nishimura T, Yun TH, Nagashima M, Morser J, Patterson AJ et al (2003) Thrombin activatable fibrinolysis inhibitor, a potential regulator of vascular inflammation. J Biol Chem 278(51):51059–51067

Naito M, Taguchi O, Kobayashi T, Takagi T, D'Alessandro-Gabazza CN, Matsushima Y et al (2013) Thrombin-activatable fibrinolysis inhibitor protects against acute lung injury by inhibiting the complement system. Am J Respir Cell Mol Biol 49(4):646–653

Nawroth PP, Stern DM, Kaplan KL, Nossel HL (1984) Prostacyclin production by perturbed bovine aortic endothelial cells in culture. Blood 64(4):801–806

Nechipurenko DY, Receveur N, Yakimenko AO, Shepelyuk TO, Yakusheva AA, Kerimov RR et al (2019) Clot contraction drives the translocation of procoagulant platelets to thrombus surface. Arterioscler Thromb Vasc Biol 39(1):37–47

Nguyen TS, Lapidot T, Ruf W (2018) Extravascular coagulation in hematopoietic stem and progenitor cell regulation Blood 132(2):123–131

Nickel KF, Long AT, Fuchs TA, Butler LM, Renne T (2017) Factor XII as a therapeutic target in thromboembolic and inflammatory diseases. Arterioscler Thromb Vasc Biol 37(1):13–20

Nishimura T, Myles T, Piliponsky AM, Kao PN, Berry GJ, Leung LL (2007) Thrombin-activatable procarboxypeptidase B regulates activated complement C5a in vivo. Blood 109(5):1992–1997

Nylander S, Schulz R (2016) Effects of P2Y12 receptor antagonists beyond platelet inhibition – comparison of ticagrelor with thienopyridines. Br J Pharmacol 173(7):1163–1178

Olie RH, van der Meijden PEJ, Ten Cate H (2018) The coagulation system in atherothrombosis: implications for new therapeutic strategies. Res Pract Thromb Haemost 2(2):188–198

Olie RH, van der Meijden PEJ, Spronk HMH, van Oerle R, Barvik S, Bonarjee VVS et al (2019) Effects of the PAR-1 antagonist vorapaxar on platelet activation and coagulation biomarkers in patients with stable coronary artery disease. TH Open 3(3):e259–ee62

Opneja A, Kapoor S, Stavrou EX (2019) Contribution of platelets, the coagulation and fibrinolytic systems to cutaneous wound healing. Thromb Res 179:56–63

Paone S, Baxter AA, Hulett MD, Poon IKH (2019) Endothelial cell apoptosis and the role of endothelial cell-derived extracellular vesicles in the progression of atherosclerosis. Cell Mol Life Sci 76(6):1093–1106

Pasterkamp G, den Ruijter HM, Libby P (2017) Temporal shifts in clinical presentation and underlying mechanisms of atherosclerotic disease. Nat Rev Cardiol 14(1):21–29

Pedicino D, Vinci R, Giglio AF, Pisano E, Porto I, Vergallo R et al (2018) Alterations of hyaluronan metabolism in acute coronary syndrome: implications for plaque erosion. J Am Coll Cardiol 72(13):1490–1503

Pingel S, Tiyerili V, Mueller J, Werner N, Nickenig G, Mueller C (2014) Thrombin inhibition by dabigatran attenuates atherosclerosis in ApoE deficient mice. Arch Med Sci 10(1):154–160

Plank F, Beyer C, Friedrich G, Stuhlinger M, Hintringer F, Dichtl W et al (2018) Influence of vitamin K antagonists and direct oral anticoagulation on coronary artery disease: a CTA analysis. Int J Cardiol 260:11–15

Posma JJ, Posthuma JJ, Spronk HM (2016) Coagulation and non-coagulation effects of thrombin. J Thromb Haemost 14(10):1908–1916

Posthuma JJ, Posma JJN, van Oerle R, Leenders P, van Gorp RH, Jaminon AMG et al (2019) Targeting coagulation factor Xa promotes regression of advanced atherosclerosis in apolipoprotein-E deficient mice. Sci Rep 9(1):3909

Preusch MR, Ieronimakis N, Wijelath ES, Cabbage S, Ricks J, Bea F et al (2015) Dabigatran etexilate retards the initiation and progression of atherosclerotic lesions and inhibits the expression of oncostatin M in apolipoprotein E-deficient mice. Drug Des Devel Ther 9:5203–5211

Price MJ, Berger PB, Teirstein PS, Tanguay JF, Angiolillo DJ, Spriggs D et al (2011) Standard- vs high-dose clopidogrel based on platelet function testing after percutaneous coronary intervention: the GRAVITAS randomized trial. JAMA 305(11):1097–1105

Quillard T, Franck G, Mawson T, Folco E, Libby P (2017) Mechanisms of erosion of atherosclerotic plaques. Curr Opin Lipidol 28(5):434–441

Relja B, Lustenberger T, Puttkammer B, Jakob H, Morser J, Gabazza EC et al (2013) Thrombin-activatable fibrinolysis inhibitor (TAFI) is enhanced in major trauma patients without infectious complications. Immunobiology 218(4):470–476

Ren M, Li R, Chen N, Pang N, Li Y, Deng X et al (2017) Platelet-derived factor V is a critical mediator of arterial thrombosis. J Am Heart Assoc 6(4):e006345

Roffi M, Patrono C, Collet JP, Mueller C, Valgimigli M, Andreotti F et al (2016) 2015 ESC guidelines for the management of acute coronary syndromes in patients presenting without persistent ST-segment elevation: Task Force for the Management of acute Coronary Syndromes in Patients Presenting without Persistent ST-Segment Elevation of the European Society of Cardiology (ESC). Eur Heart J 37(3):267–315

Ross R (1999) Atherosclerosis – an inflammatory disease. N Engl J Med 340(2):115–126

Ruf W (2018) Proteases, protease-activated receptors, and atherosclerosis. Arterioscler Thromb Vasc Biol 38(6):1252–1254

Russo I, Penna C, Musso T, Popara J, Alloatti G, Cavalot F et al (2017) Platelets, diabetes and myocardial ischemia/reperfusion injury. Cardiovasc Diabetol 16(1):71

Sanada F, Muratsu J, Otsu R, Shimizu H, Koibuchi N, Uchida K et al (2017) Local production of activated factor X in atherosclerotic plaque induced vascular smooth muscle cell senescence. Sci Rep 7(1):17172

Schirmer SH, Kratz MT, Kazakov A, Nylander S, Baumhaekel M, Laufs U et al (2012) 1357 - inhibition of the adenosine diphosphate receptor P2Y12 reduces atherosclerotic plaque size in hypercholesterolemic ApoE−/− mice. Eur Heart J 33(suppl_1):19–338

Schulz C, Massberg S (2012) Platelets in atherosclerosis and thrombosis. Handb Exp Pharmacol 210:111–133

Scridon A, Marginean A, Hutanu A, Chinezu L, Gheban D, Perian M et al (2019) Vascular protease-activated receptor 4 upregulation, increased platelet aggregation, and coronary lipid deposits induced by long-term dabigatran administration – results from a diabetes animal model. J Thromb Haemost 17(3):538–550

Seehaus S, Shahzad K, Kashif M, Vinnikov IA, Schiller M, Wang H et al (2009) Hypercoagulability inhibits monocyte transendothelial migration through protease-activated receptor-1-, phospholipase-Cbeta-, phosphoinositide 3-kinase-, and nitric oxide-dependent signaling in monocytes and promotes plaque stability. Circulation 120(9):774–784

Semple JW, Italiano JE Jr, Freedman J (2011) Platelets and the immune continuum. Nat Rev Immunol 11(4):264–274

Shao Z, Nishimura T, Leung LL, Morser J (2015) Carboxypeptidase B2 deficiency reveals opposite effects of complement C3a and C5a in a murine polymicrobial sepsis model. J Thromb Haemost 13(6):1090–1102

Shnerb Ganor R, Harats D, Schiby G, Gailani D, Levkovitz H, Avivi C et al (2016) Factor XI deficiency protects against atherogenesis in apolipoprotein E/factor XI double knockout mice. Arterioscler Thromb Vasc Biol 36(3):475–481

Shuldiner AR, O'Connell JR, Bliden KP, Gandhi A, Ryan K, Horenstein RB et al (2009) Association of cytochrome P450 2C19 genotype with the antiplatelet effect and clinical efficacy of clopidogrel therapy. JAMA 302(8):849–857

Sibbing D, Stegherr J, Latz W, Koch W, Mehilli J, Dorrler K et al (2009) Cytochrome P450 2C19 loss-of-function polymorphism and stent thrombosis following percutaneous coronary intervention. Eur Heart J 30(8):916–922

Smith P, Arnesen H, Holme I (1990) The effect of warfarin on mortality and reinfarction after myocardial infarction. N Engl J Med 323(3):147–152

Soardi F, Nicrosini F, Del Favero A, Pasotti C (1961) Experimental cholesterin atherosclerosis in the rabbit: action of a duodenal heparinoid. III. Modifications in the factors of hemocoagulation, plasmin and plasminogen, and in the thromboplastin and fibrinolytic activity of the aortic wall. Farmaco Prat 16:560–558

Spronk HM, Govers-Riemslag JW, ten Cate H (2003a) The blood coagulation system as a molecular machine. BioEssays 25(12):1220–1228

Spronk HM, Soute BA, Schurgers LJ, Thijssen HH, de Mey JG, Vermeer C (2003b) Tissue-specific utilization of menaquinone-4 results in the prevention of arterial calcification in warfarin-treated rats. J Vasc Res 40(6):531–537

Spronk HMH, Padro T, Siland JE, Prochaska JH, Winters J, van der Wal AC et al (2018) Atherothrombosis and thromboembolism: position paper from the Second Maastricht Consensus Conference on Thrombosis. Thromb Haemost 118(2):229–250

Stalker TJ, Traxler EA, Wu J, Wannemacher KM, Cermignano SL, Voronov R et al (2013) Hierarchical organization in the hemostatic response and its relationship to the platelet-signaling network. Blood 121(10) 1875–1885

Swieringa F, Spronk HMH, Heemskerk JWM, van der Meijden PEJ (2018) Integrating platelet and coagulation activation in fibrin clot formation. Res Pract Thromb Haemost 2(3):450–460

Szabo IL, Matics R, Hegyi P, Garami A, Illes A, Sarlos P et al (2017) PPIs prevent aspirin-induced gastrointestinal bleeding better than H2RAs. A systematic review and meta-analysis. J Gastrointestin Liver Dis 26(4):395–402

Takeda M, Yamashita T, Shinohara M, Sasaki N, Tawa H, Nakajima K et al (2012) Beneficial effect of anti-platelet therapies on atherosclerotic lesion formation assessed by phase-contrast X-ray CT imaging. Int J Cardiovasc Imaging 28(5):1181–1191

Tousoulis D, Oikonomou E, Economou EK, Crea F, Kaski JC (2016) Inflammatory cytokines in atherosclerosis: current therapeutic approaches. Eur Heart J 37(22):1723–1732

van Bergen PFMM et al (1994) Effect of long-term oral anticoagulant treatment on mortality and cardiovascular morbidity after myocardial infarction. Anticoagulants in the Secondary Prevention of Events in Coronary Thrombosis (ASPECT) Research Group. Lancet 343(8896):499–503

Vasina EM, Cauwenberghs S, Staudt M, Feijge MA, Weber C, Koenen RR et al (2013) Aging- and activation-induced platelet microparticles suppress apoptosis in monocytic cells and differentially signal to proinflammatory mediator release. Am J Blood Res 3(2):107–123

Veltri KT (2018) Yosprala: a fixed dose combination of aspirin and omeprazole. Cardiol Rev 26(1):50–53

von Hundelshausen P, Koenen RR, Sack M, Mause SF, Adriaens W, Proudfoot AE et al (2005) Heterophilic interactions of platelet factor 4 and RANTES promote monocyte arrest on endothelium. Blood 105(3):924–930

Wallentin L, Becker RC, Budaj A, Cannon CP, Emanuelsson H, Held C et al (2009) Ticagrelor versus clopidogrel in patients with acute coronary syndromes. N Engl J Med 361(11):1045–1057

Wang Y, Wang Y, Zhao X, Liu L, Wang D, Wang C et al (2013) Clopidogrel with aspirin in acute minor stroke or transient ischemic attack. N Engl J Med 369(1):11–19

Weitz JI, Chan NC (2019) Advances in antithrombotic therapy. Arterioscler Thromb Vasc Biol 39(1):7–12

West LE, Steiner T, Judge HM, Francis SE, Storey RF (2014) Vessel wall, not platelet, P2Y12 potentiates early atherogenesis. Cardiovasc Res 102(3):429–435

Wight TN (2018) A role for extracellular matrix in atherosclerotic plaque erosion. J Am Coll Cardiol 72(13):1504–1505

Wilcox JN (1994) Thrombotic mechanisms in atherosclerosis. Coron Artery Dis 5(3):223–229

Wilcox JN, Noguchi S, Casanova J (2003) Extrahepatic synthesis of factor VII in human atherosclerotic vessels. Arterioscler Thromb Vasc Biol 23(1):136–141

Wiviott SD, Braunwald E, McCabe CH, Montalescot G, Ruzyllo W, Gottlieb S et al (2007) Prasugrel versus clopidogrel in patients with acute coronary syndromes. N Engl J Med 357(20):2001–2015

Yin M, Loyer X, Boulanger CM (2015) Extracellular vesicles as new pharmacological targets to treat atherosclerosis. Eur J Pharmacol 763(Pt A):90–103

Zhou Q, Bea F, Preusch M, Wang H, Isermann B, Shahzad K et al (2011) Evaluation of plaque stability of advanced atherosclerotic lesions in apo E-deficient mice after treatment with the oral factor Xa inhibitor rivaroxaban. Mediat Inflamm 2011:432080

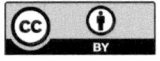

Part II

Novel Drug Developments Addressing Predefined Targets

Metabolism of Triglyceride-Rich Lipoproteins

Jan Borén and Marja-Riitta Taskinen

Contents

1	Introduction	134
2	Hepatic Formation and Secretion of VLDL	134
3	Regulators of Hepatic VLDL Secretion	136
4	Synthesis and Secretion of Chylomicrons from the Intestine	137
5	Disorders of the Synthesis of TRLs	138
6	Metabolism of Triglyceride-Rich Lipoproteins	139
7	Deciphering the Pathogenesis of Hypertriglyceridemia	140
8	Regulation of Hydrolysis of TRLs and the LPL Pathway	142
9	Role of Triglyceride-Rich Lipoproteins in Atherogenesis	144
10	Therapies to Reduce Triglyceride-Rich Lipoproteins	144
11	Development of Novel Interventions	146
12	Conclusion	147
References		147

Abstract

Triglycerides are critical lipids as they provide an energy source that is both compact and efficient. Due to its hydrophobic nature triglyceride molecules can pack together densely and so be stored in adipose tissue. To be transported in the aqueous medium of plasma, triglycerides have to be incorporated into lipoprotein particles along with other components such as cholesterol, phospholipid and

J. Borén (✉)
Institute of Medicine, Department of Molecular and Clinical Medicine, University of Gothenburg, Gothenburg, Sweden

Wallenberg Laboratory, Sahlgrenska University Hospital, Gothenburg, Sweden
e-mail: jan.boren@wlab.gu.se

M.-R. Taskinen
Research Programs Unit, Clinical and Molecular Metabolism, University of Helsinki, Helsinki, Finland

© The Author(s) 2021
A. von Eckardstein, C. J. Binder (eds.), *Prevention and Treatment of Atherosclerosis*, Handbook of Experimental Pharmacology 270, https://doi.org/10.1007/164_2021_520

associated structural and regulatory apolipoproteins. Here we discuss the physiology of normal triglyceride metabolism, and how impaired metabolism induces hypertriglyceridemia and its pathogenic consequences including atherosclerosis. We also discuss established and novel therapies to reduce triglyceride-rich lipoproteins.

Keywords

Apolipoprotein B · Chylomicrons · Hypertriglyceridemia · Metabolism · Therapies · Triglyceride-rich lipoproteins (TRL) · Very low density lipoproteins (VLDL)

1 Introduction

Interest in triglyceride-rich lipoproteins (TRLs) has for long been rather low, but recent results demonstrating that TRLs are causally associated with atherosclerotic cardiovascular disease (ASCVD) have generated major interest in these lipoproteins. Hypertriglyceridemia is quite common today and approximately 25% of US adults are estimated to have hypertriglyceridemia (triglyceride [TG] level $\geq$ 1.7 mmol/L]). TRLs are synthesized in the liver as very low-density lipoproteins (VLDL) and in the intestine as chylomicrons. During lipolysis TRLs are converted to atherogenic cholesterol-ester enriched lipoprotein remnant particles. Dysregulation of the normal metabolism of TRLs leads to excess formation of these atherogenic lipoprotein remnant particles (Chapman et al. 2011; Nordestgaard and Varbo 2014; Boren et al. 2014; Dallinga-Thie et al. 2016). Since humans are postprandial most of the day, we continuously generate atherogenic remnant particles. Consequently, the continuous generation of remnants after each meal may be an important causal risk factor for the development of atherosclerosis. Genetic studies have also identified key regulators of the metabolism of TRLs and major emphasis is now directed at evaluating their potential as novel candidate targets for dyslipidemia and premature ASCVD risk (Dallinga-Thie et al. 2016). Here we discuss how TRLs are synthesized and metabolized.

2 Hepatic Formation and Secretion of VLDL

The assembly of VLDL is a complex process and involves a stepwise lipidation of apoB100, the principal apolipoprotein on VLDL, in the liver (Olofsson et al. 2000; Olofsson and Boren 2005). ApoB100 is a large protein consisting of one globular N-terminal structure, two domains of amphipathic β-sheets and two domains of amphipathic α-helices (Segrest et al. 2001) ApoB differs from other apolipoproteins in that it is highly hydrophobic. Therefore, it cannot equilibrate between different lipoproteins but remains bound to the particle on which it was secreted into plasma. Thus, every VLDL particle contains one molecule of apoB100. This is generally thought to be explained by the presence of antiparallel β-sheets with a width of approximately 30 Å, which form very strong lipid-binding structures (Segrest et al. 2001).

The lipidation cascade starts with a cotranslational transfer of triglycerides to nascent apoB polypeptides during the assembly of nascent VLDL mediated by the microsomal triglyceride-transfer protein (MTP) in the rough endoplasmic reticulum (ER) (Fig. 1) (Boren et al. 1992; Rustaeus et al. 1998). The critical role of MTP in VLDL assembly is demonstrated by the rare, autosomal-recessive disorder abetalipoproteinemia. The disorder results from mutations in the gene encoding the large subunit of MTP and is characterized by nearly a complete absence of apoB-containing lipoproteins including VLDL. To date, over different 30 mutations

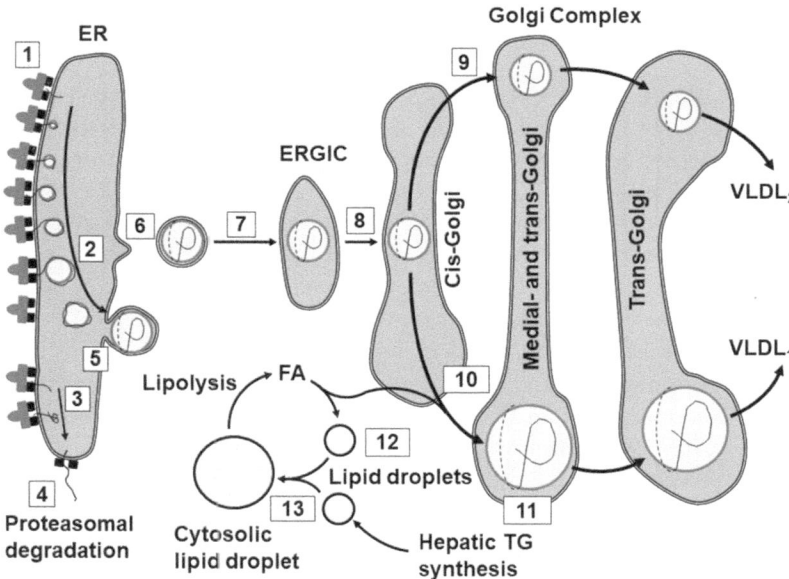

Fig. 1 *Assembly and secretion of apoB100-containing lipoproteins.* ApoB is synthesized and translocated into the lumen of the endoplasmic reticulum (ER) (1). The growing nascent apoB polypeptide is cotranslationally lipidated by the lipid transfer protein MTTP to form a partially lipidated pre-VLDL particle (2). If apoB fails to be lipidated and acquire a correct protein folding (3), it is sorted to posttranslational degradation (4). The triglyceride-poor pre-VLDL particle exits the ER by Sar1/CopII vesicles that bud off (6) from specific sites on the ER membrane (Gusarova et al. 2003). The vesicles fuse to form the ER Golgi intermediate compartment (ERGIC) (7), which then fuses with the cis-Golgi (8). The triglyceride-poor particles are either secreted as smaller VLDL$_2$ particles (9) or further lipidated (10) to form mature triglyceride-rich VLDL$_1$ particles, which are then secreted (11). The formation of triglyceride-rich VLDL$_1$ particles is highly dependent on the presence of triglyceride-containing cytosolic lipid droplets. These lipid droplets are formed as small primordial droplets from microsomal membranes (12) and increase in size by fusion (13). The triglycerides within the droplets undergo lipolysis and are re-esterified (14) before they lipidate the triglyceride-poor VLDL to form triglyceride-rich VLDL. Hepatic triglycerides originate from influx of free fatty acids, hepatic de novo lipogenesis (DNL), or hepatic uptake of lipoprotein particles

in the MTP gene have been described for ABL (Lee and Hegele 2014). Absence of MTP leads to premature proteosomal degradation of nascent apoB and therefore absence of VLDL and chylomicron production. The patients are characterized by hypocholesterolemia and the absence of apoB-containing lipoproteins (Paquette et al. 2016).

The cotranslational lipidation stabilizes the nascent apoB polypeptide and results in the formation of a nascent pre-VLDL lipoprotein particle (Bostrom et al. 1988). The immature pre-VLDL undergoes further lipidation in the secretory pathway, forming a triglyceride-poor VLDL particle (Stillemark-Billton et al. 2005). This particle can either be secreted from the liver as a smaller VLDL particle (i.e., $VLDL_2$) or undergo further lipidation to form a larger triglyceride-rich (i.e., $VLDL_1$) (Stillemark-Billton et al. 2005; Stillemark et al. 2000). The lipidation cascade is still not fully understood, but has been shown to involve several proteins including the GTP-binding protein ADP-ribosylation factor 1 (ARF-1) (Asp et al. 2005).

The conversion of smaller triglyceride-poor VLDL particles to large triglyceride-rich VLDL likely involves the fusion of cytoplasmic lipid droplets to the smaller VLDL particle. Thus, this bulk addition of triglycerides differs from the initial stepwise addition of triglycerides. The formation of the large mature VLDL particles is therefore dependent on the presence of cytosolic lipid droplets (Wiggins and Gibbons 1992; Salter et al. 1998; Gibbons et al. 2000). Therefore, it's not surprising that hepatic accumulation of triglycerides, non-alcoholic fatty liver disease (NAFLD), is linked to oversecretion of large $VLDL_1$ particles (Adiels et al. 2006a, b). However, not all forms of fatty liver disease are linked to increased hepatic secretion of $VLDL_1$, indicating that the hepatic stores of triglycerides in some genetic forms of NAFLD, like PNPLA3, are not accessible for VLDL formation. However, the molecular mechanisms are still unclear. Interestingly, the amounts of triglycerides that are added to triglyceride-rich poor VLDL seem to be constant. Thus, subjects with type 2 diabetes secrete more – not larger – $VLDL_1$ particles than non-diabetic controls (Adiels et al. 2005, 2006a, b). Thus, bulk addition of triglycerides from the cytoplasmic lipid droplets seems to be a highly regulated process.

3   Regulators of Hepatic VLDL Secretion

Hepatic triglyceride accumulation stimulates hepatic $VLDL_1$ secretion, and the sources for liver fat are: (1) plasma fatty acids generated by lipolysis of the peripheral adipose tissue; (2) fatty acids synthesized in the liver from carbohydrates through hepatic de novo lipogenesis (DNL); (3) fatty acids that come from the diet; and (4) hepatic uptake of triglyceride-rich lipoproteins (TRLs) (Parks and Hellerstein 2006; Barrows and Parks 2006). Most of the hepatic triglycerides originate from circulating fatty acids, since the hepatic uptake of fatty acids is not regulated. Thus, increased levels of circulating fatty acids are directly connected to increased hepatic uptake of fatty acids (Tamura and Shimomura 2005). Lipolysis of adipose tissue (in particular the visceral adipose tissue) is the principal contributor (approx. 80%) of the plasma NEFA pool (Tamura and Shimomura 2005). It is therefore not surprising that visceral adiposity is strongly associated with NAFLD and oversecretion of VLDL$_1$ particles (Parks and Hellerstein 2006; Barrows and Parks 2006; Farquhar et al. 1965; Parks et al. 1999; Havel 1961; Donnelly et al. 2005).

Normally the hepatic DNL plays a minor role (<5%) (Barrows and Parks 2006), but in conditions of increased plasma glucose and hyperinsulinemia it has been shown to generate ≈25% of liver triglycerides (Donnelly et al. 2005). The explanation is that glucose is the substrate for hepatic DNL and that hyperinsulinemia is linked to increased expression of factors needed for hepatic DNL such as SREBP1-c (Browning and Horton 2004; Shimomura et al. 1999), the carbohydrate response element–binding protein (ChREBP) (Koo et al. 2001), and PPARγ (Edvardsson et al. 1999; Chao et al. 2000; Westerbacka et al. 2007).

In addition, there is evidence that VLDL$_1$ and VLDL$_2$ are regulated independently. Ethanol overconsumption seems to stimulate VLDL$_1$ production in humans (Fielding et al. 2000), whereas endogenous cholesterol synthesis correlates with VLDL$_2$-apoB but not VLDL$_1$-apoB production (Prinsen et al. 2003). This finding may explain why VLDL$_2$, but not VLDL$_1$, is increased in patients with increased plasma cholesterol such as moderate hypercholesterolemia (Gaw et al. 1995) and familial hypercholesterolemia (James et al. 1989).

4 Synthesis and Secretion of Chylomicrons from the Intestine

Chylomicrons are synthesized in the enterocytes of the small intestine and each chylomicron contains one molecule of apoB48. The apoB48 protein corresponds exactly to the N-terminal 48% of apoB100. The explanation for this is that both proteins are encoded by the same gene. The mRNA for apoB48 is generated from the apoB100 mRNA by a posttranscriptional editing process during which a deamination of a cytidine (at nucleotide 6,666) to a uridine converts a glutamine codon to a stop codon. The mechanism has been extensively reviewed (Davidson and Shelness 2000; Anant and Davidson 2001; Wang et al. 2003). The assembly of chylomicrons is a highly complex multistep process, and less is still known about chylomicron assembly than VLDL assembly (Xiao et al. 2019; Hussain et al. 2005). However, it is known that in addition to MTTP, intestinal assembly of chylomicron requires Sar1 GTPase, which is critical for the intracellular transport of apoB48-containing particles from ER to the Golgi (Julve et al. 2016).

The newly synthesized chylomicrons carrying dietary lipids and fat-soluble vitamins are secreted through lacteal endothelial gaps that are present in the postprandial phase into the venous system blood system through the lymphatic system. Thus, unlike other nutrients dietary lipids bypass the hepatic portal system.

Over the last years several surprising findings have been made (Lambert and Parks 2012). First, studies have demonstrated that the intestine stores triglycerides and that lipids secreted after a meal may have been consumed in an earlier meal

(Mattes 2002; Robertson et al. 2002; Chavez-Jauregui et al. 2010). This may explain the early rise in postprandial plasma triglycerides since the intestine does not have to absorb dietary lipids and then form chylomicrons, but instead start secreting stored triglycerides in chylomicrons. We have also realized that the release of chylomicrons is linked to a taste–gut–brain axis (Khan and Besnard 2009) Interestingly, chylomicrons can be secreted when fat (Mattes 2009) or glucose (Robertson et al. 2003) is merely tasted but not consumed. Lastly, contrary to what was believed, recent studies have shown that apoB48-containing particles are secreted not only as chylomicrons but also as less triglyceride-rich lipoprotein particles (isolated in the VLDL density range) both in the fasting state and postprandially (Bjornson et al. 2019a, b).

5 Disorders of the Synthesis of TRLs

Abetalipoproteinemia (ABL) (also known as the Bassen–Kornzweig syndrome) is a rare autosomal-recessive disease that is characterized by very low plasma concentrations of TG and cholesterol (under 30 mg/dL) and undetectable levels of LDL and apoB. The rare recessive genetic disease is caused by loss-of-function mutations in the MTTP gene encoding for the microsomal triglyceride-transfer protein (MTP).

Clinic: Mutations in MTP leads to impairment of the formation of triglyceride-rich VLDL and chylomicrons. Patients with ABL (and compound heterozygous and homozygous FHBL) have therefore very low plasma total cholesterol and generally low plasma triglycerides. LDL-C when measured by direct methods, and apoB, will be absent or their concentrations will be very low. Patients may display neurological, hematological (acanthocytosis on peripheral blood smear and anemia), and gastro-intestinal symptoms due to deficiency in lipophilic vitamins and fat malabsorption (Paquette et al. 2016). The deficiency of vitamin E could lead to severe neurological disorders including spinocerebellar degeneration with ataxia and retinitis pigmentosa (Welty 2014). In addition, the impaired secretion of hepatic triglycerides may lead to hepatic steatosis (Welty 2014). The clinical phenotype and severity differs as the type and combination of MTTP mutations influence the clinical phenotype and treatment response (Paquette et al. 2016). Subjects who carry a single MTTP mutation may have normal plasma lipid levels or may have LDL-cholesterol and apoB concentrations similar to those seen in heterozygous familial hypobetalipoproteinemia (Lee and Hegele 2014; Paquette et al. 2016).

Treatment: Early diagnosis and treatment is important to prevent neurologic complications of this disease. Reversal of existing neurologic disease can also be achieved. Treatment involves a low-fat diet, supplementation with essential fatty acids and high oral doses of fat-soluble vitamins, vitamins A and E (Paquette et al. 2016; Welty 2014; Linton et al. 1993). High dose of oral fat-soluble vitamins bypasses the chylomicron pathway, and vitamins are carried via the portal circulation (Lee and Hegele 2014; Paquette et al. 2016).

Chylomicron retention disease (CRD). In addition to MTP, chylomicron formation requires Sar1 GTPase, one of the subunits of the coat protein (COPII) complex, which is critical for the vesicular transport of apoB-48-containing particles from endoplasmic reticulum to the Golgi (Julve et al. 2016). Loss-of-function mutations in SAR1B, the gene encoding Sar1 homolog B GTPase causes CRD (also known as Anderson disease) (Julve et al. 2016), a rare autosomal-recessive disorder characterized by an intestinal defect in lipid transport due to a failure of chylomicron formation in enterocytes (Julve et al. 2016).

Clinic: The failure to synthesize chylomicrons results in severe malabsorption with steatorrhea, fat-soluble vitamin deficiency, low blood cholesterol levels, and failure to thrive in infancy (Julve et al. 2016).

Treatment: Same as ABL.

Familial hypobetalipoproteinemia (FHBL) is an autosomal codominant disorder characterized by apoB <5th percentile and LDL-cholesterol usually between 20 and 50 mg/dL (Welty 2014; Linton et al. 1993). Over 60 different mutations in apoB producing truncated forms of apoB, ranging from apoB to apoB89, have been reported (Welty 2014; Linton et al. 1993). These truncated forms of apoB are named according to the percent length of the native apoB100 molecule. Truncated forms of apoB shorter than apoB30 are seldom detectable in human plasma as lipoproteins since these truncated proteins undergo intracellular degradation. Although one allele if affected only in heterozygous FBHL, the plasma levels are normally closer to one quarter to one third of normal, due to low hepatic secretion of the truncated forms of apoB combined with decreased production and increased clearance of VLDL and LDL produced by the normal allele (Welty et al. 1997; Elias et al. 1999; Aguilar-Salinas et al. 1995; Parhofer et al. 1996).

Clinic: Heterozygous FHBL is often asymptomatic and not diagnosed unless a lipid profile is obtained. In contrast, the clinical presentation of homozygous FHBL is similar to ABL. Early diagnosis of homozygous FHBL is therefore important. As the hepatic secretion of triglyceride-rich lipoproteins is impaired, FHBL has been shown to associate with hepatic steatosis and mild elevation of liver enzymes (Welty 2014). In 32 FHBL subjects, the hepatic fat content was increased to $14.0 \pm 12.0\%$ compared to $5.2 \pm 5.9\%$, respectively, for 33 controls matched for age, sex, and indices of adiposity (Tanoli et al. 2004).

Treatment: For homozygous FHBL treatment involves a low-fat diet, supplementation with essential fatty acids and high oral doses of fat-soluble vitamins, vitamins A and E (Welty 2014; Linton et al. 1993).

6   Metabolism of Triglyceride-Rich Lipoproteins

After secretion of chylomicrons and VLDL, the lipoproteins are exposed to lipoprotein lipase (LPL) on the capillary endothelial cells within adipose tissue, skeletal muscle, and the heart, leading to hydrolyzation of the triglycerides, allowing the delivery of non-esterified free fatty acids (NEFA) to adipose tissue, skeletal muscle and the heart.

As the triglycerides are removed from the particles, they shrink and their density increases (Goldberg 1996); chylomicrons become chylomicron remnants, and large triglyceride-rich VLDL$_1$ particles become smaller VLDL$_2$ and subsequently intermediate density lipoproteins (IDL). The IDL particles can be further hydrolyzed to LDL particles by action of the hepatic lipase (HL). Since all human TRLs contain a substantial amount of cholesterol esters, hydrolysis of triglycerides leads to enrichment of cholesterol esters. Consequently, TRL remnants are enriched in cholesteryl esters (Dallinga-Thie et al. 2010).

Although roughly 80% of the increase in postprandial plasma triglycerides consists of chylomicrons and their remnants (Cohn et al. 1993), the majority of particles (around 80%) comprise of liver-derived VLDL and their remnants (Karpe et al. 1995; Schneeman et al. 1993). Also, the area under the curve for apoB100 is 10-fold higher than that of apoB48 (Vakkilainen et al. 2002), and the production rate of apoB100 is 15–20 times higher than that of apoB48 (Lichtenstein et al. 1992; Welty et al. 1999). We have earlier shown that chylomicrons and VLDL particles are not cleared equally by the lipoprotein lipase pathway, and that chylomicrons seem to be the preferred substrate (Adiels et al. 2012). Therefore, the major contribution to an atherogenic lipoprotein profile from chylomicrons is likely its interference with apoB100 catabolism.

ApoB-containing particles with a diameter of about 70 nm or smaller can penetrate the arterial endothelial layer, and subsequently become retained in the artery wall. Thus, cholesterol-rich remnants (i.e., both chylomicron remnants and VLDL remnants) can lead to cholesterol deposition in growing lesions, accelerated atherosclerosis, and enhanced CVD risk in a similar manner as LDL.

Genetic deficiency of LPL leads to the rare autosomal-recessive disorder *familial LPL deficiency*. These patients usually display milky plasma (accumulation of chylomicrons) and very severe hypertriglyceridemia with episodes of abdominal pain (pancreatitis), eruptive cutaneous xanthomata, and hepatosplenomegaly.

7   Deciphering the Pathogenesis of Hypertriglyceridemia

Insulin resistance and hypertriglyceridemia are associated with an atherogenic dyslipidemia characterized by prolonged postprandial hyperlipidemia, accumulation of small dense LDL (sdLDL) and low HDL cholesterol. The mechanism that leads to the formation of sdLDL is well clarified; the cholesteryl ester transfer protein (CETP) transfers triglycerides from VLDL$_1$ to LDL. This results in formation of triglyceride-rich LDL. These lipoprotein particles are the preferred substrate for hepatic lipase (HL) that depletes triglycerides from the triglyceride-rich LDL. As large triglyceride-rich VLDL$_1$ particles are the substrate for CETP, accumulation of TRLs is a prerequisite for sdLDL formation (Adiels et al. 2006b; Packard 2003; Georgieva et al. 2004). The enzymes also act on HDL, resulting in the formation of sdHDL that are efficiently removed from circulation. The combined action of CETP and HL thus results in the formation of sdLDL and low HDL cholesterol (Verges 2005; Taskinen 2003). Several studies indicate that increased sdLDL is associated with increased CVD risk (Austin et al. 1990; Lamarche et al. 1997; Gardner et al. 1996; Vakkilainen et al. 2003). However, it is still unclear if sdLDL is a marker of an atherogenic dyslipidemia or causatively linked to the increased CVD risk (Sacks and Campos 2003).

To elucidate the pathophysiology of the hypertriglyceridemia in obese subjects we have performed a series of kinetic studies with stable isotopes. These studies have shown that the impaired lipid metabolism is caused by dual mechanisms: increased secretion of triglyceride-rich $VLDL_1$ from the liver and delayed clearance of TRLs from the circulation (Borén et al. 2015; Taskinen et al. 2011). This is illustrated in Fig. 2 by two pathways: a *synthesis pathway* and a *clearance pathway*. Interestingly, the *synthesis pathway* explained only 20% of the variation of plasma triglycerides (Borén et al. 2015). In contrast, the *clearance pathway* explained 50% of the variation in the total plasma triglycerides. Thus, the impaired catabolism of $VLDL_1$-triglycerides is the most important determinant of the plasma triglyceride concentration in subjects with abdominal obesity and dyslipidemia.

The *synthesis pathway* includes liver fat and total fat mass as these remained independent predictors of $VLDL_1$-triglyceride secretion rate in a stepwise multivariable regression analysis (Borén et al. 2015). Increased liver fat is linked to impaired regulation of VLDL production and a continuous oversecretion of $VLDL_1$ (Adiels

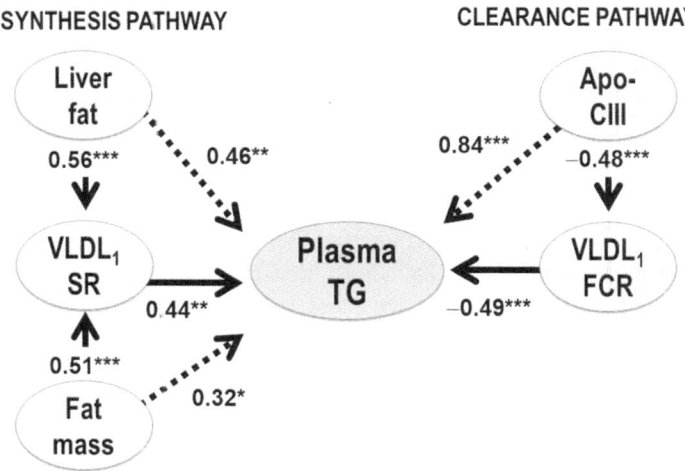

Fig. 2 *Predictors of $VLDL_1$-triglyceride secretion and catabolism.* Liver fat content ($P < 0.01$) and total fat mass ($P < 0.05$) are important independent predictors of VLDL1-TG secretion rate (SR). The plasma concentration of apoC-III correlated strongly with plasma TG and the fractional catabolism of $VLDL_1$-TG. $VLDL_1$-TG kinetics explained 76% of the variation in the total plasma triglycerides. Of these, ≈20% was explained by the secretion pathway, whereas ≈50% was explained by the clearance pathway. Thus, indices of catabolism were stronger predictors of plasma triglycerides than parameters of secretion. The associations between liver fat and fat mass vs plasma TG (dotted lines) are likely secondary and mediated via $VLDL_1$ SR. Likewise, the direct effect of apoC-III on plasma TG (dotted line) is likely explained by effect(s) of apoC-III beyond lipoprotein lipase-independent pathways of triglyceride metabolism (Borén et al. 2015)

et al. 2006b; Poulsen et al. 2016) (Fig. 2), and adipose tissue is the major source of fatty acids in the NEFA pool that determines the hepatic uptake of fatty acids. In the *clearance pathway*, the plasma concentration of apoC-III is shown to correlate strongly with plasma triglycerides and clearance of VLDL$_1$-triglycerides.

8   Regulation of Hydrolysis of TRLs and the LPL Pathway

The clearance of triglycerides is directly linked to the lipolysis of TRLs by LPL (Ginsberg et al. 1986). Full activity of LPL requires the interaction with the transport protein glycosylphosphatidylinositol anchored high density lipoprotein binding protein 1 (GPI-HBP1) and the lipase maturation factor 1 (LMF 1) present at the surface of capillaries (Sandesara et al. 2019). The LPL activity is modulated by several regulators including apoC-I, apoC-II, apoC-III, angiopoietin-like 3 (ANGPTL3), ANGPTL4 and ANGPTL8 (Kersten 2014). Insulin and apoC-III are the key regulators of LPL activity. Insulin stimulates the expression of LPL in endothelial cells whereas apoC-III inhibits LPL activity and thereby reduces the clearance of TRLs (Ginsberg and Brown 2011; Zheng et al. 2010; Yao 2012). The seminal role of LPL for the catabolic rate of TRLs and the conversion of large VLDL particles into smaller particles is demonstrated in studies in subjects with LPL gene mutations (Ooi et al. 2012). In addition, strong evidence supports the critical roles of apoC-III and apoE for suppressing or stimulating, respectively, clearance of apoB-containing lipoproteins from the circulation (Mendivil et al. 2010; Sacks 2015; Zheng et al. 2007).

ApoC-III is displacing apo-CII, an activator of LPL, from lipoprotein surfaces and thus impairing the actual lipolytic process (Sacks 2015; Gordts et al. 2016; Larsson et al. 2013). In addition, apoC-III has a wide range of actions action on triglyceride metabolism beyond its LPL-dependent effects (Taskinen and Boren 2015; Norata et al. 2015). For example, apoC-III interferes with the binding of apoB and apoE to hepatic lipoprotein receptors including heparin sulfate proteoglycan receptor (HSPG), low-density lipoprotein receptors (LDLR), and LDLR related protein 1 receptor (LRPl). This raises the option that high apoC-III would also inhibit the receptor mediated hepatic uptake of TRL remnants (Huff and Hegele 2013). The fact that an apoC-III ASO (antisense oligonucleotides) that inhibits apoC-III synthesis greatly reduced serum triglycerides in subjects with *familial LPL deficiency* demonstrates that apoC-III inhibits also hepatic clearance of remnants by LPL-independent pathways (Gaudet et al. 2014). However, recent results indicate that apoC-III inhibits turnover of TRLs primarily through a hepatic clearance mechanism mediated by the LDLR/LRPl axis, since apoC-III ASO treatment in LDLR/LRP1 deficient mice did not lower plasma TG levels (Gordts et al. 2016). Interestingly, we have recently reported that apoC-III metabolism is significantly perturbed in subjects with type 2 diabetes and that the apoC-III secretion rate was markedly higher in subjects with diabetes compared with BMI-matched non-diabetic subjects (Adiels et al. 2019). Improved glycemic control with liraglutide therapy reduced significantly apoC-III secretion rate and, thereby, apoC-III levels in type

2 diabetic subjects (Matikainen et al. 2019). These findings suggest that glucose homeostasis is a regulator of apoC-III metabolism and that the secretion rate of apoC-III seems to be an important driver for the elevation of TRLs in type 2 diabetes.

Angiopoietin-like protein (ANGPTL) family includes three members (ANGPTL3, ANGPTL4, and ANGPTL8) that are important modulators of lipoprotein metabolism (Kersten 2017; Christopoulou et al. 2019; Romeo et al. 2009; Li et al. 2020). Both ANGPTL3 and ANGPTL4 are endogenous inhibitors of LPL, and loss-of-function (LOF) mutations in ANGPTL3 and 4 associate with low triglyceride levels (Romeo et al. 2009; Minicocci et al. 2013; Zhang 2012) and reduced CVD risk (Dewey et al. 2017; Myocardial Infarction Genetics Investigators CAEC et al. 2016; Dewey et al. 2016). ANGPTL3 deficiency has been reported to reduce hepatic VLDL secretion and lower LDL-cholesterol (Wang et al. 2015a). Interestingly, ANGPTL3 gene silencing has been shown to associate not only with reduced hepatic secretion of apoB-containing lipoproteins, but also with enhanced uptake of particles via the LDL receptor. This likely explains the reduction of IDL cholesterol levels in subjects with familial hypobetalipoproteinemia (Xu et al. 2018). Consequently, targeting ANGPTL3 and ANGPTL4 genes has emerged as a promising goal for triglyceride lowering therapies (Tsimikas 2018; Gaudet et al. 2017a; Keech and Jenkins 2017; Bauer et al. 2016).

The inhibitory action of ANGPTL8 on LPL function requests the presence of ANGPTL3 (Kersten 2017; Haller et al. 2017; Luo and Peng 2018), as ANGPTL8 seems to enhance the inhibitory action of ANGPTL3 on LPL (Chi et al. 2017). Interestingly, these two proteins seem to work together to orchestrate responses of both glucose and lipid metabolism in fasting and in feeding (Wang et al. 2015b). Interestingly, ANGPTL3 is exclusively expressed in the liver being as a true hepatokine while ANGPTL8 is expressed both in adipose tissue and in the liver. The co-operative action of these two proteins seems to regulate the uptake of triglyceride-derived fatty acids either in the adipose tissue for storage or in cardiomyocytes and skeletal muscle for oxidation (Li et al. 2020; Vatner et al. 2018; Davies 2018).

ApoE plays a pivotal role in both triglyceride and cholesterol metabolism (Marais 2019). It predominantly associates with triglyceride-rich lipoproteins to mediate the clearance of their remnants after enzymatic lipolysis in the circulation (Marais 2019; Mahley and Huang 2007; Nakajima et al. 2019). Plasma levels of apoE and other lipids and lipoproteins are under strong genetic influence by *APOE* polymorphism – a combination of two genetic variants (rs429358 and rs7412) giving rise to six common *APOE* genotypes, ε22, ε32, ε33, ε42, ε43, and ε44 (Marais 2019; Mahley and Huang 2007). Both ε2 and ε4 alleles are associated with unfavorable lipid profiles, and the ε4 allele is a strong genetic risk factor for Alzheimer disease and by far the strongest hit in genome-wide association studies of longevity. The apoE variants relate to different amino acids at positions 112 and 158: cysteine in both for apoE2, arginine at both sites for apoE4, and respectively cysteine and arginine for apoE3 that is viewed as the wild type. High levels of plasma apoE have been shown to associate with increased risk of ischemic heart disease (Rasmussen et al. 2019). Hence both a quantitative importance of plasma apoE levels and a qualitative genetically determined effect appear to be important for cardiovascular disease (Rasmussen et al. 2019).

9   Role of Triglyceride-Rich Lipoproteins in Atherogenesis

It is well established that hypercholesterolemia is causatively linked to atherosclerotic cardiovascular disease and that lowering of cholesterol-rich LDL levels reduces cardiovascular events (Boren et al. 2020). However, cholesterol-lowering medication only prevents up to half of these events. Recent advances in human genetics indicate that the remaining "residual risk" of ASCVD is linked to elevated plasma triglyceride levels. Since triglyceride itself is not thought to contribute to atherogenesis, a consensus view has emerged that the remaining risk is linked to increased formation of "remnant" particles. These are derived from TRLs in the blood when the triglycerides are removed by the enzyme LPL (Boren et al. 2020). The remnant particles are not efficiently lowered by the available cholesterol-lowering medications.

To enter the artery wall, lipoproteins must cross the endothelium by transcytosis, a vesicular transport process. While chylomicrons and large VLDLs cannot undergo transcytosis because of their size, smaller chylomicron and VLDL remnants can and do penetrate the arterial wall. Thus, TRL remnants, in addition to LDL, may be retained in the arterial wall (Chapman et al. 2011). Even though remnant particles remain richer in triglycerides than cholesterol, their large size means that they contain up to twofold more cholesterol content per particle than LDL. However, the relative atherogenicity of remnants relative to LDL remains unclear.

10   Therapies to Reduce Triglyceride-Rich Lipoproteins

Lifestyle changes to lower plasma triglycerides – The first approach to lower moderately increased plasma triglycerides is to alter lifestyle (Laufs et al. 2020). Focus on a healthier diet and physical activity are cornerstones of lifestyle recommendations. Patients should reduce net caloric intake and lessen intake of sucrose, fructose, and alcohol. Diets rich in saturated fatty acids should be replaced with food enriched in monounsaturated and polyunsaturated fat (Laufs et al. 2020). It should be remembered though that scientific evidence for dietary recommendations is sparse. In addition, it is genuinely hard to persuade patients to change lifestyle and to make lifestyle changes that last. Thus, pharmaceutical approaches are often required.

Pharmacological therapies to lower plasma triglycerides – All commonly used cholesterol-lowering drugs as statins, ezetimibe, PCSK9 inhibitors only discreetly reduce triglyceride levels (around 5–15%), even though statins are somewhat more efficiently in reducing triglycerides and TRL remnants than PCSK9 inhibitors. Fibrates, omega-3-fatty acids, and niacin are somewhat more efficiently in reducing triglyceride levels (25–45%).

Fibrates are agonists of peroxisome proliferator-activated receptor-α (PPAR-α), acting via transcription factors regulating on lipid and lipoprotein metabolism. The drug has good efficacy in lowering fasting TG levels, as well as postprandial triglycerides and TRL remnants, albeit with marked interindividual variation. In addition, a small LDL-C increase may be observed in subjects with high triglyceride levels. The cardiovascular benefits have been shown to be heterogeneous and less robust than that of statins; when used as monotherapy, fibrates have been demonstrated to reduce CVD risk. However, when used in combination with statins no further reduction in CVD risk was demonstrated, although subgroup analysis indicates that hypertriglyceridemic patients with low HDL-C may benefit from such combination therapy. Results from ongoing trials using pemafibrate, a selective peroxisome proliferator-activated receptor alpha (PPARα) receptor agonist, will show if this approach will be successful (Pradhan et al. 2018).

For decades, omega-3-fatty acids have been used to lower plasma triglycerides and to prevent CVD (Bays et al. 2008). The results from two recent clinical trials using different omega-3 fatty acids have been mixed and somewhat confusing. The REDUCE-IT trial used icosapent ethyl omega-3 fatty acid (4 g daily). The results were positive and resulted in a 25% reduction in CVD and a 20% reduction in plasma triglyceride levels. Interestingly, the treatment also reduced plasma C-reactive protein by 40% (Bhatt et al. 2019). These results strengthen the link between plasma triglycerides and CVD (Myocardial Infarction Genetics Investigators CAEC et al. 2016; Do et al. 2013, 2015). However, the reduction of cardiovascular event was independent of plasma triglyceride levels both at baseline and on treatment, indicating that the reduction of cardiovascular events was only modest due to changes in TRL levels. One potential explanation for the clinical benefits could be the marked attenuation of the postprandial response by eicosapentaenoic acid, the hydrolytic product of icosapent ethyl, as 58% of the study participants had type 2 diabetes that commonly have prolonged postprandial hypertriglyceridemia (Taskinen and Boren 2015). In contrast to the positive outcome from the REDUCE-IT trial, the STRENGTH trial using another omega-3 fatty acid formulation (a combination of eicosapentaenoic acid and docosahexaenoic acid) failed to demonstrate any clinical benefit. The explanation(s) for the different outcomes is still unclear Possible reasons include that the two trials studied different type of omega-3 fatty acids, and that the REDUCE-IT trial used mineral oil as placebo which may have adverse effects, whereas STRENGTH used a corn oil placebo. A recent Cochrane review of 86 randomized controlled trials with 162,796 participants concluded "evidence suggests that increasing long-chain omega-3 slightly reduces risk of coronary heart disease mortality and events, and reduces serum triglycerides" (Abdelhamid et al. 2020).

The 2019 ESC/EAS guidelines for the management of dyslipidemias recommend that statin treatment remains the first choice for managing high triglycerides (triglycerides >200 mg/dL or 2.3 mmol/L) (Mach et al. 2020). However, the guidelines have taken account of evidence from REDUCE-IT and recommend n-3 PUFAs (particularly icosapent ethyl 2×2 g daily) in high-risk patients with persistently elevated plasma triglycerides (between 135 and 499 mg/dL or 1.5 and

5.6 mmol/L) despite statin treatment. In high-risk patients at LDL-C goal with TG >200 mg/dL or >2.3 mmol/L, fenofibrate or bezafibrate may be considered in combination with statins (Mach et al. 2020).

11 Development of Novel Interventions

Efficient interventions to reduce plasma levels of TRLs and TRL remnants are still missing, and development of the development of strategies to treat the large numbers of hypertriglyceridemic individuals who currently remain at high risk of ASCVD despite optimal treatment according to current guidelines is urgently needed. Genetic studies have demonstrated that apoC-III and angiopoietin-like protein 3 (Angptl3) are critical regulators of triglyceride metabolism, and both have been developed as drug targets.

Statins and omega-3 fatty acids modestly reduce plasma apoC-III levels by less than 20% (Ooi et al. 2008; Maki et al. 2011; Morton et al. 2016; Dunbar et al. 2015). However, development of antisense oligos and siRNA has made it possible to develop high efficiency therapies. For example, antisense therapeutic oligonucleotides conjugated with N-acetyl galactosamine-conjugated (GalNAc) adducts (i.e., the ligand of the hepatic asialoglycoprotein receptor) have been developed. These are very efficient in reducing *APOC3* expression (Graham et al. 2013). For example, results from the APPROACH trial, a 52-week randomized, double-blind, phase 3 in 66 patients with familial chylomicronemia syndrome, demonstrated that the drug resulted in an impressive 77% decrease in plasma triglyceride levels (Witztum et al. 2019). The antisense therapeutic oligonucleotides have also been shown to markedly lower plasma apoC-III and triglycerides levels in subjects with severe or uncontrolled hypertriglyceridemia (Gaudet et al. 2015; Gouni-Berthold 2017) and in subjects with diabetic dyslipidemia (Digenio et al. 2016). Intriguingly, the intervention not only improved the diabetic dyslipidemia, but also improved whole-body insulin sensitivity (by 57%).

To target Angptl3, both a monoclonal antibody and therapeutic oligonucleotides have been developed. Recent results have demonstrated that anti-ANGPTL3 therapies reduce both marked hypertriglyceridemia (around 75% reduction) and severely elevated LDL-cholesterol in subjects with familial hypercholesterolemia (around 23% reduction) (Gaudet et al. 2017b). The finding that anti-Angptl3 lowers LDL-C in subjects lacking functional LDL receptors indicates that the underlying mechanism is independent of the LDL receptor pathway. In line, a GalNac-modified antisense-oligonucleotide has recently been shown to reduce both plasma triglycerides and LDL-cholesterol (by 63.1% and 32.9%, respectively) (Graham et al. 2017). Interestingly, results from murine models indicate that the antisense-oligonucleotide seems to reduce hepatic steatosis. These results have prompted ongoing human studies.

Other ongoing projects involve lipoprotein lipase gene therapy, oral inhibitors of intestinal DGAT1 to reduce dietary fat absorption and triglyceride synthesis, and treatments targeting apoC-III and Angptl4 (Laufs et al. 2020).

12 Conclusion

Whether plasma triglycerides constitute an independent risk factor for CVD has been debated for decades, but there is now strong support for a causative role of TRLs in CVD. These studies equally indicate that cholesterol-enriched TRL remnant play a key role in the pathophysiology of atherosclerotic vascular disease. We are now beginning to understand the complex regulation of triglyceride metabolism. Hopefully, this molecular understanding will be translated into targeted treatment for the atherogenic dyslipidemia associated with hypertriglyceridemia.

References

Abdelhamid AS, Brown TJ, Brainard JS, Biswas P, Thorpe GC, Moore HJ, Deane KH, Summerbell CD, Worthington HV, Song F, Hooper L (2020) Omega-3 fatty acids for the primary and secondary prevention of cardiovascular disease. Cochrane Database Syst Rev 3:CD003177

Adiels M, Packard C, Caslake MJ, Stewart P, Soro A, Westerbacka J, Wennberg B, Olofsson SO, Taskinen MR, Boren J (2005) A new combined multicompartmental model for apolipoprotein B-100 and triglyceride metabolism in VLDL subfractions. J Lipid Res 46(1):58–67

Adiels M, Olofsson SO, Taskinen MR, Boren J (2006a) Diabetic dyslipidaemia. Curr Opin Lipidol 17(3):238–246

Adiels M, Taskinen MR, Packard C, Caslake MJ, Soro-Paavonen A, Westerbacka J, Vehkavaara S, Hakkinen A, Olofsson SO, Yki-Jarvinen H, Boren J (2006b) Overproduction of large VLDL particles is driven by increased liver fat content in man. Diabetologia 49(4):755–765

Adiels M, Matikainen N, Westerbacka J, Soderlund S, Larsson T, Olofsson SO, Boren J, Taskinen MR (2012) Postprandial accumulation of chylomicrons and chylomicron remnants is determined by the clearance capacity. Atherosclerosis 222(1):222–228

Adiels M, Taskinen MR, Bjornson E, Andersson L, Matikainen N, Soderlund S, Kahri J, Hakkarainen A, Lundbom N, Sihlbom C, Thorsell A, Zhou H, Pietilainen KH, Packard C, Boren J (2019) Role of apolipoprotein C-III overproduction in diabetic dyslipidaemia. Diabetes Obes Metab 21(8):1861–1870

Aguilar-Salinas CA, Barrett PH, Parhofer KG, Young SG, Tessereau D, Bateman J, Quinn C, Schonfeld G (1995) Apcprotein B-100 production is decreased in subjects heterozygous for truncations of apoprotein B. Arterioscler Thromb Vasc Biol 15(1):71–80

Anant S, Davidson NO (2001) Molecular mechanisms of apolipoprotein B mRNA editing. Curr Opin Lipidol 12(2):159–165

Asp L, Magnusson B, Rutberg M, Li L, Boren J, Olofsson SO (2005) Role of ADP ribosylation factor 1 in the assembly and secretion of ApoB-100-containing lipoproteins. Arterioscler Thromb Vasc Biol 25(3):566–570

Austin MA, King M-C, Vranizan KM, Krauss RM (1990) Atherogenic lipoprotein phenotype. A proposed genetic marker for coronary heart disease risk. Circulation 82:495–506

Barrows BR, Parks EJ (2006) Contributions of different fatty acid sources to very low-density lipoprotein-triacylglycerol in the fasted and fed states. J Clin Endocrinol Metab 91 (4):1446–1452

Bauer RC, Khetarpal SA, Hand NJ, Rader DJ (2016) Therapeutic targets of triglyceride metabolism as informed by human genetics. Trends Mol Med 22(4):328–340

Bays HE, Tighe AP, Sadovsky R, Davidson MH (2008) Prescription omega-3 fatty acids and their lipid effects: physiologic mechanisms of action and clinical implications. Expert Rev Cardiovasc Ther 6(3):391–409

Bhatt DL, Steg PG, Miller M, Brinton EA, Jacobson TA, Ketchum SB, Doyle RT Jr, Juliano RA, Jiao L, Granowitz C, Tardif JC, Ballantyne CM, Investigators R-I (2019) Cardiovascular risk reduction with icosapent ethyl for hypertriglyceridemia. N Engl J Med 380(1):11–22

Bjornson E, Packard CJ, Adiels M, Andersson L, Matikainen N, Soderlund S, Kahri J, Hakkarainen A, Lundbom N, Lundbom J, Sihlbom C, Thorsell A, Zhou H, Taskinen MR, Boren J (2019a) Apolipoprotein B48 metabolism in chylomicrons and very low-density lipoproteins and its role in triglyceride transport in normo- and hypertriglyceridemic human subjects. J Intern Med 288(4):422–438

Bjornson E, Packard CJ, Adiels M, Andersson L, Matikainen N, Soderlund S, Kahri J, Sihlbom C, Thorsell A, Zhou H, Taskinen MR, Boren J (2019b) Investigation of human apoB48 metabolism using a new, integrated non-steady-state model of apoB48 and apoB100 kinetics. J Intern Med 285(5):562–577

Boren J, Graham L, Wettesten M, Scott J, White A, Olofsson SO (1992) The assembly and secretion of ApoB 100-containing lipoproteins in Hep G2 cells. ApoB 100 is cotranslationally integrated into lipoproteins. J Biol Chem 267(14):9858–9867

Boren J, Matikainen N, Adiels M, Taskinen MR (2014) Postprandial hypertriglyceridemia as a coronary risk factor. Clin Chim Acta 431:131–142

Borén J, Watts GF, Adiels M, Söderlund S, Chan DC, Hakkarainen A, Lundbom N, Matikainen N, Kahri J, Vergès B, Barrett PHR, Taskinen M (2015) Kinetic and related determinants of plasma triglyceride concentration in abdominal obesity. Multicenter Tracer Kinetic Study. Arterioscler Thromb Vasc Biol 35(10):2218–2224

Boren J, Chapman MJ, Krauss RM, Packard CJ, Bentzon JF, Binder CJ, Daemen MJ, Demer LL, Hegele RA, Nicholls SJ, Nordestgaard BG, Watts GF, Bruckert E, Fazio S, Ference BA, Graham I, Horton JD, Landmesser U, Laufs U, Masana L, Pasterkamp G, Raal FJ, Ray KK, Schunkert H, Taskinen MR, van de Sluis B, Wiklund O, Tokgozoglu L, Catapano AL, Ginsberg HN (2020) Low-density lipoproteins cause atherosclerotic cardiovascular disease: pathophysiological, genetic, and therapeutic insights: a consensus statement from the European Atherosclerosis Society Consensus Panel. Eur Heart J 41(24):2313–2330

Bostrom K, Boren J, Wettesten M, Sjoberg A, Bondjers G, Wiklund O, Carlsson P, Olofsson SO (1988) Studies on the assembly of apo B-100-containing lipoproteins in HepG2 cells. J Biol Chem 263(9):4434–4442

Browning JD, Horton JD (2004) Molecular mediators of hepatic steatosis and liver injury. J Clin Invest 114(2):147–152

Chao L, Marcus-Samuels B, Mason MM, Moitra J, Vinson C, Arioglu E, Gavrilova O, Reitman ML (2000) Adipose tissue is required for the antidiabetic, but not for the hypolipidemic, effect of thiazolidinediones. J Clin Invest 106(10):1221–1228

Chapman MJ, Ginsberg HN, Amarenco P, Andreotti F, Boren J, Catapano AL, Descamps OS, Fisher E, Kovanen PT, Kuivenhoven JA, Lesnik P, Masana L, Nordestgaard BG, Ray KK, Reiner Z, Taskinen MR, Tokgozoglu L, Tybjaerg-Hansen A, Watts GF, European Atherosclerosis Society Consensus Panel (2011) Triglyceride-rich lipoproteins and high-density lipoprotein cholesterol in patients at high risk of cardiovascular disease: evidence and guidance for management. Eur Heart J 32(11):1345–1361

Chavez-Jauregui RN, Mattes RD, Parks EJ (2010) Dynamics of fat absorption and effect of sham feeding on postprandial lipema. Gastroenterology 139(5):1538–1548

Chi X, Britt EC, Shows HW, Hjelmaas AJ, Shetty SK, Cushing EM, Li W, Dou A, Zhang R, Davies BSJ (2017) ANGPTL8 promotes the ability of ANGPTL3 to bind and inhibit lipoprotein lipase. Mol Metab 6(10):1137–1149

Christopoulou E, Elisaf M, Filippatos T (2019) Effects of angiopoietin-like 3 on triglyceride regulation, glucose homeostasis, and diabetes. Dis Markers 2019:6578327

Cohn JS, Johnson EJ, Millar JS, Cohn SD, Milne RW, Marcel YL, Russell RM, Schaefer EJ (1993) Contribution of apoB-48 and apoB-100 triglyceride-rich lipoproteins (TRL) to postprandial increases in the plasma concentration of TRL triglycerides and retinyl esters. J Lipid Res 34 (12):2033–2040

Dallinga-Thie GM, Franssen R, Mooij HL, Visser ME, Hassing HC, Peelman F, Kastelein JJ, Peterfy M, Nieuwdorp M (2010) The metabolism of triglyceride-rich lipoproteins revisited: new players, new insight. Atherosclerosis 211(1):1–8

Dallinga-Thie GM, Kroon J, Boren J, Chapman MJ (2016) Triglyceride-rich lipoproteins and remnants: targets for therapy? Curr Cardiol Rep 18(7):67

Davidson NO, Shelness GS (2000) APOLIPOPROTEIN B: mRNA editing, lipoprotein assembly, and presecretory degradation. Annu Rev Nutr 20:169–193

Davies BSJ (2018) Can targeting ANGPTL proteins improve glucose tolerance? Diabetologia 61 (6):1277–1281

Dewey FE, Gusarova V, O'Dushlaine C, Gottesman O, Trejos J, Hunt C, Van Hout CV, Habegger L, Buckler D, Lai KM, Leader JB, Murray MF, Ritchie MD, Kirchner HL, Ledbetter DH, Penn J, Lopez A, Borecki IB, Overton JD, Reid JG, Carey DJ, Murphy AJ, Yancopoulos GD, Baras A, Gromada J, Shuldiner AR (2016) Inactivating variants in ANGPTL4 and risk of coronary artery disease. N Engl J Med 374(12):1123–1133

Dewey FE, Gusarova V, Dunbar RL, O'Dushlaine C, Schurmann C, Gottesman O, McCarthy S, Van Hout CV, Bruse S, Dansky HM, Leader JB, Murray MF, Ritchie MD, Kirchner HL, Habegger L, Lopez A, Penn J, Zhao A, Shao W, Stahl N, Murphy AJ, Hamon S, Bouzelmat A, Zhang R, Shumel B, Pordy R, Gipe D, Herman GA, Sheu WHH, Lee IT, Liang KW, Guo X, Rotter JI, Chen YI, Kraus WE, Shah SH, Damrauer S, Small A, Rader DJ, Wulff AB, Nordestgaard BG, Tybjaerg-Hansen A, van den Hoek AM, Princen HMG, Ledbetter DH, Carey DJ, Overton JD, Reid JG, Sasiela WJ, Banerjee P, Shuldiner AR, Borecki IB, Teslovich TM, Yancopoulos GD. Mellis SJ, Gromada J, Baras A (2017) Genetic and pharmacologic inactivation of ANGPTL3 and cardiovascular disease. N Engl J Med 377(3):211–221

Digenio A, Dunbar RL, Alexander VJ, Hompesch M, Morrow L, Lee RG, Graham MJ, Hughes SG, Yu R, Singleton W, Baker BF, Bhanot S, Crooke RM (2016) Antisense-mediated lowering of plasma apolipoprotein C-III by volanesorsen improves dyslipidemia and insulin sensitivity in type 2 diabetes. Diabetes Care 39(8):1408–1415

Do R, Willer CJ, Schmidt EM, Sengupta S, Gao C, Peloso GM, Gustafsson S, Kanoni S, Ganna A, Chen J, Buchkovich ML, Mora S, Beckmann JS, Bragg-Gresham JL, Chang HY, Demirkan A, Den Hertog HM, Donnelly LA, Ehret GB, Esko T, Feitosa MF, Ferreira T, Fischer K, Fontanillas P, Fraser RM, Freitag DF, Gurdasani D, Heikkila K, Hypponen E, Isaacs A, Jackson AU, Johansson A, Johnson T, Kaakinen M, Kettunen J, Kleber ME, Li X, Luan J, Lyytikainen LP, Magnusson PK, Mangino M, Mihailov E, Montasser ME, Muller-Nurasyid M, Nolte IM, O'Connell JR, Palmer CD, Perola M, Petersen AK, Sanna S, Saxena R, Service SK, Shah S, Shungin D, Sidore C, Song C, Strawbridge RJ, Surakka I, Tanaka T, Teslovich TM, Thorleifsson G, Van den Herik EG, Voight BF, Volcik KA, Waite LL, Wong A, Wu Y, Zhang W, Absher D, Asiki G, Barroso I, Been LF, Bolton JL, Bonnycastle LL, Brambilla P, Burnett MS, Cesana G, Dimitriou M, Doney AS, Doring A, Elliott P, Epstein SE, Eyjolfsson GI, Gigante B, Goodarzi MO, Grallert H, Gravito ML, Groves CJ, Hallmans G, Hartikainen AL, Hayward C, Hernandez D, Hicks AA, Holm H, Hung YJ, Illig T, Jones MR, Kaleebu P, Kastelein JJ, Khaw KT, Kim E, Klopp N, Komulainen P, Kumari M, Langenberg C, Lehtimaki T, Lin SY, Lindstrom J, Loos RJ, Mach F, WL MA, Meisinger C, Mitchell BD, Muller G, Nagaraja R, Narisu N, Nieminen TV, Nsubuga RN, Olafsson I, Ong KK, Palotie A, Papamarkou T, Pomilla C, Pouta A, Rader DJ, Reilly MP, Ridker PM, Rivadeneira F, Rudan I, Ruokonen A, Samani N, Scharnagl H, Seeley J, Silander K, Stancakova A, Stirrups K, Swift AJ, Tiret L, Uitterlinden AG, van Pelt LJ, Vedantam S, Wainwright N, Wijmenga C, Wild SH, Willemsen G, Wilsgaard T, Wilson JF, Young EH, Zhao JH, Adair LS, Arveiler D, Assimes TL, Bandinelli S, Bennett F, Bochud M, Boehm BO, Boomsma DI, Borecki IB, Bornstein SR, Bovet P, Burnier M, Campbell H, Chakravarti A, Chambers JC, Chen YD, Collins FS, Cooper RS, Danesh J, Dedoussis G, de Faire U, Feranil AB, Ferrieres J, Ferrucci L, Freimer NB, Gieger C, Groop LC, Gudnason V, Gyllensten U, Hamsten A, Harris TB, Hingorani A, Hirschhorn JN, Hofman A, Hovingh GK, Hsiung CA, Humphries SE, Hunt SC, Hveem K, Iribarren C, Jarvelin MR, Jula A, Kahonen M, Kaprio J, Kesaniemi A, Kivimaki M, Kooner JS,

Koudstaal PJ, Krauss RM, Kuh D, Kuusisto J, Kyvik KO, Laakso M, Lakka TA, Lind L, Lindgren CM, Martin NG, Marz W, MI MC, CA MK, Meneton P, Metspalu A, Moilanen L, Morris AD, Munroe PB, Njolstad I, Pedersen NL, Power C, Pramstaller PP, Price JF, Psaty BM, Quertermous T, Rauramaa R, Saleheen D, Salomaa V, Sanghera DK, Saramies J, Schwarz PE, Sheu WH, Shuldiner AR, Siegbahn A, Spector TD, Stefansson K, Strachan DP, Tayo BO, Tremoli E, Tuomilehto J, Uusitupa M, van Duijn CM, Vollenweider P, Wallentin L, Wareham NJ, Whitfield JB, Wolffenbuttel BH, Altshuler D, Ordovas JM, Boerwinkle E, Palmer CN, Thorsteinsdottir U, Chasman DI, Rotter JI, Franks PW, Ripatti S, Cupples LA, Sandhu MS, Rich SS, Boehnke M, Deloukas P, Mohlke KL, Ingelsson E, Abecasis GR, Daly MJ, Neale BM, Kathiresan S (2013) Common variants associated with plasma triglycerides and risk for coronary artery disease. Nat Genet 45(11):1345–1352

Do R, Stitziel NO, Won HH, Jorgensen AB, Duga S, Angelica Merlini P, Kiezun A, Farrall M, Goel A, Zuk O, Guella I, Asselta R, Lange LA, Peloso GM, Auer PL, NES P, Girelli D, Martinelli N, Farlow DN, MA DP, Roberts R, Stewart AF, Saleheen D, Danesh J, Epstein SE, Sivapalaratnam S, Hovingh GK, Kastelein JJ, Samani NJ, Schunkert H, Erdmann J, Shah SH, Kraus WE, Davies R, Nikpay M, Johansen CT, Wang J, Hegele RA, Hechter E, Marz W, Kleber ME, Huang J, Johnson AD, Li M, Burke GL, Gross M, Liu Y, Assimes TL, Heiss G, Lange EM, Folsom AR, Taylor HA, Olivieri O, Hamsten A, Clarke R, Reilly DF, Yin W, Rivas MA, Donnelly P, Rossouw JE, Psaty BM, Herrington DM, Wilson JG, Rich SS, Bamshad MJ, Tracy RP, Cupples LA, Rader DJ, Reilly MP, Spertus JA, Cresci S, Hartiala J, Tang WH, Hazen SL, Allayee H, Reiner AP, Carlson CS, Kooperberg C, Jackson RD, Boerwinkle E, Lander ES, Schwartz SM, Siscovick DS, McPherson R, Tybjaerg-Hansen A, Abecasis GR, Watkins H, Nickerson DA, Ardissino D, Sunyaev SR, O'Donnell CJ, Altshuler D, Gabriel S, Kathiresan S (2015) Exome sequencing identifies rare LDLR and APOA5 alleles conferring risk for myocardial infarction. Nature 518(7537):102–106

Donnelly KL, Smith CI, Schwarzenberg SJ, Jessurun J, Boldt MD, Parks EJ (2005) Sources of fatty acids stored in liver and secreted via lipoproteins in patients with nonalcoholic fatty liver disease. J Clin Invest 115(5):1343–1351

Dunbar RL, Nicholls SJ, Maki KC, Roth EM, Orloff DG, Curcio D, Johnson J, Kling D, Davidson MH (2015) Effects of omega-3 carboxylic acids on lipoprotein particles and other cardiovascular risk markers in high-risk statin-treated patients with residual hypertriglyceridemia: a randomized, controlled, double-blind trial. Lipids Health Dis 14:98

Edvardsson U, Bergstrom M, Alexandersson M, Bamberg K, Ljung B, Dahllof B (1999) Rosiglitazone (BRL49653), a PPARgamma-selective agonist, causes peroxisome proliferator-like liver effects in obese mice. J Lipid Res 40(7):1177–1184

Elias N, Patterson BW, Schonfeld G (1999) Decreased production rates of VLDL triglycerides and ApoB-100 in subjects heterozygous for familial hypobetalipoproteinemia. Arterioscler Thromb Vasc Biol 19(11):2714–2721

Farquhar JW, Gross RC, Wagner RM, Reaven GM (1965) Validation of an incompletely coupled two-compartment nonrecycling catenary model for turnover of liver and plasma triglyceride in man. J Lipid Res 6:119–134

Fielding BA, Reid G, Grady M, Humphreys SM, Evans K, Frayn KN (2000) Ethanol with a mixed meal increases postprandial triacylglycerol but decreases postprandial non-esterified fatty acid concentrations. Br J Nutr 83(6):597–604

Gardner CD, Fortmann SP, Krauss RM (1996) Association of small low-density lipoprotein particles with the incidence of coronary artery disease in men and women. JAMA 276:875–881

Gaudet D, Brisson D, Tremblay K, Alexander VJ, Singleton W, Hughes SG, Geary RS, Baker BF, Graham MJ, Crooke RM, Witztum JL (2014) Targeting APOC3 in the familial chylomicronemia syndrome. N Engl J Med 371(23):2200–2206

Gaudet D, Alexander VJ, Baker BF, Brisson D, Tremblay K, Singleton W, Geary RS, Hughes SG, Viney NJ, Graham MJ, Crooke RM, Witztum JL, Brunzell JD, Kastelein JJ (2015) Antisense inhibition of apolipoprotein C-III in patients with hypertriglyceridemia. N Engl J Med 373 (5):438–447

Gaudet D, Drouin-Chartier JP, Couture P (2017a) Lipid metabolism and emerging targets for lipid-lowering therapy. Can J Cardiol 33(7):872–882

Gaudet D, Gipe DA, Porcy R, Ahmad Z, Cuchel M, Shah PK, Chyu KY, Sasiela WJ, Chan KC, Brisson D, Khoury E, Banerjee P, Gusarova V, Gromada J, Stahl N, Yancopoulos GD, Hovingh GK (2017b) ANGPTL3 inhibition in homozygous familial hypercholesterolemia. N Engl J Med 377(3):296–297

Gaw A, Packard CJ, Lindsay GM, Griffin BA, Caslake MJ, Lorimer AR, Shepherd J (1995) Overproduction of small very low density lipoproteins (Sf 20-60) in moderate hypercholesterolemia: relationships between apolipoprotein B kinetics and plasma lipoproteins. J Lipid Res 36 (1):158–171

Georgieva AM, van Greevenbroek MM, Krauss RM, Brouwers MC, Vermeulen VM, Robertus-Teunissen MG, van der Kallen CJ, de Bruin TW (2004) Subclasses of low-density lipoprotein and very low-density lipoprotein in familial combined hyperlipidemia: relationship to multiple lipoprotein phenotype. Arterioscler Thromb Vasc Biol 24(4):744–749

Gibbons GF, Islam K, Pease RJ (2000) Mobilisation of triacylglycerol stores. Biochim Biophys Acta 1483(1):37–57

Ginsberg HN, Brown WV (2011) Apolipoprotein CIII: 42 years old and even more interesting. Arterioscler Thromb Vasc Biol 31(3):471–473

Ginsberg HN, Le NA, Goldberg IJ, Gibson JC, Rubinstein A, Wang-Iverson P, Norum R, Brown WV, Apolipoprotein B (1986) Metabolism in subjects with deficiency of apolipoproteins CIII and AI. Evidence that apolipoprotein CIII inhibits catabolism of triglyceride-rich lipoproteins by lipoprotein lipase in vivo. J Clin Invest 78(5):1287–1295

Goldberg IJ (1996) Lipoprotein lipase and lipolysis: central roles in lipoprotein metabolism and atherogenesis. J Lipid Res 37(4):693–707

Gordts PL, Nock R, Son NH, Ramms B, Lew I, Gonzales JC, Thacker BE, Basu D, Lee RG, Mullick AE, Graham MJ, Goldberg IJ, Crooke RM, Witztum JL, Esko JD (2016) ApoC-III inhibits clearance of triglyceride-rich lipoproteins through LDL family receptors. J Clin Invest 126(8):2855–2866

Gouni-Berthold I (2017) The role of antisense oligonucleotide therapy against apolipoprotein-CIII in hypertriglyceridemia. Atheroscler Suppl 30:19–27

Graham MJ, Lee RG, Bell TA 3rd, Fu W, Mullick AE, Alexander VJ, Singleton W, Viney N, Geary R, Su J, Baker BF, Burkey J, Crooke ST, Crooke RM (2013) Antisense oligonucleotide inhibition of apolipoprotein C-III reduces plasma triglycerides in rodents, nonhuman primates, and humans. Circ Res 112(11):1479–1490

Graham MJ, Lee RG, Brandt TA, Tai LJ, Fu W, Peralta R, Yu R, Hurh E, Paz E, McEvoy BW, Baker BF, Pham NC, Digenio A, Hughes SG, Geary RS, Witztum JL, Crooke RM, Tsimikas S (2017) Cardiovascular and metabolic effects of ANGPTL3 antisense oligonucleotides. N Engl J Med 377(3):222–232

Gusarova V, Brodsky JL, Fisher EA (2003) Apolipoprotein B100 exit from the endoplasmic reticulum (ER) is COPII-dependent, and its lipidation to very low density lipoprotein occurs post-ER. J Biol Chem 278(48):48051–48058

Haller JF, Mintah IJ, Shihanian LM, Stevis P, Buckler D, Alexa-Braun CA, Kleiner S, Banfi S, Cohen JC, Hobbs HH, Yancopoulos GD, Murphy AJ, Gusarova V, Gromada J (2017) ANGPTL8 requires ANGPTL3 to inhibit lipoprotein lipase and plasma triglyceride clearance. J Lipid Res 58(6):1166–1173

Havel RJ (1961) Conversion of plasma free fatty acids into triglycerides of plasma lipoprotein fractions in man. Metabolism 10:1031–1034

Huff MW, Hegele RA (2013) Apolipoprotein C-III: going back to the future for a lipid drug target. Circ Res 112(11):1405–1408

Hussain MM, Fatma S, Pan X, Iqbal J (2005) Intestinal lipoprotein assembly. Curr Opin Lipidol 16 (3):281–285

James RW, Martin B, Pometta D, Fruchart JC, Duriez P, Puchois P, Farriaux JP, Tacquet A, Demant T, Clegg RJ et al (1989) Apolipoprotein B metabolism in homozygous familial hypercholesterolemia. J Lipid Res 30(2):159–169

Julve J, Martin-Campos JM, Escola-Gil JC, Blanco-Vaca F (2016) Chylomicrons: advances in biology, pathology, laboratory testing, and therapeutics. Clin Chim Acta 455:134–148

Karpe F, Bell M, Bjorkegren J, Hamsten A (1995) Quantification of postprandial triglyceride-rich lipoproteins in healthy men by retinyl ester labeling and simultaneous measurement of apolipoproteins B-48 and B-100. Arterioscler Thromb Vasc Biol 15(2):199–207

Keech AC, Jenkins AJ (2017) Triglyceride-lowering trials. Curr Opin Lipidol 28(6):477–487

Kersten S (2014) Physiological regulation of lipoprotein lipase. Biochim Biophys Acta 1841 (7):919–933

Kersten S (2017) Angiopoietin-like 3 in lipoprotein metabolism. Nat Rev Endocrinol 13 (12):731–739

Khan NA, Besnard P (2009) Oro-sensory perception of dietary lipids: new insights into the fat taste transduction. Biochim Biophys Acta 1791(3):149–155

Koo SH, Dutcher AK, Towle HC (2001) Glucose and insulin function through two distinct transcription factors to stimulate expression of lipogenic enzyme genes in liver. J Biol Chem 276(12):9437–9445

Lamarche B, Tchernof A, Moorjani S, Cantin B, Dagenais GR, Lupien PJ, Despres JP (1997) Small, dense low-density lipoprotein particles as a predictor of the risk of ischemic heart disease in men. Prospective results from the Quebec Cardiovascular Study. Circulation 95(1):69–75

Lambert JE, Parks EJ (2012) Postprandial metabolism of meal triglyceride in humans. Biochim Biophys Acta 1821(5):721–726

Larsson M, Vorrsjo E, Talmud P, Lookene A, Olivecrona G (2013) Apolipoproteins C-I and C-III inhibit lipoprotein lipase activity by displacement of the enzyme from lipid droplets. J Biol Chem 288(47):33997–34008

Laufs U, Parhofer KG, Ginsberg HN, Hegele RA (2020) Clinical review on triglycerides. Eur Heart J 41(1):99–109c

Lee J, Hegele RA (2014) Abetalipoproteinemia and homozygous hypobetalipoproteinemia: a framework for diagnosis and management. J Inherit Metab Dis 37(3):333–339

Li J, Li L, Guo D, Li S, Zeng Y, Liu C, Fu R, Huang M, Xie W (2020) Triglyceride metabolism and angiopoietin-like proteins in lipoprotein lipase regulation. Clin Chim Acta 503:19–34

Lichtenstein AH, Hachey DL, Millar JS, Jenner JL, Booth L, Ordovas J, Schaefer EJ (1992) Measurement of human apolipoprotein B-48 and B-100 kinetics in triglyceride-rich lipoproteins using [5,5,5-2H3]leucine. J Lipid Res 33(6):907–914

Linton MF, Farese RV Jr, Young SG (1993) Familial hypobetalipoproteinemia. J Lipid Res 34 (4):521–541

Luo M, Peng D (2018) ANGPTL8: an important regulator in metabolic disorders. Front Endocrinol (Lausanne) 9:169

Mach F, Baigent C, Catapano AL, Koskinas KC, Casula M, Badimon L, Chapman MJ, De Backer GG, Delgado V, Ference BA, Graham IM, Halliday A, Landmesser U, Mihaylova B, Pedersen TR, Riccardi G, Richter DJ, Sabatine MS, Taskinen MR, Tokgozoglu L, Wiklund O, ESC Scientific Document Group (2020) 2019 ESC/EAS guidelines for the management of dyslipidaemias: lipid modification to reduce cardiovascular risk. Eur Heart J 41(1):111–188

Mahley RW, Huang Y (2007) Atherogenic remnant lipoproteins: role for proteoglycans in trapping, transferring, and internalizing. J Clin Invest 117(1):94–98

Maki KC, Bays HE, Dicklin MR, Johnson SL, Shabbout M (2011) Effects of prescription omega-3-acid ethyl esters, coadministered with atorvastatin, on circulating levels of lipoprotein particles, apolipoprotein CIII, and lipoprotein-associated phospholipase A2 mass in men and women with mixed dyslipidemia. J Clin Lipidol 5(6):483–492

Marais AD (2019) Apolipoprotein E in lipoprotein metabolism, health and cardiovascular disease. Pathology 51(2):165–176

Matikainen N, Soderlund S, Bjornson E, Pietilainen K, Hakkarainen A, Lundbom N, Taskinen MR, Boren J (2019) Liraglutide treatment improves postprandial lipid metabolism and cardiometabolic risk factors in humans with adequately controlled type 2 diabetes: a single-centre randomized controlled study. Diabetes Obes Metab 21(1):84–94

Mattes RD (2002) Oral fat exposure increases the first phase triacylglycerol concentration due to release of stored lipid in humans. J Nutr 132(12):3656–3662

Mattes RD (2009) Brief oral stimulation, but especially oral fat exposure, elevates serum triglycerides in humans. Am J Physiol Gastrointest Liver Physiol 296(2):G365–G371

Mendivil CO, Zheng C, Furtado J, Lel J, Sacks FM (2010) Metabolism of very-low-density lipoprotein and low-density lipoprotein containing apolipoprotein C-III and not other small apolipoproteins. Arterioscler Thromb Vasc Biol 30(2):239–245

Minicocci I, Santini S, Cantisani V, Stitziel N, Kathiresan S, Arroyo JA, Marti G, Pisciotta L, Noto D, Cefalu AB, Maranghi M, Labbadia G, Pigna G, Pannozzo F, Ceci F, Ciociola E, Bertolini S, Calandra S, Tarugi P, Averna M, Arca M (2013) Clinical characteristics and plasma lipids in subjects with familial combined hypolipidemia: a pooled analysis. J Lipid Res 54 (12):3481–3490

Morton AM, Furtado JD, Lee J, Amerine W, Davidson MH, Sacks FM (2016) The effect of omega-3 carboxylic acids on apolipoprotein CIII-containing lipoproteins in severe hypertriglyceridemia. J Clin Lipidol 10(6):1442–1451.e4

Myocardial Infarction Genetics Investigators CAEC, Stitziel NO, Stirrups KE, Masca NG, Erdmann J, Ferrario PG, Konig IR, Weeke PE, Webb TR, Auer PL, Schick UM, Lu Y, Zhang H, Dube MP, Goel A, Farrall M, Peloso GM, Won HH, Do R, van Iperen E, Kanoni S, Kruppa J, Mahajan A, Scott RA, Willenberg C, Braund PS, van Capelleveen JC, Doney AS, Donnelly LA, Asselta R, Merlini PA, Duga S, Marziliano N, Denny JC, Shaffer CM, El-Mokhtari NE, Franke A, Gottesman O, Heilmann S, Hengstenberg C, Hoffman P, Holmen OL, Hveem K, Jansson JH, Jockel KH, Kessler T, Kriebel J, Laugwitz KL, Marouli E, Martinelli N, MI MC, Van Zuydam NR, Meisinger C, Esko T, Mihailov E, Escher SA, Alver M, Moebus S, Morris AD, Muller-Nurasyid M, Nikpay M, Olivieri O, Lemieux Perreault LP, AlQarawi A, Robertson NR, Akinsanya KO, Reilly DF, Vogt TF, Yin W, Asselbergs FW, Kooperberg C, Jackson RD, Stahl E, Strauch K, Varga TV, Waldenberger M, Zeng L, Kraja AT, Liu C, Ehret GB, Newton-Cheh C, Chasman DI, Chowdhury R, Ferrario M, Ford I, Jukema JW, Kee F, Kuulasmaa K, Nordestgaard BG, Perola M, Saleheen D, Sattar N, Surendran P, Tregouet D, Young R, Howson JM, Butterworth AS, Danesh J, Ardissino D, Bottinger EP, Erbel R, Franks PW, Girelli D, Hall AS, Hovingh GK, Kastrati A, Lieb W, Meitinger T, Kraus WE, Shah SH, McPherson R, Orho-Melander M, Melander O, Metspalu A, Palmer CN, Peters A, Rader D, Reilly MP, Loos RJ, Reiner AP, Roden DM, Tardif JC, Thompson JR, Wareham NJ, Watkins H, Willer CJ, Kathiresan S, Deloukas P, Samani NJ, Schunkert H (2016) Coding variation in ANGPTL4, LPL, and SVEP1 and the risk of coronary disease. N Engl J Med 374(12):1134–1144

Nakajima K, Tokita Y, Tanaka A, Takahashi S (2019) The VLDL receptor plays a key role in the metabolism of postprandial remnant lipoproteins. Clin Chim Acta 495:382–393

Norata GD, Tsimikas S, Pirillo A, Catapano AL (2015) Apolipoprotein C-III: from pathophysiology to pharmacology. Trends Pharmacol Sci 36(10):675–687

Nordestgaard BG, Varbo A (2014) Triglycerides and cardiovascular disease. Lancet 384 (9943):626–635

Olofsson SO, Boren J (2005) Apolipoprotein B: a clinically important apolipoprotein which assembles atherogenic lipoproteins and promotes the development of atherosclerosis. J Intern Med 258(5):395–410

Olofsson SO, Stillemark-Billton P, Asp L (2000) Intracellular assembly of VLDL: two major steps in separate cell compartments. Trends Cardiovasc Med 10(8):338–345

Ooi EM, Watts GF, Chan DC, Chen MM, Nestel PJ, Sviridov D, Barrett PH (2008) Dose-dependent effect of rosuvastatin on VLDL-apolipoprotein C-III kinetics in the metabolic syndrome. Diabetes Care 31(8):1656–1661

Ooi EM, Russell BS, Olson E, Sun SZ, Diffenderfer MR, Lichtenstein AH, Keilson L, Barrett PH, Schaefer EJ, Sprecher DL (2012) Apolipoprotein B-100-containing lipoprotein metabolism in subjects with lipoprotein lipase gene mutations. Arterioscler Thromb Vasc Biol 32(2):459–466

Packard CJ (2003) Triacylglycerol-rich lipoproteins and the generation of small, dense low-density lipoprotein. Biochem Soc Trans 31(Pt 5):1066–1069

Paquette M, Dufour R, Hegele RA, Baass A (2016) A tale of 2 cousins: an atypical and a typical case of abetalipoproteinemia. J Clin Lipidol 10(4):1030–1034

Parhofer KG, Barrett PH, Aguilar-Salinas CA, Schonfeld G (1996) Positive linear correlation between the length of truncated apolipoprotein B and its secretion rate: in vivo studies in human apoB-89, apoB-75, apoB-54.8, and apoB-31 heterozygotes. J Lipid Res 37(4):844–852

Parks EJ, Hellerstein MK (2006) Thematic review series: patient-oriented research. Recent advances in liver triacylglycerol and fatty acid metabolism using stable isotope labeling techniques. J Lipid Res 47(8):1651–1660

Parks EJ, Krauss RM, Christiansen MP, Neese RA, Hellerstein MK (1999) Effects of a low-fat, high-carbohydrate diet on VLDL-triglyceride assembly, production, and clearance. J Clin Invest 104(8):1087–1096

Poulsen MK, Nellemann B, Stodkilde-Jorgensen H, Pedersen SB, Gronbaek H, Nielsen S (2016) Impaired insulin suppression of VLDL-triglyceride kinetics in nonalcoholic fatty liver disease. J Clin Endocrinol Metab 101(4):1637–1646

Pradhan AD, Paynter NP, Everett BM, Glynn RJ, Amarenco P, Elam M, Ginsberg H, Hiatt WR, Ishibashi S, Koenig W, Nordestgaard BG, Fruchart JC, Libby P, Ridker PM (2018) Rationale and design of the Pemafibrate to reduce cardiovascular outcomes by reducing triglycerides in patients with diabetes (PROMINENT) study. Am Heart J 206:80–93

Prinsen BH, Romijn JA, Bisschop PH, de Barse MM, Barrett PH, Ackermans M, Berger R, Rabelink TJ, de Sain-van der Velden MG (2003) Endogenous cholesterol synthesis is associated with VLDL-2 apoB-100 production in healthy humans. J Lipid Res 44(7):1341–1348

Rasmussen KL, Tybjaerg-Hansen A, Nordestgaard BG, Frikke-Schmidt R (2019) Plasma levels of apolipoprotein E, APOE genotype, and all-cause and cause-specific mortality in 105 949 individuals from a white general population cohort. Eur Heart J 40(33):2813–2824

Robertson MD, Henderson RA, Vist GE, Rumsey RD (2002) Extended effects of evening meal carbohydrate-to-fat ratio on fasting and postprandial substrate metabolism. Am J Clin Nutr 75 (3):505–510

Robertson MD, Parkes M, Warren BF, Ferguson DJ, Jackson KG, Jewell DP, Frayn KN (2003) Mobilisation of enterocyte fat stores by oral glucose in humans. Gut 52(6):834–839

Romeo S, Yin W, Kozlitina J, Pennacchio LA, Boerwinkle E, Hobbs HH, Cohen JC (2009) Rare loss-of-function mutations in ANGPTL family members contribute to plasma triglyceride levels in humans. J Clin Invest 119(1):70–79

Rustaeus S, Stillemark P, Lindberg K, Gordon D, Olofsson SO (1998) The microsomal triglyceride transfer protein catalyzes the post-translational assembly of apolipoprotein B-100 very low density lipoprotein in McA-RH7777 cells. J Biol Chem 273(9):5196–5203

Sacks FM (2015) The crucial roles of apolipoproteins E and C-III in apoB lipoprotein metabolism in normolipidemia and hypertriglyceridemia. Curr Opin Lipidol 26(1):56–63

Sacks FM, Campos H (2003) Clinical review 163: cardiovascular endocrinology: low-density lipoprotein size and cardiovascular disease: a reappraisal. J Clin Endocrinol Metab 88 (10):4525–4532

Salter AM, Wiggins D, Sessions VA, Gibbons GF (1998) The intracellular triacylglycerol/fatty acid cycle: a comparison of its activity in hepatocytes which secrete exclusively apolipoprotein (apo) B100 very-low-density lipoprotein (VLDL) and in those which secrete predominantly apoB48 VLDL. Biochem J 332(Pt 3):667–672

Sandesara PB, Virani SS, Fazio S, Shapiro MD (2019) The forgotten lipids: triglycerides, remnant cholesterol, and atherosclerotic cardiovascular disease risk. Endocr Rev 40(2):537–557

Schneeman BO, Kotite L, Todd KM, Havel RJ (1993) Relationships between the responses of triglyceride-rich lipoproteins in blood plasma containing apolipoproteins B-48 and B-100 to a fat-containing meal in normolipidemic humans. Proc Natl Acad Sci U S A 90(5):2069–2073

Segrest JP, Jones MK, De Loof H, Dashti N (2001) Structure of apolipoprotein B-100 in low density lipoproteins. J Lipid Res 42(9):1346–1367

Shimomura I, Bashmakov Y, Horton JD (1999) Increased levels of nuclear SREBP-1c associated with fatty livers in two mouse models of diabetes mellitus. J Biol Chem 274(42):30028–30032

Stillemark P, Boren J, Andersson M, Larsson T, Rustaeus S, Karlsson KA, Olofsson SO (2000) The assembly and secretion of apolipoprotein B-48-containing very low density lipoproteins in McA-RH7777 cells. J Biol Chem 275(14):10506–10513

Stillemark-Billton P, Beck C, Boren J, Olofsson SO (2005) Relation of the size and intracellular sorting of apoB to the formation of VLDL 1 and VLDL 2. J Lipid Res 46(1):104–114

Tamura S, Shimomura I (2005) Contribution of adipose tissue and de novo lipogenesis to nonalcoholic fatty liver disease. J Clin Invest 115(5):1139–1142

Tanoli T, Yue P, Yablonskiy D, Schonfeld G (2004) Fatty liver in familial hypobetalipoproteinemia: roles of the APOB defects, intra-abdominal adipose tissue, and insulin sensitivity. J Lipid Res 45(5):941–947

Taskinen MR (2003) Diabetic dyslipidaemia: from basic research to clinical practice. Diabetologia 46(6):733–749

Taskinen MR, Boren J (2015) New insights into the pathophysiology of dyslipidemia in type 2 diabetes. Atherosclerosis 239(2):483–495

Taskinen MR, Adiels M, Westerbacka J, Soderlund S, Kahri J, Lundbom N, Lundbom J, Hakkarainen A, Olofsson SO, Orho-Melander M, Boren J (2011) Dual metabolic defects are required to produce hypertriglyceridemia in obese subjects. Arterioscler Thromb Vasc Biol 31 (9):2144–2150

Tsimikas S (2018) RNA-targeted therapeutics for lipid disorders. Curr Opin Lipidol 29(6):459–466

Vakkilainen J, Mero N, Schweizer A, Foley JE, Taskinen MR (2002) Effects of nateglinide and glibenclamide on postprandial lipid and glucose metabolism in type 2 diabetes. Diabetes Metab Res Rev 18(6):484–490

Vakkilainen J, Steiner G, Ansquer JC, Aubin F, Rattier S, Foucher C, Hamsten A, Taskinen MR (2003) Relationships between low-density lipoprotein particle size, plasma lipoproteins, and progression of coronary artery disease: the Diabetes Atherosclerosis Intervention Study (DAIS). Circulation 107(13):1733–1737

Vatner DF, Goedeke L, Camporez JG, Lyu K, Nasiri AR, Zhang D, Bhanot S, Murray SF, Still CD, Gerhard GS, Shulman GI, Samuel VT (2018) Angptl8 antisense oligonucleotide improves adipose lipid metabolism and prevents diet-induced NAFLD and hepatic insulin resistance in rodents. Diabetologia 61(6):1435–1446

Verges B (2005) New insight into the pathophysiology of lipid abnormalities in type 2 diabetes. Diabetes Metab 31(5):429–439

Wang AB, Liu DP, Liang CC (2003) Regulation of human apolipoprotein B gene expression at multiple levels. Exp Cell Res 290(1):1–12

Wang Y, Gusarova V, Banfi S, Gromada J, Cohen JC, Hobbs HH (2015a) Inactivation of ANGPTL3 reduces hepatic VLDL-triglyceride secretion. J Lipid Res 56(7):1296–1307

Wang Y, McNutt MC, Banfi S, Levin MG, Holland WL, Gusarova V, Gromada J, Cohen JC, Hobbs HH (2015b) Hepatic ANGPTL3 regulates adipose tissue energy homeostasis. Proc Natl Acad Sci U S A 112(37):11630–11635

Welty FK (2014) Hypobetalipoproteinemia and abetalipoproteinemia. Curr Opin Lipidol 25 (3):161–168

Welty FK, Lichtenstein AH, Barrett PH, Dolnikowski GG, Ordovas JM, Schaefer EJ (1997) Decreased production and increased catabolism of apolipoprotein B-100 in apolipoprotein B-67/B-100 heterozygotes. Arterioscler Thromb Vasc Biol 17(5):881–888

Welty FK, Lichtenstein AH, Barrett PHR, Dolnikowski GG, Schaefer EJ (1999) Human apolipo-protein (Apo) B-48 and ApoB-100 kinetics with stable isotopes. Arterioscler Thromb Vasc Biol 19(12):2966–2974

Westerbacka J, Kolak M, Kiviluoto T, Arkkila P, Siren J, Hamsten A, Fisher RM, Yki-Jarvinen H (2007) Genes involved in fatty acid partitioning and binding, lipolysis, monocyte/macrophage recruitment, and inflammation are overexpressed in the human fatty liver of insulin-resistant subjects. Diabetes 56(11):2759–2765

Wiggins D, Gibbons GF (1992) The lipolysis/esterification cycle of hepatic triacylglycerol. Its role in the secretion of very-low-density lipoprotein and its response to hormones and sulphonylureas. Biochem J 284:457–462

Witztum JL, Gaudet D, Freedman SD, Alexander VJ, Digenio A, Williams KR, Yang Q, Hughes SG, Geary RS, Arca M, Stroes ESG, Bergeron J, Soran H, Civeira F, Hemphill L, Tsimikas S, Blom DJ, O'Dea L, Bruckert E (2019) Volanesorsen and triglyceride levels in familial chylomicronemia syndrome. N Engl J Med 381(6):531–542

Xiao C, Stahel P, Lewis GF (2019) Regulation of chylomicron secretion: focus on post-assembly mechanisms. Cell Mol Gastroenterol Hepatol 7(3):487–501

Xu YX, Redon V, Yu H, Querbes W, Pirruccello J, Liebow A, Deik A, Trindade K, Wang X, Musunuru K, Clish CB, Cowan C, Fizgerald K, Rader D, Kathiresan S (2018) Role of angiopoietin-like 3 (ANGPTL3) in regulating plasma level of low-density lipoprotein choles-terol. Atherosclerosis 268:196–206

Yao Z (2012) Human apolipoprotein C-III – a new intrahepatic protein factor promoting assembly and secretion of very low density lipoproteins. Cardiovasc Hematol Disord Drug Targets 12 (2):133–140

Zhang R (2012) Lipasin, a novel nutritionally-regulated liver-enriched factor that regulates serum triglyceride levels. Biochem Biophys Res Commun 424(4):786–792

Zheng C, Khoo C, Ikewaki K, Sacks FM (2007) Rapid turnover of apolipoprotein C-III-containing triglyceride-rich lipoproteins contributing to the formation of LDL subfractions. J Lipid Res 48 (5):1190–1203

Zheng C, Khoo C, Furtado J, Sacks FM (2010) Apolipoprotein C-III and the metabolic basis for hypertriglyceridemia and the dense low-density lipoprotein phenotype. Circulation 121 (15):1722–1734

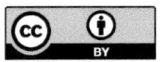

High Density Lipoproteins: Is There a Comeback as a Therapeutic Target?

Arnold von Eckardstein

Contents

1   Introduction 158
2   Possible Reasons for HDL-C's Clinical Futility 160
    2.1   Lack of Causality 160
    2.2   Epidemiology and Human Genetics Disprove "the Higher the Better" Concept 160
    2.3   Limitations of HDL Modifying Drugs 163
          2.3.1   Neither Fibrates nor Nicotinic Acid Specifically Target HDL Metabolism ... 163
          2.3.2   CETP Inhibitors Block Rather than Promote Reverse Cholesterol
                  Transport 165
          2.3.3   Combination with High-Intensity Statins: The Winner Takes it All 166
    2.4   Wrong Biomarker "the Good Cholesterol" 167
3   Consequences and Perspectives 168
    3.1   The Search for Novel HDL-Biomarkers 168
    3.2   Ongoing and Novel Drug Developments 171
          3.2.1   Reconstituted HDL, apoA-I Mimetic Peptides, and Recombinant LCAT ... 171
          3.2.2   Apabetalone 172
          3.2.3   PPAR Modulators 172
          3.2.4   ANGPTL3 and Endothelial Lipase 172
          3.2.5   ApoC-III Inhibition 173
          3.2.6   HDL-C Lowering Therapies: Probucol and Androgens 173
    3.3   Other Disease Targets 174
          3.3.1   Diabetes 175
          3.3.2   Chronic Kidney Disease 176
          3.3.3   Infections 177
          3.3.4   Autoimmune Diseases 178
          3.3.5   Cancer 179
          3.3.6   Behind the Blood Brain Barrier: Alzheimer's Disease and Age Related
                  Macular Degeneration 179
    3.4   Implications for Nowaday's Clinical Practice 180
References 181

A. von Eckardstein (✉)
Institute of Clinical Chemistry, University Hospital Zurich and University of Zurich, Zurich, Switzerland
e-mail: arnold.voneckardstein@usz.ch

© The Author(s) 2021
A. von Eckardstein, C. J. Binder (eds.), *Prevention and Treatment of Atherosclerosis*,
Handbook of Experimental Pharmacology 270, https://doi.org/10.1007/164_2021_536

Abstract

Low plasma levels of High Density Lipoprotein (HDL) cholesterol (HDL-C) are associated with increased risks of atherosclerotic cardiovascular disease (ASCVD). In cell culture and animal models, HDL particles exert multiple potentially anti-atherogenic effects. However, drugs increasing HDL-C have failed to prevent cardiovascular endpoints. Mendelian Randomization studies neither found any genetic causality for the associations of HDL-C levels with differences in cardiovascular risk. Therefore, the causal role and, hence, utility as a therapeutic target of HDL has been questioned. However, the biomarker "HDL-C" as well as the interpretation of previous data has several important limitations: First, the inverse relationship of HDL-C with risk of ASCVD is neither linear nor continuous. Hence, neither the-higher-the-better strategies of previous drug developments nor previous linear cause-effect relationships assuming Mendelian randomization approaches appear appropriate. Second, most of the drugs previously tested do not target HDL metabolism specifically so that the futile trials question the clinical utility of the investigated drugs rather than the causal role of HDL in ASCVD. Third, the cholesterol of HDL measured as HDL-C neither exerts nor reports any HDL function. Comprehensive knowledge of structure-function-disease relationships of HDL particles and associated molecules will be a pre-requisite, to test them for their physiological and pathogenic relevance and exploit them for the diagnostic and therapeutic management of individuals at HDL-associated risk of ASCVD but also other diseases, for example diabetes, chronic kidney disease, infections, autoimmune and neurodegenerative diseases.

Keywords

Apolipoprotein A-I · CETP · Cholesterol efflux · Fibrate · HDL mimetic · High density lipoproteins · Nicotinic acid

1   Introduction

Low plasma levels of high density lipoprotein (HDL) cholesterol (HDL-C) are associated with increased risks of atherosclerotic cardiovascular diseases (ASCVD), notably coronary heart disease (CHD) (Emerging Risk Factors Collaboration 2009; Madsen et al. 2021). HDL particles exert a broad spectrum of biological activities many of which are considered as anti-atherogenic, for example mediation of cholesterol efflux from macrophage foam cells and reverse transport of cholesterol to the liver, promotion of endothelial integrity and function, inhibition of inflammation by suppression of myelopoiesis and transmigration of leukocytes through the endothelium as well as macrophage activation, inhibition of lipid oxidation as well as inactivation of oxidized lipids (Fig. 1) (Von Eckardstein and Kardassis 2015; Robert et al. 2021; Rohatgi et al. 2021). Furthermore, atherosclerosis could be

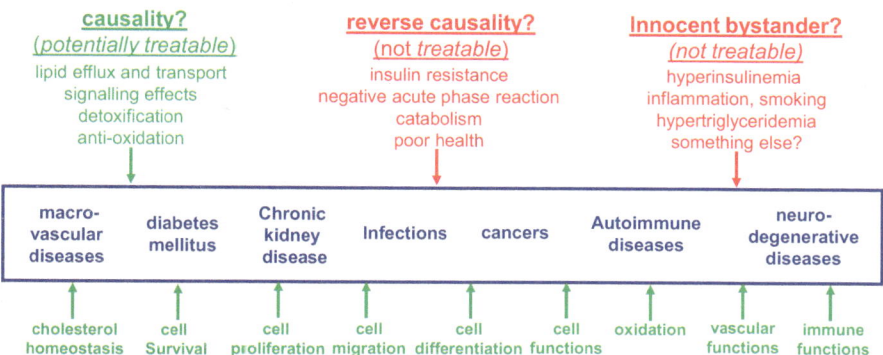

Fig. 1 Possible pathophysiological relationships of low HDL cholesterol with its associated diseases (modified from Von Eckardstein and Kardassis 2015)

decreased or even reverted in several animal models by transgenic over-expression or exogenous application of apolipoprotein (apoA-I), i.e. the most abundant protein of HDL (Hoekstra and Van Eck 2015; Lee-Rueckert et al. 2016). However, in humans, drugs increasing HDL-C such as fibrates, nicotinic acid (niacin), or inhibitors of cholesteryl ester transfer protein (CETP) have failed to prevent fatal or non-fatal cardiovascular endpoints (Keene et al. 2014; Riaz et al. 2019). Infusions of reconstituted HDL (rHDL) did not lead to regression of atherosclerosis in coronary or carotid arteries (He et al. 2021). Moreover, in several inborn errors of human HDL metabolism and genetic mouse models with altered HDL metabolism, low or high HDL-C levels were not always associated with the differences in cardiovascular risk and atherosclerotic plaque load, respectively, that were expected from epidemiology (Hoekstra and Van Eck 2015; Lee-Rueckert et al. 2016; Zanoni and von Eckardstein 2020). For example, the loss of scavenger receptor B1 (SR-BI) function aggravates the risk of ASCVD events in human carriers of SCARB1 mutations and promotes atherosclerosis in Scarb1 knock-out mice despite increasing HDL-C levels (Hoekstra and Van Eck 2015; Lee-Rueckert et al. 2016; Zanoni et al. 2016). Because of these ambiguous data, the causal role of HDL in the pathogenesis of atherosclerosis as well as the suitability of HDL-C as a therapeutic target is nowadays scrutinized if not doubted (Madsen et al. 2021; März et al. 2017). Both the previous euphoria and the current skepticism in the discussion of HDL's role in health and disease, specifically in ASCVD but also beyond, have been suffering from several misconceptions, which are described in the first part of this review. As the conclusion, several perspectives for the clinical exploitation of HDL are presented in the second part.

2 Possible Reasons for HDL-C's Clinical Futility

2.1 Lack of Causality

Mendelian randomization studies have been a successful tool to support the causality of LDL cholesterol (LDL-C) in atherosclerosis: Single nucleotide polymorphisms (SNPs) and rare genetic variants that are associated with lower or higher LDL-C levels are associated with lower and higher risk, respectively, of ASCVD events. The associations of genetically determined LDL-C with ASCVD risk are even stronger than the associations of measured LDL-C. This is because the genetic information includes both time and dosage of exposure to the harmful LDL-C whereas the measured LDL-C only records the dosage of the harm (Borén et al. 2020). Mendelian randomization studies also support causality of hypertriglyceridemia and elevated apoB levels as well as hypertension in the pathogenesis of ASCVD (Benn and Nordestgaard 2018). Conversely, this genetic strategy rather excluded genetic causality of HDL-C and apoA-I levels in the manifestation of ASCVD, at least after maximal adjustment for confounding lipid traits such as apoB and triglyceride levels (Richardson et al. 2020; Voight et al. 2012). However, it is important to note the limitations of Mendelian Randomization studies. With respect to HDL-C the most important limitation is the assumption of a continuous relationship between the risk factor and the clinical endpoint. This is true for the association of LDL-C or nonHDL-C with major cardiovascular events but not for HDL-C, where no difference in risk is observed among individuals with HDL-C levels above the 60th percentile (Emerging Risk Factors Collaboration 2009; Johannesen et al. 2020; Madsen et al. 2017; see Sect. 2.2).

HDL-C levels below the widely accepted risk thresholds of 1.0 mmol/L or 40 mg/dL are frequently confounded by other risk factors of ASCVD, notably hypertriglyceridemia, manifest diabetes mellitus type 2 (T2DM) or impaired fasting glucose, smoking, chronic inflammatory diseases (chronic obstructive lung disease, rheumatic diseases) or biomarkers of inflammation (e.g., elevated C-reactive protein), overweight or obesity (Fig. 1; Assmann et al. 1996; Damen et al. 2017). Due to the links of HDL metabolism with the metabolism of triglyceride-rich lipoproteins, it has been suggested that low HDL-C is an indirect long-term indicator of postprandial hypertriglyceridemia and hence exposure of atherogenic remnants like elevated glycated hemoglobin A1c is a long-term marker of disturbed glucose metabolism but a non-causal risk factor of glycation-induced organ damage (Langsted et al. 2020).

2.2 Epidemiology and Human Genetics Disprove "the Higher the Better" Concept

The association of HDL-C with risk of ASCVD events has been described for decades to be inverse. The resulting widespread reception of HDL-C as the "good cholesterol" led to the application of "the higher the better" strategies to both patient counselling and drug development. However, the meta-analysis of 68 population studies with more than 300,000 participants and 2,785 incident myocardial infarctions by the Emerging Risk Factors Collaboration found the unadjusted risk of myocardial infarction gradually decreasing from the first decile to the eighth decile (i.e., until about 1.5 mmol/L or 58 mg/dL) but no significant changes at higher levels of HDL-C. After adjustment for possible confounders, statistically significant dose-dependent risk decreases happen within the lower six deciles until about 50 mg/dL (1.3 mmol/L) but not above this threshold (Emerging Risk Factors Collaboration 2009). Similar observations were made in more than 110,000 and 630,000 participants of the Copenhagen General Population (CGPS) and Copenhagen City Heart Studies (CCHS) and CANHEART studies (Madsen et al. 2017; Wijeysundera et al. 2017). In Denmark, the decreases in risk of cardiovascular events reached plateaus at 1.5 mmol/L in men and 2.0 mmol/L in women (Madsen et al. 2017). In Canada, below the reference interval ranging from 50 to 60 mg/dL, the incidence of ASCVD events increased with every decreasing 10 mg/dL interval of HDL-C. Above the threshold of 60 mg/dL, the ASCVD risks were overall significantly lower compared to the reference interval, but did not differ between the increasing 10 mg/dL strata, neither in men nor in women (Wijeysundera et al. 2017). Of note, the associations of HDL-C with total as well as disease-specific mortalities including cardiovascular mortality are even parabolic (U-shaped): Both in the Danish and Canadian studies, the inverse associations of HDL-C with total mortality reached their nadirs at 1.8–1.9 mmol/L (70–75 mg/dL) and 2.3–2.4 mmol/L (90–95 mg/dL) in men and women, respectively. Beyond these thresholds, the risk of dying became gradually higher with further increasing HDL-C levels (Ko et al. 2016; Madsen et al. 2017).

The discontinuous and even parabolic associations of HDL-C with cardiovascular morbidity and mortality, respectively, have been largely ignored both in the execution of Mendelian randomization studies and in the design of randomized controlled studies that aimed at the lowering of cardiovascular risk by increasing of HDL-C: both have been based on the assumption of continuous the-higher-the-better associations. The majority of the trials on fibrates, niacin, or CETP inhibitors did not define any upper limit of HDL-C for inclusion into the trial (Table 1). No Mendelian Randomization study restricted the analysis to the ranges where changes in HDL-C are associated with changes in risk, e.g. to the lower five or six deciles (Richardson et al. 2020; Voight et al. 2012). Of note, a large register study of a lipid clinics in Boston among individuals with HDL-C below 25 mg/dL (0.8 mmol/L) found an increased prevalence of ASCVD events in carriers of mutations in the genes of APOA1, ABCA1, LCAT, and LPL (Geller et al. 2018). Also studies in Dutch and Canadian families affected by loss of function mutations in APOA1, ABCA1, or LCAT found the prevalence of ASCVD events increased among mutation carriers, but only if HDL-C was below the fifth percentile (Abdel-Razek et al. 2018; Tietjen et al. 2012). Conversely, mutations in the genes of CETP, SCARB1, and LIPG, which cause increases in HDL-C show heterogenous associations with ASCVD. Loss of function mutations in LIPG encoding endothelial lipase do not alter the risk of ASCVD (Voight et al. 2012). The associations of loss of function mutations in CETP and SCARB1 with ASCVD are controversial: Rare

Table 1 The majority of "HDL" trials did not define any cut-off level of HDL cholesterol for inclusion or exclusion of participants

Trial	Drug	Type of prevention	HDL-C inclusion criterion	HDL-C (mmol/L) at baseline
HHS	Gemfibrozil	Primary	Not defined	1.22 ± 0.28
BIP	Bezafibrate	Secondary	<1.16 mmol/L	0.89 ± 0.14
VA-HIT	Gemfibrozil	Secondary	<1.05 mmol/L	0.89 + 0.18
FIELD	Fenofibrate[a]	Diabetes mellitus	Not defined	1.10 ± 0.26
ACCORD[a]	Fenofibrate[a]	Diabetes mellitus	<1.42 mmol/L	0.98 ± 0.21
AIM-HIGH[a]	Niacin[a]	Secondary	<1.05 mmol/L	0.91 ± 0.16
HPS2-THRIVE[a]	Niacin[a]	Secondary	Not defined	1.14 ± 0.30
ILLUMINATE[a]	Torcetrapib[a]	Secondary	Not defined	1.26 ± 0.31
DALOUTCOME[a]	Dalcetrapib[a]	Secondary	Not defined	1.10 ± 0.30
ACCELERATE[a]	Evacetrapib	Secondary	<2.07 mmol/L	1.18 ± 0.30
REVEAL[a]	Anacetrapib	Secondary	Not defined	1.04 ± 0.26

HHS = Helsinki Heart Study (Frick et al. 1987), BIP = Bezafibrate Infarction Prevention (BIP) 2000, VA-HIT (Rubins et al. 1999), FIELD = Keech et al. (2005), ACCORD Study Group (2010); AIM-HIGH Investigators (2011), HPS2-THRIVE Collaborative Group (2014); ILLUMINATE (Barter et al. 2007b), Dal-OUTCOME (Schwartz et al. 2012), ACCELERATE (Lincoff et al. 2017; HPS3/TIMI55–REVEAL Collaborative Group 2017)
[a]Combined with statins vs. statins alone. *HDL-C* HDL cholesterol

SCARB1 mutations were associated with increased CVD risk in one study but not in another (Helgadottir et al. 2018; Zanoni et al. 2016). CETP deficiency was originally associated with reduced risk of ASCVD and increased life expectancy but later studies found diverse associations of loss of function mutations in CETP with ASCVD, namely increased risk in the Honolulu Heart Study but decreased risk in a Japanese population study (Moriyama et al. 1998; Yamashita and Matsuzawa 2016; Zhong et al. 1996). Likewise, the common polymorphisms in CETP which are associated with lower CETP mass and activity, LDL-C, and triglycerides but higher HDL-C were showed diverse associations with ASCVD in different studies: meta-analyses found lower risks of ASCVD associated with loss of function alleles of CETP (Kathiresan 2012; Niu and Qi 2015), but there are several individual studies which found the opposite (Agerholm-Larsen et al. 2000; Borggreve et al. 2006). Loss of function mutations in APOC3 cause higher HDL-C levels and reduce cardiovascular risk (Crosby et al. 2014; Pollin et al. 2008), but this may reflect proatherogenic features of apoC-III beyond its influence on HDL-C and triglyceride levels (Riwanto et al. 2013; Zewinger et al. 2020; Zvintzou et al. 2017) (see also Sect. 3.2).

2.3   Limitations of HDL Modifying Drugs

The futility of the most recent randomized controlled trials (RCTs) on fenofibrate (ACCORD Study Group 2010; Keech et al. 2005), nicotinic acid (AIM-HIGH Investigators 2011; HPS2-THRIVE Collaborative Group 2014), and cholesteryl ester transfer protein (CETP)-inhibitors (ILLUMINATE, Dal-OUTCOME, ACCEL-ERATE, REVEAL) (Barter et al. 2007b; HPS3/TIMI55–REVEAL Collaborative Group 2017; Lincoff et al. 2017; Schwartz et al. 2012) is frequently used as the argument to question the causality of HDL in the pathogenesis of atherosclerosis. However, this conclusion overlooks that – except the CETP inhibitor dalcetrapib (Schwartz et al. 2012) – none of these drugs is specifically altering HDL-C. Especially fibrates and nicotinic acid exert stronger effects on other lipoprotein traits than on HDL-C. Thus, their failure to reduce ASCVD events should primarily prompt to scrutinize the suitability of these pharmacological strategies rather than the causality of HDL in ASCVD. Moreover, one should be oblivious to meta-analyses that demonstrated futility of fibrates or nicotinic acid if combined with statins but efficacy if used as monotherapies (Keene et al. 2014; Riaz et al. 2019). Likewise, genetic studies indicate that potential efficacy of CETP inhibitors in ASCVD prevention may be hampered by the combination with statins (Ference et al. 2017).

2.3.1   Neither Fibrates nor Nicotinic Acid Specifically Target HDL Metabolism

Fibrates are agonists of the peroxisome proliferator agonist receptor alpha (PPARα). As such they regulate the transcription of several genes which are relevant in the metabolism of HDL metabolism (e.g., APOA1, PLTP, SCARB1) but also triglyceride-rich lipoproteins (Montaigne et al. 2021; Zandbergen and Plutzky 2007). As the result, fibrates cause increases in HDL-C of maximally 15% and decreases in triglycerides of 25–50%. The rather moderate effect on HDL-C is partially explained by the induction of APOA1 and SCARB1 genes, which enhances production and catabolism of HDL, respectively. As the result, the flux of HDL and probably reverse cholesterol transport are affected by fibrates more profoundly than reflected by changes in HDL-C. Triglycerides rather than HDL-C were the most profoundly altered lipoprotein traits. The two gemfibrozil utilizing trials – the primary prevention Helsinki Heart Study (Frick et al. 1987) and the secondary prevention study VA-HIT (Rubins et al. 1999) – were the only ones which found significant reductions of ASCVD events by the fibrate intervention vs. placebo. Only three trials (VA-HIT, BIP, and ACCORD) pre-defined plasma levels of HDL-C as inclusion criterion (ACCORD Study Group 2010; Bezafibrate Infarction Prevention Study 2000; Rubins et al. 1999). For ACCORD, the threshold was rather high with 55 mg/dL (1.42 mmol/L) (ACCORD study group 2010). Post-hoc analyses of the fibrate trials demonstrated relative risk reductions for subgroups of patients with HDL-C and triglycerides levels <35 mg/dL (0.9 mmol/L) and >200 mg/dL (2.3 mmol/L) ranging from 27% (FIELD, Keech et al. 2005) to −65% (Helsinki

Table 2 Effects of lipid modifying drug classes on lipoprotein traits and prevention of major cardiovascular events (MACE)

Drug class	LDL-C (max Δ%)	Triglycerides (max Δ%)	HDL-C (max Δ%)	MACE reduction
Statins	−50	−40	+10	Yes
Ezetimibe	−20	−10	0	Yes
Resins	−10	+20	0	Yes
PCSK9-inhibitors	−60	−20	+10	Yes
Fibrates	−10	−40	+15	Controversial: Yes, if without statins or post hoc, if HDL-C low and triglycerides elevated
Omega-3 fatty acids	+10	−35	0	Controversial
Nicotinic acid	−15	−30	+20	Controversial: Yes, if without statins
CETP inhibitors	−40	−15	+130	Anacetrapib: Yes Dalcetrapib & evacetrapib: No Torcetrapib: Adverse

CETP cholesteryl ester transfer protein, *HDL-C* High density lipoprotein cholesterol, *LDL-C* low density lipoprotein cholesterol, *MACE* major cardiovascular events, *PCSK9* proprotein subtilisin kexin type 9 convertase

Heart Study) (Sacks et al. 2010). Currently the *Pemafibrate to Reduce Cardiovascular OutcoMes by Reducing Triglycerides IN patiENts With diabeTes* (PROMINENT) trial tests prospectively the efficacy of the novel combined PPARα/PPARδ agonist pemafibrate (NCT03071692) (Pradhan et al. 2018).

Nicotinic acid (niacin) is an agonist of the G-protein coupled receptor GPR109A (HM74A or PUMA-G) (Offermanns 2014). As such, it primarily inhibits the lipolysis in adipocytes and secondarily, by reducing the free fatty acid flux, the lipogenesis and VLDL production in the liver. Reduced free fatty acid exposure may also promote ABCA1 activity in the liver and hence the production of nascent HDL (Chapman et al. 2010; KAmanna et al. 2013). In addition CETP activity was found decreased upon treatment with nicotinic acid due to direct and indirect inhibitory effects via production as well as activity of the protein and diminished pool of VLDL and hence acceptor particles, respectively (Chapman et al. 2010). In addition, nicotinic acid lowers plasma levels of LDL-C and lipoprotein(a) (Lp(a)). Despite these multiple beneficial effects on lipoproteins, in both the AIM-HIGH and HPS-THRIVE trials, the combination of statins with nicotinic acid was not superior to statin monotherapy in preventing ASCVD events (Table 2) (AIM-HIGH Investigators 2011; HPS2-THRIVE Collaborative Group 2014). Only AIM-HIGH defined inclusion criteria based on HDL-C (<1.05 mmol/L or <40 mg/dL). However, post-hoc analyses did not find any evidence that low HDL-C defines a subgroup of patients who benefit from nicotinic acid (Guyton et al. 2013; HPS2

THRIVE Collaborative Group 2014) However, in a meta-analysis monotherapy of nicotinic acid was found effective in reducing cardiovascular morbidity and mortality (Keene et al. 2014). Because of futility and the occurrence of flushes as very unpleasant and frequent side effects, nicotinic acid is no longer available for treatment in many countries.

2.3.2 CETP Inhibitors Block Rather than Promote Reverse Cholesterol Transport

CETP links the metabolism of HDL and apoB containing lipoproteins by exchanging cholesteryl esters of HDL against triglycerides of VLDL and LDL (Chapman et al. 2010). As the result of inhibiting this exchange, the most effective CETP inhibitors – torcetrapib, evacetrapib, and anacetrapib – cause increases of HDL-C by 75 (Torcetrapib) to 130% (Evacetrapib) and decreases of LDL-C by 25% (torcetrapib) to 40% (Anacetrapib) (Barter et al. 2007b; HPS3/TIMI55–REVEAL Collaborative Group 2017; Lincoff et al. 2017). The weaker CETP inhibitor dalcetrapib increases HDL-C by 30% without causing any drop in LDL-C (Schwartz et al. 2012). CETP inhibitors also decrease Lp(a) by up to 35% through an as yet unknown mechanism (Gencer and Mach 2020). Despite their at first sight beneficial effects on lipoprotein traits, three trials were prematurely stopped; the ILLUMINATE trial because of excess morbidity and mortality in the torcetrapib arm possibly due to off target effects of torcetrapib (Barter et al. 2007b). ACCELERATE and dal-OUTCOME were stopped prematurely because of futility of evacetrapib and dalcetrapib, respectively (Lincott et al. 2017; Schwartz et al. 2012). Only the combination of statin with anacetrapib in the REVEAL trial showed some superiority towards statin only therapy (HPS3/TIMI55–REVEAL Collaborative Group 2017). However, with a 9% relative risk reduction or the primary endpoint, the added value of anacetrapib was small and attributed to the decrease in LDL-C rather than to the increase in HDL-C. Because of the parallel successful development of PCSK9 inhibitors, which are much more effective in lowering LDL-C and event rates, the development of anacetrapib was stopped. Dalcetrapib, however, is further developed towards a personalized indication: post-hoc analyses of the Dal-OUTCOME study revealed that the carrier status for a mutation in the adenylate cyclase subtype 9 encoding ADCY9 gene discriminated individuals who did or did not benefit from dalcetrapib treatment by lower ASCVD event rates (Tardif et al. 2015). However, the same mutation discriminated responders and non-responders neither to anacetrapib nor to evacetrapib in the REVEAL and ACCELERATE trials, respectively (Hopewell et al. 2019; Nissen et al. 2018). Conversely, the interaction of CETP with ADCY9 was recapitulated in genetic mouse models (Rautureau et al. 2018). The Dal-GenE trial currently investigates prospectively, whether patients selected for the ADCY9 genotype benefit from treatment with dalcetrapib (NCT02525939) (Tardif et al. 2020).

At first sight the negative outcomes of the CETP inhibitor trials were surprising, not only because of the beneficial effects on the lipoprotein profile but also because several large genetic studies demonstrated lower prevalences or incidences of cardiovascular events among carriers of low activity CETP alleles (Kathiresan

2012). However, later population genetic studies showed an interaction between CETP and HMGCR alleles. In the presence of HMGCR alleles that reduce HMG-CoA reductase activity and thereby mimic treatment effects of statins, CETP alleles that cause low CETP activity and mimic the effects of CETP inhibitors did not confer any additional cardiovascular risk reduction (Ference et al. 2017). Likewise, torcetrapib treatment reduced atherosclerosis in apoE3 Leiden*CETP transgenic mice, if provided as monotherapy but not if provided in combination with statins (de Haan et al. 2008) whereas anacetrapib treatment enhanced the anti-atherogenic effect of atorvastatin (Kühnast et al. 2015). Nevertheless, the question is raised if the anti-atherogenicity of CETP inhibition depends on the capacity of the LDL receptor pathway: if this is fully functional, for example, as the result of statin treatment, CETP will promote reverse cholesterol transport and should not be blocked (von Eckardstein 2020). Only in situations, where LDL removal by the LDL receptor pathway is compromised, it may be useful to withheld cholesterol from LDL by CETP inhibition for hepatic removal through LDL receptor independent pathways involving direct HDL/receptor interactions, for example with SR-BI. As an alternative explanation, it was proposed that CETP inhibition renders HDL dysfunctional by prolonging the half-life of HDL particles and thereby making them susceptible to adverse alterations in the lipid and protein composition or oxidative and enzymatic modifications of protein or lipid components. However, the classical function of HDL, mediation of cholesterol efflux from macrophages was rather increased upon treatment of humans or animals with Evacetrapib, Anacetrapib, or Dalcetrapib (Brodeur et al. 2017; Metzinger et al. 2020; Nicholls et al. 2015; Simic et al. 2017; Tardif et al. 2015). Interestingly endothelial functions were not improved or even impaired in apoE3 Leiden*CETP transgenic mice upon treatment with evacetrapib and anacetrapib, respectively, despite increasing CEC and paraoxonase activity (Simic et al. 2017).

2.3.3 Combination with High-Intensity Statins: The Winner Takes it All

The combination of statins with fenofibrate, nicotinic acid, or CETP inhibitors was motivated by post-hoc meta-analyses of statin trials, which found the residual risk of patients treated with statins to be significantly associated with low HDL-C levels (Boekholdt et al. 2013). A closer look to post-hoc analyses of individual trials, however, reveals that these associations became weaker the lower LDLC levels were reached. For example, in the WOSCOP study, where mean levels of LDL-C were lowered from 5.0 mmol/L in the placebo arm to 3.6 mmol/L in the pravastatin arm, low baseline levels of HDL-C were associated with increased risk of ASCVD events in both treatment groups (West of Scotland Coronary Prevention Study Group 1998). However, more than 10 years later in the JUPITER study (LDL-C at baseline <3.37 mmol/L), both baseline and on-treatment levels of HDL-C were significantly associated with residual risk only in the placebo group with a mean on treatment LDL-C of 2.8 mmol/L, but not in the rosuvastatin group with an on treatment mean LDL-C level of 1.42 mmol/L (Ridker et al. 2010). Similar discrepant observations were made in the secondary prevention trials CARE and LIPID vs. TNT: HDL-C levels explained part of the residual risk in both placebo and pravastatin groups of

CARE and LIPID (mean baseline LDL-C 3.80 mmol/L, on treatment LDL-C 2.85 mmol/L) (Sacks et al. 2000). However, in the TNT trial (baseline LDL-C 2.55 mmol/L), low HDL-C increased ASCVD risk in the low-dose atorvastatin group (on treatment LDL-C 2.60 mmol/L) but not in the high dose atorvastatin group (on treatment LDL-C 2.0 mmol/L) (Barter et al. 2007a). It thus appears that the optimized control of LDL-C by high intensity statin therapy alleviates the residual risk associated with low HDL-C levels. In this regard it is also noteworthy that contemporary observational studies in general populations as well as in patients with clinically manifest ASCVD find weaker associations of HDL-C with first and recurrent cardiovascular events, respectively, than historical studies which recruited their participants in the pre-statin era (Bolibar et al. 2000; Colantonio et al. 2016; Schwartz et al. 2012). These secular trends are usually explained by the generally improved risk factor control. However, one must also be aware of the change in the methodology of HDL-C measurements that occurred in parallel with the triumphal procession of statins. Since about 1990, non-traceable and biased homogenous assays have replaced the previous cholesterol quantification after manual precipitation of apoB containing lipoproteins. One can hence not exclude that changes in the analytics affected the prognostic value of HDL-C (Miller et al. 2010).

2.4   Wrong Biomarker "the Good Cholesterol"

By contrast to the disease causing cholesterol in LDL (Borén et al. 2020), the cholesterol in HDL (that is HDL-C) neither exerts nor reflects any of the potentially anti-atherogenic activities of HDL. HDL-C is only a non-functional surrogate marker for estimating the HDL pool size without deciphering the heterogeneous composition and, hence, functionality of HDL (Rohatgi et al. 2021; Annema and von Eckardstein 2013, 2016). Differences in the molar content of apoA-I, phosphatidylcholines, cholesterol, and cholesteryl ester cause differences of HDL subclasses in shape, size, and charge. HDL particles carry hundreds of different quantitatively minor proteins and lipid species many of which are not just passive cargo (like cholesterol) but biologically active and susceptible to quantitative and qualitative modifications by diseases or interventions (Rohatgi et al. 2021, Annema and von Eckardstein 2013, 2016). These functionally active components hence have a much bigger chance than HDL-C to serve as a causal biomarker that can be exploited towards the development, targeting, and monitoring of therapies.

The most obvious candidate for a functional HDL biomarker is the plasma concentration of apoA-I which is not only a mandatory structural component of the bulk of HDL but also exerts several biological activities of HDL, for example activation of ABCA1 and LCAT to efflux and esterify cholesterol, respectively, or binding to SR-BI and other HDL receptors. In both epidemiological and clinical studies, apoA-I levels show inverse associations with ASCVD events, which however are not stronger than those of HDL-C (Emerging Risk Factors Collaboration 2009). Neither did Mendelian Randomization studies unravel any causal genetic relationship between apoA-I levels and ASCVD (Karjalainen et al. 2020; Richardson et al. 2020).

Other widely investigated HDL biomarker candidates include numbers and sizes of HDL particles. However, the outcomes of their evaluation in epidemiological and clinical studies are controversial. Some studies found HDL particle number (HDL-P) superior to HDL-C (Chandra et al. 2015; Kuller et al. 2007; Mackey et al. 2012; Otvos et al. 2006; Singh et al. 2020), others vice versa (El Harchaoui et al. 2009; Mora et al. 2009; Parish et al. 2012; Qi et al. 2015). Interestingly, within the JUPITER trial HDL-P was superior to HDL-C in the prediction of events among statin treated probands but inferior among placebo treated probands (Mora et al. 2013). Some studies found small HDL particles more strongly related with outcomes than large HDL particles (Ditah et al. 2016; Kim et al. 2016; McGarrah et al. 2016; Silbernagel et al. 2017), other studies found the opposite (Li et al. 2016; Arsenault et al. 2009). A recent meta-analysis of four studies concluded similar strong associations of small, medium, and large HDL particles with the incidence of ASCVD events (hazard ratio and 95% confidence interval 0.91 and 0.87 to 0.96) (Wu et al. 2018). With a hazard ratio and 95% confidence interval of 0.82 and 0.78 to 0.87, the total number of HDL particles showed stronger associations. Interestingly a recent Mendelian Randomization study found protective associations between the concentration of medium and – less so but also significantly – small HDL particles with coronary artery disease (Zhao et al. 2021). Drug interventions in lipoprotein metabolism result in diverse changes of HDL particle size and numbers. For example, treatment with nicotinic acid and CETP inhibitors increases HDL-C levels more profoundly than HDL-P, reflecting the shift to larger particles. Vice versa, upon treatment with fibrates, HDL-P increases more strongly than HDL-C (Rosenson et al. 2015).

3   Consequences and Perspectives

3.1   The Search for Novel HDL-Biomarkers

The further development of HDL as a therapeutic target is mainly limited by the availability of biomarkers that reflect the functional and causal role of HDL in the pathogenesis of atherosclerosis. To this end, bioassays of HDL function were recently developed and validated in population and clinical studies. Among them, cholesterol efflux capacity (CEC) has been investigated most extensively. In these studies, different macrophage cell lines treated with different drugs to enhance the cellular cholesterol efflux machinery were utilized as donors of radioactively or fluorescently labeled cholesterol. ApoB depleted plasma or serum was used as acceptors and as surrogate of HDL to avoid laborious ultracentrifugation. The heterogeneity of assays together with the heterogeneity of populations investigated has contributed to some discrepant findings (Anastasius et al. 2018). Nevertheless, a recent meta-analysis of eight prospective studies and more than 10,000 participants with more than 3,000 events found a significant inverse association of CEC with

ASCVD events (HR 0.86, 95% CI: 0.76–0.98). In a subgroup of five studies also mortality was related to CEC (HR 0.77, 95% CI: 0.80–1.0). Although CEC correlates with HDL-C, the associations of CEC with cardiovascular outcomes were independent of HDL-C (Soria-Florido et al. 2020). However, the concept of CEC as a proxy of HDL functionality has several limitations. First, as a laborious and difficult if not impossible to standardize bioassay it is a research rather than diagnostic tool, primarily for proof of concept studies and secondarily for the identification of functional molecular markers (Anastasius et al. 2018). Second, CEC should not be considered as an overall proxy of HDL functionality because other functions of HDL neither correlate nor share molecular determinants with CEC (Cardner et al. 2020). Third, although most intensively investigated, it is not clear that mediation of cholesterol efflux is the most relevant atheroprotective function of HDL. In fact, changes in CEC upon treatment with CETP inhibitors did not predict correctly the clinical outcomes of these drug interventions. They led to increases in CEC of apoB-free sera or plasmas but not to any reduction in cardiovascular event rates and coronary atherosclerosis, respectively (Brodeur et al. 2017; Metzinger et al. 2020; Nicholls et al. 2015; Simic et al. 2017; Tardif et al. 2015).

Despite these limitations, CEC has been used as the reference to develop molecular biomarkers that can be measured in clinical laboratories. One example is the derivation of an algorithm which integrates the information of differently sized HDL particles as measured by NMR. The estimated NMR-based CEC correlated very well with the in vitro measured CEC ($R^2 > 0.8$) and predicted incident CHD events with a hazards ratio of 0.86; 95% CI, 0.79–0.93, adjusted for traditional risk factors and HDL-C) (Kuusisto et al. 2019). Another example is a proteomic score integrating the information of apolipoproteins A-I, C-I, C-II, C-III, and C-IV showed good correlation with CEC as well as significant association with the presence of coronary artery disease and cardiovascular mortality independently of clinical risk factors including conventionally measured concentrations of apoA-I and apoB (Jin et al. 2019; Natarajan et al. 2019). Replication studies are needed to validate these surrogate scores of CEC.

Several laboratories have used tandem mass spectrometry to search for protein or lipid components of HDL as functional biomarkers. The most recent update of the HDL Proteome Watch data bank (http://homepages.uc.edu/~davidswm/HDLproteome.html; accessed July 15, 2021) documents more than 200 proteins which were identified in HDL by at least three of 40 independent studies and are therefore considered as highly confident components of HDL. Even higher numbers of lipid species were identified by mass spectrometry of HDL (Cardner et al. 2020; Kontush et al. 2013). The concentrations of these molecules vary from less than 1 µmol/L to more than 1 mmol/L (Annema and von Eckardstein 2013; Rohatgi et al. 2021). Already in view of the average HDL particle concentration of about 20 µmol/L it is clear that only some lipids (e.g., unesterified cholesterol, cholesteryl esters, phosphatidylcholines) or proteins (e.g., apoA-I) are present on each particle with several copies. Other low abundant lipids (e.g., sphingosine-1-phosphate, oxysterols) and proteins (apoM or LCAT) are dispersed throughout different particles. Interestingly, these molecules are non-randomly distributed among HDL particles. For example, the presence of sphingosine-1-phosphate is linked to the presence of its chaperone apoM (Christoffersen et al. 2011). By combining two immunoaffinity chromatography procedures, one with anti-apoA-I antibodies and one with an antibody against one of 16 other HDL-associated proteins, 16 HDL subclasses with distinct proteomes and little intraindividual variation over 3–24 months were identified (Furtado et al. 2018). Many proteins of each HDL subspecies exert related functions, for example in lipid transport, hemostasis, oxidation, or inflammation suggesting that specific functions beyond cholesterol efflux are exerted by distinct subspecies of HDL rather than the bulk of HDL. In agreement with this concept, a recent systems biology approach found distinct functions of HDL determined by clusters of distinct proteins and lipids carried by HDL with little overlap between the functions (Cardner et al. 2020). Moreover, in four prospective nested case–control studies, the presence or absence of distinct proteins was found to determine the association of apoA-I levels with incident cardiovascular events (Sacks et al. 2020). For example, apoA-I levels in particles that contain apoE or apoC-I but not their apoE or apoC-I- free counterparts showed the expected inverse association with incident ASCVD events. Vice versa, apoA-I levels in apoC-III-free particles but not particles containing apoC-III showed the expected inverse association with incident ASCVD events (Sacks et al. 2020). Cholesterol levels in apoC-III containing HDL even showed a positive association with incident ASCVD (Jensen et al. 2018). Moreover, apoC-III containing HDL was found to interfere with the capacity of HDL to inhibit the apoptosis of endothelial cells and to promote efflux from macrophages (Riwanto et al. 2013; Zvintzou et al. 2017). This makes apoC-III an interesting target for therapy beyond lowering of triglycerides (Zewinger et al. 2020). Other studies found the enrichment of HDL with either pulmonary surfactant protein B or serum amyloid protein A associated with increased risk of mortality in patients with diabetic end-stage nephropathy, heart failure, or CHD (Emmens et al. 2018; Kopecky et al. 2015; Zewinger et al. 2015).

Several mass spectrometric studies demonstrated gross alterations in the lipidome of HDL in patients with acute or chronic CHD as well as changes in response to statin therapy or body weight reduction (Cardner et al. 2020; Khan et al. 2018; Meikle et al. 2019; Orsoni et al. 2016; Sutter et al. 2015). However, to date, only signatures of lipid species in total plasma but not in HDL have been explored for their prognostic performance in prospective studies (Hilvo et al. 2019; Mundra et al. 2016). NMR-based studies identified some more general lipid traits of HDL to be associated with incident disease. However, they represent classes or subclasses rather than species of lipids and they are strongly intercorrelated with each other as well as measures of particle size or numbers so that they are not pursued as biomarkers beyond the latter indices (Cardner et al. 2020; Hafiane and Genest 2015; Rosenson et al. 2011).

3.2 Ongoing and Novel Drug Developments

After the failure of CETP inhibitors, only few drug developments targeting HDL have been continued or newly started. Some of the latter targets are pleiotropic and HDL is a bystander rather than the focus of these drug developments.

3.2.1 Reconstituted HDL, apoA-I Mimetic Peptides, and Recombinant LCAT

After infusions of artificially reconstituted HDL (rHDL) were found to reduce atherosclerosis in hypercholesterolemic rabbits, several formulations of rHDL were developed for investigation of their atheroprotective effects (He et al. 2021. Because rather large amounts of protein are needed, only short-term applications in acute clinical settings are feasible, for example in patients with acute coronary syndrome (ACS). rHDL containing phosphatidylcholines together with the recombinant apoA-I Milano variant (ETC-216, MDCO-216) or recombinant wild type apoA-I plus sphingomyelin (Cer001) or apoA-I isolated from plasma (CSL111, CSL112) were initially tested in phase II trials for their short-term effects on coronary atherosclerosis which was assessed by intravascular ultrasound of ACS patients. Whereas initial studies showed some regression of coronary atherosclerosis upon treatment with ETC.-216 or CSL111 (Tardif et al. 2007; Nissen et al. 2003), later larger studies with MDCO-216 or Cer001 did not (Nicholls et al. 2018a, b). Neither did Cer001 cause regression or prevent progression of carotid atherosclerosis in patients with genetic HDL deficiency (Zheng et al. 2020). Currently only one formulation – CSL112 – is further pursued by a large randomized and controlled phase III trial (ApoA-I Event Reducing in Ischemic Syndrome II = AEGIS II). Seventeen thousand four hundred patients with myocardial infarction are randomized to 4 weekly infusions of either 6 g CSL112 or placebo within 5 days of the event (Gibson et al. 2021). The primary outcome is the time to first occurrence of the composite of CV death, MI, or stroke through 90 days. Secondary outcomes include the total number of hospitalizations for coronary, cerebral, or peripheral ischemia through 90 days and time to first occurrence of the composite primary outcome through 180 and 365 days. Results are expected to become available in 2023.

In addition to rHDL containing full length apoA-I, also apoA-I mimetic peptides are developed for treatment of atherosclerosis. They showed promising results in vitro and in preclinical animal models. Three of them have been tested for safety and effects on HDL-C and HDL function. For two of them – L4F and D4F – results have been reported. They did not cause any changes in HDL-C or anti-inflammatory HDL functions. No results have been reported for ETC642. The clinical development of FX-5A is planned (Wolska et al. 2021).

Application of recombinant LCAT is an alternative strategy to increase HDL-C or promote HDL metabolism by substitution of components (Freeman et al. 2020). In a randomized controlled study 32 patients were treated with three weekly injections of different dosages of recombinant LCAT (MEDI6012) or placebo (Bonaca et al. 2021). Compared to placebo, MEDI6012 caused dose-dependent increases of

HDL-C by 66% to 144% at day 19. Interestingly the initial bolus injection led to a more than 40% increase of HDL-C within 30 min. MEDI6012 caused neither any severe side effects nor the generation of neutralizing antibodies. In an ongoing phase IIb trial (REAL-TIMI 63B), the application of 2 dosages of MEDI6012 to ACS patients is currently investigated for its effect on infarct size in more than 400 ACS patients (https://clinicaltrials.gov/ct2/show/NCT03578809). Half of the patients receive additional 4-weekly injections of MEDI6012 or placebo for 12 weeks for investigation of LCAT's effects on coronary calcification. Of note, recombinant LCAT is also attractive for the use as enzyme replacement in familial LCAT deficiency, however with the goal to prevent the development and progression of nephropathy in these patients (Freeman et al. 2020; Vaisman et al. 2019).

3.2.2   Apabetalone
Apabetalone (RVX208) is an inhibitor of bromodomain and extraterminal (BET) proteins that regulate the expression of multiple genes by interference with histone acetylation. RVX208 was initially developed because it strongly induced APOA1 gene expression in cultivated hepatocytes and caused a profound increase of HDL-C and apoA-I levels in non-human primates by 90 and 60%, respectively (Ghosh et al. 2017). Also mice responded with substantial increases of HDL cholesterol. Atherosclerosis was suppressed in apoE deficient mice. However, in humans treatment with apabetalone caused very moderate increases in HDL-C and apoA-I levels but also reduced CRP levels. The development of the drug was stopped after a recent phase III trial (BETonMACE) in patients with acute coronary syndrome and type 2 diabetes did not reveal any reduction of clinical events compared with placebo. (Ray et al. 2020).

3.2.3   PPAR Modulators
The PPARa modulator Pemafibrate is developed primarily for the treatment of hypertriglyceridemia and the related cardiovascular risk. In a phase II dose finding study, pemafibrate dose-dependently decreased triglycerides and increased HDL-C by up to 42% and 21%, respectively, compared to 30% and 14% by fenofibrate (Arai et al. 2017). In hypertriglyceridemic patients, treatment with pemafibrate caused increases of HDL-C by about 16% as well as CEC (Yamashita et al. 2018). In apoE2 knock-in mice, pemafibrate increased HDL-C, CEC as well as macrophage-to-feces reverse cholesterol transport, and reduced the extent of atherosclerotic lesions (Hennuyer et al. 2016). The PROMINENT trial investigates the effect of pemafibrate vs. placebo on cardiovascular outcomes of 10,000 participants with diabetes mellitus type 2, triglycerides 200–499 mg/dL (2.26–5.64 mmol/L), HDL-C level ≤40 mg/dL(1.03 mmol/L) during a maximal follow-up of 5 years (Pradhan et al. 2018).

3.2.4   ANGPTL3 and Endothelial Lipase
Angiopoietin-like protein 3 (ANGPTL3) is mainly produced by the liver and an endogenous inhibitor of both lipoprotein lipase and endothelial lipase (EL). After the discovery of loss of function mutations in the ANGPTL3 gene as a cause of

panhypolipoproteinemia and reduced cardiovascular risk (Arca et al. 2020), antisense oligonucleotides as well as monoclonal antibodies were developed for the treatment of hypertriglyceridemia and hypercholesterolemia. In fact, treatment of hypertriglyceridemia with the antisense oligonucleotide Vupanorsen and refractory hypercholesterolemia with the monoclonal antibody Evinacumab caused pronounced decreases of triglyceride levels and LDL-C but also HDL-C (Gaudet et al. 2020; Rosenson et al. 2020) The clinical implication of the 20–30% decrease in HDL-C is not known but very likely reflects the increased activity of EL upon ANGPTL3 inhibition (Wu et al. 2020).

Conversely, also EL inhibitors are developed with the aim to increase HDL-C. Treatment of non-human primates with the monoclonal anti-EL antibody MEDI5884 dose-dependently increased HDL-C and apoA-I levels by up to 100% and 30%, respectively (Le Lay et al. 2021). In a phase I study, human volunteers also experienced increases in HDL-C and apoA-I as well as particle number and size. CEC and anti-inflammatory activities of HDL were also improved. However, endothelial lipase inhibition also caused increases in LDL-C, albeit more profoundly in non-human primates than in humans. In non-human primates this unwanted effect could be blocked by PCSK9 inhibition. Nevertheless, one must wonder whether the risk of increasing LDL-C is well taken, especially since loss-of-function alleles of LIPG encoding EL do not confer any cardiovascular risk reduction despite increasing HDL-C thus questioning the clinical utility of EL inhibition (Voight et al. 2012).

3.2.5   ApoC-III Inhibition

Antisense oligonucleotides against apoC-III (Volanesorsen) exert pronounced triglyceride lowering effects by reducing the production of VLDL as well as by promoting lipolysis and remnant removal by disinhibiting lipoprotein lipase and remnant receptors, respectively. Probably secondarily to the lowering of triglycerides, interference with apoC-III in patients with chylomicronemia also leads to increases of HDL-C levels by 40% (Witztum et al. 2019). Although not tested, one must assume that Volanesorsen also decreases the content of apoC-III in HDL. In view of the positive rather than inverse association of apoC-III containing HDL with cardiovascular outcomes (Jensen et al. 2018; Sacks et al. 2020); as well as the noxious effects of apoC-III on HDL functionality towards cholesterol efflux and endothelial survival and inflammation (Riwanto et al. 2013; Zewinger et al. 2020; Zvintzou et al. 2017), one may hypothesize that apoC-III inhibition also exerts anti-atherogenic effects by improving HDL function. However, this hypothesis needs to be tested.

3.2.6   HDL-C Lowering Therapies: Probucol and Androgens

For a long time, lowering of HDL-C has been considered as a safety issue in drug development. This has changed as the causal role of HDL in ASCVD has been questioned. Even more so, the association of high HDL-C with increased mortality and morbidity for certain diseases (Bowe et al. 2016a; Ko et al. 2016; Madsen et al. 2017) raises the question whether under certain conditions HDL-C lowering may be useful. In view of the genetic association of loss of function mutations in SR-BI with increased cardiovascular risk (Zanoni et al. 2016) and the finding of increased atherosclerosis in Scarb1 knock-out mice (Hoekstra and van Eck 2015), especially therapies that lower HDL-C by upregulation of SR-BI in the liver may be interesting.

Probucol is an old drug which was originally developed to exploit its anti-oxidative effects on LDL. Although it was shown to induce regression of athero-sclerosis and xanthomas and has been rather widely used in Japan, the development and clinical application of probucol has not been consequently pursued (Yamashita et al. 2015). The main reason was the about 30% lowering of HDL-C. Activation of CETP and SR-BI has been elucidated as the underlying mechanism. In the most recent PROSPECTIVE trial, 876 Japanese patients with CHD and LDL-C $\geq$ 140 mg/dL without medication or those treated with lipid-lowering drugs received optimal lipid-lowering treatment together with placebo or probucol 500 mg/day. After 3 years, LDL-C and HDL-C were 8.5 mg/dL and 16.3 mg/dL, respectively, lower in the probucol than in the placebo group. The event rates did not differ significantly between the groups, although by trend, CHD events happened less frequently in the probucol group (Arai et al. 2021). Interestingly, the combined analysis of the PROMINENT and IMPACT trials showed reductions of cerebrovascular events, however in the absence of any effect on carotid atherosclerosis (Yamashita et al. 2021). Although futile, the data raise the question of whether probucol is a treatment option for patients with high HDL-C.

The stimulatory effects of testosterone on hepatic SR-BI expression are probably the main reasons for the substantial differences in HDL-C levels between males and females (Chiba-Falek et al. 2010; Langer et al. 2002). Even more so, the HDL-lowering effects of testosterone have contributed to the caution on the use of testosterone for the treatment of the aging male syndrome, transgender patients, or female sexual dysfunction as well as for male contraception (Thirumalai et al. 2015; Wu and von Eckardstein 2003). The effects of testosterone replacement on hard cardiovascular endpoints have not been investigated. However, a recent randomized controlled trial in 1007 men with overweight or obesity as well as disturbed or manifest diabetes at baseline showed benefits of 1,000 mg intramuscular testosterone vs. placebo injection on glycemic control and incidence of diabetes during 2 years of follow-up (Wittert et al. 2021).

3.3   Other Disease Targets

As late onset diseases, ASCVDs have not been rate limiting in the evolution of species. Therefore, one must envisage that the broad spectrum of HDL's protective functions has rather evolved to prevent other diseases or secure survival and healing of their victims. Such diseases or their clinical complications may serve as more appropriate targets than ASCVD for the therapeutic exploitation of HDL (Von Eckardstein and Rohrer 2016). Indeed, recent epidemiological and genetic studies unraveled several associations of HDL-C and genetic loci intimately related to HDL metabolism with non-cardiovascular diseases as well as mortality (Table 3) (Kjeldsen et al. 2021a; Madsen et al. 2021). Please note the diverse directions of

Table 3 Role of HDL in different diseases according to epidemiology, therapeutic interventions, human genetics, and animal experiments

Diseases	Association in observational studies	Clinical benefit in intervention studies	Genetic association	Animal experiments
Atherosclerotic cardiovascular diseases	Discontinuously inverse (until 60th percentile)	No (CETP inhibitors) or subgroups (fibrates)	No	Gene-dependent
Diabetes	Inverse	(yes) (post-hoc: CETP inhibitors, rHDL)	Yes (Mendelian gene scores) No (candidate genes)	Yes (ABCA1, APOA1)
Chronic kidney disease	Parabolic	Not investigated	Yes	Yes (LCAT)
Infections	Parabolic	Not investigated	Yes	Yes (APOA1, CETP, rHDL)
Autoimmune disease	Inverse	Not investigated	Not investigated	Yes (APOA1, SCARB1, S1P)
Age-related macular degeneration	Positive	Not investigated	Yes	(Yes) (ABCA1)
Alzheimer's disease	Discontinuously positive (>95th percentile)	Not investigated	No (Mendelian gene scores) Yes (GWAS, e.g., ABCA1)	(Yes) (ABCA1)

these associations which reach from inverse (diabetes, autoimmune diseases) over parabolic (infections, chronic kidney disease, mortality) to positive (Alzheimer's disease, age related macular degeneration), re-emphasizing that the kinetics of HDL metabolism and HDL function rather than the concentration of HDL particles are relevant.

3.3.1 Diabetes

Low levels of HDL-C are frequent in patients with diabetes mellitus type 2. This finding even precedes the manifestation of hyperglycemia and is hence an indicator of increased risk for incident diabetes (Haase et al. 2015; Schmidt et al. 2005; von Eckardstein et al. 2000; White et al. 2016; Wilson et al. 2007). Because of multiple effects of insulin on HDL metabolism, most of which are indirect via free fatty acids or triglyceride-rich lipoproteins, these associations have been explained for a long time by reverse causality: diabetes and pre-diabetes cause low HDL-C rather than vice versa (Parhofer 2015; Vollenweider et al. 2015; von Eckardstein and Widmann 2014). However, increasing evidence from in vitro as well as in vivo studies indicates that HDL exerts protective functions on the function and survival of pancreatic beta cells as well as on the sensitivity of target cells to insulin (Cochran et al. 2021; Manandhar et al. 2020; Vollenweider et al. 2015; von Eckardstein and Widmann 2014; Yalcinkaya et al. 2020). Also mitochondrial function and thereby cellular energy metabolism is modulated by HDL (Lehti et al. 2013). In humans, the potentially anti-diabetic effects of HDL are best illustrated by the acute glucose lowering effect of rHDL infusion (Drew et al. 2009) as well as by the findings of post-hoc analyses of the CETP inhibitor trials: Participants who received the CETP inhibitors showed better glycemic control and experienced less often new-onset diabetes as compared to the placebo treated controls (Barter et al. 2011; Masson et al. 2018; Menon et al. 2020; Schwartz et al. 2020). Mendelian randomization studies yielded controversial results on the genetic causality of HDL-C in diabetes (Fall et al. 2015; Haase et al. 2015; White et al. 2016).

3.3.2 Chronic Kidney Disease

The Veterans Administration study showed a parabolic association of HDL-C with >30% declining estimated glomerular filtration rate (eGFR) or the incidence of eGFR <60 ml/min and also provided evidence for genetic causality (Bowe et al. 2016b). Mutations in APOA1, APOE; APOL1, and LCAT are causes of genetic nephropathies (Strazzella et al. 2021). However, it is not clear whether their pathogenesis involves HDL: Certain missense mutations in APOA1 cause familial amyloidosis, which also affect other organs (Zanoni and von Eckardstein 2020). Specific mutations in APOE cause lipid glomerulopathy which however has been suggested to develop in response to disturbed interactions of apoB containing lipoproteins with the LDL receptor or due to accumulation of the structural defective apoE (Saito et al. 2020). ApoL1 is the trypanolytic factor which is transported by a minor subfraction of HDL (Friedman and Pollak 2020). Certain apoL1 variants that protect the host from infections with Trypanosoma brucei rhodesiense and gambiense dramatically increase the risk of chronic kidney disease, notably focal segmental glomerulosclerosis, in their African and Afroamerican carriers (Friedman and Pollak 2020). LCAT deficiency is a classical HDL deficiency syndrome causing a nephropathy that eventually progresses to end-stage renal disease (Pavanello and Calabresi 2020). However, the pathogenic mechanism depends on the accumulation of lipoprotein X rather than the absence of HDL (Vaisman et al. 2019). This is best illustrated by the absence of nephropathy in patients with fish-eye disease where partial loss of LCAT causes the same decrease in HDL as classical LCAT deficiency, however no nephropathy (Pavanello and Calabresi 2020).

Treatment with fibrates improves albuminuria but worsens glomerular filtration rate (Speer et al. 2021). Niacin has no effect on renal function. Small studies also indicate protective effects of probucol towards acute kidney injury, for example of patients exposed to contrast agents (Xin et al. 2019). The pleiotropic effects of these drugs on lipoprotein metabolism and the lack of association between changes in renal function and HDL-C under their treatment do not allow any conclusion on the role of HDL modifying therapies for prevention or treatment of CKD. Furthermore the exploitation of HDL towards kidney disease is also hampered by the currently unknown mechanisms how HDL exerts renal protection by HDL. Since small HDL particles are undergoing glomerular filtration and tubular re-uptake by the megalin/ cubilin co-receptors, it may be that HDL delivers protective molecules to the kidney, for example sphingosine-1-phosphate (Bisgaard and Christoffersen 2019; Strazzella et al. 2021).

3.3.3 Infections

The Copenhagen General Population study found U-shaped associations between HDL-C and the incidence of infections (Madsen et al. 2018). The associations with bacterial infections were stronger than with viral infections. Upon limited adjustment, gastroenteritis, bacterial pneumonia, skin and urinary tract infections, as well as sepsis were more prevalent among individuals with HDL-C <1.0 mmol/L as compared to individuals with higher HDL-C. Upon full adjustment the associations with gastroenteritis and pneumonia remained significant (Madsen et al. 2018). A preliminary Mendelian randomization analysis with two loci (CETP and LIPC) provided initial evidence of genetic causality (Madsen et al. 2018). Genetic causality also exists for the association of low HDL-C with the incidence of sepsis as well as with the chance of survival in patients with sepsis (Trinder et al. 2020). Evidence from population studies as well as experiments in genetic animal models points to the importance of CETP in this process (Blauw et al. 2020; Trinder et al. 2019, 2021). However also HDL particles per se as well as specific structural components of HDL exert several antibacterial activities such as binding and removal of lipopolysaccharides, protection of epithelial and endothelial barriers, or modulatory effects on leukocyte functions (Catapano et al. 2014; Meilhac et al. 2020; Pirillo et al. 2015; Robert et al. 2021; Rohatgi et al. 2021; Trakaki and Marsche 2021). The special association of HDL-C with gastroenteritis may also mirror an important role of HDL that is locally produced in the intestine (Ko et al. 2020). Similarly, the protection from pneumonia may mirror the high exposure of the lung to newly synthesized HDL due to first pass effects (Gordon et al. 2016). In sepsis models, genetically modified mice overexpressing human apoA-I showed improved survival (Meilhac et al. 2020; Morin et al. 2015). Interestingly, the clinical development of CSL111 was originally aiming at the treatment of sepsis since their infusion into volunteers exerted several beneficial effects on inflammation, coagulation, and fibrinolysis (Pajkrt et al. 1996, 1997). Most recent experiments in preclinical sepsis models demonstrated better survival of mice treated with CSL111 (Tanaka et al. 2020). The better chances of survival from sepsis by patients carrying low CETP activity alleles suggest CETP inhibitors as interesting drugs for the treatment of patients with sepsis (Trinder et al. 2019, 2021). However, an important caveat comes from the ILLUMINATE study where torcetrapib treatment was associated with excess mortality due to infections (Barter et al. 2007b).

Although the association of HDL-C with the incidence of viral infections was not statistically significant in the Copenhagen General Population Study (Madsen et al. 2018), it is noteworthy that at least in vitro HDL or apoA-I interferes with the entry or fusion of viruses with target cells (Meilhac et al. 2020; Pirillo et al. 2015). HDLs also induce viral inactivation by immune cells and protect cells from virus-induced damage (Pirillo et al. 2015). The COVID19 pandemia also raised the question of whether HDL interferes with SARS-CoV2 infections. In the UK Biobank study, a linear inverse and independent association was found between pre-infection HDL-C levels and the risk of hospitalization for severe COVID19 (Hilser et al. 2021; Lassale et al. 2021). Mendelian Randomization rather excluded any causal role of HDL in preventing SARS-CoV2 infection. (Hilser et al. 2021). Nevertheless, since SR-BI is an entry route of several viruses including SARS-CoV2 into cells (Pirillo et al. 2015; Wei et al. 2020), competition of this interaction by HDL is an intriguing hypothesis. In addition, the protective effects of HDL on the survival and function of cells may also help infected cells, for example of the lung epithelium or the endothelium (Robert et al. 2021), to combat and survive the entered viruses. Interestingly, dalcetrapib is currently tested towards its effect on the course of COVID19 infections. (Talasaz et al. 2021; https://clinicaltrials.gov/ct2/show/NCT04676867).

Finally, HDL also exerts protective activities towards infections with protozoa. The best example is the protection of humans from Trypanosoma brucei by apoL1 transported by a subfraction of HDL containing also haptoglobin related protein. This complex kills Trypanosome brucei by causing lysosomal swelling (Friedman and Pollak 2020). A similar HDL-related mechanism appears operative towards Leishmania (Samanovic et al. 2009).

3.3.4   Autoimmune Diseases

In an analysis of more than 110,000 participants of The Copenhagen General Population and the Copenhagen City Heart Study, low HDL-C concentrations were associated with elevated risk of developing the composite end point of 42 different autoimmune diseases (Madsen et al. 2019). Among them, the associations of celiac disease, idiopathic thrombocytopenic purpura, Sjögren's disease, diabetes type 1, inflammatory bowel diseases, and Graves' disease showed the strongest and individually significant associations with HDL-C. Currently, no data are available to prove or disprove causality of these associations (Madsen et al. 2021). Neither are the mechanisms understood. They may involve immunomodulatory effects of HDL which are relevant in the development of auto-immunity (Catapano et al. 2014; Pirillo et al. 2015; Rohatgi et al. 2021; Trakaki and Marsche 2021) or protective effects of HDL towards organs attacked by the immune system so that the onset of organ damage or failure and thereby the clinical diagnosis of manifest disease is delayed. For example, the anti-apoptotic effects of HDL on pancreatic beta cells may delay the loss of insulin production in the course of progressing type 1 diabetes (von Eckardstein and Widmann 2014; Yalcinkaya et al. 2020). For inflammatory bowel diseases, preclinical models generated evidence for the therapeutic potential of HDL: Intestinal inflammation was increased in Apoa1 knock-out mice but decreased in mice which overexpressed human APOA1 or were fed with apoA-I mimetic peptides (Gerster et al. 2014; Meriwether et al. 2019; Nowacki et al. 2016).

3.3.5 Cancer

Several epidemiological studies found inverse associations between HDL-C and cancer in general as well as specific cancers such as breast cancer or colorectal cancer (Ganjali et al. 2021; Madsen et al. 2021; Pirro et al. 2018). Currently, there is no evidence of causality. However, several confounders of low HDL-C are associated with increased risk of several cancers, for example smoking, overweight and obesity, type 2 diabetes, or chronic inflammatory diseases. There is hence some likelihood that low HDL-C is a confounder of other causal risk factors rather than reflecting loss of anti-cancer functions. Even if HDL is not causally related to cancer, it will offer opportunities for therapeutic or diagnostic exploitation: probably to satisfy their high need of cholesterol for growth, many cancers show a high expression of lipoprotein receptors including SR-BI (Hoekstra and Sorci-Thomas 2017; Kinslechner et al. 2018; Velagapudi et al. 2018). This can be exploited by using rHDL for the delivery of anti-cancer drugs or tracers for imaging. In fact, according experiments in preclinical models showed promising results (Morin et al. 2018; Rajora and Zheng 2016).

3.3.6 Behind the Blood Brain Barrier: Alzheimer's Disease and Age Related Macular Degeneration

Until recently, only cross-sectional studies and smaller prospective cohort studies described associations of HDL-C with neurodegenerative diseases including Alzheimer's disease (AD) and age related macular degeneration (AMD). They reported discrepant associations ranging from inverse over none to positive (Kjeldsen et al. 2021a). The situation became clearer but also surprising by recent reports of analyses in the Copenhagen General Population and Copenhagen City Heart Studies. High HDL-C levels >95th percentiles increase the risk of dementia and AD (Kjeldsen et al. 2021b). This association became even more prominent after adjustment for APOE genotypes. Also the risk of AMD was found to increase with HDL-C and even more so with apoA-I levels (Nordestgaard et al. 2021) confirming data on more than 30,000 individuals from the EYE-RISK and European Eye Epidemiology Consortia (Colijn et al. 2019). Of note, in that study higher HDL-C was most strongly associated with increased risk of early AMD. Mendelian Randomization studies found evidence for genetic causality of higher HDL-C for the higher risk of AMD but not AD (Burgess and Smith 2017; Chen et al. 2010; Fan et al. 2017; Neale et al. 2010; Ostergaard et al. 2015; Proitsi et al. 2014), the latter perhaps because of the non-linear relationship. CETP, APOE, and LIPC were important drivers of the genetic association between HDL-C and AMD (Colijn et al. 2019; Chen et al. 2010; Neale et al. 2010). However, candidate gene approaches as well as genome-wide association studies found ABCA1 as a genetic determinant of both AD and AMD risks (Bellenguez et al. 2020; Nordestgaard et al. 2015; Fritsche et al. 2016). Likewise, tissue specific knock-out experiments in mice indicate that loss of ABCA1 function in neurons and retinal pigment epithelial cells compromise neurocognitive and retinal functions, respectively (Behl et al. 2021; Storti et al. 2019). These discrepant associations of AD and AMD with high HDL-C levels in peripheral blood but locally reduced cholesterol efflux in the brain and retina probably reflect the tight separation of these compartments by the blood brain barrier. Some HDL functions in the brain are executed by HDL-like particles that contain apoE instead of apoA-I and that are produced by astrocytes within the central nervous system (Button et al. 2019). Especially the association of APOE genotypes with risk of AD, although mechanistically not resolved, has been traditionally ascribed to apoE endogenously produced by the CNS rather than supplied by the systemic circulation. Of note however, also the concentration of apoE in plasma of peripheral blood has been associated with risk of AD (Rasmussen et al. 2018). Moreover, anti-apoA-I immunoreactivity is found in the brain. These findings indicate a limiting role of the blood brain barrier for any protective role of HDL in CNS diseases such as AD and AMD. Any therapeutic exploitation of HDL for CNS diseases will have to address the interaction of HDL with the blood brain barrier, either as a target of HDL's protective actions, for example in amyloid beta clearance, or as a barrier that must be surmounted by HDL to exert protective functions within the CNS (Button et al. 2019; Robert et al. 2021). The latter is also important for the use of HDL-like nanoparticles that are currently investigated as vehicles for drug delivery into the brain (D'Arrigo 2020; Kadiyala et al. 2019; Kim et al. 2020).

3.4 Implications for Nowaday's Clinical Practice

As the result of the futile intervention trials, HDL-C unlike LDL-C has not become any treatment goal (Grundy et al. 2019; Mach et al. 2020). However, HDL-C continues to be part of ASCVD risk assessment, both directly and indirectly by using HDL-C for the calculation of nonHDL cholesterol or even LDL cholesterol (Grundy et al. 2019; Mach et al. 2020; Martin et al. 2013; Sampson et al. 2020). Especially in asymptomatic patients without any lipid modifying treatment, a low HDL-C level is considered as a risk factor of developing ASCVD. As such, HDL-C is a component of most clinical risk prediction rules that are promoted by guidelines for the prevention of ASCVD (Grundy et al. 2019; Mach et al. 2020). Unfortunately, these algorithms do not realize the discontinuous relationship of HDL-C with risk, but still de-escalate risk estimates in individuals with very high HDL-C levels. This may be a reason why, for example, in the Copenhagen City Heart study the inclusion of HDL-C impaired rather than improved the prognostic performance of SCORE promoted by ESC and EAS (Mortensen et al. 2015). With the same reasoning, clinical laboratories as well as clinicians and practitioners should stop the still widely spread clinical practice to calculate total cholesterol/HDL-C- or LDL-C/HDL-C ratios because they may underestimate the risk of individuals with high HDL-C (de Wolf et al. 2020; Nordestgaard et al. 2020). The same concern may relate to the atherogenic index – the logarithmically transformed ratio of the molar concentrations of plasma triglycerides to HDL-C – especially because some studies found the joint presence of high HDL-C and hypertriglyceridemia associated with increased ASCVD risk (Jeppesen et al. 1998; von Eckardstein et al. 1999). Finally, low HDL-C continues to be a component of definitions for the metabolic syndrome, which indicates increased risks not only for ASCVD but also for diabetes and other obesity related diseases (Alberti et al. 2009).

Whether reflecting compromised anti-atherogenic functions or indicating indirectly a proatherogenic situation, the finding of low HDL-C levels should prompt physicians and patients to optimize the control of other risk factors (März et al. 2017). The lost association of low HDL-C with increased risk upon intensive statin therapy indicates the importance of consequent LDL-C lowering in these patients. Additional important measures include cessation of smoking, correction of obesity and overweight, and treatment of hypertension. In view of the inconsistent outcomes of according randomized controlled trials it is a matter of uncertainty and controversy whether or not hypertriglyceridemia which frequently confounds low HDL-C should be targeted by drug treatment (Ginsberg et al. 2021).

The discussion on therapeutic consequences of high HDL-C levels is in its infancy. It is not clear whether the associations of high HDL-C with increased mortality and risks of CKD, infectious diseases, AD, or AMD are causal. An important potential confounder is excess alcohol consumption (Madsen et al. 2021). Potential candidates for HDL-C lowering drugs are probucol, ANGPTL3 inhibitors, or androgens. In the absence of HDL-C lowering treatments with proven efficacy, it is advisable to focus on risk factor control also in patients with high HDL-C as described for patients with low HDL-C.

References

Abdel-Razek O, Sadananda SN, Li X et al (2018) Increased prevalence of clinical and subclinical atherosclerosis in patients with damaging mutations in ABCA1 or APOA1. J Clin Lipidol 12:116–121

ACCORD Study Group, Ginsberg HN, Elam MB, Lovato LC, Crouse JR 3rd, Leiter LA, Linz P, Friedewald WT, Buse JB, Gerstein HC, Probstfield J, Grimm RH, Ismail-Beigi F, Bigger JT, Goff DC Jr, Cushman WC, Simons-Morton DG, Byington RP (2010) Effects of combination lipid therapy in type 2 diabetes mellitus. N Engl J Med 362(17):1563–1574. Erratum in: N Engl J Med. 2010 May 6;362(18):1748. https://doi.org/10.1056/NEJMoa1001282

Agerholm-Larsen B, Nordestgaard BG, Steffensen R, Jensen G, Tybjaerg-Hansen A (2000) Elevated HDL cholesterol is a risk factor for ischemic heart disease in white women when caused by a common mutation in the cholesteryl ester transfer protein gene. Circulation 101 (16):1907–1912. https://doi.org/10.1161/01.cir.101.16.1907

AIM-HIGH Investigators, Boden WE, Probstfield JL, Anderson T, Chaitman BR, Desvignes-Nickens P, Koprowicz K, McBride R, Teo K, Weintraub W (2011) Niacin in patients with low HDL cholesterol levels receiving intensive statin therapy. N Engl J Med 365 (24):2255–2267. Erratum in: N Engl J Med. 2012 Jul 12;367(2):189. https://doi.org/10.1056/NEJMoa1107579

Alberti KG, Eckel RH, Grundy SM, Zimmet PZ, Cleeman JI, Donato KA et al (2009) Harmonizing the metabolic syndrome: a joint interim statement of the International Diabetes Federation Task Force on Epidemiology and Prevention; National Heart, Lung, and Blood Institute; American Heart Association; World Heart Federation; International Atherosclerosis Society; and International Association for the Study of Obesity. Circulation 120:1640–1645

Anastasius M, Luquain-Costaz C, Kockx M, Jessup W, Kritharides L (2018) A critical appraisal of the measurement of serum 'cholesterol efflux capacity' and its use as surrogate marker of risk of cardiovascular disease. Biochim Biophys Acta Mol Cell Biol Lipids 1863(10):1257–1273. https://doi.org/10.1016/j.bbalip.2018.08.002

Annema W, von Eckardstein A (2013) High-density lipoproteins. Multifunctional but vulnerable protections from atherosclerosis. Circ J 77(10):2432–2448. https://doi.org/10.1253/circj.cj-13-1025

Annema W, von Eckardstein A (2016) Dysfunctional high-density lipoproteins in coronary heart disease: implications for diagnostics and therapy. Transl Res 173:30–57. https://doi.org/10.1016/j.trsl.2016.02.008

Arai H, Yamashita S, Yokote K, Araki E, Suganami H, Ishibashi S, K-877 Study Group (2017) Efficacy and safety of K-877, a novel selective peroxisome proliferator-activated receptor α modulator (SPPARMα), in combination with statin treatment: two randomised, double-blind, placebo-controlled clinical trials in patients with dyslipidaemia. Atherosclerosis 261:144–152. https://doi.org/10.1016/j.atherosclerosis.2017.03.032

Arai H, Bujo H, Masuda D, Ishibashi T, Nakagawa S, Tanabe K, Kagimura T, Kang HJ, Kim MH, Sung J, Kim SH, Kim CH, Park JE, Ge J, Oh BH, Kita T, Saito Y, Fukushima M, Matsuzawa Y, Yamashita S (2021) Integrated analysis of two probucol trials for the secondary prevention of atherosclerotic cardiovascular events: PROSPECTIVE and IMPACT. J Atheroscler Thromb. https://doi.org/10.5551/jat.62821

Arca M, D'Erasmo L, Minicocci I (2020) Familial combined hypolipidemia:angiopoietin-like protein-3 deficiency. Curr Opin Lipidol 31(2):41–48. https://doi.org/10.1097/MOL.0000000000000668

Arsenault BJ, Lemieux I, Després JP, Gagnon P, Wareham NJ, Stroes ES, Kastelein JJ, Khaw KT, Boekholdt SM (2009) HDL particle size and the risk of coronary heart disease in apparently healthy men and women: the EPIC-Norfolk prospective population study. Atherosclerosis 206 (1):276–281. https://doi.org/10.1016/j.atherosclerosis.2009.01.044

Assmann G, Schulte H, von Eckardstein A, Huang Y (1996) High-density lipoprotein cholesterol as a predictor of coronary heart disease risk. The PROCAM experience and pathophysiological implications for reverse cholesterol transport. Atherosclerosis 124 Suppl:S11–S20. https://doi.org/10.1016/0021-9150(96)05852-2

Barter P, Gotto AM, LaRosa JC, Maroni J, Szarek M, Grundy SM, Kastelein JJ, Bittner V, Fruchart JC, Treating to New Targets Investigators (2007a) HDL cholesterol, very low levels of LDL cholesterol, and cardiovascular events. N Engl J Med 357(13):1301–1310. https://doi.org/10.1056/NEJMoa064278

Barter PJ, Caulfield M, Eriksson M, Grundy SM, Kastelein JJ, Komajda M, Lopez-Sendon J, Mosca L, Tardif JC, Waters DD, Shear CL, Revkin JH, Buhr KA, Fisher MR, Tall AR, Brewer B, ILLUMINATE Investigators (2007b) Effects of torcetrapib in patients at high risk for coronary events. N Engl J Med 357(21):2109–2122. https://doi.org/10.1056/NEJMoa0706628

Barter PJ, Rye K-A, Tardif J-C, Waters DD, Boekholdt SM, Breazna A, Kastelein JJ (2011) Effect of torcetrapib on glucose, insulin, and hemoglobin a 1c in subjects in the investigation of lipid level management to understand its impact in atherosclerotic events (ILLUMINATE) trial. Circulation 124:555–562

Behl T, Kaur I, Sehgal A, Kumar A, Uddin MS, Bungau S (2021) The interplay of ABC transporters in Aβ translocation and cholesterol metabolism: implicating their roles in Alzheimer's disease. Mol Neurobiol 58(4):1564–1582. https://doi.org/10.1007/s12035-020-02211-x

Bellenguez C, Küçükali F, Jansen I, Andrade V, Moreno-grau S (2020) New insights on the genetic etiology of Alzheimer's and related dementia. MedRxiv:1–35. https://doi.org/10.1101/2020.10.01.20200659

Benn M, Nordestgaard BG (2018) From genome-wide association studies to Mendelian randomization: novel opportunities for understanding cardiovascular disease causality, pathogenesis, prevention, and treatment. Cardiovasc Res 114(9):1192–1208. https://doi.org/10.1093/cvr/cvy045

Bezafibrate Infarction Prevention (BIP) Study (2000) Secondary prevention by raising HDL cholesterol and reducing triglycerides in patients with coronary artery disease. Circulation 102 (1):21–27. https://doi.org/10.1161/01.cir.102.1.21

Bisgaard LS, Christoffersen C (2019) Apolipoprotein M/sphingosine-1-phosphate:novel effects on lipids, inflammation and kidney biology. Curr Opin Lipidol 30(3):212–217. https://doi.org/10.1097/MOL.0000000000000606

Blauw LL, Wang Y, Willems van Dijk K, Rensen PCN (2020) A novel role for CETP as immunological gatekeeper: raising HDL to cure sepsis? Trends Endocrinol Metab 31 (5):334–343. https://doi.org/10.1016/j.tem.2020.01.003

Boekholdt SM, Arsenault BJ, Hovingh GK, Mora S, Pedersen TR, Larosa JC, Welch KM, Amarenco P, Demicco DA, Tonkin AM, Sullivan DR, Kirby A, Colhoun HM, Hitman GA, Betteridge DJ, Durrington PN, Clearfield MB, Downs JR, Gotto AM Jr, Ridker PM, Kastelein JJ (2013) Levels and changes of HDL cholesterol and apolipoprotein A-I in relation to risk of cardiovascular events among statin-treated patients: a meta-analysis. Circulation 128 (14):1504–1512. https://doi.org/10.1161/CIRCULATIONAHA.113.002670

Bolibar I, von Eckardstein A, Assmann G, Thompson S, ECAT Angina Pectoris Study Group. European Concerted Action on Thrombosis and Disabilities (2000) Short-term prognostic value of lipid measurements in patients with angina pectoris.The ECAT Angina Pectoris Study Group: European Concerted Action on Thrombosis and Disabilities. Thromb Haemost 84(6):955–960

Bonaca MP, George RT, Morrow DA, Bergmark BA, Park JG, Abuhatzira L, Vavere AL, Karathanasis SK, Jin C, She D, Hirshberg B, Hsia J, Sabatine MS (2021) Recombinant human lecithin-cholesterol acyltransferase in patients with atherosclerosis: phase 2a primary results and phase 2b design. Eur Heart J Cardiovasc Pharmacother:pvab001. https://doi.org/10.1093/ehjcvp/pvab001

Borén J, Chapman MJ, Krauss RM, Packard CJ, Bentzon JF, Binder CJ, Daemen MJ, Demer LL, Hegele RA, Nicholls SJ, Nordestgaard BG, Watts GF, Bruckert E, Fazio S, Ference BA, Graham I, Horton JD, Landmesser U, Laufs U, Masana L, Pasterkamp G, Raal FJ, Ray KK, Schunkert H, Taskinen MR, van de Sluis B, Wiklund O, Tokgozoglu L, Catapano AL, Ginsberg HN (2020) Low-density lipoproteins cause atherosclerotic cardiovascular disease: pathophysiological, genetic, and therapeutic insights: a consensus statement from the European Atherosclerosis Society Consensus Panel. Eur Heart J 41(24):2313–2330. https://doi.org/10.1093/eurheartj/ehz962

Borggreve SE, Hillege HL, Wolffenbuttel BHR, De Jong PE, Zuurman MW, Van Der Steege G, Van Tol A, Dullaart RPF (2006) An increased coronary risk is paradoxically associated with common cholesteryl ester transfer protein gene variations that relate to higher high-density lipoprotein cholesterol: a population-based study. J Clin Endocrinol Metab 91:3382–3388

Bowe B, Xie Y, Xian H, Balasubramanian S, Zayed MA, Al-Aly Z (2016a) High density lipoprotein cholesterol and the risk of all-cause mortality among U.S. veterans. Clin J Am Soc Nephrol 11(10):1784–1793. https://doi.org/10.2215/CJN.00730116

Bowe B, Xie Y, Xian H, Balasubramanian S, Al-Aly Z (2016b) Low levels of high-density lipoprotein cholesterol increase the risk of incident kidney disease and its progression. Kidney Int 89(4):886–896. https://doi.org/10.1016/j.kint.2015.12.034

Brodeur MR, Rhainds D, Charpentier D, Mihalache-Avram T, Mecteau M, Brand G, Chaput E, Perez A, Niesor EJ, Rhéaume E, Maugeais C, Tardif JC (2017) Dalcetrapib and anacetrapib differently impact HDL structure and function in rabbits and monkeys. J Lipid Res 58 (7):1282–1291. https://doi org/10.1194/jlr.M068940

Burgess S, Smith GD (2017) Mendelian randomization implicates high-density lipoprotein cholesterol–associated mechanisms in etiology of age-related macular degeneration. Ophthalmology 124:1165–1174

Button EB, Robert J, Caffrey TM, Fan J, Zhao W, Wellington CL (2019) HDL from an Alzheimer's disease perspective. Curr Opin Lipidol 30(3):224–234. https://doi.org/10.1097/MOL. 0000000000000604

Cardner M, Yalcinkaya M, Goetze S, Luca E, Balaz M, Hunjadi M, Hartung J, Shemet A, Kraenkel N, Radosavljevic S, Keel M, Othman A, Karsai G, Hornemann T, Claassen M, Liebisch G, Carreira E, Ritsch A, Landmesser U, Krützfeldt J, Wolfrum C, Wollscheid B, Beerenwinkel N, Rohrer L, von Eckardstein A (2020) Structure-function relationships of HDL in diabetes and coronary heart disease. JCI Insight 5(1):e131491. https://doi.org/10.1172/jci. insight.131491

Catapano AL, Pirillo A, Bonacina F, Norata GD (2014) HDL in innate and adaptive immunity. Cardiovasc Res 103:372–383

Chandra A, Neeland IJ, Das SR, Khera A, Turer AT, Ayers CR, McGuire DK, Rohatgi A (2015) Relation of black race between high density lipoprotein cholesterol content, high density lipoprotein particles and coronary events (from the Dallas Heart Study). Am J Cardiol 115 (7):890–894. https://doi.org/10.1016/j.amjcard.2015.01.015

Chapman MJ, Le Goff W, Guerin M, Kontush A (2010) Cholesteryl ester transfer protein: at the heart of the action of lipid-modulating therapy with statins, fibrates, niacin, and cholesteryl ester transfer protein inhibitors. Eur Heart J 31(2):149–164. https://doi.org/10.1093/eurheartj/ehp399

Chen W, Stambolian D, Edwards AO, Branham KE, Othman M, Jakobsdottir J, Tosakulwong N, Pericak-Vance MA, Campochiaro PA, Klein ML, Tan PL, Conley YP, Kanda A, Kopplin L, Li Y, Augustaitis KJ, Karoukis AJ, Scott WK, Agarwal A, Kovach JL, Schwartz SG, Postel EA, Brooks M, Baratz KH, Brown WL, Complications of Age-Related Macular Degeneration Prevention Trial Research Group, Brucker AJ, Orlin A, Brown G, Ho A, Regillo C, Donoso L, Tian L, Kaderli B, Hadley D, Hagstrom SA, Peachey NS, Klein R, Klein BE, Gotoh N, Yamashiro K, Ferris Iii F, Fagerness JA, Reynolds R, Farrer LA, Kim IK, Miller JW, Cortón M, Carracedo A, Sanchez-Salorio M, Pugh EW, Doheny KF, Brion M, Deangelis MM, Weeks DE, Zack DJ, Chew EY, Heckenlively JR, Yoshimura N, Iyengar SK, Francis PJ, Katsanis N, Seddon JM, Haines JL, Gorin MB, Abecasis GR, Swaroop A (2010) Genetic variants near TIMP3 and high-density lipoprotein-associated loci influence susceptibility to age-related macular degeneration. Proc Natl Acad Sci U S A 107(16):7401–7406. https://doi. org/10.1073/pnas.0912702107

Chiba-Falek O, Nichols M, Suchindran S, Guyton J, Ginsburg GS, Barrett-Connor E, McCarthy JJ (2010) Impact of gene variants on sex-specific regulation of human Scavenger receptor class B type 1 (SR-BI) expression in liver and association with lipid levels in a population-based study. BMC Med Genet 11:9. https://doi.org/10.1186/1471-2350-11-9

Christoffersen C, Obinata H, Kumaraswamy SB, Galvani S, Ahnström J, Sevvana M, Egerer-Sieber C, Muller YA, Hla T, Nielsen LB, Dahlbäck B (2011) Endothelium-protective sphingo-sine-1-phosphate provided by HDL-associated apolipoprotein. MProc Natl Acad Sci U S A 108 (23):9613–9618. https://doi.org/10.1073/pnas.1103187108

Cochran BJ, Ong KL, Manandhar B, Rye KA (2021) High density lipoproteins and diabetes. Cell 10(4):850. https://doi.org/10.3390/cells10040850

Colantonio LD, Bittner V, Reynolds K, Levitan EB, Rosenson RS, Banach M, Kent ST, Derose SF, Zhou H, Safford MM, Muntner P (2016) Association of serum lipids and coronary heart disease in contemporary observational studies. Circulation 133(3):256–264. https://doi.org/10.1161/ CIRCULATIONAHA.115.011646

Colijn JM, den Hollander AI, Demirkan A, Cougnard-Grégoire A, Verzijden T, Kersten E, Meester-Smoor MA, Merle BMJ, Papageorgiou G, Ahmad S, Mulder MT, Costa MA, Benlian P, Bertelsen G, Bron AM, Claes B, Creuzot-Garcher C, Erke MG, Fauser S, Foster PJ, Hammond CJ, Hense HW, Hoyng CB, Khawaja AP, Korobelnik JF, Piermarocchi S, Segato T, Silva R, Souied EH, Williams KM, van Duijn CM, Delcourt C, Klaver CCW, European Eye Epidemiology Consortium, EYE-RISK Consortium (2019) Increased high-density lipoprotein levels associated with age-related macular degeneration: evidence from the EYE-RISK and

European eye epidemiology consortia. Ophthalmology 126(3):393–406. https://doi.org/10.1016/j.ophtha.2018.09.045

Crosby JH, Peloso GM, Auer PL, Crosslin DR, Stitziel N, Lange LA, Lu Y, Tang ZZ, Zhang H, Hindy G et al (2014) Loss-of-function mutations in APOC3, triglycerides, and coronary disease. N Engl J Med 371:22–31

Damen MSMA, Popa CD, Netea MG, Dinarello CA, Joosten LAB (2017) Interleukin-32 in chronic inflammatory conditions is associated with a higher risk of cardiovascular diseases. Atherosclerosis 264:83–91. https //doi.org/10.1016/j.atherosclerosis.2017.07.005

D'Arrigo JS (2020) Biomimetic nanocarrier targeting drug(s) to upstream-receptor mechanisms in dementia: focusing on linking pathogenic cascades. Biomimetics (Basel) 5(1):11. https://doi.org/10.3390/biomimetics5010011

de Haan W, de Vries-van der Weij J, van der Hoorn JW, Gautier T, van der Hoogt CC, Westerterp M, Romijn JA, Jukema JW, Havekes LM, Princen HM, Rensen PC (2008) Torcetrapib does not reduce atherosclerosis beyond atorvastatin and induces more proinflammatory lesions than atorvastatin. Circulation 117(19):2515–2522. https://doi.org/10.1161/CIRCULATIONAHA.107.761965

De Wolf HA, Langlois MR, Suvisaari J, Aakre KM, Baum H, Collinson P, Duff CJ, Gruson D, Hammerer-Lercher A, Pulkki K, Stankovic S, Stavljenic-Rukavina A, Laitinen P, EFLM Task Group on Cardiac Markers (2020) How well do laboratories adhere to recommended guidelines for dyslipidaemia management in Europe? The cardiac MARker guideline uptake in Europe (CAMARGUE) study. Clin Chim Acta 508:267–272. https://doi.org/10.1016/j.cca.2020.05.038

Ditah C, Otvos J, Nassar H, Shaham D, Sinnreich R, Kark JD (2016) Small and medium sized HDL particles are protectively associated with coronary calcification in a cross-sectional population-based sample. Atherosclerosis 251:124–131. https://doi.org/10.1016/j.atherosclerosis.2016.06.010

Drew BG, Duffy SJ, Formosa MF, Natoli AK, Henstridge DC, Penfold SA, Thomas WG, Mukhamedova N, de Courten B, Forbes JM et al (2009) High-density lipoprotein modulates glucose metabolism in patients with type 2 diabetes mellitus. Circulation 119:2103–2111

El Harchaoui K, Arsenault BJ, Franssen R, Després JP, Hovingh GK, Stroes ES, Otvos JD, Wareham NJ, Kastelein JJ, Khaw KT, Boekholdt SM (2009) High-density lipoprotein particle size and concentration and coronary risk. Ann Intern Med 150(2):84–93. https://doi.org/10.7326/0003-4819-150-2-200901200-00006

Emerging Risk Factors Collaboration, Di Angelantonio E, Sarwar N, Perry P, Kaptoge S, Ray KK, Thompson A, Wood AM, Lewington S, Sattar N, Packard CJ, Collins R, Thompson SG, Danesh J (2009) Major lipids, apolipoproteins, and risk of vascular disease. JAMA 302(18):1993–2000. https://doi.org/10.1001/jama.2009.1619

Emmens JE, Jones DJL, Cao TH, Chan DCS, Romaine SPR, Quinn PA, Anker SD, Cleland JG, Dickstein K, Filippatos G, Hillege HL, Lang CC, Ponikowski P, Samani NJ, van Veldhuisen DJ, Zannad F, Zwinderman AH, Metra M, de Boer RA, Voors AA, Ng LL (2018) Proteomic diversity of high-density lipoprotein explains its association with clinical outcome in patients with heart failure. Eur J Heart Fail 20(2):260–267. https://doi.org/10.1002/ejhf.1101

Fall T, Xie W, Poon W, Yaghootkar H, Mägi R, Knowles JW, Lyssenko V, Weedon M, Frayling TM, Ingelsson E (2015) Using genetic variants to assess the relationship between circulating lipids and type 2 diabetes. Diabetes 64:2676–2684

Fan Q, Maranville JC, Fritsche L, Sim X, Cheung CMG, Chen LJ, Gorski M, Yamashiro K, Ahn J, Laude A et al (2017) HDL-cholesterol levels and risk of age-related macular degeneration: a multiethnic genetic study using Mendelian randomization. Int J Epidemiol 46:1891–1902

Ference BA, Kastelein JJP, Ginsberg HN, Chapman MJ, Nicholls SJ, Ray KK, Packard CJ, Laufs U, Brook RD, Oliver-Williams C, Butterworth AS, Danesh J, Smith GD, Catapano AL, Sabatine MS (2017) Association of genetic variants related to CETP inhibitors and statins with lipoprotein levels and cardiovascular risk. JAMA 318(10):947–956. https://doi.org/10.1001/jama.2017.11467

Freeman LA, Karathanasis SK, Remaley AT (2020) Novel lecithin: cholesterol acyltransferase-based therapeutic approaches. Curr Opin Lipidol 31(2):71–79. https://doi.org/10.1097/MOL. 0000000000000673

Frick MH, Elo O, Haapa K, Heinonen OP, Heinsalmi P, Helo P, Huttunen JK, Kaitaniemi P, Koskinen P, Manninen V et al (1987) Helsinki heart study: primary-prevention trial with gemfibrozil in middle-aged men with dyslipidemia. Safety of treatment, changes in risk factors, and incidence of coronary heart disease. N Engl J Med 317(20):1237–1245. https://doi.org/10. 1056/NEJM198711123172001

Friedman DJ, Pollak MR (2020) APOL1 and kidney disease: from genetics to biology. Annu Rev Physiol 82:323–342. https://doi.org/10.1146/annurev-physiol-021119-034345

Fritsche LG, Igl W, Bailey JNC, Grassmann F, Sengupta S, Bragg-Gresham JL, Burdon KP, Hebbring SJ, Wen C, Gorski M et al (2016) A large genome-wide association study of age-related macular degeneration highlights contributions of rare and common variants. Nat Genet 48:134–143

Furtado JD, Yamamoto R, Melchior JT, Andraski AB, Gamez-Guerrero M, Mulcahy P, He Z, Cai T, Davidson WS, Sacks FM (2018) Distinct proteomic signatures in 16 HDL (high-density lipoprotein) subspecies. Arterioscler Thromb Vasc Biol 38(12):2827–2842. https://doi.org/10. 1161/ATVBAHA.118.311607

Ganjali S, Banach M, Pirro M, Fras Z, Sahebkar A (2021) HDL and cancer – causality still needs to be confirmed? Update 2020. Semin Cancer Biol 73:169–177. https://doi.org/10.1016/j. semcancer.2020.10.007

Gaudet D, Karwatowska-Prokopczuk E, Baum SJ, Hurh E, Kingsbury J, Bartlett VJ, Figueroa AL, Piscitelli P, Singleton W, Witztum JL, Geary RS, Tsimikas S, O'Dea LSL, Vupanorsen Study Investigators (2020) Vupanorsen, an N-acetyl galactosamine-conjugated antisense drug to ANGPTL3 mRNA, lowers triglycerides and atherogenic lipoproteins in patients with diabetes, hepatic steatosis, and hypertriglyceridaemia. Eur Heart J 41(40):3936–3945. https://doi.org/10. 1093/eurheartj/ehaa689

Geller AS, Polisecki EY, Diffenderfer MR et al (2018) Genetic and secondary causes of severe HDL deficiency and cardiovascular disease. J Lipid Res 59:2421–2435

Gencer B, Mach F (2020) Potential of lipoprotein(a)-lowering strategies in treating coronary artery disease. Drugs 80(3):229–239. https://doi.org/10.1007/s40265-019-01243-5

Gerster R, Eloranta JJ, Hausmann M, Ruiz PA, Cosin-Roger J, Terhalle A, Ziegler U, Kullak-Ublick GA, von Eckardstein A, Rogler G (2014) Anti-inflammatory function of high-density lipoproteins via autophagy of IκB kinase. Cell Mol Gastroenterol Hepatol 1(2):171–187.e1. https://doi.org/10.1016/j.jcmgh.2014.12.006

Ghosh GC, Bhadra R, Ghosh RK, Banerjee K, Gupta A (2017) RVX 208: a novel BET protein inhibitor, role as an inducer of apo A-I/HDL and beyond. Cardiovasc Ther 35(4). https://doi.org/ 10.1111/1755-5922.12265

Gibson CM, Kastelein JJP, Phillips AT, Aylward PE, Yee MK, Tendera M, Nicholls SJ, Pocock S, Goodman SG, Alexander JH, Lincoff AM, Bode C, Duffy D, Heise M, Berman G, Mears SJ, Tricoci P, Deckelbaum LI, Steg PG et al (2021) Rationale and design of ApoA-I event reducing in ischemic syndromes II (AEGIS-II): a phase 3, multicenter, double-blind, randomized, placebo-controlled, parallel-group study to investigate the efficacy and safety of CSL112 in subjects after acute myocardial infarction. Am Heart J 231:121–127

Ginsberg HN, Packard CJ, Chapman JM, Borén J, Aguilar-Salinas CA, Averna M, Ference BA, Gaudet D, Hegele RA, Kersten S, Lewis LF, Lichtenstein AH, Moulin P, Nordestgaard BG, Remaley AT, Staels, ESG S, Taskinen MR, Tokgözoğlu LS, Tybjaerg-Hansen A, Stock JK, Catapano AL (2021) Triglyceride-rich lipoproteins and their remnants: metabolic insights, role in atherosclerotic cardiovascular disease, and emerging therapeutic strategies. A consensus statement from the European Atherosclerosis Society. Eur Heart J. (in press)

Gordon EM, Figueroa DM, Barochia AV, Yao X, Levine SJ (2016) High-density lipoproteins and apolipoprotein A-I: potential new players in the prevention and treatment of lung disease. Front Pharmacol 7:323. https://doi.org/10.3389/fphar.2016.00323

Grundy SM, Stone NJ, Bailey AL, Beam C, Birtcher KK, Blumenthal RS, Braun LT, de Ferranti S, Faiella-Tommasino J, Forman DE, Goldberg R, Heidenreich PA, Hlatky MA, Jones DW, Lloyd-Jones D, Lopez-Pajares N, Ndumele CE, Orringer CE, Peralta CA, Saseen JJ, Smith SC Jr, Sperling L, Virani SS, Yeboah J (2019) 2018 AHA/ACC/AACVPR/AAPA/ABC/ACPM/ADA/AGS/APhA/ASPC/NLA/PCNA guideline on the management of blood cholesterol: a report of the American College of Cardiology/American Heart Association Task Force on Clinical Practice guidelines. Circulation 139(25):e1082–e1143. Erratum in: Circulation. 2019 Jun 18;139(25):e1182–e1186. https://doi.org/10.1161/CIR.0000000000000625

Guyton JR, Slee AE, Anderson T, Fleg JL, Goldberg RB, Kashyap ML, Marcovina SM, Nash SD, O'Brien KD, Weintraub WS, Xu P, Zhao XQ, Boden WE (2013) Relationship of lipoproteins to cardiovascular events: the AIM-HIGH trial (atherothrombosis intervention in metabolic syndrome with low HDL/high triglycerides and impact on global health outcomes). J Am Coll Cardiol 62(17):1580–1584. https://doi.org/10.1016/j.jacc.2013.07.023

Haase CL, Tybjærg-Hansen A, Nordestgaard BG, Frikke-Schmidt R (2015) HDL cholesterol and risk of type 2 diabetes: a Mendelian randomization study. Diabetes 64:3328–3333

Hafiane A, Genest J (2015) High density lipoproteins: measurement techniques and potential biomarkers of cardiovascular risk. BBA Clin 3:175–188. https://doi.org/10.1016/j.bbacli.2015.01.005

He H, Hong K, Liu L, Schwendeman A (2021) Artificial high-density lipoprotein mimicking nanotherapeutics for the treatment of cardiovascular diseases. Wiley Interdiscip Rev Nanomed Nanobiotechnol 14:e1737. https://doi.org/10.1002/wnan.1737

Helgadottir A, Sulem P, Thorgeirsson G, Gretarsdottir S, Thorleifsson G, Jensson BÖ, Arnadottir GA, Olafsson I, Eyjolfsson GI, Sigurdardottir O, Thorsteinsdottir U, Gudbjartsson DF, Holm H, Stefansson K (2018) Rare SCARB1 mutations associate with high-density lipoprotein cholesterol but not with coronary artery disease. Eur Heart J 39(23):2172–2178. https://doi.org/10.1093/eurheartj/ehy169

Hennuyer N, Duplan I, Paquet C, Vanhoutte J, Woitrain E, Touche V, Colin S, Vallez E, Lestavel S, Lefebvre P, Staels B (2016) The novel selective PPARα modulator (SPPARMα) pemafibrate improves dyslipidemia, enhances reverse cholesterol transport and decreases inflammation and atherosclerosis. Atherosclerosis 249:200–208. https://doi.org/10.1016/j.atherosclerosis.2016.03.003

Hilser JR, Han Y, Biswas S, Gukasyan J, Cai Z, Zhu R, Tang WHW, Deb A, Lusis AJ, Hartiala JA, Allayee H (2021) Association of serum HDL-cholesterol and apolipoprotein A1 levels with risk of severe SARS-CoV-2 infection. J Lipid Res 62:100061. https://doi.org/10.1016/j.jlr.2021.100061

Hilvo M, Meikle PJ, Pedersen ER, Tell GS, Dhar I, Brenner H, Schöttker B, Lääperi M, Kauhanen D, Koistinen KM, Jylhä A, Huynh K, Mellett NA, Tonkin AM, Sullivan DR, Simes J, Nestel P, Koenig W, Rothenbacher D, Nygård O, Laaksonen R (2019) Development and validation of a ceramide- and phospholipid-based cardiovascular risk estimation score for coronary artery disease patients. Eur Heart J. https://doi.org/10.1093/eurheartj/ehz387

Hoekstra M, Sorci-Thomas M (2017) Rediscovering scavenger receptor type BI: surprising new roles for the HDL receptor. Curr Opin Lipidol 28(3):255–260. https://doi.org/10.1097/MOL.0000000000000413

Hoekstra M, Van Eck M (2015) Mouse models of disturbed HDL metabolism. Handb Exp Pharmacol 224:301–336. https://doi.org/10.1007/978-3-319-09665-0_9

Hopewell JC, Ibrahim M, Hill M, Shaw PM, Braunwald E, Blaustein RO, Bowman L, Landray MJ, Sabatine MS, Collins R, HPS3/TIMI55 - REVEAL Collaborative Group (2019) Impact of ADCY9 genotype on response to anacetrapib. Circulation 140(11):891–898. https://doi.org/10.1161/CIRCULATIONAHA.119.041546

HPS2-THRIVE Collaborative Group, Landray MJ, Haynes R, Hopewell JC, Parish S, Aung T, Tomson J, Wallendszus K, Craig M, Jiang L, Collins R, Armitage J (2014) Effects of extended-release niacin with laropiprant in high-risk patients. N Engl J Med 371(3):203–212. https://doi.org/10.1056/NEJMoa1300955

HPS3/TIMI55–REVEAL Collaborative Group, Bowman L, Hopewell JC, Chen F, Wallendszus K, Stevens W, Collins R, Wiviott SD, Cannon CP, Braunwald E, Sammons E, Landray MJ (2017) Effects of anacetrapib in patients with atherosclerotic vascular disease. N Engl J Med 377 (13):1217–1227. https://doi.org/10.1056/NEJMoa1706444

Jensen MK, Aroner SA, Mukamal KJ, Furtado JD, Post WS, Tsai MY, Tjønneland A, Polak JF, Rimm EB, Overvad K, McClelland RL, Sacks FM (2018) High-density lipoprotein subspecies defined by presence of apolipoprotein C-III and incident coronary heart disease in four cohorts. Circulation 137(13):1364–1373. https://doi.org/10.1161/CIRCULATIONAHA.117.031276

Jeppesen J, Hein HO, Suadicani P, Gyntelberg F (1998) Triglyceride concentration and ischemic heart disease: an eight-year follow-up in the Copenhagen male study. Circulation 97 (11):1029–1036. Erratum in: Circulation 1998 May 19;97(19):1995. https://doi.org/10.1161/01.cir.97.11.1029

Jin Z, Collier TS, Dai DLY, Chen V, Hollander Z, Ng RT, McManus BM, Balshaw R, Apostolidou S, Penn MS, Bystrom C (2019) Development and validation of apolipoprotein AI-associated lipoprotein proteome panel for the prediction of cholesterol efflux capacity and coronary artery disease. Clin Chem 65(2):282–290. https://doi.org/10.1373/clinchem.2018.291922

Johannesen CDL, Langsted A, Mortensen MB, Nordestgaard BG (2020) Association between low density lipoprotein and all cause and cause specific mortality in Denmark: prospective cohort study. BMJ 371:m4266. Erratum in: BMJ. 2021 Feb 12;372:n422. https://doi.org/10.1136/bmj.m4266

Kadiyala P, Li D, Nuñez FM, Altshuler D, Doherty R, Kuai R, Yu M, Kamran N, Edwards M, Moon JJ, Lowenstein PR, Castro MG, Schwendeman A (2019) High-density lipoprotein-mimicking nanodiscs for chemo-immunotherapy against glioblastoma multiforme. ACS Nano 13(2):1365–1384. https://doi.org/10.1021/acsnano.8b06842

Kamanna VS, Ganji SH, Kashyap ML (2013) Recent advances in niacin and lipid metabolism. Curr Opin Lipidol 24(3):239–245. https://doi.org/10.1097/MOL.0b013e3283613a68

Karjalainen MK, Holmes MV, Wang Q, Anufrieva O, Kähönen M, Lehtimäki T, Havulinna AS, Kristiansson K, Salomaa V, Perola M, Viikari JS, Raitakari OT, Järvelin MR, Ala-Korpela M, Kettunen J (2020) Apolipoprotein A-I concentrations and risk of coronary artery disease: a Mendelian randomization study. Atherosclerosis 299:56–63. https://doi.org/10.1016/j.atherosclerosis.2020.02.002

Kathiresan S (2012) Will cholesteryl ester transfer protein inhibition succeed primarily by lowering low-density lipoprotein cholesterol? Insights from human genetics and clinical trials. J Am Coll Cardiol 60(20):2049–2052. https://doi.org/10.1016/j.jacc.2012.08.967

Keech A, Simes RJ, Barter P, Best J, Scott R, Taskinen MR, Forder P, Pillai A, Davis T, Glasziou P, Drury P, Kesäniemi YA, Sullivan D, Hunt D, Colman P, d'Emden M, Whiting M, Ehnholm C, Laakso M, FIELD study investigators (2005) Effects of long-term fenofibrate therapy on cardiovascular events in 9795 people with type 2 diabetes mellitus (the FIELD study): randomised controlled trial. Lancet 366(9500):1849–1861. Erratum in: Lancet. 2006 Oct 21;368(9545):1420. Erratum in: Lancet. 2006 Oct 21;368(9545):1415. https://doi.org/10.1016/S0140-6736(05)67667-2

Keene D, Price C, Shun-Shin MJ, Francis DP (2014) Effect on cardiovascular risk of high density lipoprotein targeted drug treatments niacin, fibrates, and CETP inhibitors: meta-analysis of randomised controlled trials including 117,411 patients. BMJ 349:g4379. https://doi.org/10.1136/bmj.g4379

Khan AA, Mundra PA, Straznicky NE, Nestel PJ, Wong G, Tan R, Huynh K, Ng TW, Mellett NA, Weir JM, Barlow CK, Alshehry ZH, Lambert GW, Kingwell BA, Meikle PJ (2018) Weight loss and exercise alter the high-density lipoprotein lipidome and improve high-density lipoprotein functionality in metabolic syndrome. Arterioscler Thromb Vasc Biol 38(2):438–447. https://doi.org/10.1161/ATVBAHA.117.310212

Kim DS, Li YK, Bell GA, Burt AA, Vaisar T, Hutchins PM, Furlong CE, Otvos JD, Polak JF, Arnan MK, Kaufman JD, McClelland RL, Longstreth WT Jr, Jarvik GP (2016) Concentration of smaller high-density lipoprotein particle (HDL-P) is inversely correlated with carotid intima media thickening after confounder adjustment: the multi ethnic study of atherosclerosis (MESA). J Am Heart Assoc 5(5):e002977. https://doi.org/10.1161/JAHA.115.002977

Kim J, Dey A, Malhotra A, Liu J, Ahn SI, Sei YJ, Kenney AM, MacDonald TJ, Kim Y (2020) Engineered biomimetic nanoparticle for dual targeting of the cancer stem-like cell population in sonic hedgehog medulloblastoma. Proc Natl Acad Sci U S A 117(39):24205–24212. https://doi.org/10.1073/pnas.1912229117

Kinslechner K, Schörghofer D, Schütz B, Vallianou M, Wingelhofer B, Mikulits W, Röhrl C, Hengstschläger M, Moriggl R, Stangl H, Mikula M (2018) Malignant phenotypes in metastatic melanoma are governed by SR-BI and its association with glycosylation and STAT5 activation. Mol Cancer Res 16(1) 135–146. https://doi.org/10.1158/1541-7786.MCR-17-0292

Kjeldsen EW, Nordestgaard LT, Frikke-Schmidt R (2021a) HDL cholesterol and non-cardiovascular disease: a narrative review. Int J Mol Sci 22(9):4547. https://doi.org/10.3390/ijms22094547

Kjeldsen EW, Thomassen JQ, Juul Rasmussen I, Nordestgaard BG, Tybjærg-Hansen A, Frikke-Schmidt R (2021b) Plasma HDL cholesterol and risk of dementia – observational and genetic studies. Cardiovasc Res:cvab164. https://doi.org/10.1093/cvr/cvab164

Ko DT, Alter DA, Guo H, Koh M, Lau G, Austin PC, Booth GL, Hogg W, Jackevicius CA, Lee DS, Wijeysundera HC, Wilkins JT, Tu JV (2016) High-density lipoprotein cholesterol and cause-specific mortality in individuals without previous cardiovascular conditions: the CANHEART study. J Am Coll Cardiol 68(19):2073–2083. https://doi.org/10.1016/j.jacc.2016.08.038

Ko CW, Qu J, Black DD, Tso P (2020) Regulation of intestinal lipid metabolism: current concepts and relevance to disease. Nat Rev Gastroenterol Hepatol 17(3):169–183. https://doi.org/10.1038/s41575-019-0250-7

Kontush A, Lhomme M, Chapman MJ (2013) Unraveling the complexities of the HDL lipidome. J Lipid Res 54(11):2950–2963. https://doi.org/10.1194/jlr.R036095

Kopecky C, Genser B, Drechsler C, Krane V, Kaltenecker CC, Hengstschläger M, März W, Wanner C, Säemann MD, Weichhart T (2015) Quantification of HDL proteins, cardiac events, and mortality in patients with type 2 diabetes on hemodialysis. Clin J Am Soc Nephrol 10 (2):224–231. https://doi.org/10.2215/CJN.06560714

Kühnast S, van der Tuin SJ, van der Hoorn JW, van Klinken JB, Simic B, Pieterman E, Havekes LM, Landmesser U, Lüscher TF, Willems van Dijk K, Rensen PC, Jukema JW, Princen HM (2015) Anacetrapib reduces progression of atherosclerosis, mainly by reducing non-HDL-cholesterol, improves lesion stability and adds to the beneficial effects of atorvastatin. Eur Heart J 36(1):39–48. https://doi.org/10.1093/eurheartj/ehu319

Kuller LH, Grandits G, Cohen JD, Neaton JD, Prineas R, Multiple Risk Factor Intervention Trial Research Group (2007) Lipoprotein particles, insulin, adiponectin, C-reactive protein and risk of coronary heart disease among men with metabolic syndrome. Atherosclerosis 195(1):122–128. https://doi.org/10.1016/j.atherosclerosis.2006.09.001

Kuusisto S, Holmes MV, Ohukainen P, Kangas AJ, Karsikas M, Tiainen M, Perola M, Salomaa V, Kettunen J, Ala-Korpela M (2019) Direct estimation of HDL-mediated cholesterol efflux capacity from serum. Clin Chem 65(8):1042–1050. https://doi.org/10.1373/clinchem.2018.299222

Langer C, Gansz B, Goepfert C, Engel T, Uehara Y, von Dehn G, Jansen H, Assmann G, von Eckardstein A (2002) Testosterone up-regulates scavenger receptor BI and stimulates cholesterol efflux from macrophages. Biochem Biophys Res Commun 296(5):1051–1057. https://doi.org/10.1016/s0006-291x(02)02038-7

Langsted A, Jensen AMR, Varbo A, Nordestgaard BG (2020) Low high-density lipoprotein cholesterol to monitor long-term average increased triglycerides. J Clin Endocrinol Metab 105 (4):dgz265. https://doi.org/10.1210/clinem/dgz265

Lassale C, Hamer M, Hernáez Á, Gale CR, Batty GD (2021) Association of pre-pandemic high-density lipoprotein cholesterol with risk of COVID-19 hospitalisation and death: the UK Biobank cohort study. Prev Med Rep 23:101461. https://doi.org/10.1016/j.pmedr.2021.101461

Le Lay JE, Du Q, Mehta MB, Bhagroo N, Hummer BT, Falloon J, Carlson G, Rosenbaum AI, Jin C, Kimko H, Tsai LF, Novick S, Cook B, Han D, Han CY, Vaisar T, Chait A, Karathanasis SK, Rhodes CJ, Hirshberg B, Damschroder MM, Hsia J, Grimsby JS (2021) Blocking endothelial lipase with monoclonal antibody MEDI5884 durably increases high density lipoprotein in nonhuman primates and in a phase 1 trial. Sci Transl Med 13(590):eabb0602. https://doi.org/10.1126/scitranslmed.abb0602

Lee-Rueckert M, Escola-Gil JC, Kovanen PT (2016) HDL functionality in reverse cholesterol transport--challenges in translating data emerging from mouse models to human disease. Biochim Biophys Acta 1861(7):566–583. https://doi.org/10.1016/j.bbalip.2016.03.004

Lehti M, Donelan E, Abplanalp W, Al-Massadi O, Habegger KM, Weber J, Ress C, Mansfeld J, Somvanshi S, Trivedi C, Keuper M, Ograjsek T, Striese C, Cucuruz S, Pfluger PT, Krishna R, Gordon SM, Silva RA, Luquet S, Castel J, Martinez S, D'Alessio D, Davidson WS, Hofmann SM (2013) High-density lipoprotein maintains skeletal muscle function by modulating cellular respiration in mice. Circulation 128(22):2364–2371. https://doi.org/10.1161/CIRCULATIONAHA.113.001551

Li JJ, Zhang Y, Li S, Cui CJ, Zhu CG, Guo YL, Wu NQ, Xu RX, Liu G, Dong Q, Sun J (2016) Large HDL subfraction but not HDL-C is closely linked with risk factors, coronary severity and outcomes in a cohort of nontreated patients with stable coronary artery disease: a prospective observational study. Medicine (Baltimore) 95(4):e2600. https://doi.org/10.1097/MD.0000000000002600

Lincoff AM, Nicholls SJ, Riesmeyer JS, Barter PJ, Brewer HB, Fox KAA, Gibson CM, Granger C, Menon V, Montalescot G, Rader D, Tall AR, McErlean E, Wolski K, Ruotolo G, Vangerow B, Weerakkody G, Goodman SG, Conde D, McGuire DK, Nicolau JC, Leiva-Pons JL, Pesant Y, Li W, Kandath D, Kouz S, Tahirkheli N, Mason D, Nissen SE, ACCELERATE Investigators (2017) Evacetrapib and cardiovascular outcomes in high-risk vascular disease. N Engl J Med 376(20):1933–1942. https://doi.org/10.1056/NEJMoa1609581

Mach F, Baigent C, Catapano AL, Koskinas KC, Casula M, Badimon L, Chapman MJ, De Backer GG, Delgado V, Ference BA, Graham IM, Halliday A, Landmesser U, Mihaylova B, Pedersen TR, Riccardi G, Richter DJ, Sabatine MS, Taskinen MR, Tokgozoglu L, Wiklund O, ESC Scientific Document Group (2020) 2019 ESC/EAS guidelines for the management of dyslipidaemias: lipid modification to reduce cardiovascular risk. Eur Heart J 41(1):111–188. Erratum in: Eur Heart J. 2020 Nov 21;41(44):4255. https://doi.org/10.1093/eurheartj/ehz455

Mackey RH, Greenland P, Goff DC Jr, Lloyd-Jones D, Sibley CT, Mora S (2012) High-density lipoprotein cholesterol and particle concentrations, carotid atherosclerosis, and coronary events: MESA (multi-ethnic study of atherosclerosis). J Am Coll Cardiol 60(6):508–516. https://doi.org/10.1016/j.jacc.2012.03.060

Madsen CM, Varbo A, Nordestgaard BG (2017) Extreme high high-density lipoprotein cholesterol is paradoxically associated with high mortality in men and women: two prospective cohort studies. Eur Heart J 38(32):2478–2486. https://doi.org/10.1093/eurheartj/ehx163

Madsen CM, Varbo A, Tybjærg-Hansen A, Frikke-Schmidt R, Nordestgaard BG (2018) U-shaped relationship of HDL and risk of infectious disease: two prospective population-based cohort studies. Eur Heart J 39(14):1181–1190. https://doi.org/10.1093/eurheartj/ehx665

Madsen CM, Varbo A, Nordestgaard BG (2019) Low HDL cholesterol and high risk of autoimmune disease: two population-based cohort studies including 117341 individuals. Clin Chem 65(5):644–652. https://doi.org/10.1373/clinchem.2018.299636

Madsen CM, Varbo A, Nordestgaard BG (2021) Novel insights from human studies on the role of high-density lipoprotein in mortality and noncardiovascular disease. Arterioscler Thromb Vasc Biol 41(1):128–140. https://doi.org/10.1161/ATVBAHA.120.314050

Manandhar B, Cochran BJ, Rye KA (2020) Role of high-density lipoproteins in cholesterol homeostasis and glycemic control. J Am Heart Assoc 9(1):e013531. https://doi.org/10.1161/JAHA.119.013531

Martin SS, Blaha MJ, Elshazly MB, Toth PP, Kwiterovich PO, Blumenthal RS, Jones SR (2013) Comparison of a novel method vs the Friedewald equation for estimating low-density lipoprotein cholesterol levels from the standard lipid profile. JAMA 310(19):2061–2068. https://doi.org/10.1001/jama.2013.280532

März W, Kleber ME, Scharnagl H, Speer T, Zewinger S, Ritsch A, Parhofer KG, von Eckardstein A, Landmesser U, Laufs U (2017) HDL cholesterol: reappraisal of its clinical relevance. Clin Res Cardiol 106(9):663–675. https://doi.org/10.1007/s00392-017-1106-1

Masson W, Lobo M, Siniawski D, Huerín M, Molinero G, Valéro R, Nogueira JP (2018) Therapy with cholesteryl ester transfer protein (CETP) inhibitors and diabetes risk. Diabetes Metab 44 (6):508–513. https://doi.org/10.1016/j.diabet.2018.02.005

McGarrah RW, Craig DM, Haynes C, Dowdy ZE, Shah SH, Kraus WE (2016) High-density lipoprotein subclass measurements improve mortality risk prediction, discrimination and reclassification in a cardiac catheterization cohort. Atherosclerosis 246:229–235. https://doi.org/10.1016/j.atherosclerosis.2016.01.012

Meikle PJ, Formosa MF, Mellett NA, Jayawardana KS, Giles C, Bertovic DA, Jennings GL, Childs W, Reddy M, Carey AL, Baradi A, Nanayakkara S, Wilson AM, Duffy SJ, Kingwell BA (2019) HDL phospholipids, but not cholesterol distinguish acute coronary syndrome from stable coronary artery disease. J Am Heart Assoc 8(11):e011792. https://doi.org/10.1161/JAHA.118.011792

Meilhac O, Tanaka S, Couret D (2020) High-density lipoproteins are bug scavengers. Biomol Ther 10(4):598. https://doi.org/10.3390/biom10040598

Menon V, Kumar A, Patel DR, John JS, Riesmeyer J, Weerakkody G, Ruotolo G, Wolski KE, McErlean E, Cremer PC et al (2020) Effect of CETP inhibition with evacetrapib in patients with diabetes mellitus enrolled in the ACCELERATE trial. BMJ Open Diabetes Res Care 8:e000943

Meriwether D, Sulaiman D, Volpe C, Dorfman A, Grijalva V, Dorreh N, Solorzano-Vargas RS, Wang J, O'Connor E, Pajesh J, Larauche M, Trost H, Palgunachari MN, Anantharamaiah GM, Herschman HR, Martin MG, Fogelman AM, Reddy ST (2019) Apolipoprotein A-I mimetics mitigate intestinal inflammation in COX2-dependent inflammatory bowel disease model. J Clin Invest 129(9):3670–3685. https://doi.org/10.1172/JCI123700

Metzinger MP, Saldanha S, Gulati J, Patel KV, El-Ghazali A, Deodhar S, Joshi PH, Ayers C, Rohatgi A (2020) Effect of anacetrapib on cholesterol efflux capacity: a substudy of the DEFINE trial. J Am Heart Assoc 9(24):e018136. https://doi.org/10.1161/JAHA.120.018136

Miller WG, Myers GL, Sakurabayashi I, Bachmann LM, Caudill SP, Dziekonski A, Edwards S, Kimberly MM, Korzun WJ, Leary ET, Nakajima K, Nakamura M, Nilsson G, Shamburek RD, Vetrovec GW, Warnick GR, Remaley AT (2010) Seven direct methods for measuring HDL and LDL cholesterol compared with ultracentrifugation reference measurement procedures. Clin Chem 56(6):977–986. https://doi.org/10.1373/clinchem.2009.142810

Montaigne D, Butruille L, Staels B (2021) PPAR control of metabolism and cardiovascular functions. Nat Rev Cardiol. https://doi.org/10.1038/s41569-021-00569-6

Mora S, Otvos JD, Rifai N, Rosenson RS, Buring JE, Ridker PM (2009) Lipoprotein particle profiles by nuclear magnetic resonance compared with standard lipids and apolipoproteins in predicting incident cardiovascular disease in women. Circulation 119(7):931–939. https://doi.org/10.1161/CIRCULATIONAHA.108.816181

Mora S, Glynn RJ, Ridker PM (2013) High-density lipoprotein cholesterol, size, particle number, and residual vascular risk after potent statin therapy. Circulation 128(11):1189–1197. https://doi.org/10.1161/CIRCULATIONAHA.113.002671

Morin EE, Guo L, Schwendeman A, Li XA (2015) HDL in sepsis - risk factor and therapeutic approach. Front Pharmacol 6:244. https://doi.org/10.3389/fphar.2015.00244

Morin EE, Li XA, Schwendeman A (2018) HDL in endocrine carcinomas: biomarker, drug carrier, and potential therapeutic. Front Endocrinol (Lausanne) 9:715. https://doi.org/10.3389/fendo.2018.00715

Moriyama Y, Okamura T, Inazu A, Doi M, Iso H, Mouri Y, Ishikawa Y, Suzuki H, Iida M, Koizumi J et al (1998) A low prevalence of coronary heart disease among subjects with increased high-density lipoprotein cholesterol levels, including those with plasma cholesteryl ester transfer protein deficiency. Prev Med 27:659–667

Mortensen MB, Afzal S, Nordestgaard BG, Falk E (2015) The high-density lipoprotein-adjusted SCORE model worsens SCORE-based risk classification in a contemporary population of 30,824 Europeans: the Copenhagen general population study. Eur Heart J 36(36):2446–2453. https://doi.org/10.1093/eurheartj/ehv251

Mundra PA, Shaw JE, Meikle PJ (2016) Lipidomic analyses in epidemiology. Int J Epidemiol 45 (5):1329–1338

Natarajan P, Collier TS, Jin Z, Lyass A, Li Y, Ibrahim NE, Mukai R, McCarthy CP, Massaro JM, D'Agostino RB Sr, Gaggin HK, Bystrom C, Penn MS, Januzzi JL Jr (2019) Association of an HDL apolipoproteomic score with coronary atherosclerosis and cardiovascular death. J Am Coll Cardiol 73(17):2135–2145. https://doi.org/10.1016/j.jacc.2019.01.073

Neale BM, Fagerness J, Reynolds R, Sobrin L, Parker M, Raychaudhuri S, Tan PL, Oh EC, Merriam JE, Souied E, Bernstein PS, Li B, Frederick JM, Zhang K, Brantley MA Jr, Lee AY, Zack DJ, Campochiaro B, Campochiaro P, Ripke S, Smith RT, Barile GR, Katsanis N, Allikmets R, Daly MJ, Seddon JM (2010) Genome-wide association study of advanced age-related macular degeneration identifies a role of the hepatic lipase gene (LIPC). Proc Natl Acad Sci U S A 107(16):7395–7400. https://doi.org/10.1073/pnas.0912019107

Nicholls SJ, Ruotolo G, Brewer HB, Kane JP, Wang MD, Krueger KA, Adelman SJ, Nissen SE, Rader DJ (2015) Cholesterol efflux capacity and pre-beta-1 HDL concentrations are increased in dyslipidemic patients treated with evacetrapib. J Am Coll Cardiol 66(20):2201–2210. https://doi.org/10.1016/j.jacc.2015.09.013

Nicholls SJ, Puri R, Ballantyne CM, Jukema JW, Kastelein JJP, Koenig W, Wright RS, Kallend D, Wijngaard P, Borgman M, Wolski K, Nissen SE (2018a) Effect of infusion of high-density lipoprotein mimetic containing recombinant apolipoprotein A-I milano on coronary disease in patients with an acute coronary syndrome in the MILANO-PILOT trial: a randomized clinical trial. JAMA Cardiol 3:806–814

Nicholls SJ, Andrews J, Kastelein JJP, Merkely B, Nissen SE, Ray KK, Schwartz GG, Worthley SG, Keyserling C, Dasseux JL, Griffith L, Kim SW, Janssan A, Di Giovanni G, Pisaniello AD, Scherer DJ, Psaltis PJ, Butters J (2018b) Effect of serial infusions of CER-001, a pre-β high-density lipoprotein mimetic, on coronary atherosclerosis in patients following acute coronary syndromes in the CER-001 atherosclerosis regression acute coronary syndrome trial: a randomized clinical trial. JAMA Cardiol 3:815–822

Nissen SE, Tsunoda T, Tuzcu EM, Schoenhagen P, Cooper CJ, Yasin M, Eaton GM, Lauer MA, Sheldon WS, Grines CL, Halpern S, Crowe T, Blankenship JC, Kerensky R (2003) Effect of recombinant ApoA-I Milano on coronary atherosclerosis in patients with acute coronary syndromes: a randomized controlled trial. JAMA 290:2292–2300

Nissen SE, Pillai SG, Nicholls SJ, Wolski K, Riesmeyer JS, Weerakkody GJ, Foster WM, McErlean E, Li L, Bhatnagar P, Ruotolo G, Lincoff AM (2018) ADCY9 genetic variants and cardiovascular outcomes with evacetrapib in patients with high-risk vascular disease: a nested case-control study. JAMA Cardiol 3(5):401–408. https://doi.org/10.1001/jamacardio.2018.0569

Niu W, Qi Y (2015) Circulating cholesteryl ester transfer protein and coronary heart disease: mendelian randomization meta-analysis. Circ Cardiovasc Genet 8(1):114–121. https://doi.org/10.1161/CIRCGENETICS.114.000748

Nordestgaard LT, Tybjærg-Hansen A, Nordestgaard BG, Frikke-Schmidt R (2015) Loss-of-function mutation in ABCA1 and risk of Alzheimer's disease and cerebrovascular disease. Alzheimers Dement 11(12):1430–1438. https://doi.org/10.1016/j.jalz.2015.04.006

Nordestgaard BG, Langlois MR, Langsted A, Chapman MJ, Aakre KM, Baum H, Borén J, Bruckert E, Catapano A, Cobbaert C, Collinson P, Descamps OS, Duff CJ, von Eckardstein A, Hammerer-Lercher A, Kamstrup PR, Kolovou G, Kronenberg F, Mora S, Pulkki K, Remaley AT, Rifai N, Ros E, Stankovic S, Stavljenic-Rukavina A, Sypniewska G, Watts GF, Wiklund O, Laitinen P, European Atherosclerosis Society (EAS) and the European Federation of Clinical Chemistry and Laboratory Medicine (EFLM) Joint Consensus Initiative (2020) Quantifying atherogenic lipoproteins for lipid-lowering strategies: consensus-based recommendations from EAS and EFLM. Atherosclerosis 294:46–61. https://doi.org/10.1016/j. atherosclerosis.2019.12.005

Nordestgaard LT, Tybjærg-Hansen A, Frikke-Schmidt R, Nordestgaard BG (2021) Elevated apolipoprotein A1 and HDL cholesterol associated with age-related macular degeneration: 2 population cohorts. J Clin Endocrinol Metab 106(7):e2749–e2758. https://doi.org/10.1210/ clinem/dgab095

Nowacki TM, Remaley AT, Bettenworth D, Eisenblätter M, Vowinkel T, Becker F, Vogl T, Roth J, Tietge UJ, Lügering A, Heidemann J, Nofer JR (2016) The 5A apolipoprotein A-I (apoA-I) mimetic peptide ameliorates experimental colitis by regulating monocyte infiltration. Br J Pharmacol 173(18):2730–2792. https://doi.org/10.1111/bph.13556

Offermanns S (2014) Free fatty acid (FFA) and hydroxy carboxylic acid (HCA) receptors. Annu Rev Pharmacol Toxicol 54:407–434. https://doi.org/10.1146/annurev-pharmtox-011613-135945

Orsoni A, Thérond P, Tan R, Giral P, Robillard P, Kontush A, Meikle PJ, Chapman MJ (2016) Statin action enriches HDL3 in polyunsaturated phospholipids and plasmalogens and reduces LDL-derived phospholipid hydroperoxides in atherogenic mixed dyslipidemia. J Lipid Res 57 (11):2073–2087

Ostergaard SD, Mukherjee S, Sharp SJ, Proitsi P, Lotta LA, Day FR, Perry JR, Boehme KL, Walter S, Kauwe JS et al (2015) Associations between potentially modifiable risk factors and Alzheimer disease: a Mendelian randomization study. PLoS Med 12:e1001841

Otvos JD, Collins D, Freedman DS, Shalaurova I, Schaefer EJ, McNamara JR, Bloomfield HE, Robins SJ (2006) Low-density lipoprotein and high-density lipoprotein particle subclasses predict coronary events and are favorably changed by gemfibrozil therapy in the veterans affairs high-density lipoprotein intervention trial. Circulation 113(12):1556–1563. https://doi.org/10. 1161/CIRCULATIONAHA.105.565135

Pajkrt D, Doran JE, Koster F, Lerch PG, Arnet B, van der Poll T, ten Cate JW, van Deventer SJ (1996) Antiinflammatory effects of reconstituted high-density lipoprotein during human endotoxemia. J Exp Med 184(5):1601–1608. https://doi.org/10.1084/jem.184.5.1601

Pajkrt D, Lerch PG, van der Poll T, Levi M, Illi M, Doran JE, Arnet B, van den Ende A, ten Cate JW, van Deventer SJ (1997) Differential effects of reconstituted high-density lipoprotein on coagulation, fibrinolysis and platelet activation during human endotoxemia. Thromb Haemost 77(2):303–307

Parhofer KG (2015) Interaction between glucose and lipid metabolism: more than diabetic dyslipidemia. Diabetes Metab J 39(5):353–362

Parish S, Offer A, Clarke R, Hopewell JC, Hill MR, Otvos JD, Armitage J, Collins R, Heart Protection Study Collaborative Group (2012) Lipids and lipoproteins and risk of different vascular events in the MRC/BHF heart protection study. Circulation 125(20):2469–2478. https://doi.org/10.1161/CIRCULATIONAHA.111.073684

Pavanello C, Calabresi L (2020) Genetic, biochemical, and clinical features of LCAT deficiency: update for 2020. Curr Opin Lipidol 31(4):232–237. https://doi.org/10.1097/MOL. 0000000000000697

Pirillo A, Catapano AL, Norata GD (2015) HDL in infectious diseases and sepsis. Handb Exp Pharmacol 224:483–508. https://doi.org/10.1007/978-3-319-09665-0_15

Pirro M, Ricciuti B, Rader DJ, Catapano AL, Sahebkar A, Banach M (2018) High density lipoprotein cholesterol and cancer: marker or causative? Prog Lipid Res 71:54–69. https://doi. org/10.1016/j.plipres.2013.06.001

Pollin TI, Damcott CM, Shen H, Ott SH, Shelton J, Horenstein RB, Post W, McLenithan JC, Bielak LF, Peyser PA et al (2008) A null mutation in human APOC3 confers a favorable plasma lipid profile and apparent cardioprotection. Science 322:1702–1705

Pradhan AD, Paynter NP, Everett BM, Glynn RJ, Amarenco P, Elam M, Ginsberg H, Hiatt WR, Ishibashi S, Koenig W, Nordestgaard BG, Fruchart JC, Libby P, Ridker PM (2018) Rationale and design of the pemafibrate to reduce cardiovascular outcomes by reducing triglycerides in patients with diabetes (PROMINENT) study. Am Heart J 206:80–93. https://doi.org/10.1016/j. ahj.2018.09.011

Proitsi P, Lupton MK, Velayudhan L, Newhouse S, Fogh I, Tsolaki M, Daniilidou M, Pritchard M, Kloszewska I, Soininen H et al (2014) Genetic predisposition to increased blood cholesterol and triglyceride lipid levels and risk of Alzheimer disease: a Mendelian randomization analysis. PLoS Med 11:e1001713

Qi Y, Fan J, Liu J, Wang W, Wang M, Sun J, Liu J, Xie W, Zhao F, Li Y, Zhao D (2015) Cholesterol-overloaded HDL particles are independently associated with progression of carotid atherosclerosis in a cardiovascular disease-free population: a community-based cohort study. J Am Coll Cardiol 65(4):355–363. https://doi.org/10.1016/j.jacc.2014.11.019

Rajora MA, Zheng G (2016) Targeting SR-BI for cancer diagnostics, imaging and therapy. Front Pharmacol 7:326. https://doi.org/10.3389/fphar.2016.00326

Rasmussen KL, Tybjærg-Hansen A, Nordestgaard BG, Frikke-Schmidt R (2018) Plasma apolipoprotein E levels and risk of dementia: a Mendelian randomization study of 106,562 individuals. Alzheimers Dement 14(1):71–80. https://doi.org/10.1016/j.jalz.2017.05.006

Rautureau Y, Deschambault V, Higgins MÈ, Rivas D, Mecteau M, Geoffroy P, Miquel G, Uy K, Sanchez R, Lavoie V, Brand G, Nault A, Williams PM, Suarez ML, Merlet N, Lapointe L, Duquette N, Gillis MA, Samami S, Mayer G, Pouliot P, Raignault A, Maafi F, Brodeur MR, Levesque S, Guertin MC, Dubé MP, Thorin É, Rhainds D, Rhéaume É, Tardif JC (2018) ADCY9 (adenylate cyclase type 9) inactivation protects from atherosclerosis only in the absence of CETP (cholesteryl Ester transfer protein). Circulation 138(16):1677–1692. https://doi.org/10. 1161/CIRCULATIONAHA.117.031134

Ray KK, Nicholls SJ, Buhr KA, Ginsberg HN, Johansson JO, Kalantar-Zadeh K, Kulikowski E, Toth PP, Wong N, Sweeney M, Schwartz GG, BETonMACE Investigators and Committees (2020) Effect of apabetalone added to standard therapy on major adverse cardiovascular events in patients with recent acute coronary syndrome and type 2 diabetes: a randomized clinical trial. JAMA 323(16):1565–1573. https://doi.org/10.1001/jama.2020.3308

Riaz H, Khan SU, Rahman H, Shah NP, Kaluski E, Lincoff AM, Nissen SE (2019) Effects of high-density lipoprotein targeting treatments on cardiovascular outcomes: a systematic review and meta-analysis. Eur J Prev Cardiol 26(5):533–543. https://doi.org/10.1177/2047487318816495

Richardson TG, Sanderson E, Palmer TM, Ala-Korpela M, Ference BA, Davey Smith G, Holmes MV (2020) Evaluating the relationship between circulating lipoprotein lipids and apolipoproteins with risk of coronary heart disease: a multivariable Mendelian randomisation analysis. PLoS Med 17(3):e1003062. https://doi.org/10.1371/journal.pmed.1003062

Ridker PM, Genest J, Boekholdt SM, Libby P, Gotto AM, Nordestgaard BG, Mora S, MacFadyen JG, Glynn RJ, Kastelein JJ, JUPITER Trial Study Group (2010) HDL cholesterol and residual risk of first cardiovascular events after treatment with potent statin therapy: an analysis from the JUPITER trial. Lancet 376(9738):333–339. https://doi.org/10.1016/S0140-6736(10)60713-1

Riwanto M, Rohrer L, Roschitzki B, Besler C, Mocharla P, Mueller M, Perisa D, Heinrich K, Altwegg L, von Eckardstein A, Lüscher TF, Landmesser U (2013) Altered activation of endothelial anti- and proapoptotic pathways by high-density lipoprotein from patients with coronary artery disease: role of high-density lipoprotein-proteome remodeling. Circulation 127 (8):891–904. https://doi.org/10.1161/CIRCULATIONAHA.112.108753

Robert J, Osto E, von Eckardstein A (2021) The endothelium is both a target and a barrier of HDL's protective functions. Cell 10(5):1041. https://doi.org/10.3390/cells10051041

Rohatgi A, Westerterp M, von Eckardstein A, Remaley A, Rye KA (2021) HDL in the 21st century: a multifunctional roadmap for future HDL research. Circulation 143(23):2293–2309. https:// doi.org/10.1161/CIRCULATIONAHA.120.044221

Rosenson RS, Brewer HB Jr, Chapman MJ, Fazio S, Hussain MM, Kontush A, Krauss RM, Otvos JD, Remaley AT, Schaefer EJ (2011) HDL measures, particle heterogeneity, proposed nomenclature, and relation to atherosclerotic cardiovascular events. Clin Chem 57(3):392–410. https:// doi.org/10.1373/clinchem.2010.155333

Rosenson RS, Davidson MH, Le NA, Burkle J, Pourfarzib R (2015) Underappreciated opportunities for high-density lipoprotein particles in risk stratification and potential targets of therapy. Cardiovasc Drugs Ther 29(1):41–50. https://doi.org/10.1007/s10557-014-6567-0

Rosenson RS, Burgess LJ, Ebenbichler CF, Baum SJ, Stroes ESG, Ali S, Khilla N, Hamlin R, Pordy R, Dong Y, Son V, Gaudet D (2020) Evinacumab in patients with refractory hypercholesterolemia. N Engl J Med 383(24):2307–2319. https://doi.org/10.1056/NEJMoa2031049

Rubins HB, Robins SJ, Collins D, Fye CL, Anderson JW, Elam MB, Faas FH, Linares E, Schaefer EJ, Schectman G, Wilt TJ, Wittes J (1999) Gemfibrozil for the secondary prevention of coronary heart disease in men with low levels of high-density lipoprotein cholesterol. Veterans Affairs High-Density Lipoprotein Cholesterol Intervention Trial Study Group. N Engl J Med 341 (6):410–418. https://doi.org/10.1056/NEJM199908053410604

Sacks FM, Tonkin AM, Shepherd J, Braunwald E, Cobbe S, Hawkins CM, Keech A, Packard C, Simes J, Byington R, Furberg CD (2000) Effect of pravastatin on coronary disease events in subgroups defined by coronary risk factors: the prospective pravastatin pooling project. Circulation 102(16):1893–1900. https://doi.org/10.1161/01.cir.102.16.1893

Sacks FM, Carey VJ, Fruchart JC (2010) Combination lipid therapy in type 2 diabetes. N Engl J Med 363(7):692–694; author reply 694-5. https://doi.org/10.1056/NEJMc1006407

Sacks FM, Liang L, Furtado JD, Cai T, Davidson WS, He Z, McClelland RL, Rimm EB, Jensen MK (2020) Protein-defined subspecies of HDLs (high-density lipoproteins) and differential risk of coronary heart disease in 4 prospective studies. Arterioscler Thromb Vasc Biol 40 (11):2714–2727. https://doi.org/10.1161/ATVBAHA.120.314609

Saito T, Matsunaga A, Fukunaga M, Nagahama K, Hara S, Muso E (2020) Apolipoprotein E-related glomerular disorders. Kidney Int 97(2):279–288. https://doi.org/10.1016/j.kint.2019.10.031

Samanovic M, Molina-Portela MP, Chessler AD, Burleigh BA, Raper J (2009) Trypanosome lytic factor, an antimicrobial high-density lipoprotein, ameliorates Leishmania infection. PLoS Pathog 5(1):e1000276. https://doi.org/10.1371/journal.ppat.1000276

Sampson M, Ling C, Sun Q, Harb R, Ashmaig M, Warnick R, Sethi A, Fleming JK, Otvos JD, Meeusen JW, Delaney SR, Jaffe AS, Shamburek R, Amar M, Remaley AT (2020) A new equation for calculation of low-density lipoprotein cholesterol in patients with normolipidemia and/or hypertriglyceridemia. JAMA Cardiol 5(5):540–548. Erratum in: JAMA Cardiol.2020 May 1;5(5)613. https://doi.org/10.1001/jamacardio.2020.0013

Schmidt MI, Duncan BB, Bang H, Pankow JS, Ballantyne CM, Golden SH, Folsom AR, Chambless LE (2005) Identifying individuals at high risk for diabetes: the atherosclerosis risk in communities study. Diabetes Care 28:2013–2018

Schwartz GG, Olsson AG, Abt M, Ballantyne CM, Barter PJ, Brumm J, Chaitman BR, Holme IM, Kallend D, Leiter LA, Leitersdorf E, McMurray JJ, Mundl H, Nicholls SJ, Shah PK, Tardif JC, Wright RS, dal-OUTCOMES Investigators (2012) Effects of dalcetrapib in patients with a recent acute coronary syndrome. N Engl J Med 367(22):2089–2099. https://doi.org/10.1056/NEJMoa1206797

Schwartz GG, Leiter LA, Ballantyne CM, Barter PJ, Black DM, Kallend D, Laghrissi-Thode F, Leitersdorf E, McMurray JJ, Nicholls SJ et al (2020) Dalcetrapib reduces risk of new-onset diabetes in patients with coronary heart disease. Diabetes Care 43:1077–1084

Silbernagel G, Pagel P, Pfahlert V, Genser B, Scharnagl H, Kleber ME, Delgado G, Ohrui H, Ritsch A, Grammer TB, Koenig W, März W (2017) High-density lipoprotein subclasses, coronary artery disease, and cardiovascular mortality. Clin Chem 63(12):1886–1896. https://doi.org/10.1373/clinchem.2017.275636

Simic B, Mocharla P, Crucet M, Osto E, Kratzer A, Stivala S, Kühnast S, Speer T, Doycheva P, Princen HM, van der Hoorn JW, Jukema JW, Giral H, Tailleux A, Landmesser U, Staels B, Lüscher TF (2017) Anacetrapib, but not evacetrapib, impairs endothelial function in CETP-transgenic mice in spite of marked HDL-C increase. Atherosclerosis 257:186–194. https://doi.org/10.1016/j.atherosclerosis.2017.01.011

Singh K, Chandra A, Sperry T, Joshi PH, Khera A, Virani SS, Ballantyne CM, Otvos JD, Dullaart RPF, Gruppen EG, Connelly MA, Ayers CR, Rohatgi A (2020) Associations between high-density lipoprotein particles and ischemic events by vascular domain, sex, and ethnicity: a pooled cohort analysis. Circulation 142(7):657–669. https://doi.org/10.1161/CIRCULATIONAHA.120.045713

Soria-Florido MT, Schröder H, Grau M, Fitó M, Lassale C (2020) High density lipoprotein functionality and cardiovascular events and mortality: a systematic review and meta-analysis. Atherosclerosis 302:36–42. https://doi.org/10.1016/j.atherosclerosis.2020.04.015

Speer T, Ridker PM, von Eckardstein A, Schunk SJ, Fliser D (2021) Lipoproteins in chronic kidney disease: from bench to bedside. Eur Heart J 42(22):2170–2185. https://doi.org/10.1093/eurheartj/ehaa1050

Storti F, Klee K, Todorova V, Steiner R, Othman A, van der Velde-Visser S, Samardzija M, Meneau I, Barben M, Karademir D, Pauzuolyte V, Boye SL, Blaser F, Ullmer C, Dunaief JL, Hornemann T, Rohrer L, den Hollander A, von Eckardstein A, Fingerle J, Maugeais C, Grimm C (2019) Impaired ABCA1/ABCG1-mediated lipid efflux in the mouse retinal pigment epithelium (RPE) leads to retinal degeneration. elife 8:e45100. https://doi.org/10.7554/eLife.45100

Strazzella A, Ossoli A, Calabresi L (2021) High-density lipoproteins and the kidney. Cell 10 (4):764. https://doi.org/10.3390/cells10040764

Sutter I, Velagapudi S, Othman A, Riwanto M, Manz J, Rohrer L, Rentsch K, Hornemann T, Landmesser U, von Eckardstein A (2015) Plasmalogens of high-density lipoproteins (HDL) are associated with coronary artery disease and anti-apoptotic activity of HDL. Atherosclerosis 241 (2):539–546. https://doi.org/10.1016/j.atherosclerosis.2015.05.037

Talasaz AH, Sadeghipour P, Aghakouchakzadeh M, Dreyfus I, Kakavand H, Ariannejad H, Gupta A, Madhavan MV, Van Tassell BW, Jimenez D, Monreal M, Vaduganathan M, Fanikos J, Dixon DL, Piazza G, Parikh SA, Bhatt DL, Lip GY, Stone GW, Krumholz HM, Libby P, Goldhaber SZ, Bikdeli B (2021) Lipid-modulating agents for prevention or treatment of COVID-19 in randomized trials. medRxiv. https://doi.org/10.1101/2021.05.03.21256468

Tanaka S, Genève C, Zappella N, Yong-Sang J, Planesse C, Louedec L, Viranaïcken W, Bringart M, Montravers P, Denamur E, Duranteau J, Couret D, Meilhac O (2020) Reconstituted high-density lipoprotein therapy improves survival in mouse models of sepsis. Anesthesiology 132(4):825–838. https://doi.org/10.1097/ALN.0000000000003155

Tardif JC, Grégoire J, L'Allier PL, Ibrahim R, Lespérance J, Heinonen TM, Kouz S, Berry C, Basser R, Lavoie MA, Guertin MC, Rodés-Cabau J, Effect of rHDL on Atherosclerosis-Safety and Efficacy (ERASE) Investigators (2007) Effects of reconstituted high-density lipoprotein infusions on coronary atherosclerosis: a randomized controlled trial. JAMA 297:1675–1682

Tardif JC, Rhéaume E, Lemieux Perreault LP, Grégoire JC, Feroz Zada Y, Asselin G, Provost S, Barhdadi A, Rhainds D, L'Allier PL, Ibrahim R, Upmanyu R, Niesor EJ, Benghozi R, Suchankova G, Laghrissi-Thode F, Guertin MC, Olsson AG, Mongrain I, Schwartz GG, Dubé MP (2015) Pharmacogenomic determinants of the cardiovascular effects of dalcetrapib. Circ Cardiovasc Genet 8(2):372–382. https://doi.org/10.1161/CIRCGENETICS.114.000663

Tardif JC, Dubé MP, Pfeffer MA, Waters DD, Koenig W, Maggioni AP, McMurray JJV, Mooser V, White HD, Heinonen T, Black DM, Guertin MC, dal-GenE Investigators (2020) Study design of dal-GenE, a pharmacogenetic trial targeting reduction of cardiovascular events with dalcetrapib. Am Heart J 222:157–165. https://doi.org/10.1016/j.ahj.2020.01.007

Thirumalai A, Rubinow KB, Page ST (2015) An update on testosterone, HDL and cardiovascular risk in men. Clin Lipidol 10(3):251–258. https://doi.org/10.2217/clp.15.10

Tietjen I, Hovingh GK, Singaraja R et al (2012) Increased risk of coronary artery disease in Caucasians with extremely low HDL cholesterol due to mutations in ABCA1, APOA1, and LCAT. Biochim Biophys Acta 1821:416–424

Trakaki A, Marsche G (2021) Current understanding of the immunomodulatory activities of high-density lipoproteins. Biomedicine 9(6):587. https://doi.org/10.3390/biomedicines9060587

Trinder M, Genga KR, Kong HJ, Blauw LL, Lo C, Li X, Cirstea M, Wang Y, Rensen PCN, Russell JA, Walley KR, Boyd JH, Brunham LR (2019) Cholesteryl ester transfer protein influences high-density lipoprotein levels and survival in sepsis. Am J Respir Crit Care Med 199 (7):854–862. https://doi.org/10.1164/rccm.201806-1157OC

Trinder M, Walley KR, Boyd JH, Brunham LR (2020) Causal inference for genetically determined levels of high-density lipoprotein cholesterol and risk of infectious disease. Arterioscler Thromb Vasc Biol 40(1):267–278. https://doi.org/10.1161/ATVBAHA.119.313381

Trinder M, Wang Y, Madsen CM, Ponomarev T, Bohunek L, Daisely BA, Julia Kong H, Blauw LL, Nordestgaard BG, Tybjærg-Hansen A, Wurfel MM, Russell JA, Walley KR, Rensen PCN, Boyd JH, Brunham LR (2021) Inhibition of cholesteryl ester transfer protein preserves high-density lipoprotein cholesterol and improves survival in sepsis. Circulation 143(9):921–934. https://doi.org/10.1161/CIRCULATIONAHA.120.048568

Vaisman BL, Neufeld EB, Freeman LA, Gordon SM, Sampson ML, Pryor M, Hillman E, Axley MJ, Karathanasis SK, Remaley AT (2019) LCAT enzyme replacement therapy reduces LpX and improves kidney function in a mouse model of familial LCAT deficiency. J Pharmacol Exp Ther 368(3):423–434. https://doi.org/10.1124/jpet.118.251876

Velagapudi S, Schraml P, Yalcinkaya M, Bolck HA, Rohrer L, Moch H, von Eckardstein A (2018) Scavenger receptor BI promotes cytoplasmic accumulation of lipoproteins in clear-cell renal cell carcinoma. J Lipid Res 59(11):2188–2201. https://doi.org/10.1194/jlr.M083311

Voight BF, Peloso GM, Orho-Melander M, Frikke-Schmidt R, Barbalic M, Jensen MK, Hindy G, Hólm H, Ding EL, Johnson T, Schunkert H, Samani NJ, Clarke R, Hopewell JC, Thompson JF, Li M, Thorleifsson G, Newton-Cheh C, Musunuru K, Pirruccello JP, Saleheen D, Chen L, Stewart A, Schillert A, Thorsteinsdottir U, Thorgeirsson G, Anand S, Engert JC, Morgan T, Spertus J, Stoll M, Berger K, Martinelli N, Girelli D, McKeown PP, Patterson CC, Epstein SE, Devaney J, Burnett MS, Mooser V, Ripatti S, Surakka I, Nieminen MS, Sinisalo J, Lokki ML, Perola M, Havulinna A, de Faire U, Gigante B, Ingelsson E, Zeller T, Wild P, de Bakker PI, Klungel OH, Maitland-van der Zee AH, Peters BJ, de Boer A, Grobbee DE, Kamphuisen PW, Deneer VH, Elbers CC, Onland-Moret NC, Hofker MH, Wijmenga C, Verschuren WM, Boer JM, van der Schouw YT, Rasheed A, Frossard P, Demissie S, Willer C, Do R, Ordovas JM, Abecasis GR, Boehnke M, Mohlke KL, Daly MJ, Guiducci C, Burtt NP, Surti A, Gonzalez E, Purcell S, Gabriel S, Marrugat J, Peden J, Erdmann J, Diemert P, Willenborg C, König IR, Fischer M, Hengstenberg C, Ziegler A, Buysschaert I, Lambrechts D, Van de Werf F, Fox KA, El Mokhtari NE, Rubin D, Schrezenmeir J, Schreiber S, Schäfer A, Danesh J, Blankenberg S, Roberts R, McPherson R, Watkins H, Hall AS, Overvad K, Rimm E, Boerwinkle E, Tybjaerg-Hansen A, Cupples LA, Reilly MP, Melander O, Mannucci PM, Ardissino D, Siscovick D, Elosua R, Stefansson K, O'Donnell CJ, Salomaa V, Rader DJ, Peltonen L, Schwartz SM, Altshuler D, Kathiresan S (2012) Plasma HDL cholesterol and risk of myocardial infarction: a mendelian randomisation study. Lancet 380(9841):572–580. Erratum in: Lancet. 2012 Aug 11;380(9841):564. https://doi.org/10.1016/S0140-6736(12)60312-2

Vollenweider P, Von Eckardstein A, Widmann C (2015) HDLs, diabetes and metabolic syndrome. In: High density lipoproteins: handbook of experimental pharmacology. Springer, Cham, pp 405–421

von Eckardstein A (2020) LDL contributes to reverse cholesterol transport. Circ Res 127 (6):793–795. https://doi.org/10.1161/CIRCRESAHA.120.317721

Von Eckardstein A, Kardassis DM (2015) High density lipoproteins: from biological understanding to clinical exploitation. Handbook of experimental pharmacology. Springer, Cham

Von Eckardstein A, Rohrer L (2016) HDLs in crises. Curr Opin Lipidol 27:264–273

von Eckardstein A, Widmann C (2014) High-density lipoprotein, beta cells, and diabetes. Cardiovasc Res 103(3):384–394

von Eckardstein A, Schulte H, Assmann G (1999) Increased risk of myocardial infarction in men with both hypertriglyceridemia and elevated HDL cholesterol. Circulation 99(14):1925

von Eckardstein A, Schulte H, Assmann G (2000) Risk for diabetes mellitus in middle-aged Caucasian male participants of the PROCAM study: implications for the definition of impaired fasting glucose by the American Diabetes Association. Prospective Cardiovascular Münster. J Clin Endocrinol Metab 85(9):3101–3108. https://doi.org/10.1210/jcem.85.9.6773

Wei C, Wan L, Yan Q, Wang X, Zhang J, Yang X, Zhang Y, Fan C, Li D, Deng Y, Sun J, Gong J, Yang X, Wang Y, Wang X, Li J, Yang H, Li H, Zhang Z, Wang R, Du P, Zong Y, Yin F, Zhang W, Wang N, Peng Y, Lin H, Feng J, Qin C, Chen W, Gao Q, Zhang R, Cao Y, Zhong H (2020) HDL-scavenger receptor B type 1 facilitates SARS-CoV-2 entry. Nat Metab 2 (12):1391–1400. https://doi.org/10.1038/s42255-020-00324-0

West of Scotland Coronary Prevention Study Group (1998) Influence of pravastatin and plasma lipids on clinical events in the West of Scotland Coronary Prevention Study (WOSCOPS). Circulation 97(15):1440–1445. https://doi.org/10.1161/01.cir.97.15.1440

White J, Swerdlow DI, Preiss D, Fairhurst-Hunter Z, Keating BJ, Asselbergs FW, Sattar N, Humphries SE, Hingorani AD, Holmes MV (2016) Association of lipid fractions with risks for coronary artery disease and diabetes. JAMA Cardiol 1:692–699

Wijeysundera HC, Koh M, Alter DA, Austin PC, Jackevicius CA, Tu JV, Ko DT (2017) Association of high-density lipoprotein cholesterol with non-fatal cardiac and non-cardiac events: a CANHEART substudy. Open Heart 4(2):e000731. https://doi.org/10.1136/openhrt-2017-000731

Wilson PWF, Meigs JB, Sullivan L, Fox CS, Nathan DM, D'Agostino RB (2007) Prediction of incident diabetes mellitus in middle-aged adults: the Framingham offspring study. Arch Intern Med 167:1068–1074

Wittert G, Bracken K, Robledo KP, Grossmann M, Yeap BB, Handelsman DJ, Stuckey B, Conway A, Inder W, McLachlan R, Allan C, Jesudason D, Fui MNT, Hague W, Jenkins A, Daniel M, Gebski V, Keech A (2021) Testosterone treatment to prevent or revert type 2 diabetes in men enrolled in a lifestyle programme (T4DM): a randomised, double-blind, placebo-controlled, 2-year, phase 3b trial. Lancet Diabetes Endocrinol 9(1):32–45. https://doi.org/10.1016/S2213-8587(20)30367-3

Witztum JL, Gaudet D, Freedman SD, Alexander VJ, Digenio A, Williams KR, Yang Q, Hughes SG, Geary RS, Arca M, Stroes ESG, Bergeron J, Soran H, Civeira F, Hemphill L, Tsimikas S, Blom DJ, O'Dea L, Bruckert E (2019) Volanesorsen and triglyceride levels in familial chylomicronemia syndrome. N Engl J Med 381(6):531–542. https://doi.org/10.1056/NEJMoa1715944

Wolska A, Reimund M, Sviridov DO, Amar MJ, Remaley AT (2021) Apolipoprotein mimetic peptides: potential new therapies for cardiovascular diseases. Cell 10(3):597. https://doi.org/10.3390/cells10030597

Wu FC, von Eckardstein A (2003) Androgens and coronary artery disease. Endocr Rev 24 (2):183–217. https://doi.org/10.1210/er.2001-0025

Wu Y, Fan Z, Tian Y, Liu S, Liu S (2018) Relation between high density lipoprotein particles concentration and cardiovascular events: a meta-analysis. Lipids Health Dis 17(1):142. https://doi.org/10.1186/s12944-018-0732-6

Wu L, Soundarapandian MM, Castoreno AB, Millar JS, Rader DJ (2020) LDL-cholesterol reduction by ANGPTL3 inhibition in mice is dependent on endothelial lipase. Circ Res 127 (8):1112–1114. https://doi.org/10.1161/CIRCRESAHA.120.317128

Xin W, Lin Z, Zhang T, Jia S (2019) Probucol for the prevention of contrast-induced acute kidney injury in patients undergoing coronary angiography or percutaneous coronary intervention: a meta-analysis of randomized controlled trials. Clin Nephrol 92(1):36–43. https://doi.org/10.5414/CN109701

Yalcinkaya M, Kerksiek A, Gebert K, Annema W, Sibler R, Radosavljevic S, Lütjohann D, Rohrer L, von Eckardstein A (2020) HDL inhibits endoplasmic reticulum stress-induced apoptosis of pancreatic β-cells in vitro by activation of smoothened. J Lipid Res 61 (4):492–504. https://doi.org/10.1194/jlr.RA119000509

Yamashita S, Matsuzawa Y (2016) Re-evaluation of cholesteryl ester transfer protein function in atherosclerosis based upon genetics and pharmacological manipulation. Curr Opin Lipidol 27 (5):459–472. https://doi.org/10.1097/MOL.0000000000000332

Yamashita S, Masuda D, Matsuzawa Y (2015) Did we abandon probucol too soon? Curr Opin Lipidol 26(4):304–316. https://doi.org/10.1097/MOL.0000000000000199

Yamashita S, Arai H, Yokote K, Araki E, Suganami H, Ishibashi S, K-877 Study Group (2018) Effects of pemafibrate (K-877) on cholesterol efflux capacity and postprandial hyperlipidemia in patients with atherogenic dyslipidemia. J Clin Lipidol 12(5):1267–1279.e4. https://doi.org/10. 1016/j.jacl.2018.06.010

Yamashita S, Arai H, Bujo H, Masuda D, Ohama T, Ishibashi T, Yanagi K, Doi Y, Nakagawa S, Yamashiro K, Tanabe K, Kita T, Matsuzaki M, Saito Y, Fukushima M, Matsuzawa Y, PRO-SPECTIVE Study Group (2021) Probucol trial for secondary prevention of atherosclerotic events in patients with coronary heart disease (PROSPECTIVE). J Atheroscler Thromb 28 (2):103–123. https://doi.org/10.5551/jat.55327

Zandbergen F, Plutzky J (2007) PPARalpha in atherosclerosis and inflammation. Biochim Biophys Acta 1771(8):972–982. https://doi.org/10.1016/j.bbalip.2007.04.021

Zanoni P, von Eckardstein A (2020) Inborn errors of apolipoprotein A-I metabolism: implications for disease, research and development. Curr Opin Lipidol 31(2):62–70. https://doi.org/10.1097/ MOL.0000000000000667

Zanoni P, Khetarpal SA, Larach DB, Hancock-Cerutti WF, Millar JS, Cuchel M, DerOhannessian S, Kontush A, Surendran P, Saleheen D, Trompet S, Jukema JW, De Craen A, Deloukas P, Sattar N, Ford I, Packard C, Aa M, Alam DS, Di Angelantonio E, Abecasis G, Chowdhury R, Erdmann J, Nordestgaard BG, Nielsen SF, Tybjærg-Hansen A, Schmidt RF, Kuulasmaa K, Liu DJ, Perola M, Blankenberg S, Salomaa V, Männistö S, Amouyel P, Arveiler D, Ferrieres J, Müller-Nurasyid M, Ferrario M, Kee F, Willer CJ, Samani N, Schunkert E, Butterworth AS, Howson JM, Peloso GM, Stitziel NO, Danesh J, Kathiresan S, Rader DJ, CHD Exome+ Consortium, CARDIoGRAM Exome Consortium, Global Lipids Genetics Consortium (2016) Rare variant in scavenger receptor BI raises HDL cholesterol and increases risk of coronary heart disease. Science 351(6278):1166–1171. https:// doi.org/10.1126/science.aad3517

Zewinger S, Drechsler C, Kleber ME, Dressel A, Riffel J, Triem S, Lehmann M, Kopecky C, Säemann MD, Lepper FM, Silbernagel G, Scharnagl H, Ritsch A, Thorand B, de las Heras Gala T, Wagenpfeil S, Koenig W, Peters A, Laufs U, Wanner C, Fliser D, Speer T, März W (2015) Serum amyloid A: high-density lipoproteins interaction and cardiovascular risk. Eur Heart J 36(43):3007–3016. https://doi.org/10.1093/eurheartj/ehv352

Zewinger S, Reiser J, Jankowski V, Alansary D, Hahm E, Triem S, Klug M, Schunk SJ, Schmit D, Kramann R, Körbel C, Ampofo E, Laschke MW, Selejan SR, Paschen A, Herter T, Schuster S, Silbernagel G, Sester M, Sester U, Aßmann G, Bals R, Kostner G, Jahnen-Dechent W, Menger MD, Rohrer L, März W, Böhm M, Jankowski J, Kopf M, Latz E, Niemeyer BA, Fliser D, Laufs U, Speer T (2020) Apolipoprotein C3 induces inflammation and organ damage by alternative inflammasome activation. Nat Immunol 21(1):30–41. https://doi.org/10.1038/ s41590-019-0548-1

Zhao Q, Wang J, Miao Z, Zhang NR, Hennessy S, Small DS, Rader DJ (2021) A Mendelian randomization study of the role of lipoprotein subfractions in coronary artery disease. elife 10: e58361. https://doi.org/10.7554/eLife.58361

Zheng KH, Kaiser Y, van Olden CC, Santos RD, Dasseux JL, Genest J, Gaudet D, Westerink J, Keyserling C, Verberne FJ, Leitersdorf E, Hegele RA, Descamps OS, Hopkins P, Nederveen AJ, Stroes ESG (2020) No benefit of HDL mimetic CER-001 on carotid atherosclerosis in patients with genetically determined very low HDL levels. Atherosclerosis 311:13–19

Zhong S, Sharp DS, Grove JS, Bruce C, Yano K, Curb JD, Tall AR (1996) Increased coronary heart disease in Japanese-American men with mutation in the cholesteryl ester transfer protein gene despite increased HDL levels. J Clin Invest 97(12):2917–2923. https://doi.org/10.1172/ JCI118751

Zvintzou E, Lhomme M, Chasapi S, Filou S, Theodoropoulos V, Xapapadaki E, Kontush A, Spyroulias G, Tellis CC, Tselepis AD, Constantinou C, Kypreos KE (2017) Pleiotropic effects of apolipoprotein C3 on HDL functionality and adipose tissue metabolic activity. J Lipid Res 58 (9):1869–1883. https://doi.org/10.1194/jlr.M077925

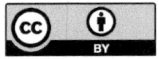

Lipoprotein(a)

Florian Kronenberg 🆔

Contents

1 Introduction 202
2 Sites of Production and Catabolism of Lp(a) 203
3 Physiology and Pathophysiology of Lp(a) 203
4 Genetic Control of Lp(a) Concentrations 206
5 Lp(a) Concentrations and Risk for CVD 208
   5.1 Searching for Lp(a) Thresholds Associated with an Increased Coronary Artery
        Disease Risk 208
   5.2 Lp(a) and Other Vascular Diseases 210
   5.3 Differences Between Primary and Secondary Prevention Studies 211
   5.4 Is Lp(a) an Independent Risk Factor for CVD? 212
6 What Evidence Do We Have for a Causal Association of High Lp(a) with CVD? ... 213
7 RNA-Targeting Therapies to Specifically Lower Lp(a) 214
   7.1 Antisense Oligonucleotides (ASO) Against Apolipoprotein(a) 214
   7.2 Short Interfering RNA (siRNA) to Target Apo(a) 215
8 Other Lipid-Lowering Drugs and Therapies with Possible Influence
   on Lp(a) Concentrations and Clinical Outcomes 216
   8.1 Lipoprotein Apheresis 216
   8.2 PCSK9 Inhibitors 217
   8.3 Statins 219
   8.4 Drugs That Are Probably No Longer Followed for Lp(a)-Lowering Potential 221
9 Therapeutic Lowering of Lipoprotein(a): How Much Is Enough? 221
10 Conclusions 223
References 223

F. Kronenberg (✉)
Department of Genetics and Pharmacology, Institute of Genetic Epidemiology, Medical University
of Innsbruck, Innsbruck, Austria
e-mail: Florian.Kronenberg@i-med.ac.at

© The Author(s) 2021
A. von Eckardstein, C. J. Binder (eds.), *Prevention and Treatment of Atherosclerosis*,
Handbook of Experimental Pharmacology 270, https://doi.org/10.1007/164_2021_504

Abstract

Lipoprotein(a) [Lp(a)] is an atherogenic lipoprotein with a strong genetic regulation. Up to 90% of the concentrations are explained by a single gene, the *LPA* gene. The concentrations show a several-hundred-fold interindividual variability ranging from less than 0.1 mg/dL to more than 300 mg/dL. Lp(a) plasma concentrations above 30 mg/dL and even more above 50 mg/dL are associated with an increased risk for cardiovascular disease including myocardial infarction, stroke, aortic valve stenosis, heart failure, peripheral arterial disease, and all-cause mortality. Since concentrations above 50 mg/dL are observed in roughly 20% of the Caucasian population and in an even higher frequency in African-American and Asian-Indian ethnicities, it can be assumed that Lp(a) is one of the most important genetically determined risk factors for cardiovascular disease.

Carriers of genetic variants that are associated with high Lp(a) concentrations have a markedly increased risk for cardiovascular events. Studies that used these genetic variants as a genetic instrument to support a causal role for Lp(a) as a cardiovascular risk factor are called Mendelian randomization studies. The principle of this type of studies has been introduced and tested for the first time ever with Lp(a) and its genetic determinants.

There are currently no approved pharmacologic therapies that specifically target Lp(a) concentrations. However, some therapies that target primarily LDL cholesterol have also an influence on Lp(a) concentrations. These are mainly PCSK9 inhibitors that lower LDL cholesterol by 60% and Lp(a) by 25–30%. Furthermore, lipoprotein apheresis lowers both, Lp(a) and LDL cholesterol, by about 60–70%. Some sophisticated study designs and statistical analyses provided support that lowering Lp(a) by these therapies also lowers cardiovascular events on top of the effect caused by lowering LDL cholesterol, although this was not the main target of the therapy. Currently, new therapies targeting RNA such as antisense oligonucleotides (ASO) or small interfering RNA (siRNA) against apolipoprotein(a), the main protein of the Lp(a) particle, are under examination and lower Lp(a) concentrations up to 90%. Since these therapies specifically lower Lp(a) concentrations without influencing other lipoproteins, they will serve the last piece of the puzzle whether a decrease of Lp(a) results also in a decrease of cardiovascular events.

Keywords

Apolipoprotein(a) · Association study · Cardiovascular disease · Copy number variation · Lipoprotein(a) · Lp(a) · Mendelian randomization · Therapy

1   Introduction

Lipoprotein(a) [Lp(a)] is one of the strongest genetically determined risk factors for cardiovascular disease (CVD) (Kronenberg and Utermann 2013). It contains besides an LDL particle an additional apolipoprotein that is called apolipoprotein

(a) [apo(a)]. This apolipoprotein shows a high homology with plasminogen. After more than 50 years of research, the physiological function of Lp(a) is still unexplained. An astonishing characteristic of Lp(a) is the more than 1,000-fold range of concentrations between individuals from almost zero to more than 300 mg/dL (Kronenberg and Utermann 2013). The distribution of Lp(a) is very skewed in most populations: for example, roughly 50% of the Europeans have concentrations below 10 mg/dL and about 25% have concentrations above 30 mg/dL.

2 Sites of Production and Catabolism of Lp(a)

Apo(a) is synthesized in the liver (Tomlinson et al. 1989; Kraft et al. 1989). Variation in Lp(a) concentrations among individuals is determined by the rate of production rather than by differences in the catalytic rate (Rader et al. 1994). After secretion of apo(a), it binds to LDL-apoB lysine-binding residues by its lysine-binding sites with subsequent forming of a disulfide bond. Whether the assembly occurs in the circulation at the hepatic surface or intracellularly is a matter of debate (Koschinsky and Marcovina 2004).

The site and mechanism of catabolism is discussed controversially. Studies in mice revealed that the liver is the main route of Lp(a) catabolism (Cain et al. 2005). The finding of an arteriovenous difference of Lp(a) concentrations in the renal circulation (Kronenberg et al. 1997), of apo(a) fragments in urine (Mooser et al. 1996), and of a disturbed Lp(a) metabolism in kidney disease (Frischmann et al. 2007) has suggested also a role of the kidney in Lp(a) catabolism. The receptors involved in the catabolic process are a matter of debate as recently comprehensively reviewed (McCormick and Schneider 2019) and include lipoprotein receptors such as the LDL receptor, VLDL receptor, LDL receptor related proteins (LRP1 and LRP2), toll-like and scavenger receptors (e.g., CD36 and SR-BI), carbohydrate receptors or lectins, and plasminogen receptors.

3 Physiology and Pathophysiology of Lp(a)

The physiological function of Lp(a) is still in the dark. It is believed that Lp(a) has proatherogenic and prothrombotic properties (Fig. 1). The apo(a) glycoprotein has a high degree of homology to plasminogen (McLean et al. 1987) suggesting that Lp(a) might not only be a link between the cholesterol transport system in plasma and the fibrinolytic system but may also act as a modulator of the balance between blood clotting and fibrinolysis. At least in vitro, Lp(a) indeed interferes with the blood clotting/fibrinolytic cascades at several steps (Boffa and Koschinsky 2016). As reviewed extensively (Koschinsky and Marcovina 2004; Boffa and Koschinsky 2016), this includes the inhibition of streptokinase and urokinase-mediated activation of plasminogen by the tissue-type plasminogen activator (t-PA), inhibition of t-PA in solution, fibrin and fibrinogen binding, competition with plasminogen and t-PA binding for soluble fibrinogen, competition with plasminogen for binding to

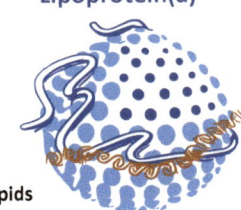

Lipoprotein(a)

Proatherogenic
- ↑ Oxidized phospholipids
- ↑ Foam cell formation
- ↑ Endothelial dysfunction
- ↑ Smooth muscle cell proliferation
- ↑ Chemoattraction of monocytes
- ↑ Inflammation of the arterial wall

Prothrombotic
- ↓ Plasminogen activation
- ↓ Fibrinolysis
- ↓ Tissue factor pathway inhibitor
- ↓ Clot permeability
- ↑ Platelet response

Fig. 1 Proatherogenic and prothrombotic properties of Lp(a)

cellular receptors, and enhancement of the plasminogen-activator-inhibitor PAI-1 activity. Considering that many individuals have low Lp(a) concentrations and some of them even almost no Lp(a) and others have concentrations far above 100 mg/dL, one might expect major effects on the balance between clotting and fibrinolysis which, however, have not convincingly been described by in vivo data. Epidemiologic and genetic studies did not provide support for a thrombogenic role and if there is any, it can only be found at very high Lp(a) values above the 95th percentile (Nordestgaard and Langsted 2016). Interestingly, there are reports that the situation might be different in childhood where high Lp(a) concentrations were found to be accompanied with venous thromboembolism (Nowak-Gottl et al. 1999).

A further property of Lp(a)/apo(a) is the interaction with components of the extracellular matrix including fibrin, fibronectin, tetranectin, proteoglycans, and β2-glycoprotein (Köchl et al. 1997). The domains in apo(a), which mediate binding to fibrin/fibrinogen, are lysine-binding sites in KIV-8 and KIV-10 (Koschinsky and Marcovina 2004). Binding of Lp(a) to fibrin has been proposed as a mechanism to deliver cholesterol to sites of injury and wound healing of the vascular wall with the negative side effect that Lp(a) also deposits cholesterol in growing atherosclerotic plaques and inhibits fibrinolysis at the plaque surface. Furthermore, high Lp(a) levels impair activation of transforming growth factor-β by downregulation of plasmin generation, thereby contributing to smooth muscle cell proliferation (Grainger et al. 1993). The published data provide clear evidence that Lp(a) can interfere with many key reactions of clotting/fibrinolysis in vitro and is deposited in atherosclerotic plaques. Moreover, effects on monocytes/macrophages result in foam cell formation (Poon et al. 1997). Lp(a) induces chemoattractant activity of monocytes and induces macrophage expression of interleucin-8 (IL-8) (Klezovitch et al. 2001).

The connection between innate immune system and Lp(a) has been further strengthened by the identification of Lp(a) as the major plasma carrier of oxidized phospholipids (OxPLs) (Bergmark et al. 2008) which can stimulate many

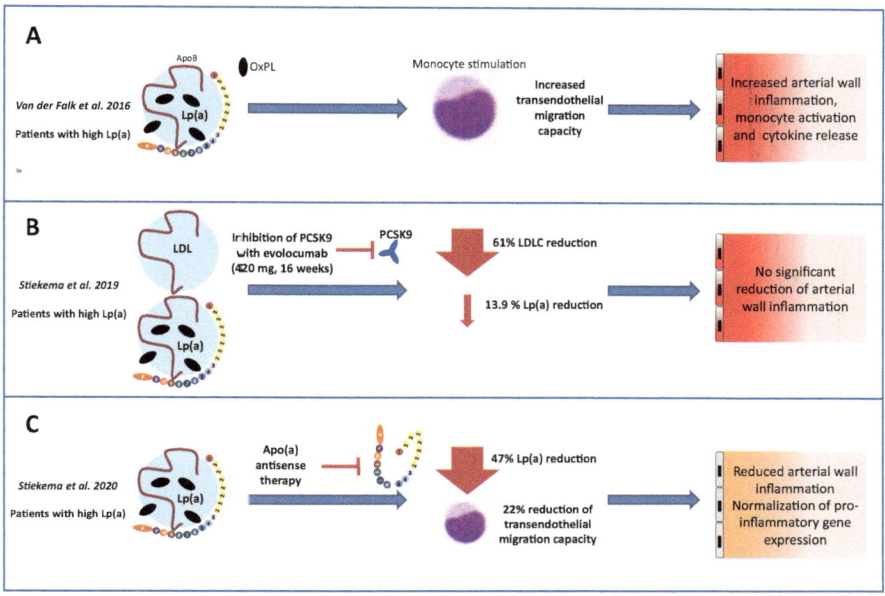

Fig. 2 Impact of Lp(a) on arterial wall inflammation. Panel (**a**) Individuals with high Lp(a) ($n = 30$, median 108 mg/dL) present significantly increased arterial wall inflammation as assessed by magnetic resonance imaging, 18-F fluorodeoxyglucose (18F-FDG) uptake PET/CT and SPECT/CT, and activated monocytes assessed by transendothelial migration and monocyte priming and challenge assays (van der Valk et al. 2016). Panel (**b**) 420 mg of the PCSK9 inhibitor evolocumab vs. placebo over 16 weeks reduced LDL-C consistently but did not improve arterial wall inflammation in individuals with high Lp(a) ($n = 129$, median ≈ 80 mg/dL), despite modest concomitant Lp(a) reduction (-13.9%) (Stiekema et al. 2019). Panel (**c**) High Lp(a) was associated with a pro-inflammatory transcriptome in monocytes. Treatment with different regimes of AKCEA-APO(a)-L$_{Rx}$ resulted in a 47% reduction of Lp(a) and in reductions of the pro-inflammatory signatures in the transcriptome, the transendothelial migration capacity, and the expression of chemokines and toll-like receptors on the monocytes surface (Stiekema et al. 2020; Coassin and Kronenberg 2020)

pro-inflammatory pathways in the arterial wall. The binding-site for oxidized phospholipids has been identified in the protein moiety of Lp(a), specifically in the KIV type 10 domain of apo(a) (Leibundgut et al. 2013). Levels of Lp(a) and OxPL in human plasma are highly correlated and it is therefore not unexpected that this also results in an association of OxPL levels with cardiovascular disease (Tsimikas et al. 2005, 2010; Kiechl et al. 2007). These oxidized lipid species are recognized by pattern recognition receptors of innate immune cells and trigger the whole cascade of inflammatory processes that can finally lead to plaque destabilization (Boffa and Koschinsky 2019). During recent years a series of publications (Fig. 2) from the group around Eric Stroes investigated the impact of Lp(a) and LDL-C on arterial wall inflammation and found that individuals with elevated Lp(a) concentrations have increased arterial inflammation and enhanced peripheral blood mononuclear cell trafficking to the arterial wall compared with subjects with normal Lp(a).

Monocytes isolated from subjects with high Lp(a) concentrations showed an increased capacity to transmigrate the endothelium and produce pro-inflammatory cytokines. This was mediated by OxPLs and subsequent blocking of the OxPLs by specific antibodies also reduced the pro-inflammatory responsiveness of the monocytes (Fig. 2a) (van der Valk et al. 2016). The subsequent publications revealed that a pronounced reduction of LDLC by PCSK9 inhibitors is not sufficient to substantially reduce the arterial wall inflammation (Fig. 2b) (Stiekema et al. 2019). In a further investigation they examined whether patients with cardiovascular disease and elevated Lp(a) concentrations experience anti-inflammatory effects following large reductions of Lp(a) by apo(a) antisense therapy. They observed in a first step that circulating monocytes of healthy individuals and patients, both having high Lp(a) concentrations, are characterized by a markedly pro-inflammatory gene expression profile with several pathways of the innate immune system being upregulated. In an intervention with apo(a) antisense therapy the authors showed that the resulting 47% lowering of Lp(a) concentrations was indeed capable of reversing the pro-inflammatory gene expression signature to levels close to that of controls with normal Lp(a) concentrations. This was accompanied with a 22% functional reduction in transendothelial migration capacity of monocytes ex vivo (Fig. 2c) (Stiekema et al. 2020; Coassin and Kronenberg 2020). These findings proposed a further mechanism how Lp(a) might mediate cardiovascular disease and added a new layer to our still shallow understanding of the exact pathophysiological mechanisms by which high Lp(a) causes cardiovascular disease.

4   Genetic Control of Lp(a) Concentrations

Lp(a) concentrations are not much influenced by age, sex, fasting state, inflammation (Kronenberg 2014a; Langsted et al. 2014) and lifestyle factors such as diet or physical activity. However, the concentrations are under strict genetic control. Family studies revealed a heritability estimate of Lp(a) concentrations of about 90% (Austin et al. 1992; Lamon-Fava et al. 1991; Utermann 1989). Lp(a) is therefore the lipoprotein with the strongest genetic control. The discovery of the size polymorphism of apo(a) in serum (Utermann et al. 1987) which is based on a variable number of the so-called kringle-IV (K-IV) repeats in the *LPA* gene (Utermann 1989; Kraft et al. 1992; Lackner et al. 1991, 1993) resulted in the identification of the *LPA* gene as the major gene for Lp(a) levels. Each of these up to more than 40 repeats has a size of 5.6 kB which results in a highly polymorphic and informative copy number variation (CNV).

There exists a pronounced inverse correlation between the number of K-IV repeats and Lp(a) concentrations. Individuals expressing a low number of K-IV repeats resulting in the so-called small apo(a) isoforms (up to 22K-IV repeats) have on average markedly higher Lp(a) concentrations than individuals carrying only large apo(a) isoforms (more than 22K-IV repeats) (Kronenberg and Utermann 2013). This K-IV size polymorphism of apo(a) explains about 20–80% of the variability of Lp(a) concentrations depending on the ethnicity (Utermann et al. 1987).

Interestingly, Lp(a) levels of unrelated individuals carrying the same isoform size combination can still vary by up to 200-fold (Cohen et al. 1993; Perombelon et al. 1994). On the other hand, same-sized alleles within families which are identical-by-descent show typically a less than 2.5-fold variation in Lp(a) concentrations (Perombelon et al. 1994). This is a clear indication that further genetic variants exist that regulate the Lp(a) concentrations in addition to the isoform size (Cohen et al. 1993; Coassin et al. 2017). The search for single nucleotide polymorphisms in the *LPA* gene region had a first peak in 2009 with the description of the two SNPs rs10455872 and rs3793220 which since then are regularly used in hundreds of association studies (Clarke et al. 2009). However, there are many more SNPs in the wider *LPA* gene region which are associated with Lp(a) concentrations and genome-wide association studies (GWAS) have explored this in a systematic way (Li et al. 2015; Mack et al. 2017; Ober et al. 2009). In a recent GWAS meta-analysis in 13,781 individuals from 5 populations we identified 2001 SNPs in a 1.76 MB large region around the *LPA* gene. 48 of these SNPs were associated independently of each other with Lp(a) concentrations (*p*-values below 5×10^{-8}) (Mack et al. 2017). However, that does not mean that each of these SNPs is causally (functionally) related to Lp(a) concentrations. Many of these SNPs are probably in linkage disequilibrium with another SNP that is causally influencing Lp(a) concentrations. A typical example is rs75692336 which showed the strongest association with Lp(a) concentrations in a statistical model in our GWAS which adjusted besides age and sex also for the apo(a) isoform size. This SNP turned out to be a proxy SNP for the real culprit, a splice-site variant (G4925A) in the kringle-IV type 2 which is not easily accessible for genotyping (Coassin et al. 2017) and therefore not found in GWAS analyses (Mack et al. 2017).

Besides the *LPA* gene region, the *APOE* gene was found to be independently associated with Lp(a) concentrations. Especially the SNP which is responsible for the APO E2 allele (rs7412) decreased Lp(a) concentrations by 3.34 mg/dL or $\approx 15\%$ of the mean values of the population (Mack et al. 2017). The recent GWAS in 293,274 White British individuals revealed two further loci, the *CETP* locus as well as the *APOH* locus, the latter encodes for beta2-glycoprotein I (Hoekstra et al. 2021).

The major part of the *LPA* gene is a so-called camouflaged gene since up to 70% of the coding sequence harboring the K-IV type 2 with up to more than 40 repeats is not easily accessible to modern sequencing technologies. Each copy of the K-IV type 2 has a size of 5.6 kb. Until recently almost no sequence information was available for that region. Our group recently developed an ultra-deep sequencing strategy for this region and a variant analysis pipeline and reported the first map of genetic variation in the KIV-2 region. By sequencing 123 Central-European individuals and reanalyzing public data of 2,504 individuals from 26 populations, we found 14 different loss-of-function and splice-site mutations, as well as >100 partially even common missense variants (Coassin et al. 2019). One of these variants is the above-mentioned splice-site variant (G4925A) which has a frequency of about 22% and tremendously decreases Lp(a) concentrations by more than 30 mg/dL

(Coassin et al. 2019). Another variant is the R21X in the KIV-2 region which was not easy to analyze until recently. It is a likely causal SNP resulting in a nonsense mutation, which leads to a truncated protein that is rapidly degraded (Parson et al. 2004). We recently developed a highly sensitive allele-specific qPCR assay and genotyped R21X in 10,910 individuals from three populations and showed that R21X carriers have significantly lower (−11.7 mg/dL) mean Lp(a) concentrations (Di Maio et al. 2020). A study by Morgan and colleagues investigated two very rare variants, R990Q (rs41259144) located in the KIV type 4 and R1771C (rs139145675) located in the kringle V which were present in four null Lp(a) individuals. These two variants are hypothesized to impair the ability of the protein folding and thereby circumventing its processing to maturity for secretion (Morgan et al. 2020). Other detected mutations are currently under investigation to explain the functional consequences of these variants. It might very well be that some of these variants explain the large ethnic and interindividual differences in Lp(a) concentrations.

5 Lp(a) Concentrations and Risk for CVD

5.1 Searching for Lp(a) Thresholds Associated with an Increased Coronary Artery Disease Risk

The evidence is quite strong that high Lp(a) concentrations are associated with an increasing risk for cardiovascular disease (Kronenberg and Utermann 2013; Cegla et al. 2019). The Copenhagen City Heart Study observed for individuals from a general population with concentrations between 30 and 76 mg/dL (corresponding to the 67th–90th percentile) a 1.60-fold increased risk for incident myocardial infarction compared to individuals with Lp(a) concentrations below 5 mg/dL (corresponding to the lower 22% of the population). This risk increased to 1.90 for persons with Lp(a) concentrations between 77 and 117 mg/dL (90th to 95th percentile) and to 2.60 for individuals with Lp(a) concentrations above 117 mg/dL (>95th percentile) (Kamstrup et al. 2009) (Fig. 3, panel (a)). The concentration threshold for an increased risk has been discussed controversially and an European Atherosclerosis Society (EAS) consensus statement proposed 50 mg/dL (Nordestgaard et al. 2010). Most importantly, such a threshold corresponds to the 80th percentile of the concentration distribution in a Caucasian population and means that 20% of the population have probably an increased risk for CVD due to elevated Lp(a) concentrations. From a standpoint of public health relevance, this makes Lp(a) a very important risk factor for CVD.

The most recent data from the UK Biobank with more than 460,000 study participants followed for more than 11 years are in line with a rather linear increase in risk for CVD with increasing Lp(a) concentrations. In that sufficiently powered study the risk started already to increase above the median of Lp(a) which was 19.6 nmol/L (corresponds to roughly 8 mg/dL) (Patel et al. 2021). Of course, this raises the question what is a clinically meaningful increase in risk? The same study revealed also that Lp(a) is not only a risk factor in non-White populations but also in

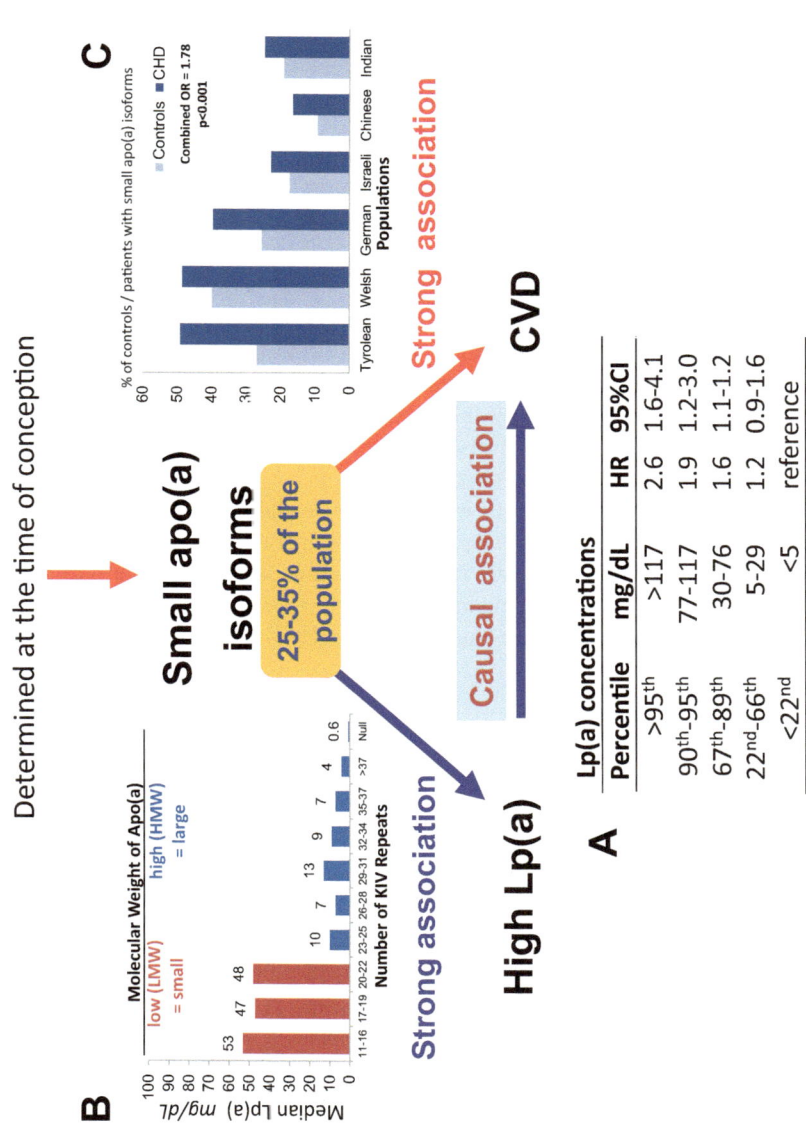

Fig. 3 Mendelian randomization approach to demonstrate a causal association between Lp(a) concentrations and cardiovascular disease. Panel (**a**) shows the association between elevated Lp(a) concentrations and cardiovascular disease (CVD) as shown in the Copenhagen City Heart Study (Kamstrup et al. 2009).

Black or Asian people (Patel et al. 2021), a matter of major discussions over the past. This is in line with earlier results from the ARIC study (Virani et al. 2012), the MESA Study (Guan et al. 2015), or the Dallas Heart Study (Lee et al. 2017), but in contrast to NHANES III or the INTERHEART Study which did not found Lp(a) to be associated with CVD in non-Hispanic Blacks (Brandt et al. 2020) or Africans (Pare et al. 2019), respectively.

The recent statement by the new ESC/EAS guidelines for the management of dyslipidemia might have introduced more confusion than clarification by stating that "Lp(a) measurement should be considered at least once in each adult person's lifetime to identify those with very high inherited Lp(a) levels >180 mg/dL (>430 nmol/L) who may have a lifetime risk of ASCVD equivalent to the risk associated with heterozygous familial hypercholesterolaemia." (Mach et al. 2019) The first part of this sentence to measure Lp(a) at least once in each individual is indeed a forward-looking advice important for risk stratification and in the near future maybe also for therapeutic interventions. However, some interpret the second part of this statement as the introduction of a new threshold for risk stratification. However, this is not the case since they mention that these values are associated with "very high inherited risk." The risk is already markedly increased at lower levels as discussed above. These very high levels are only observed in far less than 1% of White people and should not be used as an excuse either not to screen or to decline any therapeutic options to lower Lp(a) concentrations with currently available therapies such as lipid apheresis or with therapies that will become available in the future. This part of the guidelines and the cited literature did not show the data and the calculations which resulted in this threshold in a convincing and reproducible way (Mach et al. 2019). It has therefore to be considered with caution and needs further clarification.

5.2   Lp(a) and Other Vascular Diseases

Besides numerous studies on coronary artery disease, during recent years several studies found even a strong association between high Lp(a) concentrations and stroke (Erqou et al. 2009; Langsted et al. 2019a; Zhang et al. 2019), aortic valve calcification stenosis (Arsenault et al. 2014; Cairns et al. 2017; Capoulade et al. 2018; Chen et al. 2018; Kamstrup et al. 2014; Thanassoulis et al. 2013; Vongpromek et al. 2015; Vuorio et al. 2019; Perrot et al. 2019), heart failure (Kamstrup and Nordestgaard 2016) as well as peripheral arterial disease (Dieplinger et al. 2007;

Fig. 3 (continued) Panel (**b**) shows the association between the number of K-IV repeats in the *LPA* gene and Lp(a) concentrations: individuals with small apo(a) isoform have markedly higher median Lp(a) concentrations than individuals with large apo(a) isoforms (Laschkolnig et al. 2014). Panel (**c**) shows the preponderance of small apo(a) isoforms in patients with CVD when compared to controls (Sandholzer et al. 1992). Since a low number of K-IV copies (11–22 copies) is associated with high Lp(a) levels and high Lp(a) levels are associated with CVD, it follows that a low number of K-IV copies has to be associated with CVD if the association of Lp(a) with CVD is causal. Figure is taken and adapted with permission from reference (Kronenberg 2016b)

Gurdasani et al. 2012; Laschkolnig et al. 2014). A recent GWAS for peripheral arterial disease identified for the *LPA* gene region the strongest signal which was even more pronounced that for the *CDKN2B* region on chromosome 9p21 or for the LDL receptor (Klarin ɜt al. 2019). This makes Lp(a) a risk factor for many CVD endpoints although the strength of the association might differ between the various entities of endpoints. Studies that investigated the association of the *LPA* gene region with all-cause mortality (Langsted et al. 2019b) demonstrated also a significant association in case they were sufficiently powered. A sufficient study size and number of endpoints is in this context a prerequisite since the finding of an association with all-cause mortality is mainly driven by death in the wider context of CVD.

5.3   Differences Between Primary and Secondary Prevention Studies

There is strong evidencɜ for an association between high Lp(a) concentrations and future CVD events in studies in whom participants were free of CVD at baseline (primary prevention studies). However, findings are inconsistent for study populations with preexisting CVD at baseline (secondary prevention studies). A meta-analysis of 11 secondary prevention studies found that elevated Lp(a) predicted major adverse cardiovascular events with an odds ratio of 1.40 (95% CI 1.15–1.71, $p < 0.001$) with a considerable heterogeneity between studies. When the authors stratified the studies intc those with high (≥ 130 mg/dL) versus low (<130 mg/dL) average on-treatment LDL-C, the association for Lp(a) was still significant for the studies with high average LDL-C (OR $= 1.46$, 95% CI 1.23–1.73) but not for those with low average LDL-C (OR $= 1.20$, 95% CI 0.90–1.60) (O'Donoghue et al. 2014). This has raised many discussions since especially first intervention studies to specifically lower Lp(a) would target patients with established CVD. A seminal review on secondary prevention studies elucidating the reasons why some of these studies did not find an association has recently been published by Boffa and colleagues (2018). The authors distinguished between major potential general "confounders" and confounders related to Lp(a) which might have influenced the findings of some of the secondary prevention studies. As general confounders they discussed the restrictive inclusion and exclusion criteria of randomized controlled trials, the lack of statistɨcal power, differences in clinical management between primary and secondary prevention trials and finally an index event bias. Index event bias may underlie paradoxical findings whereby risk factors that are well established to contribute to pathological events do not appear to predict recurrence of these events (Dahabreh and Kent 2011). A famous example is hypertension which increases the risk for a first stroke about fourfold but is not associated with stroke recurrence (Smits et al. 2013). As confounders related to Lp(a) the authors mentioned the use of log-transformed Lp(a) levels, secondary changes in Lp(a) concentrations due to the events (consider that Lp(a) is thought to be an acute-phase protein), and issues related to the measurement of Lp(a) (e.g., standardization of the assays, isoform-dependency of the assays, or effects of sample handling and storage on Lp(a) measurement) (Boffa et al. 2018).

5.4   Is Lp(a) an Independent Risk Factor for CVD?

There is ample evidence that Lp(a) is an independent risk factor for CVD
(Kronenberg and Utermann 2013). That means that high Lp(a) can increase the
risk for CVD even if other classical risk factors are not present. And if combined
with other risk factors the entire risk of a particular person increases further. Whether
this risk increase is linear or exponential is much easier to predict on the population
level than for a given person. Risk prediction is associated with uncertainties as long
as we do not know or measure all factors that contribute to the risk of a disease. This
has recently been demonstrated quite convincingly in the Malmö Diet and Cancer
Study with almost 30,000 study participants and more than 4,122 incident coronary
artery disease cases during a long median observation period of 21.3 years. The
authors calculated polygenic risk scores for each individual using 6.24 million SNPs
and observed that the lifetime risk for coronary artery disease increased from about
16% in those 10% of the participants with the lowest polygenic risk scores to more
than 45% in the 10% of the population with the highest score. Most interestingly,
this was independent from traditional risk factors meaning that in each traditional
risk factor category (low, medium, borderline, and high) the risk increased two- to
threefold for those with a high genetic risk score category compared to a low genetic
risk score category (Hindy et al. 2020). This clearly demonstrates that a single risk
factor including Lp(a) should never be seen "isolated" without considering the other
risk factors as good as possible. This can be seen best when looking at the distribution of CVD risk contributors such as systolic blood pressure or LDL cholesterol in
individuals who remain free and those who develop CVD over the upcoming years:
there is always a substantial overlap in the distribution of these factors as already
shown in the ancient studies from the Framingham cohort (Kannel et al. 1964) and
lately by cohorts from Finland and Sweden (Ripatti et al. 2010). This explains also
why not everybody with high Lp(a) will develop CVD.

With Lp(a) and LDL-C a very special situation is present since almost each
method of LDL-C measurement (or calculation by formulas) includes also the
cholesterol content present in in the LDL particle of Lp(a). It is estimated that the
proportion of cholesterol in the Lp(a) particle is about 30% of the Lp(a) mass
(Kinpara et al. 2011), although some discuss an even higher value of 45%
(Kronenberg et al. 2004) which also depends on the apo(a) isoform size. In some
individuals with high Lp(a) concentrations the amount of cholesterol derived from
Lp(a) can be quite substantial as in the roughly 5% of the general population with an
Lp(a) concentration above 100 mg/dL. In these persons the cholesterol content
included in the LDL-C measurement but originating from Lp(a) would be 30 to
45 mg/dL. In persons with 200 mg/dL this would contribute 60 to 90 mg/dL to the
LDL-C measurement. This additional amount of LDL-C can even result in a
diagnosis (or misclassification) of hypercholesterolemia which is actually caused
by high Lp(a) concentrations (Langsted et al. 2016). A very recent study, however,
reported that the percentage of Lp(a) cholesterol relative to Lp(a) mass varied from
5.8% to 57.3% (Yeang et al. 2021). Especially this low percentage of cholesterol
might require further investigation and validation.

A further consequence from this measurement issue might become of clinical relevance, especially when a patient is given a statin and shows no response or a low response to this LDL-C-targeting treatment. A reason for this might be a high Lp(a) concentration: statins do not lower Lp(a) concentrations. If Lp(a) is very high, LDL-C might be misclassified as high which could result in a "wrong" indication for a statin under particular circumstances. When the targeted "true" LDL-C (the LDL-C without the Lp(a) cholesterol) is already in the target range, a treatment with a statin might result in a lower response than expected from the uncorrected LDL-C value (Scanu and Hinman 2002; Miltiadous et al. 2006).

6   What Evidence Do We Have for a Causal Association of High Lp(a) with CVD?

When a biomarker is changed in diseased patients, the important discussion starts whether this biomarker is a risk factor or a risk marker as illustrated recently (Kronenberg 2019a). In case of a risk factor, this parameter is causally related to disease and it might become an interesting drug target. If it is a biomarker, this parameter might be interesting for diagnostic purposes because it is changed secondarily to the disease and points the physician to the disease. It would not make sense to develop drugs which influence that parameter (see recent discussion on this issue in reference (Kronenberg 2016a). Mendelian randomization studies illustrated in Fig. 3 provide a strong support for causality. Genetic variants that are strongly associated with high Lp(a) concentrations (Fig. 3, panel (b)) show also an increased risk with CVD (Fig. 3, panel (c)) which underscores the causal link between high Lp(a) concentrations and CVD. Actually Lp(a) was the first practical example applying this approach almost a decade before the term "Mendelian randomization" has been coined: at the beginning of the 1990s data on the small apo(a) isoforms were used as genetic instrument: small isoforms with up to 22 K-IV repeats were associated with a significantly increased risk for coronary heart disease in six different populations (Sandholzer et al. 1992). A later meta-analysis including 7,382 coronary heart disease cases and 8,514 controls identified a 2.08-fold increased risk for carriers of small apo(a) isoforms (Erqou et al. 2010). Later approaches that investigated *LPA* variants on the DNA level either by the number of KIV repeats identified by pulsed-field gel electrophoresis or by the sum of KIV repeats of the two alleles by quantitative PCR or by the investigation of SNPs that are associated with high Lp(a) concentrations revealed the same finding (Clarke et al. 2009; Kamstrup et al. 2009; Kraft et al. 1996). On the other hand, genetic variants that are associated with low Lp(a) concentrations are obviously protective from CVD (Coassin et al. 2017; Di Maio et al. 2020; Lim et al. 2014). These strong associations make Lp(a) probably the most important genetic risk factor for CVD if we keep in mind the high frequency of small apo(a) isoforms or variants which go along with high Lp(a) concentrations in the population (Kronenberg 2016b).

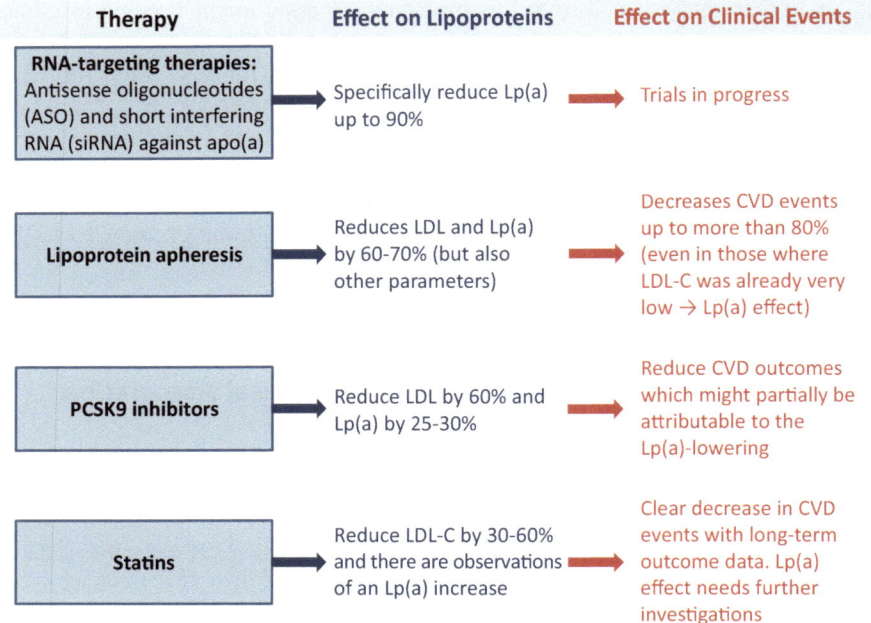

Fig. 4 Effect of therapeutic interventions on lipoproteins and clinical outcomes

7 RNA-Targeting Therapies to Specifically Lower Lp(a)

Based on the epidemiological and genetic studies the next and most consequent logical step is the therapeutic lowering of Lp(a) and the investigation whether such a therapy also decreases the number of CVD events (Fig. 4). To specifically accomplish an Lp(a)-lowering without influencing other lipoproteins, two main approaches are currently available and both selectively reduce the synthesis of apo(a) in the liver (Landmesser et al. 2020) and are therefore the optimal approach not only to lower Lp(a) but also to serve the last piece of the puzzle to demonstrate that a specific lowering of Lp(a) will also reduce CVD events.

7.1 Antisense Oligonucleotides (ASO) Against Apolipoprotein(a)

In principle, antisense oligonucleotides are 13–20 nucleic acid long and bind to the target RNA. As soon as the single-stranded ASOs are taken up by the cell, they bind directly to the mRNA creating a duplex that forms a complex with the intracellularly available RNAse H1. This finally mediates the target mRNA cleavage preventing the production of the targeted protein (Landmesser et al. 2020).

Using this principle to target apo(a), already the first phase I trial with IONIS-APO(a)$_{Rx}$ given subcutaneously in various amounts and numbers of dosages revealed a potent Lp(a)-lowering effect up to almost 80% (Tsimikas et al. 2015). In further trials it has been shown that this therapy results also in a reduction of oxidized phospholipids and a reduced monocyte inflammatory activation that returned close to baseline levels after stopping the medication. Furthermore, a new chemistry was used in this next trial in which a modified IONIS-APO(a)$_{Rx}$ antisense oligonucleotide is conjugated with a GalNAc3 complex (IONIS-APO(a)-L$_{Rx}$). This formulation targets the drug to the hepatocyte via the asialoglycoprotein receptor, making it 30 times more potent than the parent antisense oligonucleotide. This enabled the administered dose to be reduced 10-fold, thereby improving its tolerability. The highest dose administered resulted in a 92% mean reduction of Lp(a) with no serious side effects (Viney et al. 2016). The most recent trial included 286 patients with established CVD and Lp(a) concentrations of at least 60 mg/dL (Tsimikas et al. 2020a). Administration of APO(a)-L$_{Rx}$ resulted in dose-dependent decreases in Lp(a) concentrations with up to 72% at 60 mg every 4 weeks, and 80% at 20 mg every week, as compared with 6% with placebo. There were no significant differences between any APO(a)-L$_{Rx}$ dose and placebo with respect to platelet counts, liver and renal measures, or influenza-like symptoms. The most common adverse events were injection-site reactions (Tsimikas et al. 2020a).

Based on those data the Lp(a)HORIZON trial (NCT04023552: https://clinicaltrials.gov/ct2/show/study/NCT04023552) started recently and will recruit 7,680 patients with the key inclusion criteria of Lp(a) $\geq$70 mg/dL at the screening visit, an optimal LDL cholesterol lowering treatment, an optimal treatment of other CV risk factors, and a myocardial infarction or an ischemic stroke $\geq$3 months to $\leq$10 years prior to the screening visit or a clinically significant symptomatic peripheral artery disease. Patients will be injected monthly 80 mg of the drug (now called TQJ230 or Pelacarsen) or placebo subcutaneously. The estimated completion date is April 2024.

7.2   Short Interfering RNA (siRNA) to Target Apo(a)

The siRNAs are chemically synthesized and a GalNAc-siRNA conjugate selectively enters the hepatocyte via receptor-mediated endocytosis using the asialoglycoprotein receptor (similar as for ASO). After this, the double-stranded siRNA is released from the endosome and the two RNA stands dissociate into the sense and antisense strand. The antisense strand forms a highly stable complex with the RNA-induced silencing complex (RISC) which induces the cleavage of the target mRNA, degradation by exonucleases, and reduced synthesis of the protein of interest. The complex of siRNA with RISC is highly stable which results in a long-term cleavage of the targeted transcripts with a suppression of the protein production lasting more than 6 months (Landmesser et al. 2020).

Currently, two drugs under Phase I and II trials are using the siRNA principle: the first one is AMG890 (also called olpasiran) with a phase 1 (NCT03626662) and a phase 2 trial (NCT04270760). Obviously the phase 1 trial showed an Lp(a) reduction of more than 90% that persisted for 3–6 months (Abstract by Koren MJ et al.;

Circulation 2020;142:A13951). The second one is SLN360: a phase 1 trial with 88 patients is currently under way and is expected to be completed in November 2022.

8   Other Lipid-Lowering Drugs and Therapies with Possible Influence on Lp(a) Concentrations and Clinical Outcomes

Before reviewing the various other approaches of lowering Lp(a) (Fig. 4), there are two issues which should be stressed when considering the results from the trials which investigated the Lp(a) lowering effects of various interventions:

- Most previous therapeutic options were not developed and were not aiming for a specific Lp(a)-lowering but reached out for other lipoproteins and the Lp(a)-lowering is a concomitant observation. Therefore, it is hard to disentangle whether an effect observed in an intervention group is an effect of Lp(a)-lowering or an effect of the influence on other lipoproteins or risk factors which were the primary target of that intervention.
- In many cases, studies were not designed to reach out for patients with high or solely high Lp(a) concentrations but targeted other lipoproteins such as high LDL-C or low HDL-C. Therefore in many cases the median Lp(a) levels were often as low as the median in general populations and these studies do not necessarily reflect the study population one would reach out to study the therapeutic effect in a high Lp(a) group.

8.1   Lipoprotein Apheresis

The data available on lipoprotein apheresis are coming mostly from Germany and are very impressive in terms of a 60–70% lowering of LDL-C and Lp(a) concentrations as well as the massive reduction of CHD outcomes. Of course, it is a sawtooth picture of the Lp(a) changes that can be observed with a decrease of Lp (a) from before to immediately after apheresis of up to more than 70%. After the apheresis session the Lp(a) concentrations increase again and the interval mean values were calculated to be roughly 35% lower compared to the values before the session (Julius et al. 2019).

In one of the first studies patients were included whose Lp(a) concentrations were above the 90th percentile. Lipoprotein apheresis not only reduced Lp(a) by 73%, but also coronary events by 86% (Jaeger et al. 2009). Interesting was the observation that in the subgroup of patients who had a very low Lp(a)-corrected LDL-C already before the onset of apheresis, the reduction in coronary heart disease events was about the same as in the other group in which LDL-C could additionally be lowered by apheresis. This means that in the first group, the reduction of coronary heart disease events is more likely due to the decrease in Lp(a) concentrations (Jaeger et al. 2009). Similar results for reducing Lp(a) concentrations and coronary heart disease events were also shown in other investigations (Leebmann et al. 2013; Roeseler et al. 2016). A significant decline of the mean annual cardiovascular event rate was observed from 0.58 ± 0.53 in the period 2 years before regular lipoprotein apheresis to 0.11 ± 0.15 thereafter (Roeseler et al. 2016). Similar observations have been made in an US-American study (Moriarty et al. 2019).

Lipoprotein apheresis studies have been criticized since they were hard to control due to the lack of randomization and blinding. A recent small study has tried to overcome this problem in 20 patients with refractory angina pectoris and mean Lp(a) concentrations at 110 mg/dL. These patients underwent 3 months of blinded weekly lipoprotein apheresis or sham, followed by crossover. Despite the relatively short-term therapy, this resulted in a significant decrease in angina pectoris frequency, an increase in myocardial perfusion reserve, an increase in exercise capacity, and a decrease in total carotid wall volume (Khan et al. 2017).

A specific approach to study the effect of Lp(a)-lowering came from a small study applying a specific Lp(a) apheresis with sheep polyclonal monospecific antibodies against human apo(a). This intervention decreased Lp(a) on average by 73% without significant changes in true LDL-C and other risk factors. The mean percent diameter stenosis of the coronary arteries after 18 months decreased by 5% in the Lp(a) intervention group and increased by 5% in the control group that received only statins (Safarova et al. 2013).

8.2   PCSK9 Inhibitors

PCSK9 inhibitors primarily target LDL-C and lower this atherogenic lipoprotein by roughly 60%. However, Lp(a) concentrations are also lowered by 25–30% (Table 1). There are two therapeutic principles: (1) a monoclonal antibody against PCSK9 given every 2 weeks or monthly as used in evolocumab and alirocumab or (2) a small interfering RNA (siRNA) that targets the mRNA of PCSK9 as used in inclisiran which will be given twice yearly.

In a post-hoc analysis of the FOURIER Trial including 25,096 patients with established atherosclerotic CVD, the PCSK9 inhibitor evolocumab reduced the risk of CVD outcomes by 23% in patients with a baseline Lp(a) > median of 37 nmol/L ($\approx$15 mg/dL), and by 7% in those $\leq$median (p-value interaction = 0.07). The conclusion was the same when 120 nmol/L ($\approx$50 mg/dL) instead of the median was used as grouping threshold. The study observed a significant relationship with a 15% lower risk (95% CI, 2–26%; $p = 0.0199$) per 25 nmol/L ($\approx$10 mg/dL) reduction in Lp(a) after adjusting for the change in LDL-C (Table 1) (O'Donoghue et al. 2019). This would mean that even a relatively small lowering of Lp(a) should result in a clinical benefit.

Recently published data from pre-specified analysis of the ODYSSEY Outcomes trial showed that Lp(a)-lowering by alirocumab contributes to a reduction of major adverse cardiovascular events (MACE) independently of LDL-C-lowering in 18,924 patients with recent acute coronary syndrome and LDL-C $\geq$ 70 mg/dL despite intensive or maximum tolerated statin treatment (Bittner et al. 2020). Of course,

Table 1 Calculations from post-hoc analyses from PCSK9 trials as well as Mendelian randomizations studies to estimate the effect of Lp(a)-lowering on clinical outcomes

Publication	Study description	Main findings
Post-hoc analyses of PCSK9 inhibitor trials		
FOURIER trial (O'Donoghue et al. 2019)	Intervention study of 25,096 patients treated by evolocumab vs. placebo in patients with established CVD	Lp(a) > median of 37 nmol/L: HR = 0.77 (0.76–0.88) vs. ≤median: HR = 0.93 (0.80–1.08) Lp(a) >120 nmol/L: HR = 0.75 (0.64–0.88) vs. ≤120 nmol/L: HR = 0.89 (0.79–1.01)
ODYSSEY OUTCOMES trial (Bittner et al. 2020)	18,924 patients with recent acute coronary syndrome and LDL-C ≥ 70 mg/dL despite intensive or maximum tolerated statin treatment	Proportion of MACE reduction attributable to changes in Lp(a) increased from 4% to 11% to 25% for Lp(a) levels at the 25th, 50th, and 75th percentiles, respectively. Lowering of Lp(a) by 42 mg/dL would be required to lower the MACE rate by 22%
Pooled data from 10 controlled phase 3 ODYSSEY trials (Ray et al. 2019)	4,983 patients with established CVD or presence of CVD risk factors without established CVD or heterozygous familial hypercholesterolemia	Relative risk reduction per 25% reduction of Lp(a) adjusted for LDL-C changes: for group with Lp(a) ≥50 mg/dL: HR = 0.60 (95% CI 0.39–0.92), $p = 0.0201$ for group with Lp(a) <50 mg/dL: HR = 0.94 (95% CI 0.81–1.09), $p = 0.3837$
Mendelian randomization studies		
Burgess et al. (2018)	5 population-based prospective cohort and case-control studies including 20,793 individuals with CHD and 27,540 controls. Lp(a) concentrations were measured in 34,276 individuals using various assays	A 101.5-mg/dL change (95% CI, 71.0–137.0) in Lp(a) concentration had the same association with CHD risk as a 38.67-mg/dL change in LDL-C level
Lamina and Kronenberg (2019)	13,781 individuals from the Lp (a)-GWAS-consortium from 5 primarily population-based studies in whom Lp(a) was measured with the same assay	A 65.7 mg/dL change (95% CI 46.3–88.3) in Lp(a) concentration had the same association with CHD risk as a 38.67-mg/dL change in LDL-C level
Madsen et al. (2020)	2,527 individuals from the Copenhagen general population study with a history of CVD	Using data from a secondary prevention setting revealed that a ≈ 55 mg/dL change in Lp(a) concentration is required to have the same association with CHD risk as a 38.67-mg/dL change in LDL-C level. Using genetic data revealed that an absolute lowering of Lp(a) of 66 mg/dL would be required

Table is taken and updated from (Kronenberg 2019b)

the major contribution to the risk reductions comes from the reduction of Lp(a)-corrected LDL-C which is the primary target of the PCSK9 inhibitors. However, alirocumab additionally reduced Lp(a) by a median of 23%. The LDL-independent contribution to the proportion of MACE reduction attributable to changes in Lp(a) caused by alirocumab treatment increased from 4% to 11% to 25% for Lp(a) levels at the 25th, 50th, and 75th percentiles, respectively (Table 1) (Bittner et al. 2020).

Furthermore, pooled data from 10 controlled phase 3 ODYSSEY trials have been analyzed. The authors observed a 12% relative risk reduction in MACE per 25% reduction in Lp(a) which was no longer significant after adjustment for LDL-C changes. In subgroup analysis, the association between Lp(a) reduction and MACE remained significant in a fully adjusted model among participants with baseline Lp(a) ≥50 mg/dL (Table 1) (Ray et al. 2019).

The siRNA therapy inclisiran has been studied in 501 patients using different dosages and revealed median Lp(a) reductions from baseline to day 180 from −14% to −18% in the single-dose groups and −15% to −26% in the 2-dose groups. The Lp(a) reduction did not reach statistical significance in any of the dosing groups which was probably caused by the very wide interindividual variability in the Lp(a) reduction (Ray et al. 2018). It needs to be seen how pronounced the Lp(a) reductions will be in the phase III trials.

8.3   Statins

There is currently a major discussion whether statins increase Lp(a) concentrations or not. Due to the structure of Lp(a) containing an LDL particle, the LDL receptor was always an interesting candidate for Lp(a) removal. This idea was supported by the observations that Lp(a) levels are markedly elevated in patients with familial hypercholesterolemia (Utermann 1989; Utermann et al. 1989). It was therefore very surprising when first studies by Kostner et al. (1989) and later by O'Donoghue et al. (2014) observed an increase in Lp(a) concentrations after successful lowering of LDL cholesterol by statins. This is in line with the results of the JUPITER Study: patients under rosuvastatin treatment showed even a statistically significant positive shift in the overall Lp(a) distribution that was not observed in the placebo group (Khera et al. 2014; Kronenberg 2014b). Recently, Willeit and colleagues collated patient-level data from seven randomized, placebo-controlled, statin outcome trials including 29,069 patients with repeated Lp(a) measurements. 14,536 patients were randomly allocated statin treatment. The effect of statin therapy on Lp(a) concentrations was heterogeneous across studies: the pooled percentage change was −0.4% with three trials showing a mean increase (between 2 and 15%) and four trials showing a mean decrease (between −1 and −13%) in Lp(a) concentrations (Willeit et al. 2018). A further subject-level meta-analysis included 5,256 patients (1,371 on placebo and 3,885 on statin) from six randomized trials. All six trials used the same Lp(a) assay. The mean percent change from baseline ranged from 8.5% to 19.6% in the statin groups and −0.4% to −2.3% in the placebo groups. When various statins were compared, the mean percent change from baseline ranged from 11.6% to 20.4% in the pravastatin group and 18.7% to 24.2% in the atorvastatin group (Tsimikas et al. 2020b). A study in patients with dyslipidemia included 39 patients who first initiated statin treatment and a control group of 42 patients who were already on stable statin treatment for at least 4 months. Overall, Lp(a) concentrations did not increase significantly in both groups. However, when the analysis was stratified for the apo(a) isoforms, it was found that Lp(a) levels increased significantly from 66.4 to 97.4 mg/dL in patients with small apo (a) isoforms in the initiation group, but not in the control group and not in patients having only large apo(a) isoforms (Yahya et al. 2019). This interesting observation needs confirmation in larger studies.

The findings that statins might increase Lp(a) concentrations triggered discussions whether the benefit of statins by lowering LDL-C might be diminished or outweighed by the increase in Lp(a) concentrations especially in patients who have already increased Lp(a) concentrations before statin therapy is started. The JUPITER trial observed for the extended endpoint that patients with Lp(a) concentrations above the median reduced their risk for events by 28% (95% CI 3–48%) whereas those with baseline Lp(a) concentration below the median reduced the risk by 54% (95% CI 31–68%) (p-value for interaction $= 0.10$) (Khera et al. 2014). The meta-analysis by Willeit et al. found for those patients on statins a 47% higher risk when the Lp(a) levels were above compared to below 50 mg/dL (HR $= 1.48$, 95% CI 1.23–1.78). The risk was only 23% higher in the controls when Lp(a) was above compared to below 50 mg/dL (HR $= 1.23$, 95% CI 1.04–1.45%). This has been interpreted that the Lp(a)-associated risk becomes an even stronger predictor of residual risk when LDL-attributable risk is reduced with statin treatment (Willeit et al. 2018). Since this analysis did not use one of the groups as reference group for all comparisons (e.g., the controls with Lp(a) levels below 50 mg/dL), the risk estimates cannot simply be compared and might therefore be misinterpreted resulting in the idea that statins should be stopped in case of high Lp(a) concentrations. However, the probable risk benefit from lowering LDL-C by a statin outweighs the moderate increase in Lp(a) levels in most patients. This can be extrapolated from the study by Willeit et al. (see Fig. 2 of that publication): the cumulative risk was 21.7% in the placebo group (3,148 cases within 14,533 patients) which is higher compared to 17.9% in the statin-treated group (2,603 cases within 14,536 patients). This corresponds to a risk reduction to 0.83 by statins. Ethical considerations would not allow to test in a randomized controlled trial whether the avoidance of statins in patients with high Lp(a) concentrations would result in a benefit. In any case, the recent observations need careful attention and Lp(a) concentrations might better be monitored especially in patients who start statin therapy and having elevated Lp(a) concentrations since the observed increase under statin therapy in single patients can be sometimes very significant (Tsimikas et al. 2020c). In such patients a change to PCSK9 inhibitors might be an option to consider.

8.4   Drugs That Are Probably No Longer Followed for Lp(a)-Lowering Potential

There are some drugs that were not specifically designed to lower Lp(a) but showed an interesting Lp(a)-lowering effect. However, various reasons often related to the primary target and the observed side effects or efficacy revealed that they were stopped after clinical trials or they are no longer followed in extended clinical trials.

The CETP inhibitors anacetrapib (HPS3/TIMI55–REVEAL Collaborative Group et al. 2017; Thomas et al. 2017), evacetrapib (Nicholls et al. 2016), and TA-8995 (Ford et al. 2014) have in common that they not only increase HDL-C tremendously, but they also decrease Lp(a) between 25 and 40%. However, outcome studies using these drugs did not show a benefit or were even harmful in terms of CVD events. Both the thyroid analogue eprotirome (Ladenson et al. 2010) and the MTP inhibitor lomitapide (Samaha et al. 2008) lower Lp(a). Mipomersen, an antisense oligonucleotide targeting apoB mRNA lowers Lp(a) by roughly 30% but is restricted to very specific patient groups and countries due to its side effects (Raal et al. 2010).

In earlier times, niacin was thought to be a good candidate in treating Lp(a) elevation. However, in patients with optimally low levels of LDL-C, and despite favorable effects on HDL-C, triglycerides, and Lp(a), two clinical outcome trials failed to show any incremental clinical benefit on cardiovascular events with niacin when added to simvastatin (Boden et al. 2011; Landray et al. 2014). Following these trials, niacin is no longer available in most countries. However, besides other limitations these trials were not designed to examine the clinical effect in the patients with elevated Lp(a).

9   Therapeutic Lowering of Lipoprotein(a): How Much Is Enough?

On the eve of the introduction of specific Lp(a)-lowering therapies, the question has been raised, how much Lp(a) should be lowered to result in a clinical benefit. As recently discussed (Kronenberg 2019b), there are two approaches to get a rough estimate, which are a genetic estimation by using a Mendelian randomization approach or post-hoc analyses from clinical trials which target primarily LDL-C and as a "collateral yield" also lower Lp(a).

The Mendelian randomization approach uses genetic data from association studies on Lp(a) and LDL-C concentrations as well as association studies on CHD to estimate the required Lp(a)-lowering effect size to show the same association with CHD risk-lowering as a 38.67-mg/dL (1 mmol/L) therapeutic reduction in LDL-C. The latter is only used for benchmarking reasons. This intriguing idea used by Burgess and colleagues revealed that Lp(a) would have to be lowered by 101.5 mg/dL to show the same effect as lowering LDL-C by 38.67 mg/dL (Burgess et al. 2018). This number was probably markedly overestimated since the main study on which these results are based on had a median Lp(a) concentration twofold to threefold higher compared to other studies of the same ethnicity. We therefore repeated these calculations using the same approach and the same data basis except for the estimates of various SNPs on Lp(a) concentrations. For these we used our own data from almost 14.000 individuals in whom Lp(a) was measured within one laboratory and with median Lp(a) levels in the range of expectations for typical Caucasian populations (Mack et al. 2017). We calculated that an Lp(a)-lowering of roughly 65 mg/dL would be required instead of more than 100 mg/dL (Lamina and Kronenberg 2019). These data were mainly based on population-based data and it was not clear whether these hold also true for secondary prevention patients. Exactly this situation has very recently been tested in a Danish study (Madsen et al. 2020). They used population-based data from individuals with a history of CVD who were followed after their initial event. Since this equals a secondary prevention setting, they calculated that plasma Lp(a) should be lowered by 50 and 99 mg/dL for 5 years to achieve 20 and 40% MACE risk reduction in secondary prevention. Accordingly, for a 22% MACE reduction, a reduction of Lp(a) by 55 mg/dL would be required. Interestingly, when the authors used genetic data for short-term risk reduction, they found that an absolute Lp(a) reduction of 66 mg/dL would be needed to obtain a MACE reduction of 22%. This is exactly the same number as calculated by our group but using primary prevention studies (Lamina and Kronenberg 2019).

For all these studies it has to be added that the comparison with an LDL-lowering of 38.67 mg/dL was only used as a benchmark which results for LDL-C in a 22% lowering of MACE (Baigent et al. 2010). Of course, even smaller lowering might be beneficial as has been demonstrated for LDL-C.

The data from Mendelian randomization studies gave the impression that Lp(a) would have to be lowered by a higher extent than LDL-C to have the same clinical benefit. The ratio would be 2.6 to 1.0 according to Burgess and colleagues (2018) or 1.7 to 1.0 according to two other studies (Lamina and Kronenberg 2019; Madsen et al. 2020). This would mean that LDL-C would have markedly higher atherogenic properties than Lp(a) which is not necessarily supported by data. The post-hoc analyses of interventional studies with PCSK9 inhibitors provide some major hope that even a smaller Lp(a)-lowering might already show a clinical benefit (Table 1). As discussed above, the FOURIER study described a 15% lower risk per 25 nmol/L ($\approx$10 mg/dL) reduction in Lp(a) after adjusting for the change in LDL-C (O'Donoghue et al. 2019). From the recently published ODYSSEY Outcomes trial it can be calculated that a lowering of Lp(a) by 42 mg/dL would be required to lower the MACE rate by 22% (Bittner et al. 2020) which brings the above-mentioned ratio of required Lp(a)/LDL-C-lowering closer to 1.0. Furthermore, the pooled data from 10 controlled phase 3 ODYSSEY trials also showed that the relative risk reduction per 25% reduction of Lp(a) adjusted for LDL-C changes was higher for the group of patients with Lp(a) $\geq$50 mg/dL with an HR = 0.60 (95% CI 0.39–0.92, p = 0.0201) (Ray et al. 2019).

Limitations for this Mendelian randomization approach come from various assumptions which have to be considered with cautions: first, it is unclear whether Lp(a) and LDL-C particles have a similar cumulative effect on CVD over time, or with other words, whether they have the same atherogenic potential? This is not necessarily the case since there is some evidence that even Lp(a) particles of different apo(a) isoforms have different atherogenic potential (Kronenberg et al. 1999; Saleheen et al. 2017). Second, besides an atherogenic nature of Lp(a) some data point also to a thrombogenic nature (Boffa and Koschinsky 2016; Romagnuolo et al. 2018). If this is also the case in vivo, the pathogenic mechanism of Lp(a) might even be stronger than for LDL-C and the lowering of Lp(a) would have an additional benefit on the thrombogenic axis.

All the available observations from post-hoc analysis of intervention studies and from Mendelian randomization studies are helpful for the planning of future trials. These trials will have to consider the uncertainties connected with these data such as more or less wide confidence intervals of the estimates. One of these uncertainties are introduced by the insufficiently standardized Lp(a) assays used in the various studies. This became obvious when looking at the data presented by Burgess et al. with the above-mentioned very high Lp(a) concentrations in their main cohort (Burgess et al. 2018). An overestimation of the Lp(a) concentration by an insufficiently standardized assay might result in a misclassification of patients to be at high risk and an enrollment of patients which would otherwise not be appropriate for the study. Therefore, major efforts should be invested in the screening phase for suitable study patients to avoid misclassification of patients by inappropriate Lp(a) assays (Kronenberg and Tsimikas 2019; Scharnagl et al. 2019).

10   Conclusions

The causal association between high Lp(a) concentrations and CVD is strongly supported by genetic studies. Post-hoc analyses following intervention studies with PCSK9-inhibitors that targeted primarily LDL-C but additionally lower also Lp(a) provide some evidence that an additional lowering of Lp(a) besides LDL-C is beneficial. However, these studies were not designed to target patients with high Lp(a) levels and are therefore limited. Mendelian randomization studies provide further strong support that lowering Lp(a) might be beneficial.

References

Arsenault BJ, Boekholdt SM, Dube MP, Rheaume E, Wareham NJ, Khaw KT, Sandhu MS, Tardif JC (2014) Lipoprotein(a) levels, genotype, and incident aortic valve stenosis: a prospective Mendelian randomization study and replication in a case-control cohort. Circ Cardiovasc Genet 7:304–310

Austin MA, Sandholzer C, Selby JV, Newman B, Krauss RM, Utermann G (1992) Lipoprotein (a) in women twins: heritability and relationship to apolipoprotein(a) phenotypes. Am J Hum Genet 51:829–840

Baigent C, Blackwell L, Emberson J, Holland LE, Reith C, Bhala N, Peto R, Barnes EH, Keech A, Simes J, Collins R (2010) Efficacy and safety of more intensive lowering of LDL cholesterol: a meta-analysis of data from 170,000 participants in 26 randomised trials. Lancet 376:1670–1681

Bergmark C, Dewan A, Orsoni A, Merki E, Miller ER, Shin MJ, Binder CJ, Horkko S, Krauss RM, Chapman MJ, Witztum JL, Tsimikas S (2008) A novel function of lipoprotein [a] as a preferential carrier of oxidized phospholipids in human plasma. J Lipid Res 49:2230–2239

Bittner VA, Szarek M, Aylward PE, Bhatt DL, Diaz R, Edelberg JM, Fras Z, Goodman SG, Halvorsen S, Hanotin C, Harrington RA, Jukema JW, Loizeau V, Moriarty PM, Moryusef A, Pordy R, Roe MT, Sinnaeve P, Tsimikas S, Vogel R, White HD, Zahger D, Zeiher AM, Steg PG, Schwartz GG (2020) Effect of Alirocumab on lipoprotein(a) and cardiovascular risk after acute coronary syndrome. J Am Coll Cardiol 75:133–144

Boden WE, Probstfield JL, Anderson T, Chaitman BR, Desvignes-Nickens P, Koprowicz K, McBride R, Teo K, Weintraub W (2011) Niacin in patients with low HDL cholesterol levels receiving intensive statin therapy. N Engl J Med 365:2255–2267

Boffa MB, Koschinsky ML (2016) Lipoprotein (a): truly a direct prothrombotic factor in cardiovascular disease? J Lipid Res 57:745–757

Boffa MB, Koschinsky ML (2019) Oxidized phospholipids as a unifying theory for lipoprotein (a) and cardiovascular disease. Nat Rev Cardiol 16:305–318

Boffa MB, Stranges S, Klar N, Moriarty PM, Watts GF, Koschinsky ML (2018) Lipoprotein(a) and secondary prevention of atherothrombotic events: a critical appraisal. J Clin Lipidol 12:1358–1366

Brandt EJ, Mani A, Spatz ES, Desai NR, Nasir K (2020) Lipoprotein(a) levels and association with myocardial infarction and stroke in a nationally representative cross-sectional US cohort. J Clin Lipidol 14:695–706.e694

Burgess S, Ference BA, Staley JR, Freitag DF, Mason AM, Nielsen SF, Willeit P, Young R, Surendran P, Karthikeyan S, Bolton TR, Peters JE, Kamstrup PR, Tybjærg-Hansen A, Benn M, Langsted A, Schnohr P, Vedel-Krogh S, Kobylecki CJ, Ford I, Packard C, Trompet S, Jukema JW, Sattar N, Di Angelantonio E, Saleheen D, Howson JMM, Nordestgaard BG, Butterworth AS, Danesh J (2018) Association of LPA variants with risk of coronary disease and the implications for lipoprotein(a)-lowering therapies: a Mendelian randomization analysis. JAMA Cardiol 3:619–627

Cain WJ, Millar JS, Himebauch AS, Tietge UJ, Maugeais C, Usher D, Rader DJ (2005) Lipoprotein [a] is cleared from the plasma primarily by the liver in a process mediated by apolipoprotein [a]. J Lipid Res 46:2681–2691

Cairns BJ, Coffey S, Travis RC, Prendergast B, Green J, Engert JC, Lathrop M, Thanassoulis G, Clarke R (2017) A replicated, genome-wide significant association of aortic stenosis with a genetic variant for lipoprotein(a): meta-analysis of published and novel data. Circulation 135:1181–1183

Capoulade R, Yeang C, Chan KL, Pibarot P, Tsimikas S (2018) Association of mild to moderate aortic valve stenosis progression with higher lipoprotein(a) and oxidized phospholipid levels: secondary analysis of a randomized clinical trial. JAMA Cardiol 3:1212–1217

Cegla J, Neely RDG, France M, Ferns G, Byrne CD, Halcox J, Datta D, Capps N, Shoulders C, Qureshi N, Rees A, Main L, Cramb R, Viljoen A, Payne J, Soran H (2019) HEART UK consensus statement on lipoprotein(a): a call to action. Atherosclerosis 291:62–70

Chen HY, Dufresne L, Burr H, Ambikkumar A, Yasui N, Luk K, Ranatunga DK, Whitmer RA, Lathrop M, Engert JC, Thanassoulis G (2018) Association of LPA variants with aortic stenosis: a large-scale study using diagnostic and procedural codes from electronic health records. JAMA Cardiol 3:18–23

Clarke R, Peden JF, Hopewell JC, Kyriakou T, Goel A, Heath SC, Parish S, Barlera S, Franzosi MG, Rust S, Bennett D, Silveira A, Malarstig A, Green FR, Lathrop M, Gigante B, Leander K, de Faire U, Seedorf U, Hamsten A, Collins R, Watkins H, Farrall M (2009) Genetic variants associated with Lp(a) lipoprotein level and coronary disease. N Engl J Med 361:2518–2528

Coassin S, Kronenberg F (2020) Mechanistic insights into lipoprotein(a): from infamous to 'inflammous'. Eur Heart J 41:2272–2274

Coassin S, Erhart G, Weissensteiner H, de Eca Guimaraes AM, Lamina C, Schönherr S, Forer L, Haun M, Losso JL, Köttgen A, Schmidt K, Utermann G, Peters A, Gieger C, Strauch K, Finkenstedt A, Bale R, Zoller H, Paulweber B, Eckardt KU, Hüttenhofer A, Huber LA, Kronenberg F (2017) A novel but frequent variant in LPA KIV-2 is associated with a pronounced Lp(a) and cardiovascular risk reduction. Eur Heart J 38:1823–1831

Coassin S, Schoenherr S, Weissensteiner H, Erhart G, Forer L, Losso JL, Lamina C, Haun M, Utermann G, Paulweber B, Specht G, Kronenberg F (2019) A comprehensive map of single base polymorphisms in the hypervariable LPA Kringle IV-2 copy number variation region. J Lipid Res 60:186–199

Cohen JC, Chiesa G, Hobbs HH (1993) Sequence polymorphisms in the apolipoprotein (a) gene. Evidence for dissociation between apolipoprotein(a) size and plasma lipoprotein(a) levels. J Clin Invest 91:1630–1636

Dahabreh IJ, Kent DM (2011) Index event bias as an explanation for the paradoxes of recurrence risk research. JAMA 305:822–823

Di Maio S, Grüneis R, Streiter G, Lamina C, Maglione M, Schoenherr S, Öfner D, Thorand B, Peters A, Eckardt K-U, Köttgen A, Kronenberg F, Coassin S (2020) Investigation of a nonsense mutation located in the complex KIV-2 copy number variation region of apolipoprotein(a) in 10,910 individuals. Genome Med 12:74

Dieplinger B, Lingenhel A, Baumgartner N, Poelz W, Dieplinger H, Haltmayer M, Kronenberg F, Mueller T (2007) Increased serum lipoprotein(a) concentrations and low molecular weight phenotypes of apolipoprotein(a) are associated with symptomatic peripheral arterial disease. Clin Chem 53:1298–1305

Erqou S, Kaptoge S, Perry PL, Di AE, Thompson A, White IR, Marcovina SM, Collins R, Thompson SG, Danesh J (2009) Lipoprotein(a) concentration and the risk of coronary heart disease, stroke, and nonvascular mortality. JAMA 302:412–423

Erqou S, Thompson A, Di AE, Saleheen D, Kaptoge S, Marcovina S, Danesh J (2010) Apolipoprotein(a) isoforms and the risk of vascular disease: systematic review of 40 studies involving 58,000 participants. J Am Coll Cardiol 55:2160–2167

Ford J, Lawson M, Fowler D, Maruyama N, Mito S, Tomiyasu K, Kinoshita S, Suzuki C, Kawaguchi A, Round F, Boyce M, Warrington S, Weber W, van Deventer S, Kastelein JJ (2014) Tolerability, pharmacokinetics and pharmacodynamics of TA-8995, a selective cholesteryl ester transfer protein (CETP) inhibitor, in healthy subjects. Br J Clin Pharmacol 78:498–508

Frischmann ME, Kronenberg F, Trenkwalder E, Schaefer J, Schweer H, Dieplinger B, König P, Ikewaki K, Dieplinger H (2007) In vivo turnover study demonstrates diminished clearance of lipoprotein(a) in hemodialysis patients. Kidney Int 71:1036–1043

Grainger DJ, Kirschenlohr HL, Metcalfe JC, Weissberg PL, Wade DP, Lawn RM (1993) Proliferation of human smooth muscle cells promoted by lipoprotein(a). Science 260:1655–1658

Guan W, Cao J, Steffen BT, Post WS, Stein JH, Tattersall MC, Kaufman JD, McConnell JP, Hoefner DM, Warnick R, Tsai MY (2015) Race is a key variable in assigning lipoprotein (a) cutoff values for coronary heart disease risk assessment: the multi-ethnic study of atherosclerosis. Arterioscler Thromb Vasc Biol 35:996–1001

Gurdasani D, Sjouke B, Tsimikas S, Hovingh GK, Luben RN, Wainwright NW, Pomilla C, Wareham NJ, Khaw KT, Boekholdt SM, Sandhu MS (2012) Lipoprotein(a) and risk of coronary, cerebrovascular, and peripheral artery disease: the EPIC-Norfolk prospective population study. Arterioscler Thromb Vasc Biol 32:3058–3065

Hindy G, Aragam KG, Ng K, Chaffin M, Lotta LA, Baras A, Regeneron Genetics C, Drake I, Orho-Melander M, Melander O, Kathiresan S, Khera AV (2020) Genome-wide polygenic score, clinical risk factors, and long-term trajectories of coronary artery disease. Arterioscler Thromb Vasc Biol 40:2738–2746

Hoekstra M, Chen HY, Rong J, Dufresne L, Yao J, Guo X, Tsai MY, Tsimikas S, Post WS, Vasan RS, Rotter JI, Larson MG, Thanassoulis G, Engert JC (2021) Genome-wide association study highlights APOH as a novel locus for lipoprotein(a) levels. Arterioscler Thromb Vasc Biol 41: ATVBAHA120314965

HPS3/TIMI55–REVEAL Collaborative Group, Bowman L, Hopewell JC, Chen F, Wallendszus K, Stevens W, Collins R, Wiviott SD, Cannon CP, Braunwald E, Sammons E, Landray MJ (2017) Effects of anacetrapib in patients with atherosclerotic vascular disease. N Engl J Med 377:1217–1227

Jaeger BR, Richter Y, Nagel D, Heigl F, Vogt A, Roeseler E, Parhofer K, Ramlow W, Koch M, Utermann G, Labarrere CA, Seidel D (2009) Longitudinal cohort study on the effectiveness of lipid apheresis treatment to reduce high lipoprotein(a) levels and prevent major adverse coronary events. Nat Clin Pract Cardiovasc Med 6:229–239

Julius U, Tselmin S, Schatz U, Fischer S, Birkenfeld AL, Bornstein SR (2019) Actual situation of lipoprotein apheresis in patients with elevated lipoprotein(a) levels. Atheroscler Suppl 40:1–7

Kamstrup PR, Nordestgaard BG (2016) Elevated lipoprotein(a) levels, LPA risk genotypes, and increased risk of heart failure in the general population. J Am Coll Cardiol Heart Fail 4:78–87

Kamstrup PR, Tybjaerg-Hansen A, Steffensen R, Nordestgaard BG (2009) Genetically elevated lipoprotein(a) and increased risk of myocardial infarction. JAMA 301:2331–2339

Kamstrup PR, Tybjaerg-Hansen A, Nordestgaard BG (2014) Elevated lipoprotein(a) and risk of aortic valve stenosis in the general population. J Am Coll Cardiol 63:470–477

Kannel WB, Dawber TR, Friedman GD, GLENNON WE, McNamara PM (1964) Risk factors in coronary heart disease.An evaluation of several serum lipids as predictors of coronary heart disease. The Framingham study. Ann Intern Med 61:888–899

Khan TZ, Hsu LY, Arai AE, Rhodes S, Pottle A, Wage R, Banya W, Gatehouse PD, Giri S, Collins P, Pennell DJ, Barbir M (2017) Apheresis as novel treatment for refractory angina with raised lipoprotein(a): a randomized controlled cross-over trial. Eur Heart J 38:1561–1569

Khera AV, Everett BM, Caulfield MP, Hantash FM, Wohlgemuth J, Ridker PM, Mora S (2014) Lipoprotein(a) concentrations, Rosuvastatin therapy, and residual vascular risk: an analysis from the JUPITER trial (justification for the use of statins in prevention: an intervention trial evaluating Rosuvastatin). Circulation 129:635–642

Kiechl S, Willeit J, Mayr M, Viehweider B, Oberhollenzer F, Kronenberg F, Wiedermann CJ, Oberthaler S, Xu Q, Witztum JL, Tsimikas S (2007) Oxidized phospholipids, lipoprotein(a), lipoprotein-associated phospholipase A2 activity and 10-year cardiovascular outcomes: prospective results from the Bruneck study. Arterioscler Thromb Vasc Biol 27:1788–1795

Kinpara K, Okada H, Yoneyama A, Okubo M, Murase T (2011) Lipoprotein(a)-cholesterol: a significant component of serum cholesterol. Clin Chim Acta 412:1783–1787

Klarin D, Lynch J, Aragam K, Chaffin M, Assimes TL, Huang J, Lee KM, Shao Q, Huffman JE, Natarajan P, Arya S, Small A, Sun YV, Vujkovic M, Freiberg MS, Wang L, Chen J, Saleheen D, Lee JS, Miller DR, Reaven P, Alba PR, Patterson OV, DuVall SL, Boden WE, Beckman JA, Gaziano JM, Concato J, Rader DJ, Cho K, Chang KM, Wilson PWF, O'Donnell CJ, Kathiresan S, Tsao PS, Damrauer SM (2019) Genome-wide association study of peripheral artery disease in the million veteran program. Nat Med 25:1274–1279

Klezovitch O, Edelstein C, Scanu AM (2001) Stimulation of interleukin-8 production in human THP-1 macrophages by apolipoprotein (a): evidence for a critical involvement of elements in its C-terminal domain. J Biol Chem 276:46864–46869

Köchl S, Fresser F, Lobentanz E, Baier G, Utermann G (1997) Novel interaction of apolipoprotein (a) with b-2 glycoprotein I mediated by the kringle IV domain. Blood 90:1482–1489

Koschinsky ML, Marcovina SM (2004) Structure-function relationships in apolipoprotein(a): insights into lipoprotein(a) assembly and pathogenicity. Curr Opin Lipidol 15:167–174

Kostner GM, Gavish D, Leopold B, Bolzano K, Weintraub MS, Breslow JL (1989) HMG CoA reductase inhibitors lower LDL cholesterol without reducing Lp(a) levels. Circulation 80:1313–1319

Kraft HG, Menzel HJ, Hoppichler F, Vogel W, Utermann G (1989) Changes of genetic apolipoprotein phenotypes caused by liver transplantation. Implications for apolipoprotein synthesis. J Clin Invest 83:137–142

Kraft HG, Köchl S, Menzel HJ, Sandholzer C, Utermann G (1992) The apolipoprotein(a) gene: a transcribed hypervariable locus controlling plasma lipoprotein(a) concentration. Hum Genet 90:220–230

Kraft HG, Lingenhel A, Köchl S, Hoppichler F, Kronenberg F, Abe A, Mühlberger V, Schönitzer D, Utermann G (1996) Apolipoprotein(a) Kringle IV repeat number predicts risk for coronary heart disease. Arterioscler Thromb Vasc Biol 16:713–719

Kronenberg F (2014a) Lipoprotein(a) in various conditions: to keep a sense of proportions. Atherosclerosis 234:249–251

Kronenberg F (2014b) Lipoprotein(a): there's life in the old dog yet. Circulation 129:619–621

Kronenberg F (2016a) High-density lipoprotein cholesterol on a roller coaster: where will the ride end? Kidney Int 89:747–749

Kronenberg F (2016b) Human genetics and the causal role of lipoprotein(a) for various diseases. Cardiovasc Drugs Ther 30:87–100

Kronenberg F (2019a) Prediction of cardiovascular risk by Lp(a) concentrations or genetic variants within the LPA gene region. Clin Res Cardiol Suppl 14:5–12

Kronenberg F (2019b) Therapeutic lowering of lipoprotein(a): how much is enough? Atherosclerosis 288:163–165

Kronenberg F, Tsimikas S (2019) The challenges of measuring Lp(a): a fight against Hydra? Atherosclerosis 289:181–183

Kronenberg F, Utermann G (2013) Lipoprotein(a) – resurrected by genetics. J Intern Med 273:6–30

Kronenberg F, Trenkwalder E, Lingenhel A, Friedrich G, Lhotta K, Schober M, Moes N, König P, Utermann G, Dieplinger H (1997) Renovascular arteriovenous differences in Lp(a) plasma concentrations suggest removal of Lp(a) from the renal circulation. J Lipid Res 38:1755–1763

Kronenberg F, Kronenberg MF, Kiechl S, Trenkwalder E, Santer P, Oberhollenzer F, Egger G, Utermann G, Willeit J (1999) Role of lipoprotein(a) and apolipoprotein(a) phenotype in atherogenesis: prospective results from the Bruneck study. Circulation 100:1154–1160

Kronenberg F, Lingenhel A, Lhotta K, Rantner B, Kronenberg MF, König P, Thiery J, Koch M, Von Eckardstein A, Dieplinger H (2004) Lipoprotein(a)- and low-density lipoprotein-derived cholesterol in nephrotic syndrome: impact on lipid-lowering therapy? Kidney Int 66:348–354

Lackner C, Boerwinkle E, Leffert CC, Rahmig T, Hobbs HH (1991) Molecular basis of apolipoprotein (a) isoform size heterogeneity as revealed by pulsed-field gel electrophoresis. J Clin Invest 87:2153–2161

Lackner C, Cohen JC, Hobbs HH (1993) Molecular definition of the extreme size polymorphism in apolipoprotein(a). Hum Mol Genet 2:933–940

Ladenson PW, Kristensen JD, Ridgway EC, Olsson AG, Carlsson B, Klein I, Baxter JD, Angelin B (2010) Use of the thyroid hormone analogue eprotirome in statin-treated dyslipidemia. N Engl J Med 362:906–916

Lamina C, Kronenberg F (2019) Estimation of the required lipoprotein(a)-lowering therapeutic effect size for reduction in coronary heart disease outcomes: a Mendelian randomization analysis. JAMA Cardiol 4:575–579

Lamon-Fava S, Jimenez D, Christian JC, Fabsitz RR, Reed T, Carmelli D, Castelli WP, Ordovas JM, Wilson PWF, Schaefer EJ (1991) The NHLBI twin study: heritability of apolipoprotein A-I and B, and low density lipoprotein subclasses and concordance for lipoprotein(a). Atherosclerosis 91:97–106

Landmesser U, Poller W, Tsimikas S, Most P, Paneni F, Luscher TF (2020) From traditional pharmacological towards nucleic acid-based therapies for cardiovascular diseases. Eur Heart J 41:3884–3899

Landray MJ, Haynes R, Hopewell JC, Parish S, Aung T, Tomson J, Wallendszus K, Craig M, Jiang L, Collins R, Armitage J (2014) Effects of extended-release niacin with laropiprant in high-risk patients. N Engl J Med 371:203–212

Langsted A, Kamstrup PR, Nordestgaard BG (2014) Lipoprotein(a): fasting and nonfasting levels, inflammation, and cardiovascular risk. Atherosclerosis 234:95–101

Langsted A, Kamstrup PR, Benn M, Tybjaerg-Hansen A, Nordestgaard BG (2016) High lipoprotein(a) as a possible cause of clinical familial hypercholesterolaemia: a prospective cohort study. Lancet Diabetes Endocrinol 4:577–587

Langsted A, Nordestgaard BG, Kamstrup PR (2019a) Elevated lipoprotein(a) and risk of ischemic stroke. J Am Coll Cardiol 74:54–66

Langsted A, Kamstrup PR, Nordestgaard BG (2019b) High lipoprotein(a) and high risk of mortality. Eur Heart J 40:2760–2770

Laschkolnig A, Kollerits B, Lamina C, Meisinger C, Rantner B, Stadler M, Peters A, Koenig W, Stöckl A, Dähnhardt D, Böger CA, Krämer BK, Fraedrich G, Strauch K, Kronenberg F (2014) Lipoprotein(a) concentrations, apolipoprotein(a) phenotypes and peripheral arterial disease in three independent cohorts. Cardiovasc Res 103:28–36

Lee SR, Prasad A, Choi YS, Xing C, Clopton P, Witztum JL, Tsimikas S (2017) LPA gene, ethnicity, and cardiovascular events. Circulation 135:251–263

Leebmann J, Roseler E, Julius U, Heigl F, Spitthoever R, Heutling D, Breitenberger P, Maerz W, Lehmacher W, Heibges A, Klingel R (2013) Lipoprotein apheresis in patients with maximally tolerated lipid lowering therapy, Lp(a)-hyperlipoproteinemia and progressive cardiovascular disease: prospective observational multicenter study. Circulation 128:2567–2576

Leibundgut G, Scipione C, Yin H, Schneider M, Boffa MB, Green S, Yang X, Dennis E, Witztum JL, Koschinsky ML, Tsimikas S (2013) Determinants of binding of oxidized phospholipids on apolipoprotein (a) and lipoprotein (a). J Lipid Res 54:2815–2830

Li J, Lange LA, Sabourin J, Duan Q, Valdar W, Willis MS, Li Y, Wilson JG, Lange EM (2015) Genome- and exome-wide association study of serum lipoprotein (a) in the Jackson heart study. J Hum Genet 60:755–761

Lim ET, Wurtz P, Havulinna AS, Palta P, Tukiainen T, Rehnstrom K, Esko T, Magi R, Inouye M, Lappalainen T, Chan Y, Salem RM, Lek M, Flannick J, Sim X, Manning A, Ladenvall C, Bumpstead S, Hamalainen E, Aalto K, Maksimow M, Salmi M, Blankenberg S, Ardissino D, Shah S, Horne B, McPherson R, Hovingh GK, Reilly MP, Watkins H, Goel A, Farrall M, Girelli D, Reiner AP, Stitziel NO, Kathiresan S, Gabriel S, Barrett JC, Lehtimaki T, Laakso M, Groop L, Kaprio J, Perola M, McCarthy MI, Boehnke M, Altshuler DM, Lindgren CM, Hirschhorn JN, Metspalu A, Freimer NB, Zeller T, Jalkanen S, Koskinen S, Raitakari O, Durbin R, MacArthur DG, Salomaa V, Ripatti S, Daly MJ, Palotie A (2014) Distribution and medical impact of loss-of-function variants in the finnish founder population. PLoS Genet 10: e1004494

Mach F, Baigent C, Catapano AL, Koskina KC, Casula M, Badimon L, Chapman MJ, De Backer GG, Delgado V, Ference BA, Graham IM, Halliday A, Landmesser U, Mihaylova B, Pedersen TR, Riccardi G, Richter DJ, Sabatine MS, Taskinen MR, Tokgozoglu L, Wiklund O, Windecker S, Aboyans V, Collet JP, Dean V, Fitzsimons D, Gale CP, Grobbee D, Halvorsen S, Hindricks G, Iung B, Jüni P, Katus HA, Leclercq C, Lettino M, Lewis BS, Merkely B, Mueller C, Petersen S, Petronio AS, Roffi M, Shlyakhto E, Simpson IA, Sousa-Uva M, Touyz RM, Nibouche D, Zelveian PH, Siostrzonek P, Najafov R, van de Borne P, Pojskic B, Postadzhiyan A, Kypris L, Špinar J, Larsen ML, Eldin HS, Viigimaa M, Strandberg TE, Ferrières J, Agladze R, Laufs U, Rallidis L, Bajnok L, Gudjónsson T, Maher V, Henkin Y, Gulizia MM, Mussagaliyeva A, Bajraktari G, Kerimkulova A, Latkovskis G, Hamoui O, Slapikas R, Visser L, Dingli P, Ivanov V, Boskovic A, Nazzi M, Visseren F, Mitevska I, Retterstøl K, Jankowski P, Fontes-Carvalho R, Gaita D, Ezhov M, Foscoli M, Giga V, Pella D, Fras Z, Perez de Isla L, Hagström E, Lehmann R, Abid L, Ozdogan O, Mitchenko O, Patel RS (2019) ESC/EAS guidelines for the management of dyslipidaemias: lipid modification to reduce cardiovascular risk. Atherosclerosis 290:140–205

Mack S, Coassin S, Rueedi R, Yousri NA, Seppala I, Gieger C, Schoenherr S, Forer L, Erhart G, Marques-Vidal P, Ried JS, Waeber G, Bergmann S, Daehnhardt D, Stoeckl A, Raitakari OT, Khahonen M, Peters A, Meitinger T, Strauch K, Kedenko L, Paulweber B, Lehtimaki T, Hunt SC, Vollenweider P, Lamina C, Kronenberg F, Grp K-S (2017) A genome-wide association meta-analysis on lipoprotein (a) concentrations adjusted for apolipoprotein (a) isoforms. J Lipid Res 58:1834–1844

Madsen CM, Kamstrup PR, Langsted A, Varbo A, Nordestgaard BG (2020) Lp(a) (lipoprotein[a])-lowering by 50 mg/dL (105 nmol/L) may be needed to reduce cardiovascular disease 20% in secondary prevention: a population-based study. Arterioscler Thromb Vasc Biol 40:255–266

McCormick SPA, Schneider WJ (2019) Lipoprotein(a) catabolism: a case of multiple receptors. Pathology 51:155–164

McLean JW, Tomlinson JE, Kuang W-J, Eaton DL, Chen EY, Fless GM, Scanu AM, Lawn RM (1987) cDNA sequence of human apolipoprotein(a) is homologous to plasminogen. Nature 330:132–137

Miltiadous G, Saougos V, Cariolou M, Elisaf MS (2006) Plasma lipoprotein(a) levels and LDL-cholesterol lowering response to statin therapy in patients with heterozygous familial hypercholesterolemia. Ann Clin Lab Sci 36:353–355

Mooser V, Marcovina SM. White AL, Hobbs HH (1996) Kringle-containing fragments of apolipoprotein(a) circulate in human plasma and are excreted into the urine. J Clin Invest 98:2414–2424

Morgan BM, Brown AN, Deo N, Harrop TWR, Taiaroa G, Mace PD, Wilbanks SM, Merriman TR, Williams MJA, McCormick SPA (2020) Nonsynonymous SNPs in LPA homologous to plasminogen deficiency mutants represent novel null apo(a) alleles. J Lipid Res 61:432–444

Moriarty PM, Gray JV, Gorby LK (2019) Lipoprotein apheresis for lipoprotein(a) and cardiovascular disease. J Clin Lipidol 13:894–900

Nicholls SJ, Ruotolo G, Brewer HB, Wang MD, Liu L, Willey MB, Deeg MA, Krueger KA, Nissen SE (2016) Evacetrapib alone or in combination with statins lowers lipoprotein(a) and total and small LDL particle concentrations in mildly hypercholesterolemic patients. J Clin Lipidol 10:519–527

Nordestgaard BG, Langsted A (2016) Lipoprotein (a) as a cause of cardiovascular disease: insights from epidemiology, genetics, and biology. J Lipid Res 57:1953–1975

Nordestgaard BG, Chapman MJ, Ray K, Boren J, Andreotti F, Watts GF, Ginsberg H, Amarenco P, Catapano A, Descamps OS, Fisher E, Kovanen PT, Kuivenhoven JA, Lesnik P, Masana L, Reiner Z, Taskinen MR, Tokgozoglu L, Tybjaerg-Hansen A (2010) Lipoprotein(a) as a cardiovascular risk factor: current status. Eur Heart J 31:2844–2853

Nowak-Gottl U, Junker R, Hartmeier M, Koch HG, Munchow N, Assmann G, Von Eckardstein A (1999) Increased lipoprotein(a) is an important risk factor for venous thromboembolism in childhood. Circulation 100:743–748

O'Donoghue ML, Fazio S, Giugliano RP, Stroes ESG, Kanevsky E, Gouni-Berthold I, Im K, Lira PA, Wasserman SM, Ceska R, Ezhov MV, Jukema JW, Jensen HK, Tokgozoglu SL, Mach F, Huber K, Sever PS, Keech AC, Pedersen TR, Sabatine MS (2019) Lipoprotein(a), PCSK9 inhibition, and cardiovascular risk. Circulation 139:1483–1492

Ober C, Nord AS, Thompson EE, Pan L, Tan Z, Cusanovich D, Sun Y, Nicolae R, Edelstein C, Schneider DH, Billstrand C, Pfaffinger D, Phillips N, Anderson RL, Philips B, Rajagopalan R, Hatsukami TS, Rieder MJ, Heagerty PJ, Nickerson DA, Abney M, Marcovina S, Jarvik GP, Scanu AM, Nicolae DL (2009) Genome-wide association study of plasma lipoprotein(a) levels identifies multiple genes on chromosome 6q. J Lipid Res 50:798–806

O'Donoghue ML, Morrow DA, Tsimikas S, Sloan S, Ren AF, Hoffman EB, Desai NR, Solomon SD, Domanski M, Arai K, Chiuve SE, Cannon CP, Sacks FM, Sabatine MS (2014) Lipoprotein (a) for risk assessment in patients with established coronary artery disease. J Am Coll Cardiol 63:520–527

Pare G, Caku A, McQueen M, Anand SS, Enas E, Clarke R, Boffa MB, Koschinsky M, Wang X, Yusuf S (2019) Lipoprotein(a) levels and the risk of myocardial infarction among 7 ethnic groups. Circulation 139:1472–1482

Parson W, Kraft HG, Niederstatter H, Lingenhel AW, Kochl S, Fresser F, Utermann G (2004) A common nonsense mutation in the repetitive Kringle IV-2 domain of human apolipoprotein (a) results in a truncated protein and low plasma Lp(a). Hum Mutat 24:474–480

Patel AP, Wang M, Pirruccello JP, Ellinor PT, Ng K, Kathiresan S, Khera AV (2021) Lp(a) (lipoprotein[a]) concentrations and incident atherosclerotic cardiovascular disease: new insights from a large national biobank. Arterioscler Thromb Vasc Biol 41:465–474

Perombelon YFN, Soutar AK, Knight BL (1994) Variation in lipoprotein(a) concentration associated with different apolipoprotein(a) alleles. J Clin Invest 93:1481–1492

Perrot N, Theriault S, Dina C, Chen HY, Boekholdt SM, Rigade S, Despres AA, Poulin A, Capoulade R, Le TT, Messika-Zeitoun D, Trottier M, Tessier M, Guimond J, Nadeau M, Engert JC, Khaw KT, Wareham NJ, Dweck MR, Mathieu P, Pibarot P, Schott JJ, Thanassoulis G,

Clavel MA, Bosse Y, Arsenault BJ (2019) Genetic variation in LPA, calcific aortic valve stenosis in patients undergoing cardiac surgery, and familial risk of aortic valve microcalcification. JAMA Cardiol 4:620–627

Poon M, Zhang XX, Dunsky KG, Taubman MB, Harpel PC (1997) Apolipoprotein(a) induces monocyte chemotactic activity in human vascular endothelial cells. Circulation 96:2514–2519

Raal FJ, Santos RD, Blom DJ, Marais AD, Charng MJ, Cromwell WC, Lachmann RH, Gaudet D, Tan JL, Chasan-Taber S, Tribble DL, Flaim JD, Crooke ST (2010) Mipomersen, an apolipoprotein B synthesis inhibitor, for lowering of LDL cholesterol concentrations in patients with homozygous familial hypercholesterolaemia: a randomised, double-blind, placebo-controlled trial. Lancet 375:998–1006

Rader DJ, Cain W, Ikewaki K, Talley G, Zech LA, Usher D, Brewer HB (1994) The inverse association of plasma lipoprotein(a) concentrations with apolipoprotein(a) isoform size is not due to differences in Lp(a) catabolism but to differences in production rate. J Clin Invest 93:2758–2763

Ray KK, Stoekenbroek RM, Kallend D, Leiter LA, Landmesser U, Scott Wright R, Wijngaard P, Kastelein JJP (2018) Effect of an siRNA therapeutic targeting PCSK9 on atherogenic lipoproteins: prespecified secondary end points in Orion 1. Circulation 138:1304–1316

Ray KK, Vallejo-Vaz AJ, Ginsberg HN, Davidson MH, Louie MJ, Bujas-Bobanovic M, Minini P, Eckel RH, Cannon CP (2019) Lipoprotein(a) reductions from PCSK9 inhibition and major adverse cardiovascular events: pooled analysis of alirocumab phase 3 trials. Atherosclerosis 288:194–202

Ripatti S, Tikkanen E, Orho-Melander M, Havulinna AS, Silander K, Sharma A, Guiducci C, Perola M, Jula A, Sinisalo J, Lokki ML, Nieminen MS, Melander O, Salomaa V, Peltonen L, Kathiresan S (2010) A multilocus genetic risk score for coronary heart disease: case-control and prospective cohort analyses. Lancet 376:1393–1400

Roeseler E, Julius U, Heigl F, Spitthoever R, Heutling D, Breitenberger P, Leebmann J, Lehmacher W, Kamstrup PR, Nordestgaard BG, Maerz W, Noureen A, Schmidt K, Kronenberg F, Heibges A, Klingel R (2016) Lipoprotein apheresis for lipoprotein(a)-associated cardiovascular disease: prospective 5 years of follow-up and apolipoprotein(a) characterization. Arterioscler Thromb Vasc Biol 36:2019–2027

Romagnuolo R, Scipione CA, Bazzi ZA, Boffa MB, Koschinsky ML (2018) Inhibition of pericellular plasminogen activation by apolipoprotein(a): roles of urokinase plasminogen activator receptor and integrins aMb2 and aVb3. Atherosclerosis 275:11–21

Safarova MS, Ezhov MV, Afanasieva OI, Matchin YG, Atanesyan RV, Adamova IY, Utkina EA, Konovalov GA, Pokrovsky SN (2013) Effect of specific lipoprotein(a) apheresis on coronary atherosclerosis regression assessed by quantitative coronary angiography. Atheroscler Suppl 14:93–99

Saleheen D, Haycock PC, Zhao W, Rasheed A, Taleb A, Imran A, Abbas S, Majeed F, Akhtar S, Qamar N, Zaman KS, Yaqoob Z, Saghir T, Rizvi SNH, Memon A, Mallick NH, Ishaq M, Rasheed SZ, Memon FU, Mahmood K, Ahmed N, Frossard P, Tsimikas S, Witztum JL, Marcovina S, Sandhu M, Rader DJ, Danesh J (2017) Apolipoprotein(a) isoform size, lipoprotein(a) concentration, and coronary artery disease: a Mendelian randomisation analysis. Lancet Diabetes Endocrinol 5:524–533

Samaha FF, McKenney J, Bloedon LT, Sasiela WJ, Rader DJ (2008) Inhibition of microsomal triglyceride transfer protein alone or with ezetimibe in patients with moderate hypercholesterolemia. Nat Clin Pract Cardiovasc Med 5:497–505

Sandholzer C, Saha N, Kark JD, Rees A, Jaross W, Dieplinger H, Hoppichler F, Boerwinkle E, Utermann G (1992) Apo(a) isoforms predict risk for coronary heart disease: a study in six populations. Arterioscler Thromb 12:1214–1226

Scanu AM, Hinman J (2002) Issues concerning the monitoring of statin therapy in hypercholesterolemic subjects with high plasma lipoprotein(a) levels. Lipids 37:439–444

Scharnagl H, Stojakovic T, Dieplinger B, Dieplinger H, Erhart G, Kostner GM, Hermann M, März W, Grammer TB (2019) Comparison of lipoprotein(a) serum concentrations measured by six commercially available immunoassays. Atherosclerosis 289:206–213

Smits LJ, van Kuijk SM, Leffers P, Peeters LL, Prins MH, Sep SJ (2013) Index event bias-a numerical example. J Clin Epidemiol 66:192–196

Stiekema LCA, Stroes ESG, Verweij SL, Kassahun H, Chen L, Wasserman SM, Sabatine MS, Mani V, Fayad ZA (2019) Persistent arterial wall inflammation in patients with elevated lipoprotein(a) despite strong low-density lipoprotein cholesterol reduction by proprotein convertase subtilisin/kexin type 9 antibody treatment. Eur Heart J 40:2775–2781

Stiekema LCA, Prange KHM, Hoogeveen RM, Verweij SL, Kroon J, Schnitzler JG, Dzobo KE, Cupido AJ, Tsimikas S, Stroes ESG, de Winther MPJ, Bahjat M (2020) Potent lipoprotein (a) lowering following apolipoprotein(a) antisense treatment reduces the pro-inflammatory activation of circulating monocytes in patients with elevated lipoprotein(a). Eur Heart J 41:2262–2271

Thanassoulis G, Campbell CY, Owens DS, Smith JG, Smith AV, Peloso GM, Kerr KF, Pechlivanis S, Budoff MJ, Harris TB, Malhotra R, O'Brien KD, Kamstrup PR, Nordestgaard BG, Tybjaerg-Hansen A, Allison MA, Aspelund T, Criqui MH, Heckbert SR, Hwang SJ, Liu Y, Sjogren M, van der Pals J, Kalsch H, Muhleisen TW, Nothen MM, Cupples LA, Caslake M, Di AE, Danesh J, Rotter JI, Sigurdsson S, Wong Q, Erbel R, Kathiresan S, Melander O, Gudnason V, O'Donnell CJ, Post WS (2013) Genetic associations with valvular calcification and aortic stenosis. N Engl J Med 368:503–512

Thomas T, Zhou H, Karmally W, Ramakrishnan R, Holleran S, Liu Y, Jumes P, Wagner JA, Hubbard B, Previs SF, Roddy T, Johnson-Levonas AO, Gutstein DE, Marcovina SM, Rader DJ, Ginsberg HN, Millar JS, Reyes-Soffer G (2017) CETP (cholesteryl ester transfer protein) inhibition with anacetrapib decreases production of lipoprotein(a) in mildly hypercholesterolemic subjects. Arterioscler Thromb Vasc Biol 37:1770–1775

Tomlinson JE, McLean JW, Lawn RM (1989) Rhesus monkey apolipoprotein(a). Sequence, evolution, and sites of synthesis. J Biol Chem 264:5957–5965

Tsimikas S, Brilakis ES, Miller ER, McConnell JP, Lennon RJ, Kornman KS, Witztum JL, Berger PB (2005) Oxidized phospholipids, Lp(a) lipoprotein, and coronary artery disease. N Engl J Med 353:46–57

Tsimikas S, Mallat Z, Talmud PJ, Kastelein JJ, Wareham NJ, Sandhu MS, Miller ER, Benessiano J, Tedgui A, Witztum JL, Khaw KT, Boekholdt SM (2010) Oxidation-specific biomarkers, lipoprotein(a), and risk of fatal and nonfatal coronary events. J Am Coll Cardiol 56:946–955

Tsimikas S, Viney NJ, Hughes SG, Singleton W, Graham MJ, Baker BF, Burkey JL, Yang Q, Marcovina SM, Geary RS, Crooke RM, Witztum JL (2015) Antisense therapy targeting apolipoprotein(a): a randomised, double-blind, placebo-controlled phase 1 study. Lancet 386:1472–1483

Tsimikas S, Karwatowska-Prokopczuk E, Gouni-Berthold I, Tardif JC, Baum SJ, Steinhagen-Thiessen E, Shapiro MD, Stroes ES, Moriarty PM, Nordestgaard BG, Xia S, Guerriero J, Viney NJ, O'Dea L, Witztum JL (2020a) Lipoprotein(a) reduction in persons with cardiovascular disease. N Engl J Med 382:244–255

Tsimikas S, Gordts PLSM, Nora C, Yeang C, Witztum JL (2020b) Statin therapy increases lipoprotein(a) levels. Eur Heart J 41:2275–2284

Tsimikas S, Gordts PLSM, Nora C, Yeang C, Witztum JL (2020c) Statins and increases in Lp(a): an inconvenient truth that needs attention. Eur Heart J 41:192–193

Utermann G (1989) The mysteries of lipoprotein(a). Science 246:904–910

Utermann G, Menzel HJ, Kraft HG, Duba HC, Kemmler HG, Seitz C (1987) Lp(a) glycoprotein phenotypes: inheritance and relation to Lp(a)-lipoprotein concentrations in plasma. J Clin Invest 80:458–465

Utermann G, Hoppichler F, Dieplinger H, Seed M, Thompson G, Boerwinkle E (1989) Defects in the low density lipoprotein receptor gene affect lipoprotein (a) levels: multiplicative interaction of two gene loci associated with premature atherosclerosis. Proc Natl Acad Sci U S A 86:4171–4174

van der Valk FM, Bekkering S, Kroon J, Yeang C, Van den Bossche J, van Buul JD, Ravandi A, Nederveen AJ, Verberne HJ, Scipione C, Nieuwdorp M, Joosten LA, Netea MG, Koschinsky ML, Witztum JL, Tsimikas S, Riksen NP, Stroes ES (2016) Oxidized phospholipids on lipoprotein(a) elicit Arterial Wall inflammation and an inflammatory monocyte response in humans. Circulation 134:611–624

Viney NJ, van Capelleveen JC, Geary RS, Xia S, Tami JA, Yu RZ, Marcovina SM, Hughes SG, Graham MJ, Crooke RM, Crooke ST, Witztum JL, Stroes ES, Tsimikas S (2016) Antisense oligonucleotides targeting apolipoprotein(a) in people with raised lipoprotein(a): two randomised, double-blind, placebo-controlled, dose-ranging trials. Lancet 388:2239–2253

Virani SS, Brautbar A, Davis BC, Nambi V, Hoogeveen RC, Sharrett AR, Coresh J, Mosley TH, Morrisett JD, Catellier DJ, Folsom AR, Boerwinkle E, Ballantyne CM (2012) Associations between lipoprotein(a) levels and cardiovascular outcomes in black and white subjects: the atherosclerosis risk in communities (ARIC) study. Circulation 125:241–249

Vongpromek R, Bos S, Ten Kate GJ, Yahya R, Verhoeven AJ, De Feyter PJ, Kronenberg F, van Lennep JE, Sijbrands EJ, Mulder MT (2015) Lipoprotein(a) levels are associated with aortic valve calcification in asymptomatic patients with familial hypercholesterolaemia. J Intern Med 278:166–173

Vuorio A, Watts GF, Kovanen PT (2019) Lipoprotein(a) as a risk factor for calcific aortic valvulopathy in heterozygous familial hypercholesterolemia. Atherosclerosis 281:25–30

Willeit P, Ridker PM, Nestel PJ, Simes J, Tonkin AM, Pedersen TR, Schwartz GG, Olsson AG, Colhoun HM, Kronenberg F, Drechsler C, Wanner C, Mora S, Lesogor A, Tsimikas S (2018) Baseline and on-statin treatment lipoprotein(a) levels for prediction of cardiovascular events: individual patient-data meta-analysis of statin outcome trials. Lancet 392:1311–1320

Yahya R, Berk K, Verhoeven A, Bos S, van der Zee L, Touw J, Erhart G, Kronenberg F, Timman R, Sijbrands E, van Roeters LJ, Mulder M (2019) Statin treatment increases lipoprotein(a) levels in subjects with low molecular weight apolipoprotein(a) phenotype. Atherosclerosis 289:201–205

Yeang C, Witztum JL, Tsimikas S (2021) Novel method for quantification of lipoprotein(a)-cholesterol: implications for improving accuracy of LDL-C measurements. J Lipid Res 62:100053. https://doi.org/10.1016/j.jlr.2021.100053

Zhang J, Du R, Peng K, Wu X, Hu C, Li M, Xu Y, Xu M, Wang S, Bi Y, Wang W, Lu J, Chen Y (2019) Serum lipoprotein (a) is associated with increased risk of stroke in Chinese adults: a prospective study. Atherosclerosis 289:8–13

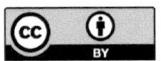

Nonalcoholic Fatty Liver Disease

Lingling Ding, Yvonne Oligschlaeger, Ronit Shiri-Sverdlov, and Tom Houben

Contents

1 Epidemiology 235
   1.1 Definition, Prevalence, and Incidence of NAFLD 235
   1.2 Association with Other Diseases 236
   1.3 Clinical, Economic, and Social Burden of NAFLD 237
2 Pathophysiology of NAFLD 239
   2.1 Intrahepatic Disturbances During NAFLD 239
   2.2 Metabolic Crosstalk in NAFLD 243
   2.3 Genetic Predisposition to NAFLD 245
3 Therapeutics 246
   3.1 Dietary/Lifestyle Intervention and Bariatric Surgery 246
   3.2 Targeting Lipotoxicity 247
   3.3 Targeting Insulin/Glucose Metabolism 248
   3.4 Targeting Hepatic Inflammation and Fibrosis 250
   3.5 Targeting Bile Acid Metabolism 251
4 Conclusion 252
References 252

Abstract

Nonalcoholic fatty liver disease (NAFLD) is considered the hepatic manifestation of the metabolic syndrome (MetS) and comprises one of the largest health threats of the twenty-first century. In this chapter, we review the current state of knowledge of NAFLD and underline the striking similarities with atherosclerosis. We first describe current epidemiological data showing the staggering increase of NAFLD numbers and its related clinical and economic costs. We then provide an overview of pathophysiological hepatic processes in NAFLD and highlight

L. Ding · Y. Oligschlaeger · R. Shiri-Sverdlov · T. Houben (✉)
Department of Molecular Genetics, School of Nutrition and Translational Research in Metabolism (NUTRIM), Maastricht University Medical Center+, Maastricht, The Netherlands
e-mail: tom.houben@maastrichtuniversity.nl

© The Author(s) 2020
A. von Eckardstein, C. J. Binder (eds.), *Prevention and Treatment of Atherosclerosis*,
Handbook of Experimental Pharmacology 270, https://doi.org/10.1007/164_2020_352

233

the systemic aspects of NAFLD that point toward metabolic crosstalk between organs as an important cause of metabolic disease. Finally, we end by highlighting the currently investigated therapeutic approaches for NAFLD, which also show strong similarities with a range of treatment options for atherosclerosis.

Keywords

Atherosclerosis · Epidemiology · NAFLD · Pathogenesis · Treatment

Abbreviations

ALT	Alanine transaminase
ASK1	Apoptosis signal-regulating kinase 1
CCR2/CCR5	C-C chemokine receptor type 2/C-C chemokine receptor 5
CKD	Chronic kidney disease
CPT-1	Carnitine palmitoyltransferase 1
DPP4	Dipeptidyl peptidase-4
ESLD	End-stage of liver disease
FXR	Farnesoid X receptor
GCKR	Glucokinase regulator
GLP1R	Glucagon-like peptide-1 receptor
HCC	Hepatocellular carcinoma
HDL	High-density lipoproteins
HmG-CoA	3-Hydroxy-3-methylglutarylcoenzyme A
HR-QOL	Health-related quality of life
KCs	Kupffer cells
LDL	Low-density lipoproteins
LPS	Lipopolysaccharide
LSECs	Liver sinusoidal endothelial cells
LXR	Liver X receptor
MetS	Metabolic syndrome
NAFLD	Nonalcoholic fatty liver disease
NASH	Nonalcoholic steatohepatitis
OCA	Obeticholic acid
oxLDL	Oxidized low-density lipoproteins
PBPLA3	Patatin-like phospholipase domain-containing 3
PCOS	Polycystic ovary syndrome
PPARα	Peroxisome proliferator-activated receptor alpha
ROS	Reactive oxygen species
SGLT2	Sodium-glucose transport protein 2
SREBP1c	Sterol regulatory element-binding protein 1
T2DM	Type 2 diabetes mellitus

THR	Thyroid hormone receptors
TM6SF2	Transmembrane 6 superfamily 2
UDCA	Ursodeoxycholic acid
VLDL	Very low-density lipoprotein

1 Epidemiology

1.1 Definition, Prevalence, and Incidence of NAFLD

Being the most prevalent chronic liver disease worldwide (Li et al. 2019), nonalcoholic fatty liver disease (NAFLD) covers a diseases spectrum, initiating with hepatic steatosis which is defined by the presence of ≥5% hepatic fat (referred to steatosis) in the absence of any secondary cause of hepatic steatosis such as chronic viral hepatitis and alcohol consumption (21 drinks/week in men and 14 drinks/week in women) (Chalasani et al. 2012, 2018). In a second, more advanced stage, hepatic steatosis may advance into nonalcoholic steatohepatitis (NASH), which is characterized by a combination of hepatic steatosis and inflammation in the presence or absence of fibrosis. Finally, NASH can progress into advanced-stage liver diseases such as cirrhosis and hepatocellular carcinoma (HCC) (Angulo 2002; Anstee and Day 2013; Calzadilla Bertot and Adams 2016; Chalasani et al. 2018; Fazel et al. 2016; Jou et al. 2008; Sayiner et al. 2016; Younossi and Henry 2016; Younossi et al. 2018a). Being the hepatic component of the metabolic syndrome (MetS) (Chalasani et al. 2012), NAFLD is commonly associated with other metabolic disorders such as obesity, which is also linked to the development of cardiovascular diseases such as atherosclerosis (Chalasani et al. 2018; Paoletti et al. 2006). Considering these links between NAFLD, obesity, and atherosclerosis, it is no surprise that NAFLD has become the most prevalent liver disease worldwide (Li et al. 2019).

Indeed, in the last three decades, the prevalence of NAFLD has increased at a constant rate. Numbers from a study from Younossi et al. showed the evolution of NAFLD prevalence in the United States from 1988 to 2008 ranging from 5.51% (1988–1994) to 9.84% (1999–2004) and 11.01% (2005–2008), indicating a twofold increase over two decades (Younossi et al. 2011a). At a global level, it is currently estimated that NAFLD affects about 25% of the general population. At the other hand, NASH has been calculated at 2–5% of the general population and so far represents the minority of NAFLD patients (10–20%) (Younossi et al. 2016a). However, while hepatic steatosis seems less harmful for the liver, patients suffering from steatosis are at increased risk for cardiac-related death (Targher et al. 2016). Therefore, steatotic patients should be monitored even at an early stage of the disease. For the future, Estes et al. predicted the NAFLD population to increase with 21% in 2030, expecting a staggering 100.9 million NAFLD patients, of which 27.00 million patients would also suffer from NASH, the latter indicating a 63% increase in prevalence compared to current numbers (Estes et al. 2018).

From a regional perspective, the pooled incidence of NAFLD in the West (being Europe and Northern America) was estimated to be 28 per 1,000 persons per year (Chalasani et al. 2018; Younossi et al. 2016b). As mentioned previously, NAFLD has been reported as the most common liver disease in the United States (Bellentani and Marino 2009). However, within the Asian population, recent metadata also indicated the global incidence rate of NAFLD at 50.9 cases per 1,000 individuals per year (Li et al. 2019). Indeed, while it was initially perceived as a "Western disease," NAFLD is now highly prevalent in all continents with the highest rates reported in South America (31%) and the Middle East (32%), followed by Asia (27%), the United States (24%), and Europe (23%), while being less common in Africa (14%) (Younossi et al. 2016b).

Taken these numbers into account, and especially those indicating the exponential increase of NASH patients, it is clear that NAFLD poses one of the largest burdens on current healthcare systems, emphasizing the urge for early and fast treatment to prevent further escalation of this disease.

1.2   Association with Other Diseases

NAFLD has been reported to be strongly linked to obesity, with a prevalence as high as 80% in obese patients and only 16% in individuals with a normal BMI and without metabolic risk factors (Bellentani et al. 2000; Williams et al. 2011). Relevantly, obesity seems to play a role in both the initial process leading to simple steatosis but also to its progression toward NASH (Polyzos et al. 2017). Indeed, it has been demonstrated that the risk of NASH development is lower in lean than overweight/obese individuals (Sookoian and Pirola 2018). Next to NASH, also patients suffering from hepatic fibrosis tend to be rather obese than non-obese (86% vs. 27%, respectively) (Fassio et al. 2004).

Besides obesity, it has been suggested that NAFLD is also tightly linked to cardiovascular diseases (Patil and Sood 2017). Recently, clinical observations indicated that NASH increases atherosclerosis and cardiovascular risks by local overexpression of inflammatory mediators, endothelial damage, and regulators of blood pressure (Targher et al. 2009, 2010). Others confirmed that NAFLD is independently associated with atherosclerosis progression (Targher et al. 2010). Additionally, other studies demonstrated that NAFLD patients have impaired flow-mediated vasodilatation (Villanova et al. 2005), increased carotid artery intimal-medial thickness and an increased prevalence of carotid atherosclerotic plaques compared to healthy subjects (Sookoian and Pirola 2008), independently of obesity and other established risk factors. These observations therefore emphasize the link between NAFLD and atherosclerosis.

Additionally, NAFLD has also been suggested as a risk factor for gastrointestinal tract malignancies, such as colorectal cancer (Lindenmeyer and McCullough 2018; Muhidin et al. 2012; Wong et al. 2011). Also, NAFLD is also associated with chronic kidney disease (CKD) (Musso et al. 2014), which is defined by the presence of kidney damage or a reduced glomerular filtration rate for 3 months or more

(Levey et al. 2005). Specifically, it has been suggested that the prevalence of CKD in NAFLD patients is between 4 and 40% (Marcuccilli and Chonchol 2016). This association has been partly explained by the NAFLD-associated microvascular alterations that also affect the kidney (Musso et al. 2016). Moreover these microvascular alterations have been linked to cerebrovascular disease, potentially contributing to cognitive impairment (Lombardi et al. 2019). Finally, polycystic ovary syndrome (PCOS), a condition that leads to the production of higher-than-normal amounts of male hormones in women, is also associated with NAFLD (Vassilatou 2014; Wu et al. 2018a). However, the clinical significance and its pathophysiological basis remain to be further investigated.

1.3   Clinical, Economic, and Social Burden of NAFLD

In spite of its increased prevalence over the last decades, to our knowledge, the clinical burden of NAFLD has not been characterized in detail (Boursier et al. 2018; Lam et al. 2016; Mullerova et al. 2019; Welte et al. 2012). Notwithstanding that all stages of NAFLD contribute to its clinical burden, the more progressive stages of NALFD are expected to have the largest impact (Sayiner et al. 2016). As a progressive form of NAFLD, NASH is currently the second leading cause for liver transplantation in the United States and even the leading cause for liver transplantation in females (Noureddin et al. 2018). Furthermore, it is known that NAFLD has become one of the leading causes for cirrhosis (Kadayifci et al. 2008), the end-stage liver disease which is associated with high risks for development of bacterial infections leading to hospitalization (Albillos et al. 2014; Li et al. 2018; Singal et al. 2014). Additionally, the presence of advanced fibrosis (stage ≥ 2) in NAFLD has been directly associated with liver-related mortality (Angulo et al. 2015; Younossi et al. 2011b). There is also accumulating evidence that NAFLD is an important risk factor for hepatocellular carcinoma (HCC), which is the fifth most common type of cancer and third most common cause of cancer mortality (El-Serag and Rudolph 2007; Piscaglia et al. 2016; Younossi et al. 2015a). Translating the latter described observations into exact numbers, a recent study showed that in 2015, 28,000 deaths (2.2% of all deaths in the NAFLD population) were related to cirrhosis, HCC, or liver transplantation, while 162,560 deaths (accounting for 12.8% of all NAFLD deaths) were due to cardiovascular diseases (Angulo et al. 2015; Ekstedt et al. 2015). Indeed, these data point toward an important role for cardiovascular diseases in NAFLD-related mortality. In line with the previously estimated increased prevalence of NAFLD in the future, reports have indicated that the total number of deaths resulting from NAFLD will increase 44%, reaching 1.83 million deaths at an annual basis by 2030 (Estes et al. 2018). Regarding to the healthcare expenditure, Lam et al. demonstrated that more frequent clinical visits are associated with improved outcomes in pediatric NAFLD patients, substantiating the importance of frequent monitoring and follow-up to manage NAFLD progression (Lam et al. 2016). Moreover, Boursier et al. evaluated the hospitalization of NAFLD-/NASH-related end-stage liver disease (ESLD) patients by a 7-year follow-up study in France. This report described that ESLD patients experience more hospitalization per year (over 400%), which are longer (400% increase in length) and are associated with a 300% increase in hospitalization costs (Boursier et al. 2018). These numbers therefore indicate the gigantic investments that are required to manage NAFLD.

In line with the increasing prevalence of NAFLD, the economic costs related to NAFLD have also been predicted to rise in the future. In the United States alone, approximately 103 billion dollars are annually spent on NAFLD-related costs, while in European countries (i.e., France, the United Kingdom, Germany, and Italy), these costs account for approximately €35 billion (Abdelmalek 2016). Of particular concern is the rising prevalence of obesity as well as the increase in general healthcare costs, which contributes to a tenfold increase in the current economic burden of NAFLD by 2025 (Abdelmalek 2016; Younossi et al. 2016a). Several studies also investigated the relationship between NAFLD patients and healthcare utilization and associated costs. These studies demonstrated that the number of outpatient visits for patients with NAFLD significantly doubled over time and underlined the fact that, between 2005 and 2010, the healthcare costs of inpatients and outpatients were increased 5% and 10%, respectively (Baumeister et al. 2008; Younossi et al. 2014, 2015b). Additionally, a study of the hepatology clinics in the West Suffolk area of the United Kingdom showed that the total annual hepatology budget for these specialized clinics was £130,000, including £58,000 for resources and £72,000 for clinic attendances. Moreover, the latest research estimating the economic burden of NASH patients by using a Markov decision analytic model demonstrated that lifetime costs of all NASH patients was approximately $222.6 billion in the United States in 2017, with $95.4 billion reflecting the advanced NASH population (Younossi et al. 2019).

From an individual perspective, NALFD patients have to contend with a range of symptoms such as fatigue, decreased physical activity, and emotional health impairment which affect their quality of life (health-related quality of life (HR-QOL)) (Golabi et al. 2016; Loria et al. 2013; Younossi and Henry 2015, 2016). Several studies have demonstrated that NAFLD patients had poorer HR-QOL compared to other chronic liver diseases and also showed that NAFLD-related fatigue associated with impairments in physical functioning (Afendy et al. 2009; Dan et al. 2007; Newton et al. 2008). Potential explanations for the decrease of HR-QOL in NAFLD patients that have been raised are related to obesity and psychological processes as well as psychiatric issues such as depression and anxiety (Stewart and Levenson 2012; Surdea-Blaga and Dumitrascu 2011; Weinstein et al. 2011). Indeed, several studies have demonstrated that depressive disorders, as well as anxiety disorders, are more frequent in patients with NAFLD/NASH and are associated with more advanced liver histological abnormalities, such as severe hepatocyte ballooning (Elwing et al. 2006; Macavei et al. 2016; Stewart et al. 2015; Weinstein et al. 2011).

Altogether, these numbers substantiate the impact of NAFLD on healthcare, economy, and also the daily life of individual patients. To prevent further escalation of the disease, it is therefore of utmost importance to increase the understanding of the disease to find approaches to diagnose and treat (and if possible prevent) the progression of NAFLD.

2   Pathophysiology of NAFLD

As NAFLD comprises a spectrum of diseases, multiple pathophysiological processes are involved including dysregulation of lipid metabolism, increased hepatic inflammation, and the presence of hepatic fibrosis. However, how patients with steatosis develop inflammation is still unclear, leaving a blind spot in the understanding of how NASH exactly arises. Nevertheless, scientists have succeeded in unraveling several disease processes in NALFD, which appear to show striking similarities with disease processes described in atherosclerosis. Furthermore, increasing evidence links different metabolic organs to NAFLD development, emphasizing the presence of metabolic crosstalk during NAFLD.

2.1   Intrahepatic Disturbances During NAFLD

The liver constitutes a key role in regulating whole body metabolism, which involves a complex interplay between different hepatic cell types ranging from hepatocytes as parenchymal cells to Kupffer cells (KCs), stellate cells, and liver sinusoidal endothelial cells (LSECs) among other cell types. As such, each of these cell types is influenced by pathophysiological processes during NAFLD, eventually leading to hepatic disturbances at whole organ level.

2.1.1   Lipo- and Glucotoxicity

Due to low physical activity and increased consumption of fats, lipotoxicity has arisen as one of the main players to contribute to NAFLD pathogenesis (Ibrahim et al. 2011). Lipotoxicity is defined by the excess generation of cytosolic lipids (mainly triglycerides and subtypes of free fatty acids) that have direct adverse effects on metabolic pathways of the cell (Schaffer 2016). Under normal conditions, triglycerides and free fatty acids are stored in adipose tissue, where they can be employed as energy source during periods of energy deprivation or during extreme exercise (Muro et al. 2014). However, in obesity, when the storage capacity of adipose tissue is exceeded, free fatty acids accumulate in ectopic organs, including the liver (but also in the arteries). As such, hepatic steatosis (Wojcik-Cichy et al. 2018) develops, resulting in the formation of adverse metabolites that hamper normal cellular physiology. For example, an excess of free fatty acids such as palmitic or stearic acids induces the generation of toxic metabolites, leading to caspase-dependent apoptosis of hepatocytes (Kakisaka et al. 2012; Pfaffenbach et al. 2010) but also of cardiomyocytes (Drosatos and Schulze 2013; Zou et al. 2017) and endothelial cells (Artwohl et al. 2008; Chinen et al. 2007). Indeed, while free fatty acid-induced apoptosis of hepatocytes is a key feature of lipotoxicity in the context of NAFLD (Trauner et al. 2010), other reports have shown that excess palmitate induces endoplasmic reticulum stress and apoptosis in the context of atherosclerosis as well (Erbay et al. 2009). Therefore, free fatty acid-induced apoptosis of parenchymal cells appears to be a shared mechanism between NAFLD and atherosclerosis development.

Besides inducing apoptosis, free fatty acid influx into hepatocytes also influences the function of key enzymes and nuclear receptors involved in hepatic de novo lipogenesis, fatty acid oxidation, and cholesterol metabolism, thereby further disturbing hepatic lipid metabolism. Indeed, expression levels of acetyl-coenzyme-A carboxylase 1, a key enzyme in fatty acid metabolism (Barber et al. 2005), were shown to decrease in advanced stages of NASH compared to individuals with steatosis (Nagaya et al. 2010). Moreover, in the transcriptional levels, liver X receptor (LXR), a nuclear receptor involved with regulation of cholesterol, fatty acid, and glucose metabolism (Kalaany and Mangelsdorf 2006), correlated with intrahepatic inflammation and fibrosis in NAFLD patients (Ahn et al. 2014; Ni et al. 2017). In line, macrophage-targeted delivery of LXR agonist inside the atherosclerotic plaque reduced atherosclerosis progression (Guo et al. 2018), pointing toward a key function of LXR in both NAFLD and atherosclerosis development.

Lipotoxic responses also affect LSECs, a type of non-parenchymal cell that is specifically involved in maintaining hepatic vascular tone and quiescence of hepatic stellate cells that are responsible for the fibrotic response. Upon treatment with oxidized lipids (Zhang et al. 2014) or palmitic acid (Matsumoto et al. 2018), LSCEs directly or indirectly triggered the release of reactive oxygen species (ROS) production (Peters et al. 2018), which influences mechanisms related to inflammation and fibrosis (Ni et al. 2017).

Increased hepatic fat accumulation has also been associated with reduced levels of high-density lipoproteins (HDL) and increased levels of total plasma cholesterol, low-density lipoproteins (LDL), and very low-density lipoprotein particles (Koruk et al. 2003), the latter being involved with hepatic lipid export. Moreover, besides triglycerides and fatty acids, it has become evident that cholesterol is a key player in inducing hepatic inflammatory responses (Caballero et al. 2009; Plat et al. 2014; van Rooyen et al. 2011). Indeed, in the context of obesity-associated diseases, it was shown that cholesterol levels are associated with hepatic inflammation (Musso et al. 2003; Puri et al. 2007) and atherosclerosis (Ference et al. 2017) in humans. In agreement with these data, it has previously been shown that omitting cholesterol from the diet was able to prevent liver inflammation in hyperlipidemic and atherosclerosis-prone mice (Wouters et al. 2008), pointing toward cholesterol as a significant risk factor for early onset of NASH and progression of atherosclerosis.

In addition to lipotoxicity, glucotoxicity is a metabolic condition linked to increased intake of dietary sugars, resulting in hyperglycemia which may cause hepatotoxic effects by increasing steatosis (Mota et al. 2016). For instance, it was shown that high carbohydrate intake plays a role in de novo lipogenesis and hepatic steatosis (Ackerman et al. 2005; Neuschwander-Tetri et al. 2012), presumably via activation of lipogenic enzymes such as fatty acid synthase and stearoyl-CoA desaturase-1 (Maslak et al. 2015). In addition, high-fructose intake was shown to correlate with the severity of fibrosis in NAFLD patients (Basaranoglu et al. 2015; Mota et al. 2016) and carbohydrate intake associated with the progression of coronary atherosclerosis (Mozaffarian et al. 2004).

Glucotoxic and lipotoxic products, including free fatty acids, cholesterol, and ceramides, among others (Han et al. 2008), are also involved in the activation of cellular stress responses. For instance, it has been shown that saturated long-chain fatty acids can disturb metabolic fluxes, thereby increasing the production of harmful lipid intermediates (Kakisaka et al. 2012). These intermediates can promote the release of ROS, leading to oxidative stress and hence the progression from steatosis to NASH (Matsuzawa et al. 2007; van Herpen and Schrauwen-Hinderling 2008) and the development of atherosclerosis (Nowak et al. 2017).

Overall, these evidences show that triglycerides, fatty acids, and cholesterol overload disturb essential processes in the liver that result in NAFLD features, placing lipids at the center of NAFLD development. Moreover, as these processes show striking similarities with disturbances present in atherosclerosis, lipotoxicity is a denominator linking NAFLD to atherosclerosis.

2.1.2 Oxidative Stress and Mitochondrial Dysfunction

As mentioned in the previous paragraph, part of the lipotoxic response involves the generation of ROS, resulting in oxidative stress. Oxidative stress comprises a state during which there is an imbalance between generation of ROS at one hand and an inability to detoxify (i.e., via antioxidant mechanisms) these oxygenated intermediates (Masarone et al. 2018). As a consequence, free radicals, peroxides, and related products are generated and react with biological components such as proteins, DNA, but also lipids (Finkel and Holbrook 2000). Indeed, considering the increased amount of lipids present during NAFLD conditions, larger quantities of lipid peroxidation products are present in the liver of NAFLD patients (Sumida et al. 2013) and contribute to the transition toward more serious stages of NAFLD (Busch et al. 2017; Feldstein et al. 2010). In addition, ROS is known to mediate endoplasmic reticulum stress, thereby causing the formation of misfolded proteins, which is a critical factor in NAFLD (Ashraf and Sheikh 2015) as well as the progression of atherosclerosis (Hotamisligil 2010; Tabas 2010). Moreover, cholesterol oxidation products that are part of oxidized low-density lipoproteins (oxLDL) are majorly involved in inflammatory and fibrotic responses in the liver (also further discussed in next section) (Bieghs et al. 2013).

Considering the key role of mitochondria in cellular oxygen consumption and production of ROS, lipotoxic influences on mitochondria have the potential to further aggravate oxidative stress (Dominguez-Perez et al. 2019). Under physiological conditions, fatty acid transport into the mitochondria is mediated via carnitine palmitoyltransferase 1 (CPT-1) in order to stimulate beta-oxidation. Nevertheless, the expression of *Cpt-1* was shown to be reduced in NAFLD (Kohjima et al. 2007), findings that were further supported by Francque et al., showing that peroxisome proliferator-activated receptor alpha (*PPARα*), an important nuclear receptor regulating CPT-1, inversely correlated with disease severity in patients with NASH (Francque et al. 2015). By using isolated mitochondria, it was also shown that short chain ceramides increase mitochondrial permeability due to the generation of ceramide channels and increased cytochrome C release (Colombini 2010), thereby mediating toxic effects. Moreover, mitochondrial cholesterol accumulation caused mitochondrial dysfunction (Balboa et al. 2017), and based on studies in the context of neurotoxicity (Barbero-Camps et al. 2014), mitochondrial cholesterol may play a role in endoplasmic reticulum stress and subsequent apoptosis.

2.1.3   Hepatic Inflammation and Fibrosis

An essential pathophysiological process during NAFLD that also unites the lipotoxic response with the generation of oxidative stress is the presence of hepatic inflammation which can progress into hepatic fibrosis. In contrast to the uptake of non-modified LDL, it has been established that the uptake of oxLDL contributes to cholesterol-induced foam cell formation and metabolic inflammation (Lara-Guzman et al. 2018) in NASH (Houben et al. 2017) but also in the context of atherosclerosis (Binder et al. 2003). Moreover, the accumulation of oxidized lipids into the lysosomal compartment of macrophages activates inflammatory cascades including inflammasome complexes and apoptosis (Bieghs et al. 2013; Grebe et al. 2018; Hendrikx et al. 2013; Jerome 2010). Indeed, recent studies show that specific inhibition of the NLRP3 inflammasome not only reverses hepatic inflammation and fibrosis (Mridha et al. 2017) but also reduces atherosclerotic lesion development (van der Heijden et al. 2017), pointing toward an important role for the inflammasome in chronic inflammatory diseases (Cai et al. 2017; Duewell et al. 2010; Pan et al. 2018). Furthermore, cholesterol-mediated activation of inflammasomes decreases cholesterol efflux, thereby disturbing the regulation of bile acid metabolism. Previously, it was indeed shown that mice lacking the bile acid receptor farnesoid X receptor (FXR) had pro-atherogenic lipoproteins (Mencarelli and Fiorucci 2010) and increased hepatic bile acid levels (Sinal et al. 2000), pointing toward a potential role for FXR in cholesterol-induced liver inflammation. Indeed, improving cholesterol efflux in hepatic macrophages by overexpressing *Cyp27a1,* an enzyme responsible for the conversion of cholesterol into bile acids, reduced hepatic inflammation and fibrosis in an experimental model (Hendrikx et al. 2015). Via accumulation of oxidized lipids into lysosomes, also disturbances in autophagy contribute to increased levels of inflammation both during NAFLD (Wu et al. 2018b) and atherosclerosis (Martinet and De Meyer 2009). Besides cholesterol, also other lipids such as phospholipids (Lee et al. 2012) and fatty acids (Reinaud et al. 1989), can (non)enzymatically interact with free radicals, triggering inflammation by a wide variety of underlying processes (Houben et al. 2017).

While macrophages play a key role in the inflammatory response, hepatic stellate cells are the main drivers of the fibrotic response (Friedman 1993). After a damaging insult, stellate cells are activated, thereby secreting collagens and related matrix proteins that lead to generation of scar tissue or fibrosis (Peters et al. 2018; Schneiderhan et al. 2001), a pathological process also described in atherosclerosis (Ostovaneh et al. 2018). Relevantly, Chu et al. recently demonstrated that exposing hepatic stellate cells to fatty acids resulted in an increased secretion of CCL20, resulting in a switch from a quiescent to an activated hepatic stellate cell. These findings were further confirmed in humans, showing increased circulating CCL20 protein levels in patients with NAFLD-related fibrosis (Chu et al. 2018). Further data based on an elegant co-culturing system using primary liver cells pointed toward CCL5 as an important hepatic stellate cell-derived chemokine capable of mediating steatosis and pro-inflammatory responses in initially healthy hepatocytes (Kim et al. 2018). Moreover, in vivo induction of CCL5 in response to high-fat diet was also shown to serve as an important regulator of vascular remodeling, revealing a role for CCL5 and its receptor in atherogenesis (Lin et al. 2018). Therefore, multiple reports indicate that lipids enable fibrotic responses by influencing hepatic stellate cells.

2.2   Metabolic Crosstalk in NAFLD

As previously mentioned, the capacity of adipose tissue to store lipids determines the quantity of free fatty acids to be released into the circulation under high lipid conditions. However, besides its storage capacity, adipose tissue is known as a "secretory" organ, releasing adipokines and adipocytokines that influence other organs (Ouchi et al. 2011). For this reason, lipid-induced adipose tissue function increases the release of adipocytokines such as TNFα, IL6, IL18, and ANGPTL, leading to inflammatory responses in other metabolic organs such as the liver (Ouchi et al. 2011; Reilly et al. 2015). Moreover, the release of these adipokines also influences circulating immune cells, contributing to a state of chronic inflammation (Bijnen et al. 2018; Mancuso 2016; Nakamura et al. 2014). Due to this systemic impact, it is not surprising that adipokines also influence atherosclerosis development. Indeed, adipose tissue-released TNFα directly influenced atherosclerosis development (Tanaka and Sata 2018). Besides modulating inflammation, the increased release of free fatty acids also hinders the anti-lipolytic role of insulin, aggravating insulin resistance (Engin 2017; Sears and Perry 2015).

Another extrahepatic organ that has been linked to NAFLD development is the thyroid. Being an endocrine organ, the thyroid secretes hormones that have a role in the regulation of energy homeostasis including the metabolism of cholesterol and fatty acids (Sinha et al. 2018). Specifically, hypothyroidism is characterized by increased serum LDL and HDL levels and decreased triglyceride levels (Duntas 2002). Besides indirectly influencing hepatic lipid metabolism by modulating circulating lipid levels, thyroid hormones also directly affect hepatic lipid metabolism mainly via the presence of hepatic thyroid hormone receptors (THR) (Sinha et al. 2018). THRs are nuclear hormone receptors that function as ligand-dependent transcription factors influencing downstream metabolic genes (Davis et al. 2016) but also disturb other metabolic transcription factors such as PPARy, LXR, and sterol regulatory element-binding protein 1 (SREBP1c) (Araki et al. 2009; Wang et al. 2015). For this regulatory role on hepatic lipid metabolism, THR agonists were also considered for the management of hepatic steatosis (Cable et al. 2009) but later observed adverse effects resulted in discontinuation of these clinical trials (Lammel Lindemann and Webb 2016). Nevertheless, thyroid hormones analogues (rather than THRs) are still considered as potential future NAFLD treatment (Perra et al. 2008).

Another organ that has gained attention in the context of NAFLD is the brain. At one hand, NAFLD-related inflammation has been demonstrated to influence microglia in the brain, leading to alterations in microvasculature of the brain (Ghareeb et al. 2011; Kim et al. 2016). Furthermore, NAFLD-associated endothelial dysfunction and the procoagulant state were linked to the same microvascular alterations, which may contribute to disturbances in brain circulation, damage, and cognitive impairment (Lombardi et al. 2019). Besides the link to the aforementioned cerebrovascular diseases (Airaghi et al. 2018), other brain-related associations have been established to NAFLD. Firstly, a recent report from Horwath et al. demonstrated that endoplasmic reticulum stress in the subfornical organ of the brain, a brain region previously linked to appetite (Matsuda et al. 2017), directly mediated hepatic steatosis, thereby directly linking the brain to the liver in the context of NAFLD. Moreover, Weinstein et al. recently linked NAFLD to lower cerebral brain volume hinting at a more profound role for the brain in NAFLD (Weinstein et al. 2018). Finally, as a regulation center for energy metabolism, brain regions such as the arcuate nucleus in the hypothalamus sense the metabolic status and govern food intake (Schwartz et al. 2000), making an obvious link to obesity-related NAFLD. An essential hormone involved with the homeostatic regulation of energy and acting via the hypothalamus is leptin (Kwon et al. 2016). Notably, variants of leptin receptors associated with increased NAFLD susceptibility, pointing toward a potential role for hypothalamic leptin sensitivity in NAFLD (Zain et al. 2013). Additional evidence linking hypothalamic inflammation to hepatic steatosis further substantiated the potential involvement of the hypothalamus in NAFLD (Valdearcos et al. 2015).

To end, multiple reports have indicated the involvement of the gastrointestinal tract to play a role in NAFLD development. Under physiological circumstances, the intestinal lining serves as a physical barrier that separates the host from contents in the gut. Disruption of this barrier leads to intestinal permeability (Winer et al. 2016), allowing for leakage of intestinal bacteria and other products into the circulation. Indeed, leakage of lipopolysaccharide (LPS) derived from intestinal bacteria into the circulation (Kitabatake et al. 2017) can activate KCs in the liver (Ye et al. 2012), thereby directly resulting in NASH development (Kitabatake et al. 2017; Wigg et al. 2001). Relevantly, gut-derived serum LPS was similarly associated with atherosclerosis development, reaffirming the tight link between NASH and atherosclerosis (Pastori et al. 2017). Though there are limited studies providing a causal role of the gut microbiome in NAFLD pathogenesis, the current amount of evidence suggests that the gut microbiota are at least involved with the development of NAFLD (Gregory et al. 2015; Kaden-Volynets et al. 2018; Martinez-Guryn et al. 2018; Turnbaugh et al. 2006) (Wang et al. 2018). Other well-known factors linking the gut to NAFLD are bile acid metabolism (Dumas et al. 2006; Tremaroli and Backhed 2012), bacterial-derived short-chain fatty acids (Canfora et al. 2019), and the toxic compounds dimethylamine and trimethylamine that were converted by bacteria from choline (Spencer et al. 2011; Wang et al. 2011). In line with our other descriptions, each of these compounds has also been associated with atherosclerosis development (Chambers et al. 2018; Charach et al. 2018; Tang et al. 2013).

Based on these evidences, it is clear that the development of NAFLD is linked to pathophysiological processes that arise in other (metabolic) organs. This information fuels a view of NAFLD being a complex, systemic disease influenced by a range of other organs. It is therefore likely that future management of NAFLD will require a systemic rather than a liver-specific approach.

2.3   Genetic Predisposition to NAFLD

NAFLD is considered a polygenic disease, implying the involvement of a variety of genetic factors in predisposing individuals to disease onset. While mutations in the patatin-like phospholipase domain-containing 3 (PNPLA3) gene were initially associated with hepatic steatosis (Romeo et al. 2008), other reports have also correlated the PNPLA3 variation to NASH progression (BasuRay et al. 2019; Valenti et al. 2010). Similarly, PNPLA3 genetic variants are also associated with carotid atherosclerosis in younger patients NAFLD (Petta et al. 2013). Though PNPLA3 variants were recently linked to the ubiquitylation processes (BasuRay et al. 2017), the exact underlying mechanism explaining the onset of NAFLD is still unclear.

Additionally, based on several population studies, it was recently described that mutations in the transmembrane 6 superfamily 2 (TM6SF2), a key regulator of very low-density lipoprotein (VLDL) export, correlated with NASH progression (Manne et al. 2018) and cardiovascular disease (Li et al. 2018), most likely via changes in plasma lipids. Indeed, plasma lipids appear to be one of the common denominators predicting severity of both NAFLD and coronary artery disease (Brouwers et al. 2019).

Further genetic screenings for NAFLD revealed that glucokinase regulator (*GCKR*) (Santoro et al. 2012) and lysophospholipid acyltransferase 7 (known as MBOAT7) (Mancina et al. 2016), key enzymes for glucose metabolism and reacetylation of phospholipids, respectively, as well as neurocan were associated with NAFLD development (Speliotes et al. 2011). Yet, a more recent study focusing on the aforementioned NAFLD-risk alleles (*PNPLA3, TM6SF2, GCKR,* and *LYPLAL1*) substantiated the heterogeneity of the NAFLD phenotype between patients, emphasizing the complexity of the disease (Sliz et al. 2018). As such, though genetic predisposition may influence disease onset, other pathophysiological factors that are independent of genetic predisposition are likely a stronger contributor to explain NAFLD development.

A line of research that has received increased attention is the influence of epigenetic changes on NAFLD development (Eslam et al. 2018). Epigenetic changes are induced by modifications in the regulators of DNA such as DNA methylation reactions, histone proteins, chromatin structure, and RNA-based mechanisms resulting in changes in genes expression (Eslam et al. 2018). These epigenetic modifications influence aging-related processes which contribute to NALFD (Horvath et al. 2014) but can also be transmitted to the progeny, thereby combining genetic and environmental factors involved in the development of disease. Mice that were rechallenged with a high-fat diet after being exposed to this diet during fetal life showed more several hepatic steatosis, inflammation, and fibrosis (Bruce et al. 2009). This influence of a detrimental fetal environment on NAFLD has been further substantiated by studies linking intrauterine growth retardation to increased risk of developing NAFLD (Nobili et al. 2007; Suomela et al. 2016; Valenti and Romeo 2016). Furthermore, methylation patterns of genes involved insulin signaling associated with the presence of NASH, which disappeared after bariatric surgery (Ahrens et al. 2013). As such, though being in its infancy, epigenetic modifications are expected to have an important role on NAFLD progression (Eslam et al. 2018).

3 Therapeutics

The involvement of different mechanisms in the pathogenesis of NAFLD also adds a level of complexity in finding appropriate therapeutic options to improve the different aspects of NAFLD. While therapies to reduce hepatic steatosis are known, a major problem is reversing the inflammatory component in the liver. Indeed, at present, no effective therapeutic approaches exist for reducing hepatic inflammation (Houben et al. 2017). From market size perspective, NASH-related therapeutics generated $1,179 million in 2017 and is estimated to reach $21,478 million by 2025 (Shinde 2018), pointing toward the huge demand for NASH treatments. Due to the magnitude of this health concern and its potential impact on healthcare, multiple treatments are currently being investigated with the aim to decrease inflammation and fibrosis (Oh et al. 2016). In this section, we provide a selection of currently investigated therapeutic approaches for NAFLD and demonstrate that these approaches are also investigated in the context of atherosclerosis (see Fig. 1). From this perspective, we further highlight the link between NAFLD and atherosclerosis.

3.1 Dietary/Lifestyle Intervention and Bariatric Surgery

Dietary changes and lifestyle interventions resulting in weight reduction are currently the first-line therapy for NAFLD patients (Sumida and Yoneda 2018). Indeed, dietary restriction is the most effective way to reduce liver fat (Marchesini et al. 2016; Patel et al. 2015). Furthermore, it has been suggested that hepatic triglyceride content normalizes after a few weeks under a strictly hypocaloric diet (Patel et al. 2015), i.e., low fat and low carbohydrate, which has been proposed as the optimal composition of a diet for NAFLD patients (Asrih and Jornayvaz 2014). Apart from dietary changes, lifestyle modification

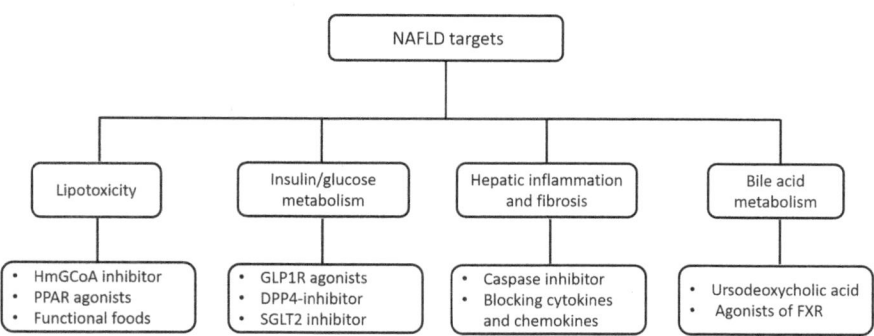

Fig. 1 Targets for NAFLD therapy. Besides exercise, changing the dietary pattern or surgical intervention and pharmacological intervention to improve NAFLD targets the pathological mechanisms of lipotoxicity, insulin/glucose metabolism, hepatic inflammation, fibrosis, as well as bile acid metabolism. *HmG-CoA* 3-hydroxy-3-methylglutarylcoenzyme A, *PPAR* peroxisome proliferator-activated receptor, *GLP1R* glucagon-like peptide-1 receptor, *DPP4* dipeptidyl peptidase-4, *SGLT2* sodium-glucose transport protein 2, *FXR* farnesoid X receptor

is another way to lose weight, for instance, via physical activity instead of sedentariness (Fabricatore 2007). However, compared to dietary restriction, physical activity is less effective in losing weight due to reduced caloric consumption as compared with dietary restriction (Marchesini et al. 2016; Zou et al. 2018). While dietary change and lifestyle intervention are able to reduce body weight, many patients cannot achere to these interventions. Therefore, bariatric surgery, and more recently termed metabolic surgery (Sasaki et al. 2014), typically results in massive weight loss and in concordant improvements in liver histology (Dixon et al. 2004). Indeed, Mummadi et al. reported that the resolution rates of steatosis, steatohepatitis, and fibrosis were 91.6%, 81.3%, and 65.5% in 15 studies using paired liver biopsies after bariatric surgery (Mummadi et al. 2008). Recently, a 1-year follow-up study by Nickel et al. also supported bariatric surgery as an effective treatment for NAFLD (Nickel et al. 2018). However, as not all NAFLD patients qualify for bariatric surgery, other interventions are necessary to combat NAFLD and related symptoms.

3.2   Targeting Lipotoxicity

As accumulation of lipids inside the liver comprises an essential component in the development of NAFLD, multiple therapeutic approaches have aimed to reduce hepatic lipids with the objective to concordantly reduce hepatic inflammation and fibrosis. The best known example of cholesterol-reducing agents are statins, which are drugs aimed at inhibiting 3-hydroxy-3-methylglutarylcoenzyme A (HmG-CoA) reductase, the rate-limiting enzyme in the cholesterol biosynthesis pathway (Stancu and Sima 2001). Showing beneficial results in the context of atherosclerosis (Bittencourt and Cerci 2015), statins were also investigated in

NAFLD progression. Though some improvements were observed in hepatic damage and inflammation (Kargiotis et al. 2014), other reports declare only minor improvements or even increasing levels of inflammation and fibrosis when statins are administered over a longer period of time (Hyogo et al. 2008). Moreover, recent observations pointing toward the detrimental effects of statins on aging and associated processes (Cholesterol Treatment Trialists 2019; Izadpanah et al. 2015) raise drawbacks for using these drugs under certain conditions.

Finally, and potentially, the most promising pharmacological compound currently under investigation to regress NASH are agonists of PPAR. PPARs are nuclear receptor proteins exerting key regulatory functions as transcription factors on metabolism, among other physiological processes (Dubois et al. 2017). Currently, three types of PPARs (being PPARα, PPARβ/δ, and PPARγ) are known and used as targets to improve MetS-related symptoms. In the context of NAFLD, and specifically NASH, the PPARγ agonist class thiazolidinediones has been shown to improve hepatic inflammation and advanced fibrosis (Bril et al. 2018; Musso et al. 2017). Furthermore, a new agonist, named elafibranor (or GFT505) that targets PPARα and PPARδ, was recently shown to improve hepatic inflammation and fibrosis, along with improvements in systemic inflammation, lipid, and glucose metabolism (Ratziu et al. 2016; Staels et al. 2013).

Due to these positive results, both thiazolidinediones and elafibranor are currently under clinical investigation for the treatment of NASH (Connolly et al. 2018). With regard to their application in atherosclerosis, thiazolidinediones have also been proven to slow progression of atherosclerosis in patients (Saremi et al. 2013), while elafibranor was so far not tested in this context. However, preliminary results in an atherosclerotic mouse model suggest that this latter PPARα/δ dual agonist might also be beneficial in the context of atherosclerosis (Graham et al. 2005).

Besides pharmacological intervention, a more convenient manner of reducing lipids is by means of dietary intervention. Apart from following dietary regimens in which the composition of lipids, protein, and carbohydrates is modulated and caloric intake is minimized (Ratziu et al. 2015) in order to achieve improvements in energy metabolism (Kargulewicz et al. 2014; Perumpail et al. 2017), another approach is to increase the intake of food components named functional foods. Plant sterol and stanol esters are examples of such functional foods that have been proven to reduce serum total and LDL cholesterol (Lichtenstein and Deckelbaum 2001; Plat et al. 2019), leading to improvements in atherosclerosis (Kohler et al. 2017) and NAFLD (Plat et al. 2014). However, more studies are necessary to prove the potential benefit of plant sterol and stanol esters in NAFLD patients.

3.3   Targeting Insulin/Glucose Metabolism

As diabetes has been associated with several stages of NAFLD (Hazlehurst et al. 2016), researchers have investigated the impact of improving insulin and glucose metabolism in order to improve aspects of NAFLD. Firstly, glucagon-like peptide-1 receptor (GLP1R) agonists, which mimic the function of incretins, are currently investigated in NAFLD (Gastaldelli and Marchesini 2016). GLP is a peptide derived from the L cells of the lower gastrointestinal tract (the small intestine and proximal colon) and known to enhance insulin secretion from pancreatic β cells and inhibit glucagon release from pancreatic α cells (Campbell and Drucker 2013; Ratziu et al. 2015). Whereas the GLP1R agonist exenatide enhanced hepatic steatosis (Tanaka et al. 2014), hepatic oxidative stress, and hepatic inflammation (Shao et al. 2018) and improved adipose tissue lipolysis in different in vivo models, the application of dulaglutide, lixisenatide, liraglutide, and, recently, semaglutide also shows promising results in terms of improvements in hepatic fat, damage, inflammation, and fibrosis (Armstrong et al. 2016; Cusi et al. 2018; Ipsen et al. 2018; Koutsovasilis et al. 2018; Petit et al. 2017; Rakipovski et al. 2018). As such, liraglutide (Armstrong et al. 2016) and semaglutide were under extensive clinical investigation. While liraglutide will not be further evaluated in phase 3 development, Novo Nordisk has initiated a phase 2b trial (NCT02970942) evaluating semaglutide versus placebo in 372 participants with stage F2-F3 fibrosis and NAS ≥ 4 with a score of at least 1 for each of the components (steatosis, ballooning, and lobular inflammation) (Connolly et al. 2018). Relevantly, as diabetes has also been linked to formation and progression of the atherosclerotic plaque (Beckman et al. 2002; Chait and Bornfeldt 2009; Katakami 2018), several GLP1R agonists have also been shown to improve atherosclerosis including exenatide, liraglutide, and semaglutide (Li et al. 2017; Marso et al. 2013; Rakipovski et al. 2018; Yang et al. 2017).

Besides the GLRP1 agonists, another approach to improve the GLP1-related effects on insulin and glucose metabolism is by administration of dipeptidyl peptidase-4 (DPP4) inhibitors. DPP4 (also referred to as CD26) is an enzyme known to degrade GLP1. Hence, inhibition of DPP4 enhances the activity of GLP1. While administration of the DPP4 inhibitor sitagliptin has been successfully applied in diabetic patients (Derosa et al. 2015; Drucker and Nauck 2006), several reports demonstrated only minor to no beneficial effects on hepatic fat content or hepatic fibrosis (Cui et al. 2016; Joy et al. 2017). Relevantly, these negative results in the context of NAFLD were also confirmed in atherosclerosis, showing only minor effects on coronary artery plaque improvement (Katakami et al. 2018; Nozue et al. 2016).

Another class of pharmacological compounds that specifically improve glucose metabolism is inhibitors for sodium-glucose transport protein 2 (SGLT2), a transporter protein in the kidney responsible for the reabsorption of glucose (Hsia et al. 2017; Marshall 2018; van Baar et al. 2018). In contrast to the minor effects of the DPP4 inhibitors on NAFLD, the SGLT2 inhibitors canagliflozin, ipragliflozin, and luseogliflozin all show substantial improvements in hepatic steatosis, apoptosis, and fibrosis in in vivo models and NAFLD patients (Ito et al. 2017; Kabil and Mahmoud 2018; Shiba et al. 2018; Shibuya et al. 2018; Sumida et al. 2019). In line with the previously described similarities between NAFLD and atherosclerosis, SGLT2 inhibitors were shown to also positively impact atherosclerosis progression and development (Nakatsu et al. 2017; Nasiri-Ansari et al. 2018; Tanaka et al. 2016; Zelniker et al. 2019).

Together, several treatments aimed at improving insulin or glucose metabolism have positive effects on several aspects of NAFLD, substantiating the role of insulin and glucose metabolism in the progression of NAFLD. Moreover, therapeutic products that improve features of NAFLD also positively impact atherosclerosis, providing further evidence for the similarities between NAFLD and atherosclerosis.

3.4 Targeting Hepatic Inflammation and Fibrosis

Another therapeutic approach to ameliorate NAFLD is to directly target components of the inflammatory and/or fibrotic pathway, as these features are the main cause for hepatic symptoms in NAFLD patients and are also responsible for the development toward advanced liver diseases (Schuster et al. 2018). The caspase inhibitor, emricasan, is one of those investigated compounds targeting the inflammatory aspect of NAFLD. Specifically, caspases are enzymes involved with several physiological processes including inflammation, making them an attractive inflammatory drug target. Administration of emricasan to NAFLD patients showed improvements in hepatic damage (as evidenced by reductions in alanine transaminase (ALT) levels) (Shiffman et al. 2019). However, recent negative results with this compound have questioned its continuation for further clinical investigation (Garcia-Tsao et al. 2019). Another potential caspase-related target for inflammatory drugs is blocking the activation of inflammasomes (Schuster et al. 2018). Indeed, inhibition of the P2X7 receptor, which is known to activate the NLRP3 inflammasome (Amores-Iniesta et al. 2017), via SGM-1019 resulted in improvements in hepatic inflammation and fibrosis in mouse models and NASH patients (Dabbagh et al. 2018), substantiating its further clinical investigation in NAFLD.

Another way to reduce inflammation and fibrosis is by blocking the effect of cytokines and chemokines that propagate the inflammatory reaction. With this regard, the C-C chemokine receptor type 2/C-C chemokine receptor 5 (CCR2/CCR5) inhibitor cenicriviroc has been successfully created. Specifically, cenicriviroc reduced hepatic fibrosis, inflammation, as well as systemic inflammatory parameters in NAFLD patients and animal models (Friedman et al. 2018; Lefebvre et al. 2016; Tacke 2018). Currently, cenicriviroc is being evaluated in phase 3 trials, targeting patients with F2-F3 fibrosis and having an anticipated enrollment of 2,000 participants (Connolly et al. 2018). Additionally, inhibition of galectin-3, a protein belonging to the lectin family and previously linked to NASH severity, has provided promising first results (Harrison et al. 2016), which need to be further validated. Finally, inhibition of apoptosis signal-regulating kinase 1 (ASK1) has also been investigated as drug target to reduce hepatic inflammation and fibrosis. ASK1 is part of the mitogen-activated protein kinase family and has been shown an essential role in NASH development in patients and mouse models (Wang et al. 2017; Xiang et al. 2016; Zhang et al. 2018). In line with this observation, inhibition of ASK1 using selonsertib has shown impressive improvements in hepatic inflammation and fibrosis

(Loomba et al. 2017; Younossi et al. 2018b). Selonsertib is currently under evaluation in two phase 3 clinical trials (STELLAR-3 [NCT03053050] and STELLAR-4 [NCT03053063]) for the treatment of NASH (Connolly et al. 2018).

Similar to the dual therapeutic effects of approaches targeting insulin and glucose metabolism, therapeutic approaches targeting inflammation and fibrosis also show dual positive influences in atherosclerosis and NASH. Galectin-3 has, for example, been linked atherosclerotic plaque progression (Papaspyridonos et al. 2008), and its inhibition results in reductions of atherosclerotic lesion size in vivo (MacKinnon et al. 2013). However, compared to drugs targeting insulin and glucose metabolism, targeting inflammation and fibrosis pathways is less investigated in the context of atherosclerosis, as exemplified by no described clinical studies for selonsertib, emricasan, ASK1 inhibitors, or cenicriviroc.

3.5   Targeting Bile Acid Metabolism

Hepatic components that have been extensively linked to different aspects of NAFLD include bile acids. Bile acids have regulatory functions on lipid and glucose metabolism, impact gut microbiota composition, and influence hepatic inflammation and damage (Schuster et al. 2018), explaining why modulation of bile acid metabolism has been an attractive therapeutic target for NAFLD. Firstly, the hepatoprotective natural bile acid ursodeoxycholic acid (UDCA) has been shown to exert beneficial effects on immune function, has anti-apoptotic and insulin-sensitizing effects, and reduces harmful effects of reactive oxygen species (Kars et al. 2010; Ljubuncic et al. 1996; Rodrigues et al. 1998), all aspects present during NAFLD. Indeed, besides improvements in hepatic steatosis, inflammation, and damage in NASH animal models, two randomized controlled trials showed improvements in lobular inflammation and hepatic fibrosis along with reductions in ALT levels upon UDCA administration (Leuschner et al. 2010; Ratziu et al. 2011). However, other studies showed no effect of UDCA administration in NASH patients (Liechti and Dufour 2012), emphasizing the need for further investigation. In addition, agonists of FXR, a nuclear receptor that has been linked to NAFLD (Zhang et al. 2009), have also been tested in NAFLD. Obeticholic acid (OCA), a semisynthetic variant of chenodeoxycholic acid, showed reductions in steatosis and fibrosis (Fiorucci et al. 2005; Goto et al. 2018), and recently, the first promising results were published from the FLINT study, investigated OCA in NAFLD patients (Neuschwander-Tetri et al. 2015). Currently, OCA is being evaluated in the phase 3 study REGENERATE (NCT02548351) for the treatment of NASH (Connolly et al. 2018).

Strikingly, though bile acids are produced by the liver, multiple evidences have pointed toward their systemic effects on inflammation, cell death, and apoptosis (Chiang 2013). As such, recent evidences have also shown beneficial effects of UDCA (Bode et al. 2016) and OCA (Hageman et al. 2010; Moris et al. 2017) in atherosclerotic models.

4 Conclusion

As the hepatic component of the MetS, NAFLD comprises one of the largest global health threats of the twenty-first century. Though the exact etiology of why NAFLD patients progress from hepatic steatosis to hepatic inflammation and fibrosis is unclear, several studies have established key pathophysiological processes contributing to hepatic inflammation. Considering this large amount of processes involved with NAFLD (which have intra- and extrahepatic origins), it is clear that NAFLD is a complex, systemic disease with high interindividual variation, pointing toward combination therapies or personalized medicine as potential future directions for NAFLD. Moreover, due to this systemic nature, it is clear that NAFLD and atherosclerosis are very closely linked (Bieghs et al. 2012), implying the liver as a potential target to manage atherosclerosis.

References

Abdelmalek MF (2016) NAFLD: the clinical and economic burden of NAFLD: time to turn the tide. Nat Rev Gastroenterol Hepatol 13:685–686

Ackerman Z, Oron-Herman M, Grozovski M, Rosenthal T, Pappo O, Link G, Sela BA (2005) Fructose-induced fatty liver disease: hepatic effects of blood pressure and plasma triglyceride reduction. Hypertension 45:1012–1018

Afendy A, Kallman JB, Stepanova M, Younoszai Z, Aquino RD, Bianchi G, Marchesini G, Younossi ZM (2009) Predictors of health-related quality of life in patients with chronic liver disease. Aliment Pharmacol Ther 30:469–476

Ahn SB, Jang K, Jun DW, Lee BH, Shin KJ (2014) Expression of liver X receptor correlates with intrahepatic inflammation and fibrosis in patients with nonalcoholic fatty liver disease. Dig Dis Sci 59:2975–2982

Ahrens M, Ammerpohl O, von Schonfels W, Kolarova J, Bens S, Itzel T, Teufel A, Herrmann A, Brosch M, Hinrichsen H, Erhart W, Egberts J, Sipos B, Schreiber S, Hasler R, Stickel F, Becker T, Krawczak M, Rocken C, Siebert R, Schafmayer C, Hampe J (2013) DNA methylation analysis in nonalcoholic fatty liver disease suggests distinct disease-specific and remodeling signatures after bariatric surgery. Cell Metab 18:296–302

Airaghi L, Rango M, Maira D, Barbieri V, Valenti L, Lombardi R, Biondetti P, Fargion S, Fracanzani AL (2018) Subclinical cerebrovascular disease in NAFLD without overt risk factors for atherosclerosis. Atherosclerosis 268:27–31

Albillos A, Lario M, Alvarez-Mon M (2014) Cirrhosis-associated immune dysfunction: distinctive features and clinical relevance. J Hepatol 61:1385–1396

Amores-Iniesta J, Barbera-Cremades M, Martinez CM, Pons JA, Revilla-Nuin B, Martinez-Alarcon L, di Virgilio F, Parrilla P, Baroja-Mazo A, Pelegrin P (2017) Extracellular ATP activates the NLRP3 inflammasome and is an early danger signal of skin allograft rejection. Cell Rep 21:3414–3426

Angulo P (2002) Nonalcoholic fatty liver disease. N Engl J Med 346:1221–1231

Angulo P, Kleiner DE, Dam-Larsen S, Adams LA, Bjornsson ES, Charatcharoenwitthaya P, Mills PR, Keach JC, Lafferty HD, Stahler A, Haflidadottir S, Bendtsen F (2015) Liver fibrosis, but no other histologic features, is associated with long-term outcomes of patients with nonalcoholic fatty liver disease. Gastroenterology 149:389–97.e10

Anstee QM, Day CP (2013) The genetics of NAFLD. Nat Rev Gastroenterol Hepatol 10:645–655

Araki O, Ying H, Zhu XG, Willingham MC, Cheng SY (2009) Distinct dysregulation of lipid metabolism by unliganded thyroid hormone receptor isoforms. Mol Endocrinol 23:308–315

Armstrong MJ, Gaunt P, Aithal GP, Barton D, Hull D, Parker R, Hazlehurst JM, Guo K, Team LT, Abouda G, Aldersley MA, Stocken D, Gough SC, Tomlinson JW, Brown RM, Hubscher SG, Newsome PN (2016) Liraglutide safety and efficacy in patients with non-alcoholic steatohepatitis (LEAN): a multicentre, double-blind, randomised, placebo-controlled phase 2 study. Lancet 387:679–690

Artwohl M, Lindenmair A, Sexl V, Maier C, Rainer G, Freudenthaler A, Huttary N, Wolzt M, Nowotny P, Luger A, Baumgartner-Parzer SM (2008) Different mechanisms of saturated versus polyunsaturated FFA-induced apoptosis in human endothelial cells. J Lipid Res 49:2627–2640

Ashraf NU, Sheikh TA (2015) Endoplasmic reticulum stress and oxidative stress in the pathogenesis of non-alcoholic fatty liver disease. Free Radic Res 49:1405–1418

Asrih M, Jornayvaz FR (2014) Diets and nonalcoholic fatty liver disease: the good and the bad. Clin Nutr 33:186–190

Balboa E, Castro J, Pinochet MJ, Cancino GI, Matias N, Saez PJ, Martinez A, Alvarez AR, Garcia-Ruiz C, Fernandez-Checa JC, Zanlungo S (2017) MLN64 induces mitochondrial dysfunction associated with increased mitochondrial cholesterol content. Redox Biol 12:274–284

Barber MC, Price NT, Travers MT (2005) Structure and regulation of acetyl-CoA carboxylase genes of metazoa. Biochim Biophys Acta 1733:1–28

Barbero-Camps E, Fernandez A, Baulies A, Martinez L, Fernandez-Checa JC, Colell A (2014) Endoplasmic reticulum stress mediates amyloid beta neurotoxicity via mitochondrial cholesterol trafficking. Am J Pathol 184:2066–2081

Basaranoglu M, Basaranoglu G, Bugianesi E (2015) Carbohydrate intake and nonalcoholic fatty liver disease: fructose as a weapon of mass destruction. Hepatobiliary Surg Nutr 4:109–116

BasuRay S, Smagris E, Cohen JC, Hobbs HH (2017) The PNPLA3 variant associated with fatty liver disease (I148M) accumulates on lipid droplets by evading ubiquitylation. Hepatology 66:1111–1124

BasuRay S, Wang Y, Smagris E, Cohen JC, Hobbs HH (2019) Accumulation of PNPLA3 on lipid droplets is the basis of associated hepatic steatosis. Proc Natl Acad Sci U S A 116:9521–9526

Baumeister SE, Volzke H, Marschall P, John U, Schmidt CO, Flessa S, Alte D (2008) Impact of fatty liver disease on health care utilization and costs in a general population: a 5-year observation. Gastroenterology 134:85–94

Beckman JA, Creager MA, Libby P (2002) Diabetes and atherosclerosis: epidemiology, pathophysiology, and management. JAMA 287:2570–2581

Bellentani S, Marino M (2009) Epidemiology and natural history of non-alcoholic fatty liver disease (NAFLD). Ann Hepatol 8(Suppl 1):S4–S8

Bellentani S, Saccoccio G, Masutti F, Croce LS, Brandi G, Sasso F, Cristanini G, Tiribelli C (2000) Prevalence of and risk factors for hepatic steatosis in northern Italy. Ann Intern Med 132:112–117

Bieghs V, Rensen PC, Hofker MH, Shiri-Sverdlov R (2012) NASH and atherosclerosis are two aspects of a shared disease: central role for macrophages. Atherosclerosis 220:287–293

Bieghs V, Walenbergh SM, Hendrikx T, van Gorp PJ, Verheyen F, Olde Damink SW, Masclee AA, Koek GH, Hofker MH, Binder CJ, Shiri-Sverdlov R (2013) Trapping of oxidized LDL in lysosomes of Kupffer cells is a trigger for hepatic inflammation. Liver Int 33:1056–1061

Bijnen M, Josefs T, Cuijpers I, Maalsen CJ, van de Gaar J, Vroomen M, Wijnands E, Rensen SS, Greve JWM, Hofker MH, Biessen EAL, Stehouwer CDA, Schalkwijk CG, Wouters K (2018) Adipose tissue macrophages induce hepatic neutrophil recruitment and macrophage accumulation in mice. Gut 67:1317–1327

Binder CJ, Horkko S, Dewan A, Chang MK, Kieu EP, Goodyear CS, Shaw PX, Palinski W, Witztum JL, Silverman GJ (2003) Pneumococcal vaccination decreases atherosclerotic lesion formation: molecular mimicry between Streptococcus pneumoniae and oxidized LDL. Nat Med 9:736–743

Bittencourt MS, Cerci RJ (2015) Statin effects on atherosclerotic plaques: regression or healing? BMC Med 13:260

Bode N, Grebe A, Kerksiek A, Lutjohann D, Werner N, Nickenig G, Latz E, Zimmer S (2016) Ursodeoxycholic acid impairs atherogenesis and promotes plaque regression by cholesterol crystal dissolution in mice. Biochem Biophys Res Commun 478:356–362

Boursier J, Fabron C, Lafuma A, Bureau I (2018) NASH/NAFLD patients with end stage liver disease experienced high inpatient hospitalization costs and substantial disease progression: results of a French national database on hospital care analysis. J Hepatol 68:S238–S239

Bril F, Kalavalapalli S, Clark VC, Lomonaco R, Soldevila-Pico C, Liu IC, Orsak B, Tio F, Cusi K (2018) Response to pioglitazone in patients with nonalcoholic steatohepatitis with vs without type 2 diabetes. Clin Gastroenterol Hepatol 16:558–566.e2

Brouwers M, Simons N, Stehouwer CDA, Koek GH, Schaper NC, Isaacs A (2019) Relationship between nonalcoholic fatty liver disease susceptibility genes and coronary artery disease. Hepatol Commun 3:587–596

Bruce KD, Cagampang FR, Argenton M, Zhang J, Ethirajan PL, Burdge GC, Bateman AC, Clough GF, Poston L, Hanson MA, McConnell JM, Byrne CD (2009) Maternal high-fat feeding primes steatohepatitis in adult mice offspring, involving mitochondrial dysfunction and altered lipogenesis gene expression. Hepatology 50:1796–1808

Busch CJ, Hendrikx T, Weismann D, Jackel S, Walenbergh SM, Rendeiro AF, Weisser J, Puhm F, Hladik A, Goderle L, Papac-Milicevic N, Haas G, Millischer V, Subramaniam S, Knapp S, Bennett KL, Bock C, Reinhardt C, Shiri-Sverdlov R, Binder CJ (2017) Malondialdehyde epitopes are sterile mediators of hepatic inflammation in hypercholesterolemic mice. Hepatology 65:1181–1195

Caballero F, Fernandez A, de Lacy AM, Fernandez-Checa JC, Caballeria J, Garcia-Ruiz C (2009) Enhanced free cholesterol, SREBP-2 and StAR expression in human NASH. J Hepatol 50:789–796

Cable EE, Finn PD, Stebbins JW, Hou J, Ito BR, van Poelje PD, Linemeyer DL, Erion MD (2009) Reduction of hepatic steatosis in rats and mice after treatment with a liver-targeted thyroid hormone receptor agonist. Hepatology 49:407–417

Cai C, Zhu X, Li P, Li J, Gong J, Shen W, He K (2017) NLRP3 deletion inhibits the non-alcoholic steatohepatitis development and inflammation in Kupffer cells induced by palmitic acid. Inflammation 40:1875–1883

Calzadilla Bertot L, Adams LA (2016) The natural course of non-alcoholic fatty liver disease. Int J Mol Sci 17:774

Campbell JE, Drucker DJ (2013) Pharmacology, physiology, and mechanisms of incretin hormone action. Cell Metab 17:819–837

Canfora EE, Meex RCR, Venema K, Blaak EE (2019) Gut microbial metabolites in obesity, NAFLD and T2DM. Nat Rev Endocrinol 15:261–273

Chait A, Bornfeldt KE (2009) Diabetes and atherosclerosis: is there a role for hyperglycemia? J Lipid Res 50(Suppl):S335–S339

Chalasani N, Younossi Z, Lavine JE, Diehl AM, Brunt EM, Cusi K, Charlton M, Sanyal AJ (2012) The diagnosis and management of non-alcoholic fatty liver disease: practice guideline by the American Association for the Study of Liver Diseases, American College of Gastroenterology, and the American Gastroenterological Association. Hepatology 55:2005–2023

Chalasani N, Younossi Z, Lavine JE, Charlton M, Cusi K, Rinella M, Harrison SA, Brunt EM, Sanyal AJ (2018) The diagnosis and management of nonalcoholic fatty liver disease: practice guidance from the American Association for the Study of Liver Diseases. Hepatology 67:328–357

Chambers ES, Preston T, Frost G, Morrison DJ (2018) Role of gut microbiota-generated short-chain fatty acids in metabolic and cardiovascular health. Curr Nutr Rep 7:198–206

Charach G, Argov O, Geiger K, Charach L, Rogowski O, Grosskopf I (2018) Diminished bile acids excretion is a risk factor for coronary artery disease: 20-year follow up and long-term outcome. Ther Adv Gastroenterol 11. https://doi.org/10.1177/1756283X17743420

Chiang JY (2013) Bile acid metabolism and signaling. Compr Physiol 3:1191–1212

Chinen I, Shimabukuro M, Yamakawa K, Higa N, Matsuzaki T, Noguchi K, Ueda S, Sakanashi M, Takasu N (2007) Vascular lipotoxicity: endothelial dysfunction via fatty-acid-induced reactive oxygen species overproduction in obese Zucker diabetic fatty rats. Endocrinology 148:160–165

Cholesterol Treatment Trialists (2019) Efficacy and safety of statin therapy in older people: a meta-analysis of individual participant data from 28 randomised controlled trials. Lancet 393:407–415

Chu X, Jin Q, Chen H, Wood GC, Petrick A, Strodel W, Gabrielsen J, Benotti P, Mirshahi T, Carey DJ, Still CD, DiStefano JK, Gerhard GS (2018) CCL20 is up-regulated in non-alcoholic fatty liver disease fibrosis and is produced by hepatic stellate cells in response to fatty acid loading. J Transl Med 16:108

Colombini M (2010) Ceramide channels and their role in mitochondria-mediated apoptosis. Biochim Biophys Acta 1797:1239–1244

Connolly JJ, Ooka K, Lim JK (2018) Future pharmacotherapy for non-alcoholic steatohepatitis (NASH): review of phase 2 and 3 trials. J Clin Transl Hepatol 6:264–275

Cui J, Philo L, Nguyen P, Hofflich H, Hernandez C, Bettencourt R, Richards L, Salotti J, Bhatt A, Hooker J, Haufe W, Hooker C, Brenner DA, Sirlin CB, Loomba R (2016) Sitagliptin vs. placebo for non-alcoholic fatty liver disease: a randomized controlled trial. J Hepatol 65:369–376

Cusi K, Sattar N, Garcia-Perez LE, Pavo I, Yu M, Robertson KE, Karanikas CA, Haupt A (2018) Dulaglutide decreases plasma aminotransferases in people with type 2 diabetes in a pattern consistent with liver fat reduction: a post hoc analysis of the AWARD programme. Diabet Med 35:1434–1439

Dabbagh K, Dodson GS, Yamamoto L, Baeza-Raja B, Goodyear AW (2018) Preclinical and first-in human development of SGM-1019, a first-in-class novel small molecule modulator of inflammasome activity for the treatment of nonalcoholic steatohepatitis (NASH). J Hepatol 68:S60–S60

Dan AA, Kallman JB, Wheeler A, Younoszai Z, Collantes R, Bondini S, Gerber L, Younossi ZM (2007) Health-related quality of life in patients with non-alcoholic fatty liver disease. Aliment Pharmacol Ther 26:815–820

Davis PJ, Goglia F, Leonard JL (2016) Nongenomic actions of thyroid hormone. Nat Rev Endocrinol 12:111–121

Derosa G, D'Angelo A, Maffioli P (2015) Sitagliptin in type 2 diabetes mellitus: efficacy after five years of therapy. Pharmacol Res 100:127–134

Dixon JB, Bhathal PS, Hughes NR, O'Brien PE (2004) Nonalcoholic fatty liver disease: improvement in liver histological analysis with weight loss. Hepatology 39:1647–1654

Dominguez-Perez M, Simoni-Nieves A, Rosales P, Nuno-Lambarri N, Rosas-Lemus M, Souza V, Miranda RU, Bucio L, Uribe Carvajal S, Marquardt JU, Seo D, Gomez-Quiroz LE, Gutierrez-Ruiz MC (2019) Cholesterol burden in the liver induces mitochondrial dynamic changes and resistance to apoptosis. J Cell Physiol 234:7213–7223

Drosatos K, Schulze PC (2013) Cardiac lipotoxicity: molecular pathways and therapeutic implications. Curr Heart Fail Rep 10:109–121

Drucker DJ, Nauck MA (2006) The incretin system: glucagon-like peptide-1 receptor agonists and dipeptidyl peptidase-4 inhibitors in type 2 diabetes. Lancet 368:1696–1705

Dubois V, Eeckhoute J, Lefebvre P, Staels B (2017) Distinct but complementary contributions of PPAR isotypes to energy homeostasis. J Clin Invest 127:1202–1214

Duewell P, Kono H, Rayner KJ, Sirois CM, Vladimer G, Bauernfeind FG, Abela GS, Franchi L, Nunez G, Schnurr M, Espevik T, Lien E, Fitzgerald KA, Rock KL, Moore KJ, Wright SD, Hornung V, Latz E (2010) NLRP3 inflammasomes are required for atherogenesis and activated by cholesterol crystals. Nature 464:1357–1361

Dumas ME, Barton RH, Toye A, Cloarec O, Blancher C, Rothwell A, Fearnside J, Tatoud R, Blanc V, Lindon JC, Mitchell SC, Holmes E, McCarthy MI, Scott J, Gauguier D, Nicholson JK (2006) Metabolic profiling reveals a contribution of gut microbiota to fatty liver phenotype in insulin-resistant mice. Proc Natl Acad Sci U S A 103:12511–12516

Duntas LH (2002) Thyroid disease and lipids. Thyroid 12:287–293

Ekstedt M, Hagstrom H, Nasr P, Fredrikson M, Stal P, Kechagias S, Hultcrantz R (2015) Fibrosis stage is the strongest predictor for disease-specific mortality in NAFLD after up to 33 years of follow-up. Hepatology 61:1547–1554

El-Serag HB, Rudolph KL (2007) Hepatocellular carcinoma: epidemiology and molecular carcinogenesis. Gastroenterology 132:2557–2576

Elwing JE, Lustman PJ, Wang HL, Clouse RE (2006) Depression, anxiety, and nonalcoholic steatohepatitis. Psychosom Med 68:563–569

Engin AB (2017) What is lipotoxicity? Adv Exp Med Biol 960:197–220

Erbay E, Babaev VR, Mayers JR, Makowski L, Charles KN, Snitow ME, Fazio S, Wiest MM, Watkins SM, Linton MF, Hotamisligil GS (2009) Reducing endoplasmic reticulum stress through a macrophage lipid chaperone alleviates atherosclerosis. Nat Med 15:1383–1391

Eslam M, Valenti L, Romeo S (2018) Genetics and epigenetics of NAFLD and NASH: clinical impact. J Hepatol 68:268–279

Estes C, Razavi H, Loomba R, Younossi Z, Sanyal AJ (2018) Modeling the epidemic of nonalcoholic fatty liver disease demonstrates an exponential increase in burden of disease. Hepatology 67:123–133

Fabricatore AN (2007) Behavior therapy and cognitive-behavioral therapy of obesity: is there a difference? J Am Diet Assoc 107:92–99

Fassio E, Alvarez E, Dominguez N, Landeira G, Longo C (2004) Natural history of nonalcoholic steatohepatitis: a longitudinal study of repeat liver biopsies. Hepatology 40:820–826

Fazel Y, Koenig AB, Sayiner M, Goodman ZD, Younossi ZM (2016) Epidemiology and natural history of non-alcoholic fatty liver disease. Metabolism 65:1017–1025

Feldstein AE, Lopez R, Tamimi TA, Yerian L, Chung YM, Berk M, Zhang R, McIntyre TM, Hazen SL (2010) Mass spectrometric profiling of oxidized lipid products in human nonalcoholic fatty liver disease and nonalcoholic steatohepatitis. J Lipid Res 51:3046–3054

Ference BA, Ginsberg HN, Graham I, Ray KK, Packard CJ, Bruckert E, Hegele RA, Krauss RM, Raal FJ, Schunkert H, Watts GF, Boren J, Fazio S, Horton JD, Masana L, Nicholls SJ, Nordestgaard BG, van de Sluis B, Taskinen MR, Tokgozoglu L, Landmesser U, Laufs U, Wiklund O, Stock JK, Chapman MJ, Catapano AL (2017) Low-density lipoproteins cause atherosclerotic cardiovascular disease. 1. Evidence from genetic, epidemiologic, and clinical studies. A consensus statement from the European Atherosclerosis Society Consensus Panel. Eur Heart J 38:2459–2472

Finkel T, Holbrook NJ (2000) Oxidants, oxidative stress and the biology of ageing. Nature 408:239–247

Fiorucci S, Rizzo G, Antonelli E, Renga B, Mencarelli A, Riccardi L, Morelli A, Pruzanski M, Pellicciari R (2005) Cross-talk between farnesoid-X-receptor (FXR) and peroxisome proliferator-activated receptor gamma contributes to the antifibrotic activity of FXR ligands in rodent models of liver cirrhosis. J Pharmacol Exp Ther 315:58–68

Francque S, Verrijken A, Caron S, Prawitt J, Paumelle R, Derudas B, Lefebvre P, Taskinen MR, van Hul W, Mertens I, Hubens G, van Marck E, Michielsen P, van Gaal L, Staels B (2015) PPARalpha gene expression correlates with severity and histological treatment response in patients with non-alcoholic steatohepatitis. J Hepatol 63:164–173

Friedman SL (1993) Seminars in medicine of the Beth Israel Hospital, Boston. The cellular basis of hepatic fibrosis. Mechanisms and treatment strategies. N Engl J Med 328:1828–1835

Friedman SL, Ratziu V, Harrison SA, Abdelmalek MF, Aithal GP, Caballeria J, Francque S, Farrell G, Kowdley KV, Craxi A, Simon K, Fischer L, Melchor-Khan L, Vest J, Wiens BL, Vig P, Seyedkazemi S, Goodman Z, Wong VW, Loomba R, Tacke F, Sanyal A, Lefebvre E (2018) A randomized, placebo-controlled trial of cenicriviroc for treatment of nonalcoholic steatohepatitis with fibrosis. Hepatology 67:1754–1767

Garcia-Tsao G, Bosch J, Kayali Z, Harrison S, Abdelmalek M, Lawitz E, Satapathy S, Ghabril M, Shiffman M, Younes ZH, Thuluvath PJ, Berzigotti A, Albillos A, Robinson J, Chan JL, Hagerty D, Sanyal A (2019) Multicenter, double-blind, placebo-controlled, randomized trial of emricasan in subjects with NASH cirrhosis and severe portal hypertension. J Hepatol 70:E127–E127

Gastaldelli A, Marchesini G (2016) Time for glucagon like peptide-1 receptor agonists treatment for patients with NAFLD? J Hepatol 64:262–264

Ghareeb DA, Hafez HS, Hussien HM, Kabapy NF (2011) Non-alcoholic fatty liver induces insulin resistance and metabolic disorders with development of brain damage and dysfunction. Metab Brain Dis 26:253–267

Golabi P, Otgonsuren M, Cable R, Felix S, Koenig A, Sayiner M, Younossi ZM (2016) Non-alcoholic fatty liver disease (NAFLD) is associated with impairment of health related quality of life (HRQOL). Health Qual Life Outcomes 14:18

Goto T, Itoh M, Suganami T, Kanai S, Shirakawa I, Sakai T, Asakawa M, Yoneyama T, Kai T, Ogawa Y (2018) Obeticholic acid protects against hepatocyte death and liver fibrosis in a murine model of nonalcoholic steatohepatitis. Sci Rep 8:8157

Graham TL, Mookherjee C, Suckling KE, Palmer CN, Patel L (2005) The PPARdelta agonist GW0742X reduces atherosclerosis in LDLR(−/−) mice. Atherosclerosis 181:29–37

Grebe A, Hoss F, Latz E (2018) NLRP3 inflammasome and the IL-1 pathway in atherosclerosis. Circ Res 122:1722–1740

Gregory JC, Buffa JA, Org E, Wang Z, Levison BS, Zhu W, Wagner MA, Bennett BJ, Li L, DiDonato JA, Lusis AJ, Hazen SL (2015) Transmission of atherosclerosis susceptibility with gut microbial transplantation. J Biol Chem 290:5647–5660

Guo Y, Yuan W, Yu B, Kuai R, Hu W, Morin EE, Garcia-Barrio MT, Zhang J, Moon JJ, Schwendeman A, Eugene Chen Y (2018) Synthetic high-density lipoprotein-mediated targeted delivery of liver x receptors agonist promotes atherosclerosis regression. EBioMedicine 28:225–233

Hageman J, Herrema H, Groen AK, Kuipers F (2010) A role of the bile salt receptor FXR in atherosclerosis. Arterioscler Thromb Vasc Biol 30:1519–1528

Han MS, Park SY, Shinzawa K, Kim S, Chung KW, Lee JH, Kwon CH, Lee KW, Lee JH, Park CK, Chung WJ, Hwang JS, Yan JJ, Song DK, Tsujimoto Y, Lee MS (2008) Lysophosphatidylcholine as a death effector in the lipoapoptosis of hepatocytes. J Lipid Res 49:84–97

Harrison SA, Marri SR, Chalasani N, Kohli R, Aronstein W, Thompson GA, Irish W, Miles MV, Xanthakos SA, Lawitz E, Noureddin M, Schiano TD, Siddiqui M, Sanyal A, Neuschwander-Tetri BA, Traber PG (2016) Randomised clinical study: GR-MD-02, a galectin-3 inhibitor, vs. placebo in patients having non-alcoholic steatohepatitis with advanced fibrosis. Aliment Pharmacol Ther 44:1183–1198

Hazlehurst JM, Woods C, Marjot T, Cobbold JF, Tomlinson JW (2016) Non-alcoholic fatty liver disease and diabetes. Metabolism 65:1096–1108

Hendrikx T, Bieghs V, Walenbergh SM, van Gorp PJ, Verheyen F, Jeurissen ML, Steinbusch MM, Vaes N, Binder CJ, Koek GH, Stienstra R, Netea MG, Hofker MH, Shiri-Sverdlov R (2013) Macrophage specific caspase-1/11 deficiency protects against cholesterol crystallization and hepatic inflammation in hyperlipidemic mice. PLoS One 8:e78792

Hendrikx T, Jeurissen ML, Bieghs V, Walenbergh SM, van Gorp PJ, Verheyen F, Houben T, Guichot YD, Gijbels MJ, Leitersdorf E, Hofker MH, Lutjohann D, Shiri-Sverdlov R (2015) Hematopoietic overexpression of Cyp27a1 reduces hepatic inflammation independently of 27-hydroxycholesterol levels in Ldlr(−/−) mice. J Hepatol 62:430–436

Horvath S, Erhart W, Brosch M, Ammerpohl O, von Schonfels W, Ahrens M, Heits N, Bell JT, Tsai PC, Spector TD, Deloukas P, Siebert R, Sipos B, Becker T, Rocken C, Schafmayer C, Hampe J (2014) Obesity accelerates epigenetic aging of human liver. Proc Natl Acad Sci U S A 111:15538–15543

Hotamisligil GS (2010) Endoplasmic reticulum stress and the inflammatory basis of metabolic disease. Cell 140:900–917

Houben T, Brandsma E, Walenbergh SMA, Hofker MH, Shiri-Sverdlov R (2017) Oxidized LDL at the crossroads of immunity in non-alcoholic steatohepatitis. Biochim Biophys Acta Mol Cell Biol Lipids 1862:416–429

Hsia DS, Grove O, Cefalu WT (2017) An update on sodium-glucose co-transporter-2 inhibitors for the treatment of diabetes mellitus. Curr Opin Endocrinol Diabetes Obes 24:73–79

Hyogo H, Tazuma S, Arihiro K, Iwamoto K, Nabeshima Y, Inoue M, Ishitobi T, Nonaka M, Chayama K (2008) Efficacy of atorvastatin for the treatment of nonalcoholic steatohepatitis with dyslipidemia. Metabolism 57:1711–1718

Ibrahim SH, Kohli R, Gores GJ (2011) Mechanisms of lipotoxicity in NAFLD and clinical implications. J Pediatr Gastroenterol Nutr 53:131–140

Ipsen DH, Rolin B, Rakipovski G, Skovsted GF, Madsen A, Kolstrup S, Schou-Pedersen AM, Skat-Rordam J, Lykkesfeldt J, Tveden-Nyborg P (2018) Liraglutide decreases hepatic inflammation and injury in advanced lean non-alcoholic steatohepatitis. Basic Clin Pharmacol Toxicol 123:704–713

Ito D, Shimizu S, Inoue K, Saito D, Yanagisawa M, Inukai K, Akiyama Y, Morimoto Y, Noda M, Shimada A (2017) Comparison of ipragliflozin and pioglitazone effects on nonalcoholic fatty liver disease in patients with type 2 diabetes: a randomized, 24-week, open-label, active-controlled trial. Diabetes Care 40:1364–1372

Izadpanah R, Schachtele DJ, Pfnur AB, Lin D, Slakey DP, Kadowitz PJ, Alt EU (2015) The impact of statins on biological characteristics of stem cells provides a novel explanation for their pleiotropic beneficial and adverse clinical effects. Am J Physiol Cell Physiol 309:C522–C531

Jerome WG (2010) Lysosomes, cholesterol and atherosclerosis. Clin Lipidol 5:853–865

Jou J, Choi SS, Diehl AM (2008) Mechanisms of disease progression in nonalcoholic fatty liver disease. Semin Liver Dis 28:370–379

Joy TR, McKenzie CA, Tirona RG, Summers K, Seney S, Chakrabarti S, Malhotra N, Beaton MD (2017) Sitagliptin in patients with non-alcoholic steatohepatitis: a randomized, placebo-controlled trial. World J Gastroenterol 23:141–150

Kabil SL, Mahmoud NM (2018) Canagliflozin protects against non-alcoholic steatohepatitis in type-2 diabetic rats through zinc alpha-2 glycoprotein up-regulation. Eur J Pharmacol 828:135–145

Kadayifci A, Tan V, Ursell PC, Merriman RB, Bass NM (2008) Clinical and pathologic risk factors for atherosclerosis in cirrhosis: a comparison between NASH-related cirrhosis and cirrhosis due to other aetiologies. J Hepatol 49:595–599

Kaden-Volynets V, Basic M, Neumann U, Pretz D, Rings A, Bleich A, Bischoff SC (2018) Lack of liver steatosis in germ-free mice following hypercaloric diets. Eur J Nutr 58:1933–1945

Kakisaka K, Cazanave SC, Fingas CD, Guicciardi ME, Bronk SF, Werneburg NW, Mott JL, Gores GJ (2012) Mechanisms of lysophosphatidylcholine-induced hepatocyte lipoapoptosis. Am J Physiol Gastrointest Liver Physiol 302:G77–G84

Kalaany NY, Mangelsdorf DJ (2006) LXRS and FXR: the yin and yang of cholesterol and fat metabolism. Annu Rev Physiol 68:159–191

Kargiotis K, Katsiki N, Athyros VG, Giouleme O, Patsiaoura K, Katsiki E, Mikhailidis DP, Karagiannis A (2014) Effect of rosuvastatin on non-alcoholic steatohepatitis in patients with metabolic syndrome and hypercholesterolaemia: a preliminary report. Curr Vasc Pharmacol 12:505–511

Kargulewicz A, Stankowiak-Kulpa H, Grzymislawski M (2014) Dietary recommendations for patients with nonalcoholic fatty liver disease. Przeglad Gastroenterol 9:18–23

Kars M, Yang L, Gregor MF, Mohammed BS, Pietka TA, Finck BN, Patterson BW, Horton JD, Mittendorfer B, Hotamisligil GS, Klein S (2010) Tauroursodeoxycholic acid may improve liver and muscle but not adipose tissue insulin sensitivity in obese men and women. Diabetes 59:1899–1905

Katakami N (2018) Mechanism of development of atherosclerosis and cardiovascular disease in diabetes mellitus. J Atheroscler Thromb 25:27–39

Katakami N, Mita T, Irie Y, Takahara M, Matsuoka TA, Gosho M, Watada H, Shimomura I, Sitagliptin Preventive study of Intima-media thickness Evaluation C (2018) Effect of sitagliptin on tissue characteristics of the carotid wall in patients with type 2 diabetes: a post hoc sub-analysis of the sitagliptin preventive study of intima-media thickness evaluation (SPIKE). Cardiovasc Diabetol 17:24

Kim DG, Krenz A, Toussaint LE, Maurer KJ, Robinson SA, Yan A, Torres L, Bynoe MS (2016) Non-alcoholic fatty liver disease induces signs of Alzheimer's disease (AD) in wild-type mice and accelerates pathological signs of AD in an AD model. J Neuroinflammation 13:1

Kim BM, Abdelfattah AM, Vasan R, Fuchs BC, Choi MY (2018) Hepatic stellate cells secrete Ccl5 to induce hepatocyte steatosis. Sci Rep 8:7499

Kitabatake H, Tanaka N, Fujimori N, Komatsu M, Okubo A, Kakegawa K, Kimura T, Sugiura A, Yamazaki T, Shibata S, Ichikawa Y, Joshita S, Umemura T, Matsumoto A, Koinuma M, Sano K, Aoyama T, Tanaka E (2017) Association between endotoxemia and histological features of nonalcoholic fatty liver disease. World J Gastroenterol 23:712–722

Kohjima M, Enjoji M, Higuchi N, Kato M, Kotoh K, Yoshimoto T, Fujino T, Yada M, Yada R, Harada N, Takayanagi R, Nakamuta M (2007) Re-evaluation of fatty acid metabolism-related gene expression in nonalcoholic fatty liver disease. Int J Mol Med 20:351–358

Kohler J, Teupser D, Elsasser A, Weingartner O (2017) Plant sterol enriched functional food and atherosclerosis. Br J Pharmacol 174:1281–1289

Koruk M, Savas MC, Yilmaz O, Taysi S, Karakok M, Gundogdu C, Yilmaz A (2003) Serum lipids, lipoproteins and apolipoproteins levels in patients with nonalcoholic steatohepatitis. J Clin Gastroenterol 37:177–182

Koutsovasilis A, Sotiropoulos A, Papadaki D, Bletsa E, Kokotos G, Kounelakis I, Bousboulas S, Peppas T (2018) Qualitative and quantitative effect of IDegLira compared with the nonfixed administration of degludec and liraglutide. Diabetes 67. https://doi.org/10.2337/db18-1104-P

Kwon O, Kim KW, Kim MS (2016) Leptin signalling pathways in hypothalamic neurons. Cell Mol Life Sci 73:1457–1477

Lam C, Bandsma R, Ling S, Mouzaki M (2016) More frequent clinic visits are associated with improved outcomes for children with NAFLD. Can J Gastroenterol Hepatol 2016:8205494

Lammel Lindemann J, Webb P (2016) Sobetirome: the past, present and questions about the future. Expert Opin Ther Targets 20:145–149

Lara-Guzman OJ, Gil-Izquierdo A, Medina S, Osorio E, Alvarez-Quintero R, Zuluaga N, Oger C, Galano JM, Durand T, Munoz-Durango K (2018) Oxidized LDL triggers changes in oxidative stress and inflammatory biomarkers in human macrophages. Redox Biol 15:1–11

Lee S, Birukov KG, Romanoski CE, Springstead JR, Lusis AJ, Berliner JA (2012) Role of phospholipid oxidation products in atherosclerosis. Circ Res 111:778–799

Lefebvre E, Moyle G, Reshef R, Richman LP, Thompson M, Hong F, Chou HI, Hashiguchi T, Plato C, Poulin D, Richards T, Yoneyama H, Jenkins H, Wolfgang G, Friedman SL (2016) Antifibrotic effects of the dual CCR2/CCR5 antagonist cenicriviroc in animal models of liver and kidney fibrosis. PLoS One 11(6):e0158156

Leuschner UF, Lindenthal B, Herrmann G, Arnold JC, Rossle M, Cordes HJ, Zeuzem S, Hein J, Berg T, Group NS (2010) High-dose ursodeoxycholic acid therapy for nonalcoholic steatohepatitis: a double-blind, randomized, placebo-controlled trial. Hepatology 52:472–479

Levey AS, Eckardt KU, Tsukamoto Y, Levin A, Coresh J, Rossert J, de Zeeuw D, Hostetter TH, Lameire N, Eknoyan G (2005) Definition and classification of chronic kidney disease: a position statement from kidney disease: improving global outcomes (KDIGO). Kidney Int 67:2089–2100

Li J, Liu X, Fang Q, Ding M, Li C (2017) Liraglutide attenuates atherosclerosis via inhibiting ER-induced macrophage derived microvesicles production in T2DM rats. Diabetol Metab Syndr 9:94

Li B, Zhang C, Zhan YT (2018) Nonalcoholic fatty liver disease cirrhosis: a review of its epidemiology, risk factors, clinical presentation, diagnosis, management, and prognosis. Can J Gastroenterol 2018:2784537

Li J, Zou B, Yeo YH, Feng Y, Xie X, Lee DH, Fujii H, Wu Y, Kam LY, Ji F, Li X, Chien N, Wei M, Ogawa E, Zhao C, Wu X, Stave CD, Henry L, Barnett S, Takahashi H, Furusyo N, Eguchi Y, Hsu YC, Lee TY, Ren W, Qin C, Jun DW, Toyoda H, Wong VW, Cheung R, Zhu Q, Nguyen MH (2019) Prevalence, incidence, and outcome of non-alcoholic fatty liver disease in Asia, 1999-2019: a systematic review and meta-analysis. Lancet Gastroenterol Hepatol 4:389–398

Lichtenstein AH, Deckelbaum RJ (2001) AHA science advisory. Stanol/sterol ester-containing foods and blood cholesterol levels. A statement for healthcare professionals from the Nutrition Committee of the Council on nutrition, physical activity, and metabolism of the American Heart Association. Circulation 103:1177–1179

Liechti F, Dufour JF (2012) Treatment of NASH with ursodeoxycholic acid: cons. Clin Res Hepatol Gastroenterol 36(Suppl 1):S46–S52

Lin CS, Hsieh PS, Hwang LL, Lee YH, Tsai SH, Tu YC, Hung YW, Liu CC, Chuang YP, Liao MT, Chien S, Tsai MC (2018) The CCL5/CCR5 axis promotes vascular smooth muscle cell proliferation and atherogenic phenotype switching. Cell Physiol Biochem 47:707–720

Lindenmeyer CC, McCullough AJ (2018) The natural history of nonalcoholic fatty liver disease-an evolving view. Clin Liver Dis 22:11–21

Ljubuncic P, Fuhrman B, Oiknine J, Aviram M, Bomzon A (1996) Effect of deoxycholic acid and ursodeoxycholic acid on lipid peroxidation in cultured macrophages. Gut 39:475–478

Lombardi R, Fargion S, Fracanzani AL (2019) Brain involvement in non-alcoholic fatty liver disease (NAFLD): a systematic review. Dig Liver Dis 51(9):1214–1222

Loomba R, Lawitz E, Mantry PS, Jayakumar S, Caldwell SH, Arnold H, Diehl AM, Djedjos CS, Han L, Myers RP, Subramanian GM, McHutchison JG, Goodman ZD, Afdhal NH, Charlton MR, Investigators G.U (2017) The ASK1 inhibitor selonsertib in patients with nonalcoholic steatohepatitis: a randomized, phase 2 trial. Hepatology 67:549–559

Loria A, Escheik C, Gerber NL, Younossi ZM (2013) Quality of life in cirrhosis. Curr Gastroenterol Rep 15:301

Macavei B, Baban A, Dumitrascu DL (2016) Psychological factors associated with NAFLD/ NASH: a systematic review. Eur Rev Med Pharmacol Sci 20:5081–5097

MacKinnon AC, Liu X, Hadoke PW, Miller MR, Newby DE, Sethi T (2013) Inhibition of galectin-3 reduces atherosclerosis in apolipoprotein E-deficient mice. Glycobiology 23:654–663

Mancina RM, Dongiovanni P, Petta S, Pingitore P, Meroni M, Rametta R, Boren J, Montalcini T, Pujia A, Wiklund O, Hindy G, Spagnuolo R, Motta BM, Pipitone RM, Craxi A, Fargion S, Nobili V, Kakela P, Karja V, Mannisto V, Pihlajamaki J, Reilly DF, Castro-Perez J, Kozlitina J, Valenti L, Romeo S (2016) The MBOAT7-TMC4 variant rs641738 increases risk of nonalcoholic fatty liver disease in individuals of European descent. Gastroenterology 150(1219–1230):e6

Mancuso P (2016) The role of adipokines in chronic inflammation. Immunotargets Ther 5:47–56

Manne V, Handa P, Kowdley KV (2018) Pathophysiology of nonalcoholic fatty liver disease/ nonalcoholic steatohepatitis. Clin Liver Dis 22:23–37

Marchesini G, Petta S, Dalle Grave R (2016) Diet, weight loss, and liver health in nonalcoholic fatty liver disease: pathophysiology, evidence, and practice. Hepatology 63:2032–2043

Marcuccilli M, Chonchol M (2016) NAFLD and chronic kidney disease. Int J Mol Sci 17:562

Marshall SM (2018) The bark giving diabetes therapy some bite: the SGLT inhibitors. Diabetologia 61:2075–2078

Marso SP, Poulter NR, Nissen SE, Nauck MA, Zinman B, Daniels GH, Pocock S, Steinberg WM, Bergenstal RM, Mann JF, Ravn LS, Frandsen KB, Moses AC, Buse JB (2013) Design of the liraglutide effect and action in diabetes: evaluation of cardiovascular outcome results (LEADER) trial. Am Heart J 166:823–30.e5

Martinet W, de Meyer GR (2009) Autophagy in atherosclerosis: a cell survival and death phenomenon with therapeutic potential. Circ Res 104:304–317

Martinez-Guryn K, Hubert N, Frazier K, Urlass S, Musch MW, Ojeda P, Pierre JF, Miyoshi J, Sontag TJ, Cham CM, Reardon CA, Leone V, Chang EB (2018) Small intestine microbiota regulate host digestive and absorptive adaptive responses to dietary lipids. Cell Host Microbe 23:458–469.e5

Masarone M, Rosato V, Dallio M, Gravina AG, Aglitti A, Loguercio C, Federico A, Persico M (2018) Role of oxidative stress in pathophysiology of nonalcoholic fatty liver disease. Oxidative Med Cell Longev 2018:9547613

Maslak E, Buczek E, Szumny A, Szczepnski W, Franczyk-Zarow M, Kopec A, Chlopicki S, Leszczynska T, Kostogrys RB (2015) Individual CLA isomers, c9t11 and t10c12, prevent excess liver glycogen storage and inhibit lipogenic genes expression induced by high-fructose diet in rats. Biomed Res Int 2015:535982

Matsuda T, Hiyama TY, Niimura F, Matsusaka T, Fukamizu A, Kobayashi K, Kobayashi K, Noda M (2017) Distinct neural mechanisms for the control of thirst and salt appetite in the subfornical organ. Nat Neurosci 20:230–241

Matsumoto M, Zhang J, Zhang X, Liu J, Jiang JX, Yamaguchi K, Taruno A, Katsuyama M, Iwata K, Ibi M, Cui W, Matsuno K, Marunaka Y, Itoh Y, Torok NJ, Yabe-Nishimura C (2018) The NOX1 isoform of NADPH oxidase is involved in dysfunction of liver sinusoids in nonalcoholic fatty liver disease. Free Radic Biol Med 115:412–420

Matsuzawa N, Takamura T, Kurita S, Misu H, Ota T, Ando H, Yokoyama M, Honda M, Zen Y, Nakanuma Y, Miyamoto K, Kaneko S (2007) Lipid-induced oxidative stress causes steatohepatitis in mice fed an atherogenic diet. Hepatology 46:1392–1403

Mencarelli A, Fiorucci S (2010) FXR an emerging therapeutic target for the treatment of atherosclerosis. J Cell Mol Med 14:79–92

Moris D, Giaginis C, Tsourouflis G, Theocharis S (2017) Farnesoid-X receptor (FXR) as a promising pharmaceutical target in atherosclerosis. Curr Med Chem 24:1147–1157

Mota M, Banini BA, Cazanave SC, Sanyal AJ (2016) Molecular mechanisms of lipotoxicity and glucotoxicity in nonalcoholic fatty liver disease. Metabolism 65:1049–1061

Mozaffarian D, Rimm EB, Herrington DM (2004) Dietary fats, carbohydrate, and progression of coronary atherosclerosis in postmenopausal women. Am J Clin Nutr 80:1175–1184

Mridha AR, Wree A, Robertson AAB, Yeh MM, Johnson CD, van Rooyen DM, Haczeyni F, Teoh NC, Savard C, Ioannou GN, Masters SL, Schroder K, Cooper MA, Feldstein AE, Farrell GC (2017) NLRP3 inflammasome blockade reduces liver inflammation and fibrosis in experimental NASH in mice. J Hepatol 66:1037–1046

Muhidin SO, Magan AA, Osman KA, Syed S, Ahmed MH (2012) The relationship between nonalcoholic fatty liver disease and colorectal cancer: the future challenges and outcomes of the metabolic syndrome. J Obes 2012:637538

Mullerova H, Meeraus WH, Galkin DV, Albers FC, Landis SH (2019) Clinical burden of illness among patients with severe eosinophilic COPD. Int J Chron Obstruct Pulmon Dis 14:741–755

Mummadi RR, Kasturi KS, Chennareddygari S, Sood GK (2008) Effect of bariatric surgery on nonalcoholic fatty liver disease: systematic review and meta-analysis. Clin Gastroenterol Hepatol 6:1396–1402

Muro E, Atilla-Gokcumen GE, Eggert US (2014) Lipids in cell biology: how can we understand them better? Mol Biol Cell 25:1819–1823

Musso G, Gambino R, de Michieli F, Cassader M, Rizzetto M, Durazzo M, Faga E, Silli B, Pagano G (2003) Dietary habits and their relations to insulin resistance and postprandial lipemia in nonalcoholic steatohepatitis. Hepatology 37:909–916

Musso G, Gambino R, Tabibian JH, Ekstedt M, Kechagias S, Hamaguchi M, Hultcrantz R, Hagstrom H, Yoon SK, Charatcharoenwitthaya P, George J, Barrera F, Hafliethadottir S, Bjornsson ES, Armstrong MJ, Hopkins LJ, Gao X, Francque S, Verrijken A, Yilmaz Y, Lindor KD, Charlton M, Haring R, Lerch MM, Rettig R, Volzke H, Ryu S, Li G, Wong LL, Machado M, Cortez-Pinto H, Yasui K, Cassader M (2014) Association of non-alcoholic fatty liver disease with chronic kidney disease: a systematic review and meta-analysis. PLoS Med 11:e1001680

Musso G, Cassader M, Cohney S, de Michieli F, Pinach S, Saba F, Gambino R (2016) Fatty liver and chronic kidney disease: novel mechanistic insights and therapeutic opportunities. Diabetes Care 39:1830–1845

Musso G, Cassader M, Paschetta E, Gambino R (2017) Thiazolidinediones and advanced liver fibrosis in nonalcoholic steatohepatitis: a meta-analysis. JAMA Intern Med 177:633–640

Nagaya T, Tanaka N, Suzuki T, Sano K, Horiuchi A, Komatsu M, Nakajima T, Nishizawa T, Joshita S, Umemura T, Ichijo T, Matsumoto A, Yoshizawa K, Nakayama J, Tanaka E, Aoyama T (2010) Down-regulation of SREBP-1c is associated with the development of burned-out NASH. J Hepatol 53:724–731

Nakamura K, Fuster JJ, Walsh K (2014) Adipokines: a link between obesity and cardiovascular disease. J Cardiol 63:250–259

Nakatsu Y, Kokubo H, Bumdelger B, Yoshizumi M, Yamamotoya T, Matsunaga Y, Ueda K, Inoue Y, Inoue MK, Fujishiro M, Kushiyama A, Ono H, Sakoda H, Asano T (2017) The SGLT2 inhibitor luseogliflozin rapidly normalizes aortic mRNA levels of inflammation-related but not lipid-metabolism-related genes and suppresses atherosclerosis in diabetic ApoE KO mice. Int J Mol Sci 18:1704

Nasiri-Ansari N, Dimitriadis GK, Agrogiannis G, Perrea D, Kostakis ID, Kaltsas G, Papavassiliou AG, Randeva HS, Kassi E (2018) Canagliflozin attenuates the progression of atherosclerosis and inflammation process in APOE knockout mice. Cardiovasc Diabetol 17:106

Neuschwander-Tetri BA, Ford DA, Acharya S, Gilkey G, Basaranoglu M, Tetri LH, Brunt EM (2012) Dietary trans-fatty acid induced NASH is normalized following loss of trans-fatty acids from hepatic lipid pools. Lipids 47:941–950

Neuschwander-Tetri BA, Loomba R, Sanyal AJ, Lavine JE, van Natta ML, Abdelmalek MF, Chalasani N, Dasarathy S, Diehl AM, Hameed B, Kowdley KV, McCullough A, Terrault N, Clark JM, Tonascia J, Brunt EM, Kleiner DE, Doo E, Network NCR (2015) Farnesoid X nuclear receptor ligand obeticholic acid for non-cirrhotic, non-alcoholic steatohepatitis (FLINT): a multicentre, randomised, placebo-controlled trial. Lancet 385:956–965

Newton JL, Jones DE, Henderson E, Kane L, Wilton K, Burt AD, Day CP (2008) Fatigue in non-alcoholic fatty liver disease (NAFLD) is significant and associates with inactivity and excessive daytime sleepiness but not with liver disease severity or insulin resistance. Gut 57:807–813

Ni Y, Li JM, Liu MK, Zhang TT, Wang DP, Zhou WH, Hu LZ, Lv WL (2017) Pathological process of liver sinusoidal endothelial cells in liver diseases. World J Gastroenterol 23:7666–7677

Nickel F, Tapking C, Benner L, Sollors J, Billeter AT, Kenngott HG, Bokhary L, Schmid M, von Frankenberg M, Fischer L, Mueller S, Muller-Stich BP (2018) Bariatric surgery as an efficient treatment for non-alcoholic fatty liver disease in a prospective study with 1-year follow-up: BariScan study. Obes Surg 28:1342–1350

Nobili V, Marcellini M, Marchesini G, Vanni E, Manco M, Villani A, Bugianesi E (2007) Intrauterine growth retardation, insulin resistance, and nonalcoholic fatty liver disease in children. Diabetes Care 30:2638–2640

Noureddin M, Vipani A, Bresee C, Todo T, Kim IK, Alkhouri N, Setiawan VW, Tran T, Ayoub WS, Lu SC, Klein AS, Sundaram V, Nissen NN (2018) NASH leading cause of liver transplant in women: updated analysis of indications for liver transplant and ethnic and gender variances. Am J Gastroenterol 113:1649–1659

Nowak WN, Deng J, Ruan XZ, Xu Q (2017) Reactive oxygen species generation and atherosclerosis. Arterioscler Thromb Vasc Biol 37:e41–e52

Nozue T, Fukui K, Koyama Y, Fujii H, Kunishima T, Hikita H, Hibi K, Miyazawa A, Michishita I, Investigators FT (2016) Effects of sitagliptin on coronary atherosclerosis in patients with type 2 diabetes-A serial integrated backscatter-intravascular ultrasound study. Am J Cardiovasc Dis 6:153–162

Oh H, Jun DW, Saeed WK, Nguyen MH (2016) Non-alcoholic fatty liver diseases: update on the challenge of diagnosis and treatment. Clin Mol Hepatol 22:327–335

Ostovaneh MR, Ambale-Venkatesh B, Fuji T, Bakhshi H, Shah R, Murthy VL, Tracy RP, Guallar E, Wu CO, Bluemke DA, Lima JAC (2018) Association of liver fibrosis with cardiovascular diseases in the general population: the multi-ethnic study of atherosclerosis (MESA). Circ Cardiovasc Imaging 11:e007241

Ouchi N, Parker JL, Lugus JJ, Walsh K (2011) Adipokines in inflammation and metabolic disease. Nat Rev Immunol 11:85–97

Pan J, Ou Z, Cai C, Li P, Gong J, Ruan XZ, He K (2018) Fatty acid activates NLRP3 inflammasomes in mouse Kupffer cells through mitochondrial DNA release. Cell Immunol 332:111–120

Paoletti R, Bolego C, Poli A, Cignarella A (2006) Metabolic syndrome, inflammation and atherosclerosis. Vasc Health Risk Manag 2:145–152

Papaspyridonos M, McNeill E, de Bono JP, Smith A, Burnand KG, Channon KM, Greaves DR (2008) Galectin-3 is an amplifier of inflammation in atherosclerotic plaque progression through macrophage activation and monocyte chemoattraction. Arterioscler Thromb Vasc Biol 28:433–440

Pastori D, Carnevale R, Nocella C, Novo M, Santulli M, Cammisotto V, Menichelli D, Pignatelli P, Violi F (2017) Gut-derived serum lipopolysaccharide is associated with enhanced risk of major adverse cardiovascular events in atrial fibrillation: effect of adherence to Mediterranean diet. J Am Heart Assoc 6:e005784

Patel NS, Doycheva I, Peterson MR, Hooker J, Kisselva T, Schnabl B, Seki E, Sirlin CB, Loomba R (2015) Effect of weight loss on magnetic resonance imaging estimation of liver fat and volume in patients with nonalcoholic steatohepatitis. Clin Gastroenterol Hepatol 13:561–568.e1

Patil R, Sood GK (2017) Non-alcoholic fatty liver disease and cardiovascular risk. World J Gastrointest Pathophysiol 8:51–58

Perra A, Simbula G, Simbula M, Pibiri M, Kowalik MA, Sulas P, Cocco MT, Ledda-Columbano GM, Columbano A (2008) Thyroid hormone (T3) and TRbeta agonist GC-1 inhibit/reverse nonalcoholic fatty liver in rats. FASEB J 22:2981–2989

Perumpail BJ, Cholankeril R, Yoo ER, Kim D, Ahmed A (2017) An overview of dietary interventions and strategies to optimize the management of non-alcoholic fatty liver disease. Diseases 5:23

Peters KM, Wilson RB, Borradaile NM (2018) Non-parenchymal hepatic cell lipotoxicity and the coordinated progression of non-alcoholic fatty liver disease and atherosclerosis. Curr Opin Lipidol 29:417–422

Petit JM, Cercueil JP, Loffroy R, Denimal D, Bouillet B, Fourmont C, Chevallier O, Duvillard L, Verges B (2017) Effect of liraglutide therapy on liver fat content in patients with inadequately controlled type 2 diabetes: the Lira-NAFLD study. J Clin Endocrinol Metab 102:407–415

Petta S, Valenti L, Marchesini G, di Marco V, Licata A, Camma C, Barcellona MR, Cabibi D, Donati B, Fracanzani A, Grimaudo S, Parrinello G, Pipitone RM, Torres D, Fargion S, Licata G, Craxi A (2013) PNPLA3 GG genotype and carotid atherosclerosis in patients with non-alcoholic fatty liver disease. PLoS One 8:e74089

Pfaffenbach KT, Gentile CL, Nivala AM, Wang D, Wei Y, Pagliassotti MJ (2010) Linking endoplasmic reticulum stress to cell death in hepatocytes: roles of C/EBP homologous protein and chemical chaperones in palmitate-mediated cell death. Am J Physiol Endocrinol Metab 298:E1027–E1035

Piscaglia F, Svegliati-Baroni G, Barchetti A, Pecorelli A, Marinelli S, Tiribelli C, Bellentani S, Group H-NIS (2016) Clinical patterns of hepatocellular carcinoma in nonalcoholic fatty liver disease: a multicenter prospective study. Hepatology 63:827–838

Plat J, Hendrikx T, Bieghs V, Jeurissen ML, Walenbergh SM, van Gorp PJ, de Smet E, Konings M, Vreugdenhil AC, Guichot YD, Rensen SS, Buurman WA, Greve JW, Lutjohann D, Mensink RP, Shiri-Sverdlov R (2014) Protective role of plant sterol and stanol esters in liver inflammation: insights from mice and humans. PLoS One 9:e110758

Plat J, Baumgartner S, Vanmierlo T, Lutjohann D, Calkins KL, Burrin DG, Guthrie G, Thijs C, Te Velde AA, Vreugdenhil ACE, Sverdlov R, Garssen J, Wouters K, Trautwein EA, Wolfs TG, van Gorp C, Mulder MT, Riksen NP, Groen AK, Mensink RP (2019) Plant-based sterols and stanols in health & disease: "consequences of human development in a plant-based environment?". Prog Lipid Res 74:87–102

Polyzos SA, Kountouras J, Mantzoros CS (2017) Adipose tissue, obesity and non-alcoholic fatty liver disease. Minerva Endocrinol 42:92–108

Puri P, Baillie RA, Wiest MM, Mirshahi F, Choudhury J, Cheung O, Sargeant C, Contos MJ, Sanyal AJ (2007) A lipidomic analysis of nonalcoholic fatty liver disease. Hepatology 46:1081–1090

Rakipovski G, Rolin B, Nohr J, Klewe I, Frederiksen KS, Augustin R, Hecksher-Sorensen J, Ingvorsen C, Polex-Wolf J, Knudsen LB (2018) The GLP-1 analogs liraglutide and semaglutide reduce atherosclerosis in ApoE(−/−) and LDLr(−/−) mice by a mechanism that includes inflammatory pathways. JACC Basic Transl Sci 3:844–857

Ratziu V, de Ledinghen V, Oberti F, Mathurin P, Wartelle-Bladou C, Renou C, Sogni P, Maynard M, Larrey D, Serfaty L, Bonnefont-Rousselot D, Bastard JP, Riviere M, Spenard J, FRESGUN (2011) A randomized controlled trial of high-dose ursodesoxycholic acid for nonalcoholic steatohepatitis. J Hepatol 54:1011–1019

Ratziu V, Goodman Z, Sanyal A (2015) Current efforts and trends in the treatment of NASH. J Hepatol 62:S65–S75

Ratziu V, Harrison SA, Francque S, Bedossa P, Lehert P, Serfaty L, Romero-Gomez M, Boursier J, Abdelmalek M, Caldwell S, Drenth J, Anstee QM, Hum D, Hanf R, Roudot A, Megnien S, Staels B, Sanyal A, Group G-IS (2016) Elafibranor, an agonist of the peroxisome proliferator-activated receptor-alpha and −delta, induces resolution of nonalcoholic steatohepatitis without fibrosis worsening. Gastroenterology 150:1147–1159.e5

Reilly SM, Ahmadian M, Zamarron BF, Chang L, Uhm M, Poirier B, Peng X, Krause DM, Korytnaya E, Neidert A, Liddle C, Yu RT, Lumeng CN, Oral EA, Downes M, Evans RM, Saltiel AR (2015) A subcutaneous adipose tissue-liver signalling axis controls hepatic gluconeogenesis. Nat Commun 6:6047

Reinaud O, Delaforge M, Boucher JL, Rocchiccioli F, Mansuy D (1989) Oxidative metabolism of linoleic acid by human leukocytes. Biochem Biophys Res Commun 161:883–891

Rodrigues CM, Fan G, Ma X, Kren BT, Steer CJ (1998) A novel role for ursodeoxycholic acid in inhibiting apoptosis by modulating mitochondrial membrane perturbation. J Clin Invest 101:2790–2799

Romeo S, Kozlitina J, Xing C, Pertsemlidis A, Cox D, Pennacchio LA, Boerwinkle E, Cohen JC, Hobbs HH (2008) Genetic variation in PNPLA3 confers susceptibility to nonalcoholic fatty liver disease. Nat Genet 40:1461–1465

Santoro N, Zhang CK, Zhao H, Pakstis AJ, Kim G, Kursawe R, Dykas DJ, Bale AE, Giannini C, Pierpont B, Shaw MM, Groop L, Caprio S (2012) Variant in the glucokinase regulatory protein (GCKR) gene is associated with fatty liver in obese children and adolescents. Hepatology 55:781–789

Saremi A, Schwenke DC, Buchanan TA, Hodis HN, Mack WJ, Banerji M, Bray GA, Clement SC, Henry RR, Kitabchi AE, Mudaliar S, Ratner RE, Stentz FB, Musi N, Tripathy D, DeFronzo RA, Reaven PD (2013) Pioglitazone slows progression of atherosclerosis in prediabetes independent of changes in cardiovascular risk factors. Arterioscler Thromb Vasc Biol 33:393–399

Sasaki A, Nitta H, Otsuka K, Umemura A, Baba S, Obuchi T, Wakabayashi G (2014) Bariatric surgery and non-alcoholic fatty liver disease: current and potential future treatments. Front Endocrinol (Lausanne) 5:164

Sayiner M, Koenig A, Henry L, Younossi ZM (2016) Epidemiology of nonalcoholic fatty liver disease and nonalcoholic steatohepatitis in the United States and the rest of the world. Clin Liver Dis 20:205–214

Schaffer JE (2016) Lipotoxicity: many roads to cell dysfunction and cell death: introduction to a thematic review series. J Lipid Res 57:1327–1328

Schneiderhan W, Schmid-Kotsas A, Zhao J, Grunert A, Nussler A, Weidenbach H, Menke A, Schmid RM, Adler G, Bachem MG (2001) Oxidized low-density lipoproteins bind to the scavenger receptor, CD36, of hepatic stellate cells and stimulate extracellular matrix synthesis. Hepatology 34:729–737

Schuster S, Cabrera D, Arrese M, Feldstein AE (2018) Triggering and resolution of inflammation in NASH. Nat Rev Gastroenterol Hepatol 15:349–364

Schwartz MW, Woods SC, Porte D Jr, Seeley RJ, Baskin DG (2000) Central nervous system control of food intake. Nature 404:661–671

Sears B, Perry M (2015) The role of fatty acids in insulin resistance. Lipids Health Dis 14:121

Shao N, Yu XY, Ma XF, Lin WJ, Hao M, Kuang HY (2018) Exenatide delays the progression of nonalcoholic fatty liver disease in C57BL/6 mice, which may involve inhibition of the NLRP3 inflammasome through the mitophagy pathway. Gastroenterol Res Pract 2018:1864307

Shiba K, Tsuchiya K, Komiya C, Miyachi Y, Mori K, Shimazu N, Yamaguchi S, Ogasawara N, Katoh M, Itoh M, Suganami T, Ogawa Y (2018) Canagliflozin, an SGLT2 inhibitor, attenuates the development of hepatocellular carcinoma in a mouse model of human NASH. Sci Rep 8:2362

Shibuya T, Fushimi N, Kawai M, Yoshida Y, Hachiya H, Ito S, Kawai H, Ohashi N, Mori A (2018) Luseogliflozin improves liver fat deposition compared to metformin in type 2 diabetes patients with non-alcoholic fatty liver disease: a prospective randomized controlled pilot study. Diabetes Obes Metab 20:438–442

Shiffman M, Freilich B, Vuppalanchi R, Watt K, Chan JL, Spada A, Hagerty DT, Schiff E (2019) Randomised clinical trial: emricasan versus placebo significantly decreases ALT and caspase 3/7 activation in subjects with non-alcoholic fatty liver disease. Aliment Pharmacol Ther 49:64–73

Shinde PJS (2018) Non-alcoholic steatohepatitis (NASH) market by drug type (vitamin E & pioglitazone, ocaliva, elafibranor, and selonsertib & cenicriviroc), and sales channel (Hospital pharmacy, online provider, and retail pharmacy) – global opportunity analysis and industry forecast, 2021–2025, p 155

Sinal CJ, Tohkin M, Miyata M, Ward JM, Lambert G, Gonzalez FJ (2000) Targeted disruption of the nuclear receptor FXR/BAR impairs bile acid and lipid homeostasis. Cell 102:731–744

Singal AK, Salameh H, Kamath PS (2014) Prevalence and in-hospital mortality trends of infections among patients with cirrhosis: a nationwide study of hospitalised patients in the United States. Aliment Pharmacol Ther 40:105–112

Sinha RA, Singh BK, Yen PM (2018) Direct effects of thyroid hormones on hepatic lipid metabolism. Nat Rev Endocrinol 14:259–269

Sliz E, Sebert S, Wurtz P. Kangas AJ, Soininen P, Lehtimaki T, Kahonen M, Viikari J, Mannikko M, Ala-Korpela M, Raitakari OT, Kettunen J (2018) NAFLD risk alleles in PNPLA3, TM6SF2, GCKR and LYPLAL1 show divergent metabolic effects. Hum Mol Genet 27:2214–2223

Sookoian S, Pirola CJ (2008) Non-alcoholic fatty liver disease is strongly associated with carotid atherosclerosis: a systematic review. J Hepatol 49:600–607

Sookoian S, Pirola CJ (2018) Systematic review with meta-analysis: the significance of histological disease severity in lean patients with nonalcoholic fatty liver disease. Aliment Pharmacol Ther 47:16–25

Speliotes EK, Yerges-Armstrong LM, Wu J, Hernaez R, Kim LJ, Palmer CD, Gudnason V, Eiriksdottir G, Garcia ME, Launer LJ, Nalls MA, Clark JM, Mitchell BD, Shuldiner AR, Butler JL, Tomas M, Hoffmann U, Hwang SJ, Massaro JM, O'Donnell CJ, Sahani DV, Salomaa V, Schadt EE, Schwartz SM, Siscovick DS, Nash CRN, Consortium G, Investigators M, Voight BF, Carr JJ, Feitosa MF, Harris TB, Fox CS, Smith AV, Kao WH, Hirschhorn JN, Borecki IB, Consortium G (2011) Genome-wide association analysis identifies variants associated with nonalcoholic fatty liver disease that have distinct effects on metabolic traits. PLoS Genet 7:e1001324

Spencer MD, Hamp TJ, Reid RW, Fischer LM, Zeisel SH, Fodor AA (2011) Association between composition of the human gastrointestinal microbiome and development of fatty liver with choline deficiency. Gastroenterology 140:976–986

Staels B, Rubenstrunk A, Noel B, Rigou G, Delataille P, Millatt LJ, Baron M, Lucas A, Tailleux A, Hum DW, Ratziu V, Cariou B, Hanf R (2013) Hepatoprotective effects of the dual peroxisome proliferator-activated receptor alpha/delta agonist, GFT505, in rodent models of nonalcoholic fatty liver disease/nonalcoholic steatohepatitis. Hepatology 58:1941–1952

Stancu C, Sima A (2001) Statins: mechanism of action and effects. J Cell Mol Med 5:378–387

Stewart KE, Levenson JL (2012) Psychological and psychiatric aspects of treatment of obesity and nonalcoholic fatty liver disease. Clin Liver Dis 16:615–629

Stewart KE, Haller DL, Sargeant C, Levenson JL, Puri P, Sanyal AJ (2015) Readiness for behaviour change in non-alcoholic fatty liver disease: implications for multidisciplinary care models. Liver Int 35:936–943

Sumida Y, Yoneda M (2018) Current and future pharmacological therapies for NAFLD/NASH. J Gastroenterol 53:362–376

Sumida Y, Niki E, Naito Y, Yoshikawa T (2013) Involvement of free radicals and oxidative stress in NAFLD/NASH. Free Radic Res 47:869–880

Sumida Y, Murotani K, Saito M, Tamasawa A, Osonoi Y, Yoneda M, Osonoi T (2019) Effect of luseogliflozin on hepatic fat content in type 2 diabetes patients with non-alcoholic fatty liver disease: a prospective, single-arm trial (LEAD trial). Hepatol Res 49:64–71

Suomela E, Oikonen M, Pitkanen N, Ahola-Olli A, Virtanen J, Parkkola R, Jokinen E, Laitinen T, Hutri-Kahonen N, Kahonen M, Lehtimaki T, Taittonen L, Tossavainen P, Jula A, Loo BM, Mikkila V, Telama R, Viikari JSA, Juonala M, Raitakari OT (2016) Childhood predictors of adult fatty liver. The cardiovascular risk in Young Finns study. J Hepatol 65:784–790

Surdea-Blaga T, Dumitrascu DL (2011) Depression and anxiety in nonalcoholic steatohepatitis: is there any association? Rom J Intern Med 49:273–280

Tabas I (2010) Macrophage death and defective inflammation resolution in atherosclerosis. Nat Rev Immunol 10:36–46

Tacke F (2018) Cenicriviroc for the treatment of non-alcoholic steatohepatitis and liver fibrosis. Expert Opin Investig Drugs 27:301–311

Tanaka K, Sata M (2018) Roles of perivascular adipose tissue in the pathogenesis of atherosclerosis. Front Physiol 9:3

Tanaka K, Masaki Y, Tanaka M, Miyazaki M, Enjoji M, Nakamuta M, Kato M, Nomura M, Inoguchi T, Kotoh K, Takayanagi R (2014) Exenatide improves hepatic steatosis by enhancing lipid use in adipose tissue in nondiabetic rats. World J Gastroenterol 20:2653–2663

Tanaka A, Murohara T, Taguchi I, Eguchi K, Suzuki M, Kitakaze M, Sato Y, Ishizu T, Higashi Y, Yamada H, Nanasato M, Shimabukuro M, Teragawa H, Ueda S, Kodera S, Matsuhisa M, Kadokami T, Kario K, Nishio Y, Inoue T, Maemura K, Oyama J, Ohishi M, Sata M, Tomiyama H, Node K, Investigators PS (2016) Rationale and design of a multicenter randomized controlled study to evaluate the preventive effect of ipragliflozin on carotid atherosclerosis: the PROTECT study. Cardiovasc Diabetol 15:133

Tang WH, Wang Z, Levison BS, Koeth RA, Britt EB, Fu X, Wu Y, Hazen SL (2013) Intestinal microbial metabolism of phosphatidylcholine and cardiovascular risk. N Engl J Med 368:1575–1584

Targher G, Chonchol M, Miele L, Zoppini G, Pichiri I, Muggeo M (2009) Nonalcoholic fatty liver disease as a contributor to hypercoagulation and thrombophilia in the metabolic syndrome. Semin Thromb Hemost 35:277–287

Targher G, Day CP, Bonora E (2010) Risk of cardiovascular disease in patients with nonalcoholic fatty liver disease. N Engl J Med 363:1341–1350

Targher G, Byrne CD, Lonardo A, Zoppini G, Barbui C (2016) Non-alcoholic fatty liver disease and risk of incident cardiovascular disease: a meta-analysis. J Hepatol 65:589–600

Trauner M, Arrese M, Wagner M (2010) Fatty liver and lipotoxicity. Biochim Biophys Acta 1801:299–310

Tremaroli V, Backhed F (2012) Functional interactions between the gut microbiota and host metabolism. Nature 489:242–249

Turnbaugh PJ, Ley RE, Mahowald MA, Magrini V, Mardis ER, Gordon JI (2006) An obesity-associated gut microbiome with increased capacity for energy harvest. Nature 444:1027–1031

Valdearcos M, Xu AW, Koliwad SK (2015) Hypothalamic inflammation in the control of metabolic function. Annu Rev Physiol 77:131–160

Valenti L, Romeo S (2016) Destined to develop NAFLD? The predictors of fatty liver from birth to adulthood. J Hepatol 65:668–670

Valenti L, Al-Serri A, Daly AK, Galmozzi E, Rametta R, Dongiovanni P, Nobili V, Mozzi E, Roviaro G, Vanni E, Bugianesi E, Maggioni M, Fracanzani AL, Fargion S, Day CP (2010) Homozygosity for the patatin-like phospholipase-3/adiponutrin I148M polymorphism influences liver fibrosis in patients with nonalcoholic fatty liver disease. Hepatology 51:1209–1217

van Baar MJB, van Ruiten CC, Muskiet MHA, van Bloemendaal L, IJzerman RG, van Raalte DH (2018) SGLT2 inhibitors in combination therapy: from mechanisms to clinical considerations in type 2 diabetes management. Diabetes Care 41:1543–1556

van der Heijden T, Kritikou E, Venema W, van Duijn J, van Santbrink PJ, Slutter B, Foks AC, Bot I, Kuiper J (2017) NLRP3 inflammasome inhibition by MCC950 reduces atherosclerotic lesion development in apolipoprotein E-deficient mice-brief report. Arterioscler Thromb Vasc Biol 37:1457–1461

van Herpen NA, Schrauwen-Hinderling VB (2008) Lipid accumulation in non-adipose tissue and lipotoxicity. Physiol Behav 94:231–241

van Rooyen DM, Larter CZ, Haigh WG, Yeh MM, Ioannou G, Kuver R, Lee SP, Teoh NC, Farrell GC (2011) Hepatic free cholesterol accumulates in obese, diabetic mice and causes nonalcoholic steatohepatitis. Gastroenterology 141:1393–1403.e1-5

Vassilatou E (2014) Nonalcoholic fatty liver disease and polycystic ovary syndrome. World J Gastroenterol 20:8351–8363

Villanova N, Moscatiello S, Ramilli S, Bugianesi E, Magalotti D, Vanni E, Zoli M, Marchesini G (2005) Endothelial dysfunction and cardiovascular risk profile in nonalcoholic fatty liver disease. Hepatology 42:473–480

Wang Z, Klipfell E, Bennett BJ, Koeth R, Levison BS, Dugar B, Feldstein AE, Britt EB, Fu X, Chung YM, Wu Y, Schauer P, Smith JD, Allayee H, Tang WH, DiDonato JA, Lusis AJ, Hazen SL (2011) Gut flora metabolism of phosphatidylcholine promotes cardiovascular disease. Nature 472:57–63

Wang Y, Viscarra J, Kim SJ, Sul HS (2015) Transcriptional regulation of hepatic lipogenesis. Nat Rev Mol Cell Biol 16 678–689

Wang PX, Ji YX, Zhang XJ, Zhao LP, Yan ZZ, Zhang P, Shen LJ, Yang X, Fang J, Tian S, Zhu XY, Gong J, Zhang X, Wei QF, Wang Y, Li J, Wan L, Xie Q, She ZG, Wang Z, Huang Z, Li H (2017) Targeting CASP8 and FADD-like apoptosis regulator ameliorates nonalcoholic steatohepatitis in mice and nonhuman primates. Nat Med 23:439–449

Wang R, Li H, Yang X, Xue X, Deng L, Shen J, Zhang M, Zhao L, Zhang C (2018) Genetically obese human gut microbiota induces liver steatosis in germ-free mice fed on normal diet. Front Microbiol 9:1602

Weinstein AA, Kallman Price J, Stepanova M, Poms LW, Fang Y, Moon J, Nader F, Younossi ZM (2011) Depression in patients with nonalcoholic fatty liver disease and chronic viral hepatitis B and C. Psychosomatics 52:127–132

Weinstein G, Zelber-Sagi S, Preis SR, Beiser AS, DeCarli C, Speliotes EK, Satizabal CL, Vasan RS, Seshadri S (2018) Association of nonalcoholic fatty liver disease with lower brain volume in healthy middle-aged adults in the Framingham study. JAMA Neurol 75:97–104

Welte T, Torres A, Nathwani D (2012) Clinical and economic burden of community-acquired pneumonia among adults in Europe. Thorax 67:71–79

Wigg AJ, Roberts-Thomson IC, Dymock RB, McCarthy PJ, Grose RH, Cummins AG (2001) The role of small intestinal bacterial overgrowth, intestinal permeability, endotoxaemia, and tumour necrosis factor alpha in the pathogenesis of non-alcoholic steatohepatitis. Gut 48:206–211

Williams CD, Stengel J, Asike MI, Torres DM, Shaw J, Contreras M, Landt CL, Harrison SA (2011) Prevalence of nonalcoholic fatty liver disease and nonalcoholic steatohepatitis among a largely middle-aged population utilizing ultrasound and liver biopsy: a prospective study. Gastroenterology 140:124–131

Winer DA, Luck H, Tsai S, Winer S (2016) The intestinal immune system in obesity and insulin resistance. Cell Metab 23:413–426

Wojcik-Cichy K, Koslinska-Berkan E, Piekarska A (2018) The influence of NAFLD on the risk of atherosclerosis and cardiovascular diseases. Clin Exp Hepatol 4:1–6

Wong VW, Wong GL, Tsang SW, Fan T, Chu WC, Woo J, Chan AW, Choi PC, Chim AM, Lau JY, Chan FK, Sung JJ, Chan HL (2011) High prevalence of colorectal neoplasm in patients with non-alcoholic steatohepatitis. Gut 60:829–836

Wouters K, van Gorp PJ, Bieghs V, Gijbels MJ, Duimel H, Lutjohann D, Kerksiek A, van Kruchten R, Maeda N, Staels B, van Bilsen M, Shiri-Sverdlov R, Hofker MH (2008) Dietary cholesterol, rather than liver steatosis, leads to hepatic inflammation in hyperlipidemic mouse models of nonalcoholic steatohepatitis. Hepatology 48:474–486

Wu J, Yao XY, Shi RX, Liu SF, Wang XY (2018a) A potential link between polycystic ovary syndrome and non-alcoholic fatty liver disease: an update meta-analysis. Reprod Health 15:77

Wu WKK, Zhang L, Chan MTV (2018b) Autophagy, NAFLD and NAFLD-related HCC. Adv Exp Med Biol 1061:127–138

Xiang M, Wang PX, Wang AB, Zhang XJ, Zhang Y, Zhang P, Mei FH, Chen MH, Li H (2016) Targeting hepatic TRAF1-ASK1 signaling to improve inflammation, insulin resistance, and hepatic steatosis. J Hepatol 64:1365–1377

Yang G, Lei Y, Inoue A, Piao L, Hu L, Jiang H, Sasaki T, Wu H, Xu W, Yu C, Zhao G, Ogasawara S, Okumura K, Kuzuya M, Cheng XW (2017) Exenatide mitigated diet-induced vascular aging and atherosclerotic plaque growth in ApoE-deficient mice under chronic stress. Atherosclerosis 264:1–10

Ye D, Li FY, Lam KS, Li H, Jia W, Wang Y, Man K, Lo CM, Li X, Xu A (2012) Toll-like receptor-4 mediates obesity-induced non-alcoholic steatohepatitis through activation of X-box binding protein-1 in mice. Gut 61:1058–1067

Younossi ZM, Henry L (2015) Economic and quality-of-life implications of non-alcoholic fatty liver disease. PharmacoEconomics 33:1245–1253

Younossi Z, Henry L (2016) Contribution of alcoholic and nonalcoholic fatty liver disease to the burden of liver-related morbidity and mortality. Gastroenterology 150:1778–1785

Younossi ZM, Stepanova M, Afendy M, Fang Y, Younossi Y, Mir H, Srishord M (2011a) Changes in the prevalence of the most common causes of chronic liver diseases in the United States from 1988 to 2008. Clin Gastroenterol Hepatol 9:524–530.e1; quiz e60

Younossi ZM, Stepanova M, Rafiq N, Makhlouf H, Younoszai Z, Agrawal R, Goodman Z (2011b) Pathologic criteria for nonalcoholic steatohepatitis: interprotocol agreement and ability to predict liver-related mortality. Hepatology 53:1874–1882

Younossi ZM, Zheng L, Stepanova M, Venkatesan C, Mishra A (2014) Clinical outcomes and resource utilisation in medicare patients with chronic liver disease: a historical cohort study. BMJ Open 4:e004318

Younossi ZM, Otgonsuren M, Henry L, Venkatesan C, Mishra A, Erario M, Hunt S (2015a) Association of nonalcoholic fatty liver disease (NAFLD) with hepatocellular carcinoma (HCC) in the United States from 2004 to 2009. Hepatology 62:1723–1730

Younossi ZM, Zheng L, Stepanova M, Henry L, Venkatesan C, Mishra A (2015b) Trends in outpatient resource utilizations and outcomes for medicare beneficiaries with nonalcoholic fatty liver disease. J Clin Gastroenterol 49:222–227

Younossi ZM, Blissett D, Blissett R, Henry L, Stepanova M, Younossi Y, Racila A, Hunt S, Beckerman R (2016a) The economic and clinical burden of nonalcoholic fatty liver disease in the United States and Europe. Hepatology 64:1577–1586

Younossi ZM, Koenig AB, Abdelatif D, Fazel Y, Henry L, Wymer M (2016b) Global epidemiology of nonalcoholic fatty liver disease-meta-analytic assessment of prevalence, incidence, and outcomes. Hepatology 64:73–84

Younossi Z, Tacke F, Arrese M, Sharma BC, Mostafa I, Bugianesi E, Wong VW, Yilmaz Y, George J, Fan J, Vos MB (2018a) Global perspectives on non-alcoholic fatty liver disease and non-alcoholic steatohepatitis. Hepatology 69:2672–2682

Younossi ZM, Stepanova M, Lawitz E, Charlton M, Loomba R, Myers RP, Subramanian M, McHutchison JG, Goodman Z (2018b) Improvement of hepatic fibrosis and patient-reported outcomes in non-alcoholic steatohepatitis treated with selonsertib. Liver Int 38:1849–1859

Younossi ZM, Tampi R, Priyadarshini M, Nader F, Younossi IM, Racila A (2019) Burden of illness and economic model for patients with nonalcoholic steatohepatitis in the United States. Hepatology 69:564–572

Zain SM, Mohamed Z, Mahadeva S, Cheah PL, Rampal S, Chin KF, Mahfudz AS, Basu RC, Tan HL, Mohamed R (2013) Impact of leptin receptor gene variants on risk of non-alcoholic fatty liver disease and its interaction with adiponutrin gene. J Gastroenterol Hepatol 28:873–879

Zelniker TA, Wiviott SD, Raz I, Im K, Goodrich EL, Bonaca MP, Mosenzon O, Kato ET, Cahn A, Furtado RHM, Bhatt DL, Leiter LA, McGuire DK, Wilding JPH, Sabatine MS (2019) SGLT2 inhibitors for primary and secondary prevention of cardiovascular and renal outcomes in type 2 diabetes: a systematic review and meta-analysis of cardiovascular outcome trials. Lancet 393:31–39

Zhang S, Wang J, Liu Q, Harnish DC (2009) Farnesoid X receptor agonist WAY-362450 attenuates liver inflammation and fibrosis in murine model of non-alcoholic steatohepatitis. J Hepatol 51:380–388

Zhang Q, Liu J, Liu J, Huang W, Tian L, Quan J, Wang Y, Niu R (2014) oxLDL induces injury and defenestration of human liver sinusoidal endothelial cells via LOX1. J Mol Endocrinol 53:281–293

Zhang P, Wang PX, Zhao LP, Zhang X, Ji YX, Zhang XJ, Fang C, Lu YX, Yang X, Gao MM, Zhang Y, Tian S, Zhu XY, Gong J, Ma XL, Li F, Wang Z, Huang Z, She ZG, Li H (2018) The deubiquitinating enzyme TNFAIP3 mediates inactivation of hepatic ASK1 and ameliorates nonalcoholic steatohepatitis. Nat Med 24:84–94

Zou L, Li X, Wu N, Jia P, Liu C, Jia D (2017) Palmitate induces myocardial lipotoxic injury via the endoplasmic reticulum stressmediated apoptosis pathway. Mol Med Rep 16:6934–6939

Zou TT, Zhang C, Zhou YF, Han YJ, Xiong JJ, Wu XX, Chen YP, Zheng MH (2018) Lifestyle interventions for patients with nonalcoholic fatty liver disease: a network meta-analysis. Eur J Gastroenterol Hepatol 30:747–755

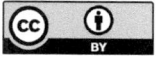

Prevention and Treatment of Atherosclerosis: The Use of Nutraceuticals and Functional Foods

Francesco Visioli and Andrea Poli

Contents

1 Introduction 272
2 Red Yeast Rice 273
   2.1 Untoward Effects 274
3 Phytosterols and Phytostanols 274
   3.1 Untoward Effects 276
4 Berberine 276
   4.1 Untoward Effects 277
5 Fiber 277
   5.1 Untoward Effects 278
6 Supplements in the Pipeline 278
   6.1 Astaxanthin 278
   6.2 Hydroxytyrosol 279
   6.3 Probiotics 279
   6.4 Bergamot 280
7 Conclusions 281
References 281

Abstract

Nutritional interventions are effective and – in theory – easy to implement primary and secondary prevention strategies that reduce several risk factors of atherosclerosis and cardiovascular disease (CVD). Yet, because of (a) the severe impact of CVD in terms of mortality, morbidity, quality of life, and economy, (b) the proved role of LDL plasma concentrations as the most critical risk factor,

F. Visioli
Department of Molecular Medicine, University of Padova, Padua, Italy

IMDEA-Food, CEI UAM+CSIC, Madrid, Spain

A. Poli (✉)
Nutrition Foundation of Italy, Milan, Italy
e-mail: poli@nutrition-foundation.it

© The Author(s) 2019
A. von Eckardstein, C. J. Binder (eds.), *Prevention and Treatment of Atherosclerosis*,
Handbook of Experimental Pharmacology 270, https://doi.org/10.1007/164_2019_341

and (c) the obstacles found both in terms of biological effects and compliance of the patient by an exclusively dietary intervention, food supplements or *nutraceuticals* are now valuable resources for physicians. As regards cholesterol control, several preparations are available in the market, and we will critically review them in this chapter.

Keywords

Atherosclerosis · Cardiovascular disease · Cholesterol · Diet · Functional foods · Nutraceuticals

1 Introduction

Atherosclerosis is multifactorial in nature and leads to various clinical forms of cardiovascular disease (CVD). Risk factors are manifold, but inflammation and elevated low-density lipoprotein (LDL) cholesterol are thought to be among the most important contributors (Alenghat and Davis 2019). In particular, Mendelian randomization studies and many intervention trials demonstrated that modifications of plasma LDL cholesterol concentrations are *casually* associated with cardiovascular risk (Ference 2015). As discussed in other parts of this book, variations of LDL predict cardiovascular risk in terms of amplitude and direction. Indeed, clinical trials have not yet allowed finding a lower limit of LDL concentrations to be achieved for optimal cardiovascular protection (Cholesterol Treatment Trialists et al. 2015).

Nutritional interventions are effective and – in theory – easy to implement primary and secondary prevention strategies that reduce several risk factors of atherosclerosis and CVD (Visioli and Poli 2019; Visioli et al. 2008). Focus on healthful food items, namely, fruit and vegetables and, hence, fiber, vitamins, (poly)phenols, and healthy fats (from extra virgin olive oil, vegetable oils, nuts, fatty fish) and low sodium improves diets and lessens CVD risk (Visioli and Hagen 2007; Visioli and Poli 2019). One notable example is the Mediterranean diet, which is associated with a significant improvement in health status and a significant reduction in overall mortality, as well as in morbidity and mortality from CVD and other major chronic diseases (Rees et al. 2019). Several systematic reviews of observational prospective studies have confirmed that greater adherence to such diet is associated with better health and greater longevity. Finally, the PREDIMED study provided important experimental proof of the cardioprotective properties of the Mediterranean diet (Martinez-Gonzalez et al. 2019). Consequently, physicians should pay particular attention to their patients' diets – even though curricular training is often suboptimal – and insist they preferentially adopt a plant-based regimen, enriched with fish and seafoods and with dairy products. Two limitations of dietary interventions are worth discussing. The first one is that the most commonly prescribed dietary and physical interventions have a limited (-1.5 to 5%) direct impact on LDL cholesterol levels, i.e., the foremost risk factor (Visioli and Poli 2019). The second and, perhaps, most important one is that extensive modifications of dietary habits are difficult to implement in real-life settings. It is worth reminding that humans are hardwired to maximize energy intake and limit expenditure (i.e., the "thrifty" genotype). New neurocognitive training methods are being investigated to lose weight and reduce sweets and fats consumption more effectively. However, translation of such results to clinical practice will require time.

Because of (a) the severe impact of CVD in terms of mortality, morbidity, quality of life, and economy, (b) the proved role of LDL plasma levels as the most critical risk factor among a large collection of others, and (c) the obstacles found both in terms of biological effects and compliance of the patient by an exclusively dietary intervention, food supplements or *nutraceuticals* deserve an in-depth analysis because they are valuable resources for physicians (Poli et al. 2018; Poli and Visioli 2019). As regards cholesterol control, several preparations are available in the market, and we will critically review them in this chapter.

2   Red Yeast Rice

The most popular supplement for cholesterol control is red yeast rice (RYR), which originates from the fermentation of rice performed by the fungus *Monascus purpureus*. Its denomination comes from color of the fermenting rice, *Oryza sativa*. With fermentation, a group of molecules identified as monacolin K is synthesized in both lactone (K) and open ring acid forms (Ka). Both molecules undergo interconversion in the body (Poli et al. 2013). Fermentations can take place in liquid and solid mediums. The latter is less efficient than the former, where the overall production of monacolin K is lower (5–130 mg/L) but is also relatively simpler (Vendruscolo et al. 2016). Some studies have shown that environmental factors affect the production of secondary metabolites by *Monascus*. Examples include nitrogen sources and glutamic acid, which improve (from 48.4 to 215.4 mg/L) the production of monacolin K (Vendruscolo et al. 2016). Glutamic acid also increases the production of acetyl coenzyme A, which is a substrate for monacolin K. This line of research stems from the similarities with lovastatin synthetic genes (LNKS) in *Aspergillus*. Indeed, often unbeknownst to the lay public, monacolin K is chemically identical to lovastatin and, thus, strongly inhibits HMG-CoA reductase. RYR also contains monacolins J, L, X, and M that contribute to the inhibitory process to a lesser extent. A possible difference between RYR and lovastatin is their relative bioavailability: the former, according to a single study (Chen et al. 2013), is more bioavailable than the latter and, therefore, more effective on an mg-per-mg basis. Administered at doses of 3–10 mg/day, monacolin K reduces LDL cholesterol concentrations by 20–25% (Fogacci et al. 2019; Li et al. 2014). Its effects on HDL cholesterol are negligible; triglyceridemia is mildly reduced unless plasma triglyceride concentrations are elevated, in which case the effects of RYR are stronger (Li et al. 2014; Sahebkar et al. 2016).

As with statins, probably due to their effects on LDL plasma levels, monacolin K improves endothelial function, with a number of favorable consequences: from systolic blood pressure reduction to plaque stabilization (Strazzullo et al. 2007).

2.1 Untoward Effects

Even though RYR is perceived as "natural" and, hence, intrinsically safe, adverse effects of monacolin K are similar to those of statins, namely, lovastatin. These include elevated hepatic enzyme levels, gastrointestinal distress, and statin-associated myalgias (SAMs), i.e., muscle pain and weakness. Myositis (elevated creatinine phosphokinase [CPK] level) and rhabdomyolysis are more serious albeit highly infrequent complications of statin therapy (Stroes et al. 2015). Indeed, a recent review concluded that RYR is overall relatively tolerable and safe (Fogacci et al. 2019). Quite illogically, patients who experience statin-induced untoward effects often shift to RYR without telling their physicians. Some patients do experience a reduction of side effects, which could be explained by a "nocebo" effect. An alternative explanation for the higher tolerability of RYR products as compared with statins and observed in some studies (Becker et al. 2009) could be the lower doses of the active ingredient (2.5–3 mg) that are usually found in supplements sold in Europe. Indeed, patients who are truly intolerant to statins are not many, and the safety profile of this class of drugs is excellent.

One often overlooked issue is that monacolin K can interact with other drugs, as in the case of statin therapy. RYR should not be co-administered with drugs containing itraconazole, ketoconazole, erythromycin, clarithromycin, telithromycin, HIV protease inhibitors, cyclosporine, nefazodone, green tea, and grapefruit juice (≥ 0.2 L/day) because monacolin K and statins are metabolized by cytochrome P450 and – in particular – by isoenzyme 3A4. Finally, the co-administration of statins and RYR should be avoided for pharmacodynamic reasons (both have the same mechanism of action) and comparable side effects (Cicero et al. 2017; Fogacci et al. 2019).

As a final cautionary note, the quality of commercial RYR-based products is rather heterogeneous (Gordon et al. 2010). The amount of active principle was found to vary by up to 100 times; recently, moreover, in an EFSA document, highly variable amounts of monacolin K in the lactone and in the open ring form were found in RYR-based products found on the market (EFSA 2018). The open ring form usually accounts for about one third of the total monacolins in RYR, whereas synthetic lovastatin is almost 100% lactone. Considering that open ring monacolin K levels as low as 0.1% were found in some samples, the possibility that synthetic monacolin is fraudulently sold as RYR cannot be excluded (Gordon et al. 2010).

Because nutraceuticals are not regulated as drugs, red rice supplements are not always subjected to strict adverse event monitoring programs. Physicians should make patients aware of potential risk factors related to the use of RYR nutraceuticals to ensure safety, lack of allergenic compounds, and potential untoward effects (Dujovne 2017).

3 Phytosterols and Phytostanols

Phytosterols (PS) are triterpenes that are usually classified as *sterols* or *stanols*, according to the presence or absence of a double bond in position 5. PS are found in free or esterified forms: free sterols are integral part of the cellular wall of plants, where they play important structural functions, whereas sterol esters represent storage products within the cell (Mamode Cassim et al. 2019). The only structural difference between sitosterol and cholesterol consists of an additional ethyl group present at position C-24 in sitosterol, which is probably at least in part responsible for its relatively poor intestinal absorption (Marangoni and Poli 2010).

There are more than 250 different PS molecules identified to date, β-sitosterol being the most abundant of them. Other plant sterols are present in vegetables and vegetable oils and include campesterol, stigmasterol, and dihydrobrassicasterol, at concentrations much lower than those of β-sitosterol; the saturated derivatives campestanol and sitostanol are found in almost negligible amounts in the vegetal kingdom (Marangoni and Poli 2010).

As mentioned, PS are mostly found in vegetables and derivatives such as vegetable oils; nuts, grains, and grain-derived products; and also sprouts, cabbages, cauliflowers, and green and black olives. Non-vegetable sources of PS include egg yolks, mammalian liver, and crustaceans. Commercially, PS are obtained from tall oil – which contains up to 80% of β-sitosterol – and the by-products of soybean oil production. Phytosterols are usually used as esterified forms to increase their solubility and allow for their incorporation into lipid-based foods (Marangoni and Poli 2010).

Considering that PS cannot be synthesized by humans, their circulating concentrations depend upon diet and absorption efficiency, as well as by its secretion in the gut by ABCG5-G5 transmembrane transporters. Depending on the type and amount of plant foods consumed, PS consumption and, in turn, PS blood concentrations vary within and between populations yet remain usually very low. Intervention studies report that higher phytosterols' intake as food supplements increases their circulating levels, while plant stanols supplementation decreases them. The absorption process is that of cholesterol and includes solubilized in mixed micelles, after the hydrolyzation of esters by a pancreatic ester hydroxylase. The specific carrier of cholesterol and PS is the Niemann-Pick C1-Like 1 (NPC1L1), i.e., the one that is specifically blocked by ezetimibe as discussed in other chapters of this book (Davis and Altmann 2009). Plasma levels of PS in humans are normally about 0.5% of those of cholesterol, because (1) the latter is synthesized in the liver, (2) PS is less efficiently absorbed by the small intestine, and (3) PS are rapidly excreted. Plant stanols concentrations in plasma are only 0.05% that of cholesterol (de Jong et al. 2003). Of note, PS play no known biological or functional role.

The main mechanisms responsible for the PS-induced reduction in cholesterol are their competition with cholesterol for incorporation into mixed micelles in the intestinal tract (Ras et al. 2014). As compared with cholesterol, PS are more readily hydrolyzed, and this process leads to a lower solubilization of cholesterol into micelles, which decreases their absorption and, in turn, increases fecal excretion of cholesterol and its metabolites. Co-crystallization of cholesterol and PS, leading to increased fecal excretion of cholesterol, may play a minor role.

Since PS absorbed from the gut are rapidly re-excreted in the gut lumen through the ATP-binding cassette transporters ABCG-5 and ABCG-8, located at the apical surface of the enterocyte, PS can have a rather long duration of action. This may explain why similar effects can be obtained by administering PS in a single dose or divided into three canonical meals (Plat et al. 2000). If this is true, the daily intake pattern would not affect PS efficacy, and the reduced incorporation of cholesterol into mixed micelles may only partially be responsible for the cholesterol-lowering effect of PS taken with meals. On the other hand, administration of PS without a meal is less effective (-30%) than the same dose administered after a main meal (Doornbos et al. 2006). Patients need hence to be instructed to take PS after lunch or dinner.

In general, the cholesterol-lowering effect of PS is noticeable within few weeks and remains stable if supplementation is continuous (Ras et al. 2014). However, interruption of regular intakes reverses the effects of PS and brings cholesterol concentrations back to basal conditions. This is obvious, but patients are often satisfied with the results and stop taking PS without telling their physician. Finally, PS can be used as ad hoc preparations (beverages) or as functional ingredients of spreads, margarines, etc. (Ras et al. 2014).

This effect is additive to that of cholesterol synthesis inhibitors (statins), which compensatively tend to increase cholesterol absorption from the gut (Miettinen and Gylling 2003).

3.1 Untoward Effects

PS are safe, except for patients with homozygous sitosterolemia, who absorb between 15 and 60% of the ingested sitosterol compared to <5% of normal subjects. The only proven untoward effect of PS is the reduction of circulating fat-soluble vitamins. Physicians should, therefore, reinforce the advice to consume five or more servings of fruit and vegetables per day, which effectively maintains carotenoid levels in the normal range.

4   Berberine

Berberine is the active component of barberry (*Berberis vulgaris* L. family Berberidaceae), which grows in Asia and Europe. Barberry is an integral part of Iranian traditional medicine (Dong et al. 2013). Among its many purported actions, hypotensive activity, gastric secretory stimulation, choleretic activity, increased tone of the digestive tract, anti-inflammatory activity, complement alternative pathway inhibition, delayed-type cutaneous hypersensitivity inhibition, antibacterial effects, antifungal effects, narcotic antagonist activity, and sedation have been suggested yet poorly investigated (Koppen et al. 2017). Of note, berberine is poorly bioavailable, i.e., ~1%, and pharmaceutical research is studying absorption enhancers and the use of nanoparticles or microemulsions to overcome this issue (Li et al. 2009; Liu et al. 2016).

Berberine is being mostly studied in Asian subjects and is being marketed in the West for its hypocholesterolemic activities. Indeed, some reviews indicate that berberine can lower plasma cholesterol to an extent similar to that of statins, i.e., 20–30% (Johnston et al. 2017). This effect is greater in subjects with higher basal cholesterolemia and also depends on individual genetics.

In terms of mechanisms of action, berberine upregulates hepatic LDL receptor expression, likely by stabilizing LDL receptor mRNA through activation of extracellular signal-regulated kinase (ERK) pathways. Other studies suggest that berberine promotes LDL receptor expression through the inhibition of the proprotein PCSK9, which is also – likely – ERK-dependent (Dong et al. 2015). Another mechanism proposed for berberine is that it might interfere with intraluminal cholesterol micellarization, decreasing enterocyte cholesterol uptake, as shown in vitro in Caco-2 cells (Wang et al. 2014).

The effect of berberine on PCSK9 levels (which are compensatively increased during statin treatment) may explain the additive effect of berberine when administered with statins (Cicero et al. 2007). Nutraceuticals containing RYR and berberine are, in fact, quite popular.

The possibility that berberine also exerts a prebiotic effect, leading to a microbiota-mediated anti-atherosclerotic action, has recently been put forward based on animal studies (Zhu et al. 2018). Such effect would lead to reconsider the role of the amount of berberine unabsorbed from the gut.

4.1 Untoward Effects

Barberry per se is thought to be mildly toxic, but berberine is safe at therapeutic dosages. Gastrointestinal problems such as [chiefly] constipation, diarrhea, nausea, and abdominal distension are the most commonly reported side effects of berberine (Pirro et al. 2017). However, these effects diminish after reducing the dose of berberine. No other serious adverse events were reported in the trials that reported safety data, mainly obtained in Eastern countries. As with any other herbal treatment, herb-drug interactions should be carefully assessed in light of mutual cytochrome metabolism. Of note, repeated oral administration of berberine (0.3 g three times daily) decreases CYP2D6, CYP2C9, and CYP3A4 activities in healthy subjects (Guo et al. 2012).

5 Fiber

An adequate intake of fiber has multiple beneficial effects on human health that transcend their mere actions on plasma cholesterol (Rubin 2019).

In terms of cholesterol control, some meta-analyses did quantify the actions of beta-glucan (a class of non-starch polysaccharides: $(1 \rightarrow 3)(1 \rightarrow 4)$-β-D-glucan, which are highly viscous nondigestible fiber). A daily beta-glucan dose of 3 g reduces LDL cholesterol by 5–6%; no effects on other blood lipids have been reported (Cloetens et al. 2012). In addition to grains and cereals, namely, barley and oats, beta-glucan is available as ingredient of functional foods or as plain supplement. Glucomannan, psyllium (a predominantly gelling polysaccharide mixture), and chitosan are other cholesterol-lowering kinds of fiber.

The mechanisms of action of soluble fibers such as beta-glucan are still elusive (Ho et al. 2016). The most plausible hypothesis is that fiber increases fecal excretion of cholesterol, bile acids, and other dietary fats via formation of gels in the intestine. It is therefore advisable to tell patients to increase their intake of water during supplementation with fiber to facilitate the formation of such gel-like substances. The high molecular weight fraction of beta-glucan appears to be the most effective one.

A prebiotic effect cannot on the other hand be ruled out, leading to an increased synthesis of SCFA (especially propionate), which, after absorption, may act as an inhibitor of cholesterol synthesis in the liver (Reis et al. 2017). At high dosage, beta-glucan also improves postprandial glycemic response (Ho et al. 2016).

5.1   Untoward Effects

The most frequently reported side effects of high fiber intake are gastrointestinal in nature and there is no tolerable upper limit for fiber. Precisely because fiber is nondigestible, it reaches the colon quite intact and undergoes fermentation by the microbiota. This can cause bloating and intestinal distress ranging from diarrhea to constipation (if water intake is inadequate). Co-administration of drugs also calls for caution because fiber can sequester active molecules and alter (usually decrease) bioavailability (Poli et al. 2018; Poli and Visioli 2019). Patients should be told to avoid such practice and to get used to fiber gradually.

6   Supplements in the Pipeline

After the policosanol fiasco, some molecules are being actively investigated for their potential role in hypercholesterolemia and dyslipidemia. We will briefly and critically review them here.

6.1   Astaxanthin

In light of its multiple biological actions, the xanthophyll carotenoid astaxanthin has been proposed as a suitable preventive and therapeutic agent in cardiovascular disease (Kishimoto et al. 2016). Astaxanthin exhibited lipid-lowering activity in laboratory mice supplemented diet with >0.03% of astaxanthin from *H. pluvialis* for 12 weeks, namely, lowering plasma TG concentrations. No significant differences in plasma TC and HDL-C concentrations between the control and treatment groups were reported (Yang et al. 2014). In a murine model of metabolic syndrome, a significant increase in HDL-C and a significant decrease of plasma TG levels and nonesterified fatty acids were induced by astaxanthin given at 50 mg/kg/day for

22 weeks. Moreover, astaxanthin decreased the size of the fat cells of white adipose tissue. In addition, lower adiponectin concentrations were recorded in the serum of obese, insulin-resistant type 2 diabetic rodents and humans, indicating a possible correlation between adiponectin concentrations and insulin resistance and fat accumulation (Stern et al. 2016).

The purported hypolipidemic effects of astaxanthin require further investigation, and its mechanisms of action are still unclear (Visioli and Artaria 2017). A meta-analysis by Ursoniu et al. (2015) indeed concluded that astaxanthin does not exert any significant effect in terms of plasma lipid profile. Of note, astaxanthin sourced from the microalgae *H. pluvialis* is the only one currently authorized for direct human consumption (Visioli and Artaria 2017), and consumers should be aware of possible contaminations with other sources of this carotenoid (as in the case of monacolin K). Further ad hoc investigations will eventually allow (or not) the addition of astaxanthin to the array of nutraceuticals for cholesterol control.

6.2   Hydroxytyrosol

Hydroxytyrosol (HT)'s activities on cholesterol and TGs are still equivocal and, likely, quantitatively irrelevant (Crespo et al. 2018). However, it is worth noting that HT has manifold biological actions that might prove useful to hypercholesterolemic patients (Tome-Carneiro and Visioli 2016). Such activities include thrombogenic potential reduction, anti-inflammatory actions, and inhibition of LDL oxidation as per an EFSA-authorized health claim (Crespo et al. 2018). Despite the hype, this last activity is of dubious relevance to human physiology, also in light of the antioxidant therapy debacle and the lack of appropriate and validated tests (Visioli et al. 2018). In any case, HT is being actively studied for its molecular actions, and accumulated data are strongly suggestive of its cardioprotective actions, regardless of the effects on cholesterol (Visioli et al. 2018).

6.3   Probiotics

Despite the lack of strong scientific evidence, the use of probiotics is increasing, and this includes the cardiovascular arena (Cavalcanti Neto et al. 2018).

Several possible mechanisms for cholesterol's intestinal removal by probiotics have been proposed (Shimizu et al. 2015). Examples include binding of cholesterol to cell surface (in a fashion similar to that of PS of fiber), uptake of cholesterol by growing cells, deconjugation of bile via bile salt hydrolase and subsequent coprecipitation of cholesterol, and some unclear physiological actions of short-chain fatty acid fermentation (Reis et al. 2017).

Prebiotics such as inulin and fructooligosaccharides are soluble, indigestible, viscous, and fermentable compounds that might play hypocholesterolemic actions either by decreasing cholesterol absorption and increasing its fecal excretion (similar to fiber as discussed above) or via production of short-chain fatty acids after their fermentation by the microbiota. The use of synbiotics is, thus, often advocated for cholesterol control (Mahboobi et al. 2018).

We would like to make the readers aware of the fact that no health claim has been awarded for any probiotic strain as related to lowering cholesterol. The use of probiotics rests on theoretical grounds and some in vitro experiments. Future, well-controlled and large-scale human experiments will eventually support the use of probiotics in hypercholesterolemic patients.

6.4   Bergamot

Bergamot is a citrus fruit belonging to the genus *Citrus*, endemic to the Southern coastal area of Calabria (Italy). The derivatives of bergamot traditionally come from the essential oil contained in the peel and were obtained manually, by pressing. This process is now industrialized and allows the marketing of large quantities of preparations. The main use of bergamot essential oil (after de-furocumarinization) is still in the food industry (for the flavoring of Earl Grey tea) and in the perfumery field, for its particular aroma. From a biomedical viewpoint, the most interesting phytochemical components of bergamot are the (poly)phenolic molecules present in its juice (commercially called bergamot polyphenolic fraction (BPF)) and the volatile terpenes that characterize the essential oil (Nauman and Johnson 2019).

The BPF exercises various actions on glycolipid metabolism, including the ability to reduce the hepatic accumulation of triglycerides, the partial inhibition of their synthesis, and the ability to inhibit the action of acyl-CoA cholesterol acyltransferase (ACAT) (Janda et al. 2016). The result is a lower production of apoB-containing lipoproteins. More recently, it has also been observed that the BPF is able to efficiently inhibit the pancreatic cholesterol ester hydrolase (pCEH), which leads to a reduction in the absorption of dietary cholesterol (Giglio et al. 2016).

Furthermore, the (poly)phenolic components of bergamot activate AMPK. AMPK is an important regulator of the metabolic pathways involved in the production of ATP in mammalian cells and acts as a sensor of AMP/ATP levels. The intracellular AMP increases when the energy state is low and binds to the AMPK to allow activation.

Finally, it is important to emphasize that the BPF can act directly as an HMG-CoA reductase inhibitor, thus exerting effects potentially similar to those of statins (Leopoldini et al. 2010).

In randomized, double-blind studies carried out in hyperlipemic and type 2 diabetes subjects, a remarkable effect of BPF was found in terms of reducing fasting blood glucose, LDL cholesterol, and triglycerides and increasing HDL cholesterol (Cai et al. 2017; Toth et al. 2015). In another study, a lecithin formulation (to increase bioavailability) of BPF, already successfully tested at the preclinical level, was used at a daily dose of 1,000 mg (corresponding to 400 mg of BPF) (Mollace et al. 2019). Lipid-lowering and hypoglycemic effects similar to those of BPF at a dose of 1,300 mg were recorded (Mollace et al. 2019). All these data must be, obviously, confirmed in other randomized clinical trials before the BPF can become part of the therapeutic armamentarium (Nauman and Johnson 2019).

7 Conclusions

The decision to recommend a functional food or supplement/nutraceutical is integral part of the therapy and should be taken by physicians, not patients or other health professionals. This process includes the decision of which supplement to prescribe and at which dose, as well as timely checkups in order to monitor the safety and efficacy of treatment.

Furthermore, physicians should instruct patients on the importance and role of supplements, removing the "natural" halo with which they are often marketed. Because most supplements are not reimbursed by national healthcare systems, physicians should make sure their patients can sustain costs over time, considering that such treatment is often lengthy and in theory lifelong.

In this framework, some supplements and functional foods can effectively reduce plasma LDL cholesterol levels by 5–25%, either alone or in combination. As with pharmacological treatments, physicians must monitor the use of nutraceuticals and verify their regular use, their effects on lipid profile, as well as the eventual occurrence of untoward effects, many of which are typical of classic drugs. Should cardiovascular risk worsen remarkably, inclusion of ethical drugs is mandatory.

In conclusion, many effective and relatively safe nutraceuticals and functional foods are available and are backed by solid scientific evidence. Their use in cholesterol control and dyslipidemia is warranted in the frame of a comprehensive therapeutic strategy.

Acknowledgments Supported in part by POR FESR 3S4H.

Conflict of Interest None.

References

Alenghat FJ, Davis AM (2019) Management of Blood Cholesterol. JAMA 321:800–801

Becker DJ, Gordon RY, Halbert SC, French B, Morris PB, Rader DJ (2009) Red yeast rice for dyslipidemia in statin-intolerant patients: a randomized trial. Ann Intern Med 150:830–839, W147–9

Cai Y, Xing G, Shen T, Zhang S, Rao J, Shi R (2017) Effects of 12-week supplementation of Citrus bergamia extracts-based formulation CitriCholess on cholesterol and body weight in older adults with dyslipidemia: a randomized, double-blind, placebo-controlled trial. Lipids Health Dis 16:251

Cavalcanti Neto MP, Aquino JS, Romao da Silva LF, de Oliveira Silva R, Guimaraes KSL, de Oliveira Y, de Souza EL, Magnani M, Vidal H, de Brito Alves JL (2018) Gut microbiota and probiotics intervention: a potential therapeutic target for management of cardiometabolic disorders and chronic kidney disease? Pharmacol Res 130:152–163

Chen CH, Yang JC, Uang YS, Lin CJ (2013) Improved dissolution rate and oral bioavailability of lovastatin in red yeast rice products. Int J Pharm 444:18–24

Cholesterol Treatment Trialists C, Fulcher J, O'Connell R, Voysey M, Emberson J, Blackwell L, Mihaylova B, Simes J, Collins R, Kirby A, Colhoun H, Braunwald E, La Rosa J, Pedersen TR, Tonkin A, Davis B, Sleight P, Franzosi MG, Baigent C, Keech A (2015) Efficacy and safety of LDL-lowering therapy among men and women: meta-analysis of individual data from 174,000 participants in 27 randomised trials. Lancet 385:1397–1405

Cicero AF, Rovati LC, Setnikar I (2007) Eulipidemic effects of berberine administered alone or in combination with other natural cholesterol-lowering agents. A single-blind clinical investigation. Arzneimittelforschung 57:26–30

Cicero AFG, Colletti A, Bajraktari G, Descamps O, Djuric DM, Ezhov M, Fras Z, Katsiki N, Langlois M, Latkovskis G, Panagiotakos DB, Paragh G, Mikhailidis DP, Mitchenko O, Paulweber B, Pella D, Pitsavos C, Reiner Z, Ray KK, Rizzo M, Sahebkar A, Serban MC, Sperling LS, Toth PP, Vinereanu D, Vrablik M, Wong ND, Banach M (2017) Lipid-lowering nutraceuticals in clinical practice: position paper from an International Lipid Expert Panel. Nutr Rev 75:731–767

Cloetens L, Ulmius M, Johansson-Persson A, Akesson B, Onning G (2012) Role of dietary beta-glucans in the prevention of the metabolic syndrome. Nutr Rev 70:444–458

Crespo MC, Tome-Carneiro J, Davalos A, Visioli F (2018) Pharma-nutritional properties of olive oil phenols. Transfer of new findings to human nutrition. Foods 7

Davis HR Jr, Altmann SW (2009) Niemann-Pick C1 Like 1 (NPC1L1) an intestinal sterol transporter. Biochim Biophys Acta 1791:679–683

de Jong A, Plat J, Mensink RP (2003) Metabolic effects of plant sterols and stanols (review). J Nutr Biochem 14:362–369

Dong H, Zhao Y, Zhao L, Lu F (2013) The effects of berberine on blood lipids: a systemic review and meta-analysis of randomized controlled trials. Planta Med 79:437–446

Dong B, Li H, Singh AB, Cao A, Liu J (2015) Inhibition of PCSK9 transcription by berberine involves down-regulation of hepatic HNF1alpha protein expression through the ubiquitin-proteasome degradation pathway. J Biol Chem 290:4047–4058

Doornbos AM, Meynen EM, Duchateau GS, van der Knaap HC, Trautwein EA (2006) Intake occasion affects the serum cholesterol lowering of a plant sterol-enriched single-dose yoghurt drink in mildly hypercholesterolaemic subjects. Eur J Clin Nutr 60:325–333

Dujovne CA (2017) Red yeast rice preparations: are they suitable substitutions for statins? Am J Med 130:1148–1150

EFSA Panel on Food Additives and Sources Added to Food (2018) Scientific opinion on the safety of monacolins in red yeast rice. EFSA J 16:5368

Ference BA (2015) Mendelian randomization studies: using naturally randomized genetic data to fill evidence gaps. Curr Opin Lipidol 26:566–571

Fogacci F, Banach M, Mikhailidis DP, Bruckert E, Toth PP, Watts GF, Reiner Z, Mancini J, Rizzo M, Mitchenko O, Pella D, Fras Z, Sahebkar A, Vrablik M, Cicero AFG, Lipid, Blood Pressure Meta-analysis Collaboration Group the International Lipid Expert P (2019) Safety of red yeast rice supplementation: a systematic review and meta-analysis of randomized controlled trials. Pharmacol Res 143:1–16

Giglio RV, Patti AM, Nikolic D, Li Volti G, Al-Rasadi K, Katsiki N, Mikhailidis DP, Montalto G, Ivanova E, Orekhov AN, Rizzo M (2016) The effect of bergamot on dyslipidemia. Phytomedicine 23:1175–1181

Gordon RY, Cooperman T, Obermeyer W, Becker DJ (2010) Marked variability of monacolin levels in commercial red yeast rice products: buyer beware! Arch Intern Med 170:1722–1727

Guo Y, Chen Y, Tan ZR, Klaassen CD, Zhou HH (2012) Repeated administration of berberine inhibits cytochromes P450 in humans. Eur J Clin Pharmacol 68:213–217

Ho HV, Sievenpiper JL, Zurbau A, Blanco Mejia S, Jovanovski E, Au-Yeung F, Jenkins AL, Vuksan V (2016) The effect of oat beta-glucan on LDL-cholesterol, non-HDL-cholesterol and apoB for CVD risk reduction: a systematic review and meta-analysis of randomised-controlled trials. Br J Nutr 116:1369–1382

Janda E, Lascala A, Martino C, Ragusa S, Nucera S, Walker R, Gratteri S, Mollace V (2016) Molecular mechanisms of lipid- and glucose-lowering activities of bergamot flavonoids. PharmaNutrition 4:S8–S18

Johnston TP, Korolenko TA, Pirro M, Sahebkar A (2017) Preventing cardiovascular heart disease: promising nutraceutical and non-nutraceutical treatments for cholesterol management. Pharmacol Res 120:219–225

Kishimoto Y, Yoshida H, Kondo K (2016) Potential anti-atherosclerotic properties of astaxanthin. Mar Drugs 14

Koppen LM, Whitaker A, Rosene A, Beckett RD (2017) Efficacy of berberine alone and in combination for the treatment of hyperlipidemia: a systematic review. J Evid Based Complementary Altern Med 22:956–968

Leopoldini M, Malaj N, Toscano M, Sindona G, Russo N (2010) On the inhibitor effects of bergamot juice flavonoids binding to the 3-hydroxy-3-methylglutaryl-CoA reductase (HMGR) enzyme. J Agric Food Chem 58:10768–10773

Li YH, Yang P, Kong WJ, Wang YX, Hu CQ, Zuo ZY, Wang YM, Gao H, Gao LM, Feng YC, Du NN, Liu Y, Song DQ, Jiang JD (2009) Berberine analogues as a novel class of the low-density-lipoprotein receptor up-regulators: synthesis, structure-activity relationships, and cholesterol-lowering efficacy. J Med Chem 52:492–501

Li Y, Jiang L, Jia Z, Xin W, Yang S, Yang Q, Wang L (2014) A meta-analysis of red yeast rice: an effective and relatively safe alternative approach for dyslipidemia. PLoS One 9:e98611

Liu CS, Zheng YR, Zhang YF, Long XY (2016) Research progress on berberine with a special focus on its oral bioavailability. Fitoterapia 109:274–282

Mahboobi S, Rahimi F, Jafarnejad S (2018) Effects of prebiotic and synbiotic supplementation on glycaemia and lipid profile in type 2 diabetes: a meta-analysis of randomized controlled trials. Adv Pharm Bull 8:565–574

Mamode Cassim A, Gouguet P, Gronnier J, Laurent N, Germain V, Grison M, Boutte Y, Gerbeau-Pissot P, Simon-Plas F, Mongrand S (2019) Plant lipids: key players of plasma membrane organization and function. Prog Lipid Res 73:1–27

Marangoni F, Poli A (2010) Phytosterols and cardiovascular health. Pharmacol Res 61:193–199

Martinez-Gonzalez MA, Gea A, Ruiz-Canela M (2019) The Mediterranean diet and cardiovascular health. Circ Res 124:779–798

Miettinen TA, Gylling H (2003) Synthesis and absorption markers of cholesterol in serum and lipoproteins during a large dose of statin treatment. Eur J Clin Investig 33:976–982

Mollace V, Scicchitano M, Paone S, Casale F, Calandruccio C, Gliozzi M, Musolino V, Carresi C, Maiuolo J, Nucera S, Riva A, Allegrini P, Ronchi M, Petrangolini G, Bombardelli E (2019) Hypoglycemic and hypolipemic effects of a new lecithin formulation of bergamot polyphenolic fraction: a double blind, randomized, placebo-controlled study. Endocr Metab Immune Disord Drug Targets 19:136–143

Nauman MC, Johnson JJ (2019) Clinical application of bergamot (Citrus bergamia) for reducing high cholesterol and cardiovascular disease markers. Integr Food Nutr Metab 6

Pirro M, Vetrani C, Bianchi C, Mannarino MR, Bernini F, Rivellese AA (2017) Joint position statement on "nutraceuticals for the treatment of hypercholesterolemia" of the Italian Society of Diabetology (SID) and of the Italian Society for the Study of Arteriosclerosis (SISA). Nutr Metab Cardiovasc Dis 27:2–17

Plat J, van Onselen EN, van Heugten MM, Mensink RP (2000) Effects on serum lipids, lipoproteins and fat soluble antioxidant concentrations of consumption frequency of margarines and shortenings enriched with plant stanol esters. Eur J Clin Nutr 54:671–677

Poli A, Visioli F (2019) Pharmacology of nutraceuticals with lipid lowering properties. High Blood Press Cardiovasc Prev 26:113–118

Poli A, Marangoni F, Avogaro A, Barba G, Bellentani S, Bucci M, Cambieri R, Catapano AL, Costanzo S, Cricelli C, de Gaetano G, Di Castelnuovo A, Faggiano P, Fattirolli F, Fontana L, Forlani G, Frattini S, Giacco R, La Vecchia C, Lazzaretto L, Loffredo L, Lucchin L, Marelli G, Marrocco W, Minisola S, Musicco M, Novo S, Nozzoli C, Pelucchi C, Perri L, Pieralli F, Rizzoni D, Sterzi R, Vettor R, Violi F, Visioli F (2013) Moderate alcohol use and health: a consensus document. Nutr Metab Cardiovasc Dis 23:487–504

Poli A, Barbagallo CM, Cicero AFG, Corsini A, Manzato E, Trimarco B, Bernini F, Visioli F, Bianchi A, Canzone G, Crescini C, de Kreutzenberg S, Ferrara N, Gambacciani M, Ghiselli A, Lubrano C, Marelli G, Marrocco W, Montemurro V, Parretti D, Pedretti R, Perticone F, Stella R, Marangoni F (2018) Nutraceuticals and functional foods for the control of plasma cholesterol levels. An intersociety position paper. Pharmacol Res 134:51–60

Ras RT, Geleijnse JM, Trautwein EA (2014) LDL-cholesterol-lowering effect of plant sterols and stanols across different dose ranges: a meta-analysis of randomised controlled studies. Br J Nutr 112:214–219

Rees K, Takeda A, Martin N, Ellis L, Wijesekara D, Vepa A, Das A, Hartley L, Stranges S (2019) Mediterranean-style diet for the primary and secondary prevention of cardiovascular disease. Cochrane Database Syst Rev 3:CD009825

Reis SA, Conceicao LL, Rosa DD, Siqueira NP, Peluzio MCG (2017) Mechanisms responsible for the hypocholesterolaemic effect of regular consumption of probiotics. Nutr Res Rev 30:36–49

Rubin R (2019) High-fiber diet might protect against range of conditions. JAMA 321:1653–1655

Sahebkar A, Serban MC, Gluba-Brzozka A, Mikhailidis DP, Cicero AF, Rysz J, Banach M (2016) Lipid-modifying effects of nutraceuticals: an evidence-based approach. Nutrition 32:1179–1192

Shimizu M, Hashiguchi M, Shiga T, Tamura HO, Mochizuki M (2015) Meta-analysis: effects of probiotic supplementation on lipid profiles in normal to mildly hypercholesterolemic individuals. PLoS One 10:e0139795

Stern JH, Rutkowski JM, Scherer PE (2016) Adiponectin, leptin, and fatty acids in the maintenance of metabolic homeostasis through adipose tissue crosstalk. Cell Metab 23:770–784

Strazzullo P, Kerry SM, Barbato A, Versiero M, D'Elia L, Cappuccio FP (2007) Do statins reduce blood pressure?: a meta-analysis of randomized, controlled trials. Hypertension 49:792–798

Stroes ES, Thompson PD, Corsini A, Vladutiu GD, Raal FJ, Ray KK, Roden M, Stein E, Tokgozoglu L, Nordestgaard BG, Bruckert E, De Backer G, Krauss RM, Laufs U, Santos RD, Hegele RA, Hovingh GK, Leiter LA, Mach F, Marz W, Newman CB, Wiklund O, Jacobson TA, Catapano AL, Chapman MJ, Ginsberg HN, European Atherosclerosis Society Consensus P (2015) Statin-associated muscle symptoms: impact on statin therapy-European Atherosclerosis Society Consensus Panel statement on assessment, aetiology and management. Eur Heart J 36:1012–1022

Tome-Carneiro J, Visioli F (2016) Polyphenol-based nutraceuticals for the prevention and treatment of cardiovascular disease: review of human evidence. Phytomedicine 23:1145–1174

Toth PP, Patti AM, Nikolic D, Giglio RV, Castellino G, Biancucci T, Geraci F, David S, Montalto G, Rizvi A, Rizzo M (2015) Bergamot reduces plasma lipids, atherogenic small dense LDL, and subclinical atherosclerosis in subjects with moderate hypercholesterolemia: a 6 months prospective study. Front Pharmacol 6:299

Ursoniu S, Sahebkar A, Serban MC, Banach M (2015) Lipid profile and glucose changes after supplementation with astaxanthin: a systematic review and meta-analysis of randomized controlled trials. Arch Med Sci 11:253–266

Vendruscolo F, Meinicke Buhler RM, Cesar de Carvalho J, de Oliveira D, Moritz DE, Schmidell W, Ninow JL (2016) Monascus: a reality on the production and application of microbial pigments. Appl Biochem Biotechnol 178:211–223

Visioli F, Artaria C (2017) Astaxanthin in cardiovascular health and disease: mechanisms of action, therapeutic merits, and knowledge gaps. Food Funct 8:39–63

Visioli F, Hagen TM (2007) Nutritional strategies for healthy cardiovascular aging: focus on micronutrients. Pharmacol Res 55:199–206

Visioli F, Poli A (2019) Dietary advice to cardiovascular patients. A brief update for physicians. Monaldi Arch Chest Dis 89

Visioli F, Poli A, Richard D, Paoletti R (2008) Modulation of inflammation by nutritional interventions. Curr Atheroscler Rep 10:451–453

Visioli F, Franco M, Toledo E, Luchsinger J, Willett WC, Hu FB, Martinez-Gonzalez MA (2018) Olive oil and prevention of chronic diseases: summary of an international conference. Nutr Metab Cardiovasc Dis 28:649–656

Wang Y, Yi X, Ghanam K, Zhang S, Zhao T, Zhu X (2014) Berberine decreases cholesterol levels in rats through multiple mechanisms, including inhibition of cholesterol absorption. Metabolism 63:1167–1177

Yang Y, Pham TX, Wegner CJ, Kim B, Ku CS, Park YK, Lee JY (2014) Astaxanthin lowers plasma TAG concentrations and increases hepatic antioxidant gene expression in diet-induced obesity mice. Br J Nutr 112:1797–1804

Zhu L, Zhang D, Zhu H, Zhu J, Weng S, Dong L, Liu T, Hu Y, Shen X (2018) Berberine treatment increases Akkermansia in the gut and improves high-fat diet-induced atherosclerosis in Apoe(−/−) mice. Atherosclerosis 268:117–126

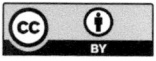

Part III

Hypothesis Based Approaches to Unravel Novel Targets

.

Novel Adipose Tissue Targets to Prevent and Treat Atherosclerosis

Ludger Scheja and Joerg Heeren

Contents

1 Introduction 290
2 Types of Adipose Tissue and Their Impact on Cardiovascular Disease 292
   2.1 White Adipose Tissue 292
   2.2 Thermogenic Adipose Tissue 294
   2.3 Perivascular Adipose Tissue 295
3 Therapies Targeting Adipose Tissue with Proven Clinical Efficacy in the Treatment
   of Atherosclerosis 296
   3.1 Peroxisome Proliferator-Activated Receptor-γ (PPARγ) Agonists 296
   3.2 Niacin 296
   3.3 Renin-Angiotensin System Blockade 297
4 Novel Therapeutic Targets in Adipose Tissue for Treatment of Atherosclerosis 297
   4.1 Promoting Lipoprotein Disposal and Lipid Storage in Adipose Tissues 297
   4.2 Boosting Thermogenic Activation 299
   4.3 Targeting Inflammation in Adipose Tissue 299
   4.4 Hormones Derived from Thermogenic Adipose Tissue 300
   4.5 De Novo Lipogenesis-Derived Lipokines 301
5 Future Directions 302
References 303

Abstract

Adipose tissue as a major organ of lipid and lipoprotein metabolism has a major impact on metabolic homeostasis and thus influences the development of atherosclerosis and related cardiometabolic diseases. Unhealthy adipose tissue, which is often associated with obesity and systemic insulin resistance, promotes the development of diabetic dyslipidemia and can negatively affect vascular tissue

L. Scheja (✉) · J. Heeren
Department of Biochemistry and Molecular Cell Biology, University Medical Center Hamburg-Eppendorf, Hamburg, Germany
e-mail: l.scheja@uke.de

© The Author(s) 2020   289
A. von Eckardstein, C. J. Binder (eds.), *Prevention and Treatment of Atherosclerosis*,
Handbook of Experimental Pharmacology 270, https://doi.org/10.1007/164_2020_363

homeostasis by secreting pro-inflammatory peptides and lipids. Conversely, paracrine and endocrine factors that are released from healthy adipose tissue can preserve metabolic balance and a functional vasculature. In this chapter, we describe adipose tissue types relevant for atherosclerosis and address the question how lipid metabolism as well as regulatory molecules produced in these fat depots can be targeted to counteract atherogenic processes in the vessel wall and improve plasma lipids. We discuss the role of adipose tissues in the action of approved drugs with anti-atherogenic activity. In addition, we present potential novel targets and therapeutic approaches aimed at increasing lipoprotein disposal in adipose tissue, boosting the activity of heat-producing (thermogenic) adipocytes, reducing adipose tissue inflammation, and improving or replacing beneficial hormones released from adipose tissues. Furthermore, we describe the future potential of innovative drug delivery technologies.

Keywords

Adipokines · Atherosclerosis · Brown adipose tissue · Diabetic dyslipidemia · Hyperlipidemia · Inflammation · Insulin resistance · Lipid-lowering therapy · Lipoproteins · Obesity · Perivascular adipose tissue · Thermogenesis · Vascular remodeling · White adipose tissue

1   Introduction

Adipocytes are triglyceride-storing cells present in anatomically distinct adipose tissue depots throughout the mammalian body (Cinti 2001). Originally, two major subtypes, white and brown adipocytes, were identified, both playing an important role in energy metabolism. White adipocytes in white adipose tissue (WAT) store large amounts of triglycerides, typically in a single large lipid droplet, which can be hydrolyzed to provide other organs with free fatty acids (FFA) (Young and Zechner 2013). Brown adipocytes in brown adipose tissue (BAT) also store triglycerides, albeit in lower quantities, and, in many, smaller lipid droplets. When BAT is activated, for example, by exposure to a cold environment, brown adipocytes oxidize fatty acids, glucose, and other fuels in their numerous mitochondria to generate heat (Cannon and Nedergaard 2004). Under chronic cold exposure, adipocytes that are morphologically and functionally very similar to brown adipocytes, referred to as beige adipocytes, develop in WAT depots in a process called WAT browning (Bartelt and Heeren 2014). The number of thermogenic adipocytes thus increases when demand is high. As summarized in Fig. 1, white, brown, and beige adipocytes influence whole-body energy metabolism, lipoprotein levels (Scheja and Heeren 2016), and, through secretion of regulatory molecules, tissue homeostasis in other organs (Scheja and Heeren 2019). How these systemic effects of adipose tissues modulate the development of cardiovascular disease (CVD), and how they can be targeted therapeutically, is the topic of this chapter. Furthermore, local effects exerted by adipocytes found next to blood vessels (perivascular adipocytes) will be described and discussed.

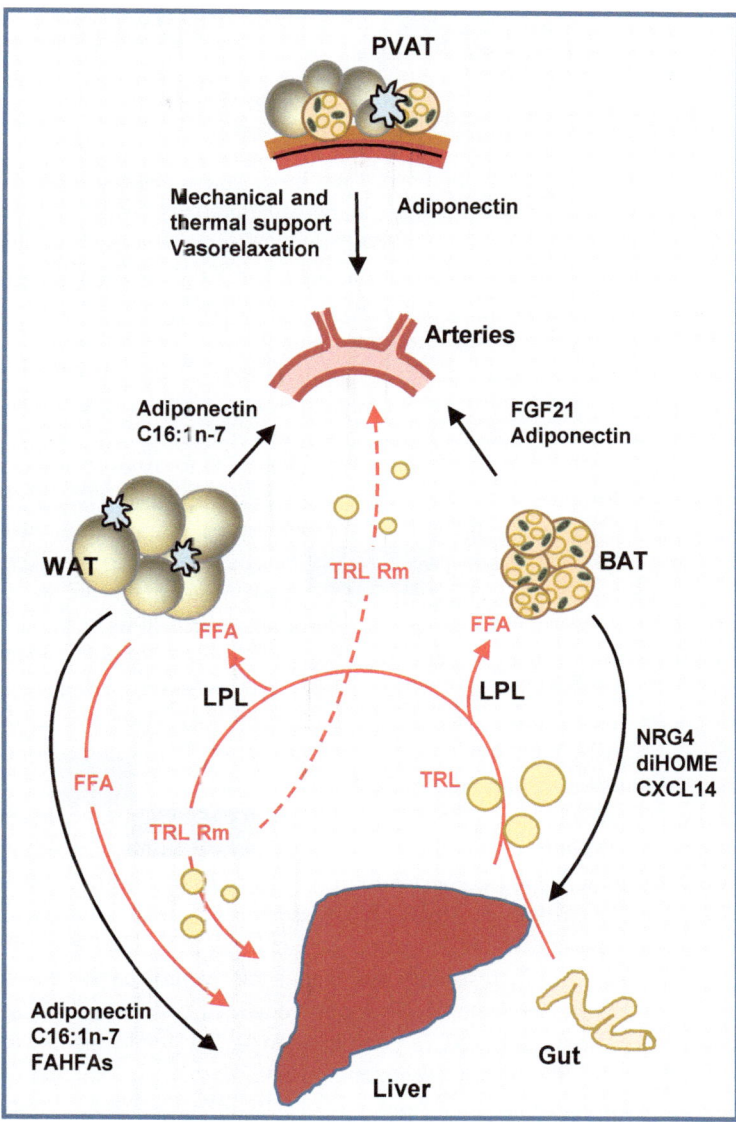

Fig. 1 Role of adipose tissues for cardiometabolic homeostasis under healthy conditions. In metabolic health, white and brown adipose can control systemic lipid homeostasis by regulating both the efficient clearance of triglyceride-rich lipoproteins and the release of fatty acids under catabolic conditions. Healthy adipose tissues harbor mostly anti-inflammatory immune cells (indicated by blue-colored immune cells) that are important to maintain tissue homeostasis. Under this condition, adipocytes mostly release beneficial hormones such as anti-inflammatory lipokines, adiponectin, and FGF21 that support vascular health by direct effects on arteries or indirectly by regulating hepatic lipid metabolism. Overall, healthy adipose tissues are associated with a state of metabolic flexibility that prevents atherosclerosis. *BAT* brown adipose tissue, *FFA* free fatty acids, *FGF21* fibroblast growth factor 21, *LPL* lipoprotein lipase, *NRG4* neuregulin 4, *PVAT* perivascular adipose tissue, *Rm* remnants, *TRL* triglyceride-rich lipoproteins, *WAT* white adipose tissue

2   Types of Adipose Tissue and Their Impact on Cardiovascular Disease

2.1   White Adipose Tissue

The bulk of triglycerides in the body is stored in subcutaneous and intra-abdominal WAT depots. The stored fatty acids can be released from white adipocytes by intracellular triglyceride lipolysis (Young and Zechner 2013). Norepinephrine, which is secreted by sympathetic nerves and signals through β-adrenergic receptors, is the major physiological trigger of lipolysis. β-Adrenergic stimulation elevates cyclic AMP, thereby activating adipose tissue triglyceride lipase (ATGL) and hormone-sensitive lipase (HSL). This regulation ensures that in catabolic states such as fasting or endurance exercise, WAT releases FFA into the circulation to provide other organs with energy. In contrast, after feeding, intracellular lipolysis is suppressed by insulin, and WAT takes up dietary fatty acids from circulating triglyceride-rich lipoproteins (TRL). In this anabolic process, TRL triglycerides are hydrolyzed by lipoprotein lipase (LPL) bound to the luminal side of the capillary endothelium, and the FFA then pass through the endothelium to be taken up and esterified by the adipocytes (Kersten 2014). Apart from their role in fatty acid metabolism, white adipocytes are also an important source of adipokines (adipose peptide hormones) and other secreted regulatory molecules. Notably, only a few of them such as leptin and adiponectin are exclusively expressed in adipose tissue and act at the same time as a true endocrine hormone. In other words, most adipokines are also expressed by cells other than adipocytes and may act predominantly in a paracrine fashion (Scheja and Heeren 2019).

In prolonged periods of caloric surplus, i.e., when energy uptake exceeds energy expenditure, WAT depots expand by increasing adipocyte number (hyperplasia) and adipocyte size (hypertrophy). The resulting overweight or obesity is detrimental when adipocyte hypertrophy prevails (Klöting et al. 2010). In this state of unhealthy obesity, chronic low-grade inflammation occurs in WAT (Crewe et al. 2017), adipocytes become insulin resistant, and fatty acids cannot be stored efficiently any longer. Hence, they are ectopically deposited as part of various lipid species in other organs, a process believed to contribute to the systemic insulin resistance typically associated with obesity (Petersen and Shulman 2018). Another important consequence of limited WAT lipid storage in obesity is liver steatosis. Among other effects, this causes increased secretion of very low-density lipoproteins (VLDL) and thus promotes diabetic dyslipidemia (Scheja and Heeren 2016). Together with pro-inflammatory changes in adipokine patterns, dyslipidemia links expanded WAT depots, especially abdominal visceral fat (Lim and Meigs 2014), to the increased atherosclerosis risk observed in obese individuals (Fig. 2).

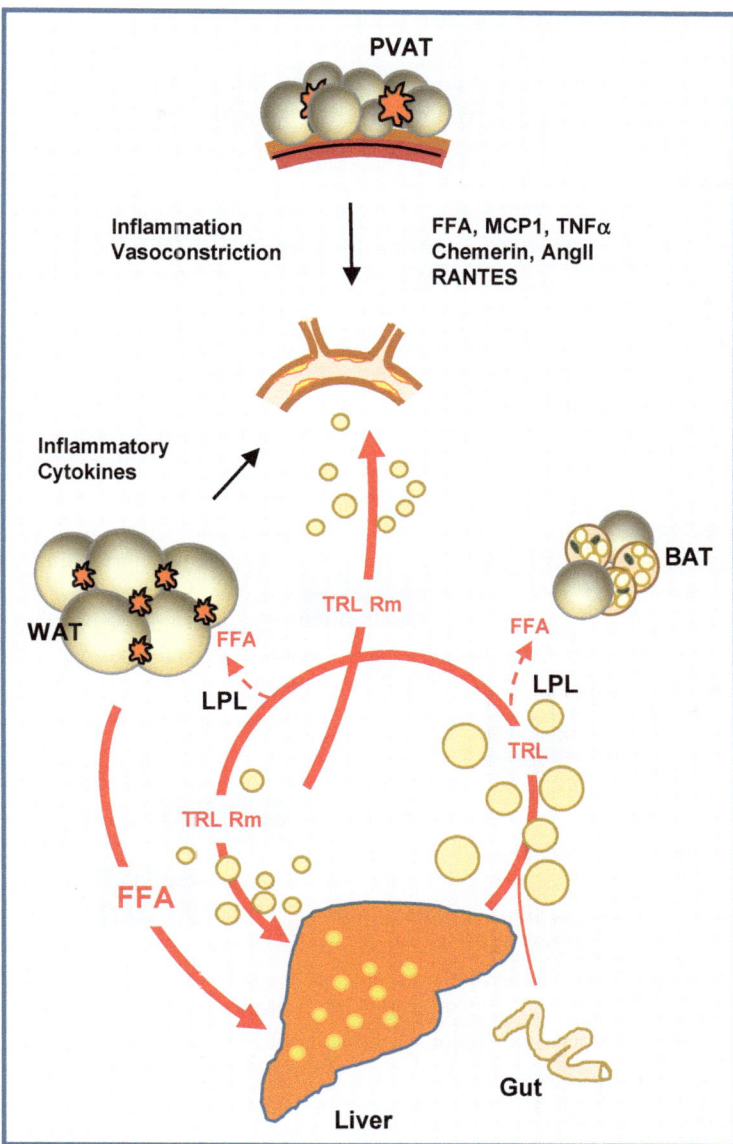

Fig. 2 Hypertrophy and inflammation in adipose tissues cause dyslipidemia and promote athero-sclerosis. Chronic caloric surplus and low energy expenditure result in obesity, which is characterized by inflamed (indicated by red-colored immune cells) and hypertrophic adipose tissues as well as dysfunctional brown adipose tissues. Eventually, this causes atherogenic dyslipidemia due to impaired TRL clearance and enhanced fatty acid flux to the liver leading to increased lipoprotein secretion. The lower release of adipocyte-derived anti-inflammatory molecules (see Fig. 1) and pro-inflammatory cytokines in particular those released by PVAT promote inflammation and vasoconstriction. Overall, this creates an immunometabolic state that promotes atherosclerotic plaque formation

2.2   Thermogenic Adipose Tissue

Brown adipocytes present in distinct BAT depots (Zhang et al. 2018) generate heat
to maintain body temperature by non-shivering thermogenesis (NST), a process that
depends on the mitochondrial proton transporter uncoupling protein-1 (UCP1) that
disconnects the respiratory chain from ATP synthesis (Cannon and Nedergaard
2004). NST is triggered by activation of lipolysis through increased β-adrenergic
signaling and other catabolic stimuli (Bordicchia et al. 2012). Fatty acids released
from the lipid droplets allosterically activate UCP1 and serve as mitochondrial fuel.
During prolonged thermogenic stimulation by cold exposure, or other sustained
catabolic stimuli such as burn trauma (Sidossis et al. 2015), mitochondria-rich
beige adipocytes appear in WAT, a phenomenon called WAT browning (Bartelt
and Heeren 2014). Although these adipocytes appear to be developmentally distinct,
they are very similar to brown adipocytes with regard to gene expression, morphology, and function. Both brown and beige adipocytes exhibit a very high metabolic
capacity and can combust large quantities of triglycerides and other sources of
energy when activated. In cold-treated mice, BAT internalizes high amounts of
triglycerides from circulating TRL (Bartelt et al. 2011). Under this condition,
cholesterol-enriched TRL remnants are efficiently cleared by the liver where bile
acid synthesis from cholesterol is increased (Worthmann et al. 2017). Furthermore,
the flux of high-density lipoprotein (HDL) cholesterol from the periphery to the liver
is enhanced (Bartelt et al. 2017). Consistent with the observed improved lipoprotein
profiles, the size of atherosclerotic plaques was reduced in BAT-activated mice fed a
cholesterol-rich diet compared to controls (Chang et al. 2012, Berbée et al. 2015). Of
note, this beneficial outcome on atherosclerosis depends on lowering of plasma
remnant cholesterol, as it was not observed in experiments with mouse models of
severely compromised hepatic remnant clearance (LDL receptor (LDLR)- or apolipoprotein (apo) E-deficient mice) where BAT activation and thus TRL processing
resulted in elevation of plasma remnant cholesterol (Berbée et al. 2015; Sui et al.
2019). Whether activated BAT or beige WAT has enough metabolic capacity to
reduce atherosclerosis in humans needs to be shown. However, a recent, large
epidemiological study indicates that high BAT mass inversely correlates with the
risk of type 2 diabetes and major cardiometabolic diseases (Becher et al. 2020).
Relative to body weight, BAT mass is smaller in humans than in rodents, and it
apparently declines in obesity (van Marken Lichtenbelt et al. 2009). However,
humans usually live under thermoneutrality, defined as an environmental temperature where the basal metabolic rate generates sufficient heat to maintain body core
temperature. When mice are kept under thermoneutral conditions (ca. 30 °C; in
dressed humans approximately 24 °C), BAT accumulates lipid and partially loses
mitochondria, UCP1, and other determinants of thermogenic capacity (Kotzbeck
et al. 2018). Thus, it is likely that in humans, reactivation of BAT and induction of
beige WAT, for example, by repeated cold treatments, would profoundly increase
metabolic rate and hence the capacity to metabolize atherogenic lipoproteins.
Another issue is that metabolic imaging studies to quantify BAT activity in humans
are usually done with radioactive glucose analogues. Suitable tracer analogues of

TRL, the major physiological fuel of BAT, still need to be developed. Most adipokines are expressed by both WAT and BAT, and due to its smaller size, BAT is probably less important. However, several adipokines are enriched in thermogenic adipose tissue, and some are induced and released from BAT under thermogenic stimulation or stress conditions (Villarroya et al. 2017). Overall, dysfunctional BAT is likely to influence atherosclerotic development especially by promoting dyslipidemia and inflammation (Fig. 2).

2.3   Perivascular Adipose Tissue

The adventitial layer of arteries is in close contact with adipocytes that form the perivascular adipose tissue (PVAT). PVAT is an important regulator of arterial function. It supports the blood vessel mechanically, by clearing FFA and by releasing paracrine factors that regulate vascular tone, inflammation, redox state, and smooth muscle cell proliferation (Costa et al. 2018). Given these multiple roles, it is not surprising that experimental stripping of arteries in rodents by mechanical or genetic means accelerates the development of atherosclerosis (Chang et al. 2012; Tian et al. 2013; Manka et al. 2014). Perivascular adipocytes may resemble white or brown adipocytes, depending on the anatomical location and the physiological state. For example, PVAT surrounding mesenteric arteries in mice was found to be similar to WAT (Gálvez-Prieto et al. 2008), whereas PVAT associated with the thoracic aorta contains brown-like adipocytes (Fitzgibbons et al. 2011). Of note, the latter adipocytes are functionally thermogenic, as they influence intravascular temperature in mice exposed to cold (Chang et al. 2012).

The quantity of PVAT in humans increases in obesity and is associated with cardiovascular disease (Britton et al. 2012). Mechanistic studies indicate that not only the volume but also altered properties of PVAT in obesity influence the development of atherosclerosis (Costa et al. 2018; Nosalski and Guzik 2017). One important alteration accelerating atheroma formation appears to be increased inflammation and infiltration of macrophages into PVAT (Henrichot et al. 2005; Skiba et al. 2017). Supporting this notion, expression of the pro-inflammatory molecule monocyte chemo-attractant protein-1 in transplanted PVAT is a determinant of neointima formation in a wire injury atherosclerosis model (Manka et al. 2014). Furthermore, PVAT-derived tumor necrosis factor-α is a causal factor for mitochondrial ROS production leading to aortic vasoconstriction in obese mice (Menezes da Costa et al. 2017). Inflammation promotes changes in the secretion of paracrine hormones from PVAT. For example, the release of adiponectin is reduced in obese, diabetic mice, leading to impaired insulin-dependent vasorelaxation (Meijer et al. 2013), whereas expression of the adipokine chemerin in PVAT confers vasoconstriction, and this is linked to obesity-induced hypertension (Ferland et al. 2018; Weng et al. 2017). These and several other hormones secreted by PVAT act as paracrine regulators of vascular tone, hypertension, and atherosclerosis (Nosalski and Guzik 2017) and thereby determine the health of arteries both under homeostatic and inflammatory circumstances (Figs. 1 and 2).

3 Therapies Targeting Adipose Tissue with Proven Clinical Efficacy in the Treatment of Atherosclerosis

3.1 Peroxisome Proliferator-Activated Receptor-γ (PPARγ) Agonists

PPARγ agonists of the thiazolidinedione (TZD) class are insulin-sensitizing drugs used for the treatment of type 2 diabetes. PPARγ is a transcription factor critical for adipocyte differentiation, and WAT and BAT are the tissues with the highest expression. The main target for TZD-based diabetes therapy is dysfunctional hypertrophic adipose tissue where TZDs improve insulin signaling and lipid storage while inducing an anti-inflammatory adipokine profile. Together, these actions lead to less ectopic lipid deposition in liver and muscle and improved systemic insulin sensitivity (Yau et al. 2013). TZDs also have anti-atherogenic activity Saremi et al. 2013; Thorp et al. 2007. Whether these protective cardiovascular effects are mediated by PPARγ expressed in adipocytes, for example, through improved thermogenesis and anti-inflammation (Chang et al. 2018), is unclear as the transcription factor is also expressed and mediates anti-atherosclerotic effects in immune, smooth muscle and endothelial cells (Murakami-Nishida et al. 2019; Subramanian et al. 2010; Qu et al. 2012, Ozasa et al. 2011). Nevertheless, several prospective clinical studies showed an improved plasma lipoprotein profile, reduced carotid artery intima media thickness, fewer cardiovascular disease events, and lower mortality in patients treated with the TZD pioglitazone compared to controls (Hanefeld 2009; Yau et al. 2013, Sartemi et al. 2013). Unfortunately, adverse effects, especially fluid retention, congestive heart failure, and bladder cancer, at least some of them target-related (Yau et al. 2013, Devchand et al. 2018), can offset the desired actions of the drug.

3.2 Niacin

Niacin (nicotinic acid) is a vitamin that, when applied orally at high doses, reduces atherosclerosis and cardiovascular mortality, especially in patients with metabolic syndrome (Superko et al. 2017). One anti-atherosclerotic mechanism of niacin is the improvement of diabetic dyslipidemia, including reduction in triglycerides and small dense LDL as well as the raising of HDL cholesterol (Kühnast et al. 2013). Signaling through the most important niacin receptor HCA2 (GPR109A, HM74) in adipocytes lowers cyclic AMP and reduces lipolysis and, hence, release of FFA. A longstanding hypothesis is that this improves diabetic dyslipidemia, as the decreased FFA flux to the liver entails reduced hepatic VLDL triglyceride secretion (Zeman et al. 2016). This notion has, however, been challenged by a paper describing that in both mice and humans, niacin and synthetic HCA2 ligands acutely lower plasma FFA whereas only niacin reduces plasma triglycerides and LDL cholesterol while elevating HDL (Lauring et al. 2012). Thus, the beneficial effects of niacin on diabetic dyslipidemia are at least in part independent of HCA2-mediated lipolysis. Of note, HCA2 is expressed and mediates anti-inflammatory effects in other artery wall cell types, in particular macrophages, endothelial cells, and vascular smooth muscle cells (Graff et al. 2016). An important role of macrophages was suggested by a bone marrow transplantation study with LDLR-deficient ($Ldlr^{-/-}$) mice. In this study, niacin was not able to suppress intimal macrophage recruitment and atheroma formation in wild-type acceptor mice that received HCA2-deficient cells, whereas transplantation of HCA2 wild-type hematopoietic cells restored niacin efficacy. This effect was independent of plasma lipid levels (Lukasova et al. 2011). Taken together, niacin has anti-atherogenic properties by improving plasma lipoprotein concentrations especially under diabetic conditions and probably by direct anti-inflammatory effects on immune cells. In addition, niacin may exert anti-atherosclerotic effects through HCA2 by increasing the secretion of adiponectin (Plaisance et al. 2009) and by suppressing pro-inflammatory mediators in adipocytes (Digby et al. 2010).

3.3 Renin-Angiotensin System Blockade

Inhibitors of the renin-angiotensin system (RAS) are widely prescribed drugs for hypertension, known to reduce atherosclerosis in humans and preclinical models, to some degree through their anti-inflammatory activity (Ranjbar et al. 2019). Of note, all components of the RAS are expressed in PVAT (Gálvez-Prieto et al. 2008), and pre-clinical models indicate a role of PVAT RAS in atherosclerosis. For example, angiotensin II was increased in periaortic adipose tissue but not in the circulation or other adipose tissues of $Apoe^{-/-}$ mice with unilateral nephrectomy, a model of accelerated atherosclerosis. Of note, no increase in PVAT inflammatory markers was observed in the nephrectomized mice, and angiotensin receptor blockers (ARBs) reduced atheroma (Kawahito et al. 2013). In another study, aortic transplantation of PVAT from $Apoe^{-/-}$ mice fed a high cholesterol diet increased atherosclerosis in acceptor mice, whereas transplantation of PVAT from angiotensin II type 1 receptor knockout mice or PVAT from ARB-treated mice reduced atheroma (Irie et al. 2015). Taken together, it is plausible that PVAT in part mediates the anti-atherosclerotic efficacy of RAS inhibitors.

4 Novel Therapeutic Targets in Adipose Tissue for Treatment of Atherosclerosis

4.1 Promoting Lipoprotein Disposal and Lipid Storage in Adipose Tissues

WAT is a major site of TRL fatty acid disposal after a meal, and human studies showed that this process is frequently impaired in obese and diabetic subjects (Jacome-Sosa and Parks 2014; Kersten 2014). Improving TRL processing and lipid storage in white adipocytes is, therefore, a suitable approach to reduce plasma triglycerides and hence diabetic dyslipidemia. LPL is the gatekeeper of TRL disposal in adipose tissue. The activity of the dimeric enzyme is controlled in a complex manner at the level of gene expression, assembly, translocation from adipocytes to the capillary lumen, and interaction of LPL with TRL particles (Kersten 2014). Insulin is the most important positive regulator of LPL activity, whereas angiopoietin-like-4 (ANGPTL4) and APOC3 are prominent negative regulators in adipose tissues (Kersten 2014). APOC3 has attracted a lot of attention in recent years, because plasma concentrations of this abundant apolipoprotein are a major determinant of plasma triglycerides and cardiovascular risk in the human population (Jørgensen et al. 2014; Crosby et al. 2014), explained by APOC3 inhibiting LPL as well as hepatic endocytosis of TRL remnants (Ramms and Gordts 2018; Taskinen et al. 2019). Recently, it became clear that the effect of APOC3 on lipoprotein receptor inactivation seems to be more relevant than its anti-lipolytic action (Gordts et al. 2016), especially as antisense-based reduction of APOC3 substantially lowered triglyceride levels in LPL-deficient patients (Gaudet et al. 2014). In addition to its role in dyslipidemia, APOC3 appears to directly act on arteries and to facilitate subendothelial accumulation of atherogenic particles (Taskinen et al. 2019). Overall, downregulation of APOC3 in the liver efficiently lowers triglycerides, and in part this effect is mediated via TRL disposal in adipose tissue.

ANGPTL4 negatively regulates LPL activity by preventing assembly of LPL and destabilizing the enzyme already during secretion from adipocytes (Dijk et al. 2018). Population-based genetic studies have consistently found reduced plasma triglycerides and reduced coronary artery disease risk in humans with a loss-of-function ANGPTL4 mutation (Bailetti et al. 2018; Stitziel et al. 2016; Dewey et al. 2016). A monoclonal antibody against ANGPTL4 suppressed plasma triglycerides in mice and monkeys (Dewey et al. 2016). Selective knockout of *Angptl4* in brown adipocytes of mice reduced TRL disposal only in BAT (Singh et al. 2018), supporting the notion that targeting ANGPTL4 in adipose tissue can be a means to specifically control organ-specific LPL activity. Importantly, LPL itself is also a drug target. Small molecules that bind to and activate LPL were identified in pharmaceutical screening efforts (Tsutsumi et al. 1993; Geldenhuys et al. 2014).

Another method to increase TRL disposal in adipose tissue is fibroblast growth factor (FGF) 21. FGF21 is an endocrine FGF isoform that fine-tunes systemic glucose and lipid metabolism (Bondurant and Potthoff 2018). At pharmacological doses, it increases insulin sensitivity and lowers blood glucose as well as lipids in mice (Kharitonenkov et al. 2005). Of note, lowering of triglycerides, but not glucose, was the most prominent effect of FGF21 in phase 1b clinical studies (Gaich et al. 2013; Talukdar et al. 2016). Mechanistic studies in mice showed that pharmacologically administered FGF21 acutely lowers plasma triglycerides and FFA. Tracer studies with labeled lipids demonstrated that this was due to higher uptake into WAT and BAT but not into other organs (Schlein et al. 2016). This effect was observed for both TRL-associated and albumin-bound fatty acids, indicating that FGF21 acts at least in part through stimulating fatty acid transport into adipocytes (Schlein et al. 2016).

An alternative target to boost lipoprotein disposal in adipose tissue is C-X-C chemokine motif receptor-7 (CXCR7). CXCR7 is also known as atypical chemokine receptor-3, because it is not expressed in leukocytes (Berahovich et al. 2010). $Cxcr7^{-/-}$ $Apoe^{-/-}$ mice on Western-type diet had exacerbated hypercholesterolemia and atherosclerosis, whereas the selective CXCR7 agonist CCX771 attenuated plaque formation in $Apoe^{-/-}$ mice (Li et al. 2014). CCX771 treatment lowered plasma triglycerides and VLDL cholesterol, which could be explained by increased VLDL clearance in visceral WAT but not BAT or other organs. This depot specifically exhibited increased LPL activity and reduced ANGPTL4 (Li et al. 2014).

Taken together, several targets and therapeutic approaches have been identified for the stimulation of lipoprotein clearance in adipose tissue with the aim to lower the plasma levels of atherogenic lipoproteins.

4.2 Boosting Thermogenic Activation

Activated thermogenic adipose tissue takes up energy at a high rate, and, at least in mice, a majority of calories is provided by TRL (Heine et al. 2018). BAT activation was shown to improve diabetic dyslipidemia, to increase reverse cholesterol transport and reduce atherosclerosis in APOE3-Leiden-CETP mice, an atherosclerosis-prone mouse model with humanized lipoprotein metabolism (Berbée et al. 2015; Bartelt et al. 2017). Reduction in atherosclerosis could be achieved by chronic β3-adrenergic receptor (β3-AR) stimulation using a synthetic agonist (Berbée et al. 2015), demonstrating feasibility of pharmacological intervention. Of note, the β3-AR agonist mirabegron, an approved drug for overactive bladder, activates BAT in humans (Cypess et al. 2015), and chronic dosing with mirabegron induces WAT browning (Finlin et al. 2018). β3-AR is highly expressed in adipocytes, and cardiovascular side effects of currently available β3 agonists such as hypertension occur only at high doses and are in part due to cross-reactivity on β1-ARs (Hainer 2016; Loh et al. 2019). Whether chronic BAT activation or induction of beige adipocytes by β3-AR agonists is sufficient to improve diabetic dyslipidemia in humans needs to be shown and is currently under investigation. Importantly, boosting thermogenic adipocytes by β3-AR agonists may counteract atherosclerosis independently of systemic lipoprotein metabolism via local activation of thermogenic adipocytes in PVAT. For example, a recent study demonstrated increased vascular temperature and reduced local inflammation in transgenic mice with higher thermogenic activity in PVAT (Xiong et al. 2017). Given that the common presence of BAT in adult humans has only been recognized recently (Celi 2009), it is likely that drugs directed at thermogenic adipose tissue targets other than β3-AR, such as adenosine A_{2A} agonists (Gnad et al. 2014), will be developed in the future.

4.3 Targeting Inflammation in Adipose Tissue

Chronic, subclinical inflammation is a hallmark of insulin-resistant WAT in unhealthy obesity. Anti-inflammatory interventions in adipose tissue may slow or prevent the development of atherosclerosis by improving lipoprotein disposal, normalizing systemic glucose homeostasis, and changing the secretome of adipose tissues in a favorable way. General anti-inflammatory therapies can have beneficial cardiovascular effects, as demonstrated by neutralizing antibodies directed against TNFα that reduce cardiovascular events in rheumatoid arthritis patients (Jacobsson et al. 2005) and raise plasma adiponectin levels (Nishida et al. 2008). Although immune cells are not organ-specific and found throughout the body, positive effects of many anti-inflammation therapies are likely to be at least in part mediated via inflammation in adipose tissue. This is especially true for PVAT that is in close proximity with atherosclerosis-prone arteries and exhibits a profound infiltration of macrophages, T-lymphocytes, and other immune cells during initiation and progression of atherosclerosis (Akoumianakis et al. 2017). Many anti-inflammatory proteins can be targeted in PVAT and have the potential to prevent and reduce atherosclerosis, as suggested by rodent studies. For example, the angiotensin 1–7 analogue AVE0991 that signals through the receptor Mas was demonstrated to selectively suppress inflammation in PVAT and reduce atherosclerosis in $Apoe^{-/-}$ mice (Skiba et al. 2017). Receptors of the chemokine RANTES (CCL5) are associated with PVAT inflammation, and $Ccl5^{-/-}$ mice are protected from perivascular inflammation (Mikolajczyk et al. 2016), while the RANTES receptor antagonist met-RANTES suppresses atherosclerosis in $Ldlr^{-/-}$ mice (Veillard et al. 2004). Similarly, CXCL10 signaling regulates T cell infiltration in atherosclerosis, and genetic deficiency of the CXCL10 receptor CXCR3 (Veillard et al. 2005) or treatment with the CXCR3 antagonist NBI-74330 (van Wanrooij et al. 2008) attenuates atherosclerosis in hypercholesterolemic mice. Several other chemokines appear to play an important role in PVAT inflammation and atherosclerosis (Nosalski and Guzik 2017). Taken together, several promising targets to tackle atherosclerosis by reducing inflammation in adipose tissue depots have been identified in mouse experiments. Whether anti-atherosclerotic approaches targeting adipose tissue inflammation with proof of concept in rodents can be translated into human therapies needs, however, to be shown.

4.4   Hormones Derived from Thermogenic Adipose Tissue

Compared to WAT, BAT and other thermogenic fat depots have a small mass and thus are probably a minor source of most circulating adipokines. However, there are exceptions to the rule, and some hormones are enriched in BAT (Villarroya et al. 2017). Recent studies suggest that some of these hormones are potential targets to prevent or treat atherosclerosis. For example, transplantation of BAT into the visceral cavity of $Apoe^{-/-}$ mice led to reduction in atherosclerotic plaque size. This was accompanied by increased plasma FGF21 and adiponectin, and the beneficial effect of BAT transplantation in this study could be blocked by β3-AR antagonists (Kikai et al. 2018). Many anti-atherogenic activities of FGF21 have been identified in rodents (Jin et al. 2016; Domouzoglou et al. 2015). Therefore, it is plausible that elevated FGF21 mediates at least some of the effects in this model. Of note, adenosine A_{2A} receptor agonists, molecules that activate thermogenic adipocytes in mice and humans (Gnad et al. 2014), were found to trigger FGF21 expression and secretion from BAT, and this was important to prevent hypertension-induced cardiac hypertrophy (Ruan et al. 2018). Thus, at least in mice, activated BAT is a meaningful source of cardio-protective and anti-atherosclerotic FGF21.

Moreover, the peptide neuregulin-4 and the linoleic acid derivative 12,13-dihydroxy-9Z-octadecenoic acid (diHOME) have recently been described as hormones enriched in and released by activated thermogenic adipocytes. They act in a paracrine fashion to potentiate thermogenic function and appear to exhibit beneficial metabolic functions in the liver and muscle (Nugroho et al. 2018; Stanford et al. 2018; Pellegrinelli et al. 2018; Guo et al. 2017; Lynes et al. 2017; Wang et al. 2014). It is tempting to speculate that these, and other pro-thermogenic hormones secreted by brown and beige adipocytes such as C-X-C motif chemokine ligand-14 (Cereijo et al. 2018), have a protective effect in atherosclerosis, for example, by increasing lipoprotein disposal or by modulating inflammation.

4.5 De Novo Lipogenesis-Derived Lipokines

Adipose tissue is a quantitatively relevant site of de novo lipogenesis (DNL), the endogenous synthesis of fatty acids from non-lipid precursors. One important feature of unhealthy obesity is increased DNL in the liver accompanied by decreased DNL in WAT (Eissing et al. 2013). Elevated hepatic DNL promotes insulin resistance and is a mechanism that worsens diabetic dyslipidemia by increasing triglyceride availability for VLDL production (Scheja and Heeren 2016). How decreased WAT DNL contributes to the development of metabolic disease has long been elusive. Research of the recent years has provided strong evidence that DNL-associated lipids secreted from adipocytes, coined lipokines, are part of the mechanism. The first lipokine to be identified was the FFA variant of palmitoleate (C16:1n-7), a major fatty acid produced by DNL that was found to be reduced in WAT of obese mice. Palmitoleate FFA turned out to be an anti-inflammatory, insulin-sensitizing molecule that improves systemic glucose homeostasis in mice (Cao et al. 2008). Palmitoleate was identified to reduce atherosclerosis via suppressing pro-inflammatory differentiation of macrophages, and $Apoe^{-/-}$ mice on a Western-type diet supplemented with palmitoleate had significantly reduced plaque size compared to control mice (Çimen et al. 2016; Yang et al. 2019). Thus, WAT-derived palmitoleate can reduce atherosclerosis risk by modulating inflammation. It is important to note that WAT-derived palmitoleate is not or only marginally lower in obese, insulin-resistant compared to healthy humans (Eissing et al. 2013; Stefan et al. 2010). Nevertheless, dietary palmitoleate supplementation decreased inflammation and lowered LDL in human subjects (Bueno-Hernández et al. 2017; Bernstein et al. 2014), highlighting the anti-atherosclerosis potential of palmitoleate.

Other lipids proposed as adipose tissue-derived DNL-associated lipokines are fatty acid esters of hydroxy fatty acids (FAHFAs), a novel class of lipids (Yore et al. 2014). WAT levels of certain FAHFA species were shown to depend on DNL. Moreover, circulating levels of DNL-linked FAHFA were shown to be tightly associated with insulin sensitivity in mice and in humans (Yore et al. 2014; Hammarstedt et al. 2018). In addition, oral FAHFA supplementation was demonstrated to improve glucose tolerance in mice (Yore et al. 2014), an FAHFA effect that has, however, been questioned by another group (Pflimlin et al. 2018). More research is warranted, especially with regard to FAHFA synthesis and degradation as well as FAHFA signaling mechanisms to better understand the role of this novel lipid class in metabolic regulation. Furthermore, studies addressing the association of DNL-derived FAHFAs with cardiovascular risk markers are needed to find out whether FAHFAs modulate the development of cardiovascular disease.

5   Future Directions

In the past decades, many adipokines, chemokines, and other regulatory molecules acting on or derived from adipose tissues that affect the development and progression of atherosclerosis have been identified. One major task will be to successfully translate these findings into the clinics. In some cases such as pioglitazone, cardiovascular clinical benefit is evident; however, adverse effects in other organs have precluded more widespread use or even led to the retraction of the drug. Here, adipose tissue targeted delivery using advanced drug delivery technologies could be a solution. Peptides that selectively bind to endothelium in WAT (Kolonin et al. 2004) and BAT (Azhdarinia et al. 2013), respectively, have been identified, and the WAT-selective peptide was successfully used for WAT-specific drug delivery (Xue et al. 2016). Although this WAT-directed drug delivery system is not suitable for oral application, proof of concept that adipose tissue depots can be targeted specifically was delivered.

Methods to achieve adipose-directed delivery of nucleic acids with the goal to overexpress a beneficial protein, or to modulate endogenous RNA levels, have been considerably advanced in the past years. For example, adipose tissue-directed expression of genes, or suppression using small hairpin RNAs, can be achieved by the means of adeno-associated virus vectors (O'Neill et al. 2014). Another promising approach is the delivery of silencing RNAs encapsulated by glucan shells, a method that specifically delivers the regulatory RNA species to WAT macrophages (Aouadi et al. 2013).

An alternative approach to molecular interventions in unhealthy adipose tissues would be the development of regenerative medicines based on bioelectric stimulation devices to increase the sympathetic tone in specific adipose depots or gene therapy and cell transplantation to restore functional adipocytes. Such innovative concepts and highly advanced technologies would provide a novel therapeutic strategy to target obesity-associated cardiovascular disease.

References

Akoumianakis I, Tarun A, Antoniades C (2017) Perivascular adipose tissue as a regulator of vascular disease pathogenesis: identifying novel therapeutic targets. Br J Pharmacol 174:3411–3424

Aouadi M, Tencerova M, Vangala P, Yawe JC, Nicoloro SM, Amano SU, Cohen JL, Czech MP (2013) Gene silencing in adipose tissue macrophages regulates whole-body metabolism in obese mice. Proc Natl Acad Sci U S A 110:8278–8283

Azhdarinia A, Daquinag AC, Tseng C, Ghosh SC, Ghosh P, Amaya-Manzanares F, Sevick-Muraca E, Kolonin MG (2013) A peptide probe for targeted brown adipose tissue imaging. Nat Commun 4:2472

Bailetti D, Bertoccini L, Mancina RM, Barchetta I, Capoccia D, Cossu E, Pujia A, Lenzi A, Leonetti F, Cavallo MG, Romeo S, Baroni MG (2018) ANGPTL4 gene E40K variation protects against obesity-associated dyslipidemia in participants with obesity. Obes Sci Pract 5:83–90

Bartelt A, Heeren J (2014) Adipose tissue browning and metabolic health. Nat Rev Endocrinol 10:24–36

Bartelt A, Bruns OT, Reimer R, Hohenberg H, Ittrich H, Peldschus K, Kaul MG, Tromsdorf UI, Weller H, Waurisch C, Eychmüller A, Gordts PL, Rinninger F, Bruegelmann K, Freund B, Nielsen P, Merkel M, Heeren J (2011) Brown adipose tissue activity controls triglyceride clearance. Nat Med 17:200–205

Bartelt A, John C, Schaltenberg N, Berbée JFP, Worthmann A, Cherradi ML, Schlein C, Piepenburg J, Boon MR, Rinninger F, Heine M, Toedter K, Niemeier A, Nilsson SK, Fischer M, Wijers SL, van Marken LW, Scheja L, Rensen PCN, Heeren J (2017) Thermogenic adipocytes promote HDL turnover and reverse cholesterol transport. Nat Commun 8:15010

Becher T, Palanisamy S, Kramer DJ, Marx SJ, Wibmer AG, Del Gaudio I, Butler SD, Jiang CS, Vaughan R, Schöder H et al (2020) Brown adipose tissue is associated with improved cardiometabolic health and regulates blood pressure. bioRxiv, 2020.2002.2008.933754

Berahovich RD, Zabel BA, Penfold ME, Lewén S, Wang Y, Miao Z, Gan L, Pereda J, Dias J, Slukvin II, McGrath KE, Jaen JC, Schall TJ (2010) CXCR7 protein is not expressed on human or mouse leukocytes. J Immunol 185:5130–5139

Berbée JF, Boon MR, Khedoe PP, Bartelt A, Schlein C, Worthmann A, Kooijman S, Hoeke G, Mol IM, John C, Jung C, Vazirpanah N, Brouwers LP, Gordts PL, Esko JD, Hiemstra PS, Havekes LM, Scheja L, Heeren J, Rensen PC (2015) Brown fat activation reduces hypercholesterolaemia and protects from atherosclerosis development. Nat Commun 6:6356

Bernstein AM, Roizen MF, Martinez L (2014) Purified palmitoleic acid for the reduction of high-sensitivity C-reactive protein and serum lipids: a double-blinded, randomized, placebo controlled study. J Clin Lipidol 8:612–617

BonDurant LD, Potthoff MJ (2018) Fibroblast growth factor 21: a versatile regulator of metabolic homeostasis. Annu Rev Nutr 38:173–196

Bordicchia M, Liu D, Amri EZ, Ailhaud G, Dessì-Fulgheri P, Zhang C, Takahashi N, Sarzani R, Collins S (2012) Cardiac natriuretic peptides act via p38 MAPK to induce the brown fat thermogenic program in mouse and human adipocytes. J Clin Invest 122:1022–1036

Britton KA, Pedley A, Massaro JM, Corsini EM, Murabito JM, Hoffmann U, Fox CS (2012) Prevalence, distribution, and risk factor correlates of high thoracic periaortic fat in the Framingham heart study. J Am Heart Assoc 1:e004200

Bueno-Hernández N, Sixtos-Alonso MS, Milke García MDP, Yamamoto-Furusho JK (2017) Effect of Cis-palmitoleic acid supplementation on inflammation and expression of HNF4γ, HNF4α and IL6 in patients with ulcerative colitis. Minerva Gastroenterol Dietol 63:257–263

Cannon B, Nedergaard J (2004) Brown adipose tissue: function and physiological significance. Physiol Rev 84:277–359

Cao H, Gerhold K, Mayers JR, Wiest MM, Watkins SM, Hotamisligil GS (2008) Identification of a lipokine, a lipid hormone linking adipose tissue to systemic metabolism. Cell 134:933–944

Celi FS (2009) Brown adipose tissue--when it pays to be inefficient. N Engl J Med 360:1553–1556

Cereijo R, Gavalda-Navarro A, Cairo M, Quesada-López T, Villarroya J, Morón-Ros S, Sánchez-Infantes D, Peyrou M, Iglesias R, Mampel T, Turatsinze JV, Eizirik DL, Giralt M, Villarroya F (2018) CXCL14, a brown adipokine that mediates brown-fat-to-macrophage communication in thermogenic adaptation. Cell Metab 28:750–763

Chang L, Villacorta L, Li R, Hamblin M, Xu W, Dou C, Zhang J, Wu J, Zeng R, Chen YE (2012) Loss of perivascular adipose tissue on peroxisome proliferator-activated receptor-γ deletion in smooth muscle cells impairs intravascular thermoregulation and enhances atherosclerosis. Circulation 126:1067–1078

Chang L, Zhao X, Garcia-Barrio M, Zhang J, Eugene Chen Y (2018) MitoNEET in perivascular adipose tissue prevents arterial stiffness in aging mice. Cardiovasc Drugs Ther 32:531–539

Çimen I, Kocatürk B, Koyuncu S, Tufanlı Ö, Onat UI, Yıldırım AD, Apaydın O, Demirsoy Ş, Aykut ZG, Nguyen UT, Watkins SM, Hotamışlıgil GS, Erbay E (2016) Prevention of athero-sclerosis by bioactive palmitoleate through suppression of organelle stress and inflammasome activation. Sci Transl Med 8:358ra126

Cinti S (2001) The adipose organ: morphological perspectives of adipose tissues. Proc Nutr Soc 60:319–328

Costa RM, Neves KB, Tostes RC, Lobato NS (2018) Perivascular adipose tissue as a relevant fat depot for cardiovascular risk in obesity. Front Physiol 9:253

Crewe C, An YA, Scherer PE (2017) The ominous triad of adipose tissue dysfunction: inflamma-tion, fibrosis, and impaired angiogenesis. J Clin Invest 127:74–82

Crosby J, Peloso GM, Auer PL, Crosslin DR, Stitziel NO, Lange LA, Lu Y, Tang ZZ, Zhang H, Hindy G, Masca N, Stirrups K, Kanoni S, Do R, Jun G, Hu Y, Kang HM, Xue C, Goel A, Farrall M, Duga S, Merlini PA, Asselta R, Girelli D, Olivieri O, Martinelli N, Yin W, Reilly D, Speliotes E, Fox CS, Hveem K, Holmen OL, Nikpay M, Farlow DN, Assimes TL, Franceschini N, Robinson J, North KE, Martin LW, DePristo M, Gupta N, Escher SA, Jansson JH, Van Zuydam N, Palmer CN, Wareham N, Koch W, Meitinger T, Peters A, Lieb W, Erbel R, Konig IR, Kruppa J, Degenhardt F, Gottesman O, Bottinger EP, O'Donnell CJ, Psaty BM, Ballantyne CM, Abecasis G, Ordovas JM, Melander O, Watkins H, Orho-Melander M, Ardissino D, Loos RJ, McPherson R, Willer CJ, Erdmann J, Hall AS, Samani NJ, Deloukas P, Schunkert H, Wilson JG, Kooperberg C, Rich SS, Tracy RP, Lin DY, Altshuler D, Gabriel S, Nickerson DA, Jarvik GP, Cupples LA, Reiner AP, Boerwinkle E, Kathiresan S (2014) Loss-of-function mutations in APOC3, triglycerides, and coronary disease. N Engl J Med 371:22–31

Cypess AM, Weiner LS, Roberts-Toler C, Franquet Elía E, Kessler SH, Kahn PA, English J, Chatman K, Trauger SA, Doria A, Kolodny GM (2015) Activation of human brown adipose tissue by a β3-adrenergic receptor agonist. Cell Metab 21:33–38

Devchand PR, Liu T, Altman RB, FitzGerald GA, Schadt EE (2018) The pioglitazone trek via human PPAR gamma: from discovery to a medicine at the FDA and beyond. Front Pharmacol 9:1093

Dewey FE, Gusarova V, O'Dushlaine C, Gottesman O, Trejos J, Hunt C, Van Hout CV, Habegger L, Buckler D, Lai KM, Leader JB, Murray MF, Ritchie MD, Kirchner HL, Ledbetter DH, Penn J, Lopez A, Borecki IB, Overton JD, Reid JG, Carey DJ, Murphy AJ, Yancopoulos GD, Baras A, Gromada J, Shuldiner AR (2016) Inactivating variants in ANGPTL4 and risk of coronary artery disease. N Engl J Med 374:1123–1133

Digby JE, McNeill E, Dyar OJ, Lam V, Greaves DR, Choudhury RP (2010) Anti-inflammatory effects of nicotinic acid in adipocytes demonstrated by suppression of fractalkine, RANTES, and MCP-1 and upregulation of adiponectin. Atherosclerosis 209:89–95

Dijk W, Ruppert PMM, Oost LJ, Kersten S (2018) Angiopoietin-like 4 promotes the intracellular cleavage of lipoprotein lipase by PCSK3/furin in adipocytes. J Biol Chem 293:14134–14145

Domouzoglou EM, Naka KK, Vlahos AP, Papafaklis MI, Michalis LK, Tsatsoulis A, Maratos-Flier E (2015) Fibroblast growth factors in cardiovascular disease: the emerging role of FGF21. Am J Physiol Heart Circ Physiol 309:H1029–H1038

Eissing L, Scherer T, Tödter K, Knippschild U, Greve JW, Buurman WA, Pinnschmidt HO, Rensen SS, Wolf AM, Bartelt A, Heeren J, Buettner C, Scheja L (2013) De novo lipogenesis in human fat and liver is linked to ChREBP-β and metabolic health. Nat Commun 4:1528

Ferland DJ, Seitz B, Darics ES, Thompson JM, Yeh ST, Mullick AE, Watts SW (2018) Whole-body but not hepatic knockdown of Chemerin by antisense oligonucleotide decreases blood pressure in rats. J Pharmacol Exp Ther 365:212–218

Finlin BS, Memetimin H, Confides AL, Kasza I, Zhu B, Vekaria HJ, Harfmann B, Jones KA, Johnson ZR, Westgate PM, Alexander CM, Sullivan PG, Dupont-Versteegden EE, Kern PA (2018) Human adipose beiging in response to cold and mirabegron. JCI Insight 3:121510

Fitzgibbons TP, Kogan S, Aouadi M, Hendricks GM, Straubhaar J, Czech MP (2011) Similarity of mouse perivascular and brown adipose tissues and their resistance to diet-induced inflammation. Am J Physiol Heart Circ Physiol 301:H1425–H1437

Gaich G, Chien JY, Fu H, Glass LC, Deeg MA, Holland WL, Kharitonenkov A, Bumol T, Schilske HK, Moller DE (2013) The effects of LY2405319, an FGF21 analog, in obese human subjects with type 2 diabetes. Cell Metab 18:333–340

Gálvez-Prieto B, Bolbrinker J, Stucchi P, de Las Heras AI, Merino B, Arribas S, Ruiz-Gayo M, Huber M, Wehland M, Kreutz R, Fernandez-Alfonso MS (2008) Comparative expression analysis of the renin-angiotensin system components between white and brown perivascular adipose tissue. J Endocrinol 197:55–64

Gaudet D, Brisson D, Tremblay K, Alexander VJ, Singleton W, Hughes SG, Geary RS, Baker BF, Graham MJ, Crooke RM, Witztum JL (2014) Targeting APOC3 in the familial chylomicronemia syndrome. N Engl J Med 371:2200–2206

Geldenhuys WJ, Aring D, Sadana P (2014) A novel lipoprotein lipase (LPL) agonist rescues the enzyme from inhibition by angiopoietin-like 4 (ANGPTL4). Bioorg Med Chem Lett 24:2163–2167

Gnad T, Scheibler S, von Kügelgen I, Scheele C, Kilić A, Glöde A, Hoffmann LS, Reverte-Salisa L, Horn P, Mutlu S, El-Tayeb A, Kranz M, Deuther-Conrad W, Brust P, Lidell ME, Betz MJ, Enerbäck S, Schrader J, Yegutkin GG, Müller CE, Pfeifer A (2014) Adenosine activates brown adipose tissue and recruits beige adipocytes via A2A receptors. Nature 516:395–399

Gordts PL, Nock R, Son NH, Ramms B, Lew I, Gonzales JC, Thacker BE, Basu D, Lee RG, Mullick AE, Graham MJ, Goldberg IJ, Crooke RM, Witztum JL, Esko JD (2016) ApoC-III inhibits clearance of triglyceride-rich lipoproteins through LDL family receptors. J Clin Invest 126:2855–2866

Graff EC, Fang H, Wanders D, Judd RL (2016) Anti-inflammatory effects of the hydroxycarboxylic acid receptor 2. Metabolism 65:102–113

Guo L, Zhang P, Chen Z, Xia H, Li S, Zhang Y, Kobberup S, Zou W, Lin JD (2017) Hepatic neuregulin 4 signaling defines an endocrine checkpoint for steatosis-to-NASH progression. J Clin Invest 127:4449–4461

Hainer V (2016) Beta3-adrenoreceptor agonist mirabegron - a potential antiobesity drug? Expert Opin Pharmacother 17:2125–2127

Hammarstedt A, Syed I, Vijayakumar A, Eliasson B, Gogg S, Kahn BB, Smith U (2018) Adipose tissue dysfunction is associated with low levels of the novel palmitic acid hydroxystearic acids. Sci Rep 8:15757

Hanefeld M (2009) The role of pioglitazone in modifying the atherogenic lipoprotein profile. Diabetes Obes Metab 11:742–756

Heine M, Fischer AW, Schlein C, Jung C, Straub LG, Gottschling K, Mangels N, Yuan Y, Nilsson SK, Liebscher G, Chen O, Schreiber R, Zechner R, Scheja L, Heeren J (2018) Lipolysis triggers a systemic insulin response essential for efficient energy replenishment of activated brown adipose tissue in mice. Cell Metab 28:644–655

Henrichot E, Juge-Aubry CE, Pernin A, Pache JC, Velebit V, Dayer JM, Meda P, Chizzolini C, Meier CA (2005) Production of chemokines by perivascular adipose tissue: a role in the pathogenesis of atherosclerosis? Arterioscler Thromb Vasc Biol 25:2594–2599

Irie D, Kawahito H, Wakana N, Kato T, Kishida S, Kikai M, Ogata T, Ikeda K, Ueyama T, Matoba S, Yamada H (2015) Transplantation of periaortic adipose tissue from angiotensin receptor blocker-treated mice markedly ameliorates atherosclerosis development in apoE−/− mice. J Renin-Angiotensin-Aldosterone Syst 16:67–78

Jacobsson LT, Turesson C, Gülfe A, Kapetanovic MC, Petersson IF, Saxne T, Geborek P (2005) Treatment with tumor necrosis factor blockers is associated with a lower incidence of first cardiovascular events in patients with rheumatoid arthritis. J Rheumatol 32:1213

Jacome-Sosa MM, Parks EJ (2014) Fatty acid sources and their fluxes as they contribute to plasma triglyceride concentrations and fatty liver in humans. Curr Opin Lipidol 25:213–220

Jin L, Lin Z, Xu A (2016) Fibroblast growth factor 21 protects against atherosclerosis via fine-tuning the multiorgan crosstalk. Diabetes Metab J 40:22–31

Jørgensen AB, Frikke-Schmidt R, Nordestgaard BG, Tybjærg-Hansen A (2014) Loss-of-function mutations in APOC3 and risk of ischemic vascular disease. N Engl J Med 371:32–41

Kawahito H, Yamada H, Irie D, Kato T, Akakabe Y, Kishida S, Takata H, Wakana N, Ogata T, Ikeda K, Ueyama T, Matoba S, Mori Y, Matsubara H (2013) Periaortic adipose tissue-specific activation of the renin-angiotensin system contributes to atherosclerosis development in uninephrectomized apoE−/− mice. Am J Physiol Heart Circ Physiol 305:H667–H675

Kersten S (2014) Physiological regulation of lipoprotein lipase. Biochim Biophys Acta 1841:919–933

Kharitonenkov A, Shiyanova TL, Koester A, Ford AM, Micanovic R, Galbreath EJ, Sandusky GE, Hammond LJ, Moyers JS, Owens RA, Gromada J, Brozinick JT, Hawkins ED, Wroblewski VJ, Li DS, Mehrbod F, Jaskunas SR, Shanafelt AB (2005) FGF-21 as a novel metabolic regulator. J Clin Invest 115:1627–1635

Kikai M, Yamada H, Wakana N, Terada K, Yamamoto K, Wada N, Motoyama S, Saburi M, Sugimoto T, Irie D, Kato T, Kawahito H, Ogata T, Matoba S (2018) Adrenergic receptor-mediated activation of FGF-21-adiponectin axis exerts atheroprotective effects in brown adipose tissue-transplanted apoE−/− mice. Biochem Biophys Res Commun 497:1097–1103

Klöting N, Fasshauer M, Dietrich A, Kovacs P, Schön MR, Kern M, Stumvoll M, Blüher M (2010) Insulin-sensitive obesity. Am J Physiol Endocrinol Metab 299:E506–E515

Kolonin MG, Saha PK, Chan L, Pasqualini R, Arap W (2004) Reversal of obesity by targeted ablation of adipose tissue. Nat Med 10:625–632

Kotzbeck P, Giordano A, Mondini E, Murano I, Severi I, Venema W, Cecchini MP, Kershaw EE, Barbatelli G, Haemmerle G, Zechner R, Cinti S (2018) Brown adipose tissue whitening leads to brown adipocyte death and adipose tissue inflammation. J Lipid Res 59:784–794

Kühnast S, Louwe MC, Heemskerk MM, Pieterman EJ, van Klinken JB, van den Berg SA, Smit JW, Havekes LM, Rensen PC, van der Hoorn JW, Princen HM, Jukema JW (2013) Niacin reduces atherosclerosis development in APOE*3Leiden.CETP mice mainly by reducing NonHDL-cholesterol. PLoS One 8:e66467

Lauring B, Taggart AK, Tata JR, Dunbar R, Caro L, Cheng K, Chin J, Colletti SL, Cote J, Khalilieh S, Liu J, Luo WL, Maclean AA, Peterson LB, Polis AB, Sirah W, Wu TJ, Liu X, Jin L, Wu K, Boatman PD, Semple G, Behan DP, Connolly DT, Lai E, Wagner JA, Wright SD, Cuffie C, Mitchel YB, Rader DJ, Paolini JF, Waters MG, Plump A (2012) Niacin lipid efficacy is independent of both the niacin receptor GPR109A and free fatty acid suppression. Sci Transl Med 4:148ra115

Li X, Zhu M, Penfold ME, Koenen RR, Thiemann A, Heyll K, Akhtar S, Koyadan S, Wu Z, Gremse F, Kiessling F, van Zandvoort M, Schall TJ, Weber C, Schober A (2014) Activation of CXCR7 limits atherosclerosis and improves hyperlipidemia by increasing cholesterol uptake in adipose tissue. Circulation 129:1244–1253

Lim S, Meigs JB (2014) Links between ectopic fat and vascular disease in humans. Arterioscler Thromb Vasc Biol 34:1820–1826

Loh RKC, Formosa MF, La Gerche A, Reutens AT, Kingwell BA, Carey AL (2019) Acute metabolic and cardiovascular effects of mirabegron in healthy individuals. Diabetes Obes Metab 21:276–284

Lukasova M, Malaval C, Gille A, Kero J, Offermanns S (2011) Nicotinic acid inhibits progression of atherosclerosis in mice through its receptor GPR109A expressed by immune cells. J Clin Invest 121:1163–1173

Lynes MD, Leiria LO, Lurdh M, Bartelt A, Shamsi F, Huang TL, Takahashi H, Hirshman MF, Schlein C, Lee A, Baer LA, May FJ, Gao F, Narain NR, Chen EY, Kiebish MA, Cypess AM, Blüher M, Goodyear LJ, Hotamisligil GS, Stanford KI, Tseng YH (2017) The cold-induced lipokine 12,13-diHOME promotes fatty acid transport into brown adipose tissue. Nat Med 23:631–637

Manka D, Chatterjee TK, Stoll LL, Basford JE, Konaniah ES, Srinivasan R, Bogdanov VY, Tang Y, Blomkalns AL, Hui DY, Weintraub NL (2014) Transplanted perivascular adipose tissue accelerates injury-induced neointimal hyperplasia: role of monocyte chemoattractant protein-1. Arterioscler Thromb Vasc Biol 34:1723–1730

Meijer RI, Bakker W, Alta CL, Sipkema P, Yudkin JS, Viollet B, Richter EA, Smulders YM, van Hinsbergh VW, Serné EH, Eringa EC (2013) Perivascular adipose tissue control of insulin-induced vasoreactivity in muscle is impaired in db/db mice. Diabetes 62:590–598

Menezes da Costa R, Fais RS, Dechandt CRP, Louzada-Junior P, Alberici LC, Lobato NS, Tostes RC (2017) Increased mitochondrial ROS generation mediates the loss of the anti-contractile effects of perivascular adipose tissue in high-fat diet obese mice. Br J Pharmacol 174:3527–3541

Mikolajczyk TP, Nosalski R, Szczepaniak P, Budzyn K, Osmenda G, Skiba D, Sagan A, Wu J, Vinh A, Marvar PJ, Guzik B, Podolec J, Drummond G, Lob HE, Harrison DG, Guzik TJ (2016) Role of chemokine RANTES in the regulation of perivascular inflammation, T-cell accumulation, and vascular dysfunction in hypertension. FASEB J 30:1987–1999

Murakami-Nishida S, Matsumura T, Senokuchi T, Ishii N, Kinoshita H, Yamada S, Morita Y, Nishida S, Motoshima H, Kondo T, Komohara Y, Araki E (2019) Pioglitazone suppresses macrophage proliferation in apolipoprotein-E deficient mice by activating PPARγ. Atherosclerosis 286:30–39

Nishida K, Okada Y, Nawata M, Saito K, Tanaka Y (2008) Induction of hyperadiponectinemia following long-term treatment of patients with rheumatoid arthritis with infliximab (IFX), an anti-TNF-alpha antibody. Endocr J 55:213–216

Nosalski R, Guzik TJ (2017) Perivascular adipose tissue inflammation in vascular disease. Br J Pharmacol 174:3496–3513

Nugroho DB, Ikeda K, Barinda AJ, Wardhana DA, Yagi K, Miyata K, Oike Y, Hirata KI, Emoto N (2018) Neuregulin-4 is an angiogenic factor that is critically involved in the maintenance of adipose tissue vasculature. Biochem Biophys Res Commun 503:378–384

O'Neill SM, Hinkle C, Chen SJ, Sandhu A, Hovhannisyan R, Stephan S, Lagor WR, Ahima RS, Johnston JC, Reilly MP (2014) Targeting adipose tissue via systemic gene therapy. Gene Ther 21:653–661

Ozasa H, Ayaori M, Iizuka M, Terao Y, Uto-Kondo H, Yakushiji E, Takiguchi S, Nakaya K, Hisada T, Uehara Y, Ogura M, Sasaki M, Komatsu T, Horii S, Mochizuki S, Yoshimura M, Ikewaki K (2011) Pioglitazone enhances cholesterol efflux from macrophages by increasing ABCA1/ABCG1 expressions via PPARγ/LXRα pathway: findings from in vitro and ex vivo studies. Atherosclerosis 219:141–150

Pellegrinelli V, Peirce VJ, Howard L, Virtue S, Türei D, Senzacqua M, Frontini A, Dalley JW, Horton AR, Bidault G, Severi I, Whittle A, Rahmouni K, Saez-Rodriguez J, Cinti S, Davies AM, Vidal-Puig A (2018) Adipocyte-secreted BMP8b mediates adrenergic-induced remodeling of the neuro-vascular network in adipose tissue. Nat Commun 9:4974

Petersen MC, Shulman GI (2018) Mechanisms of insulin action and insulin resistance. Physiol Rev 98:2133–2223

Pflimlin E, Bielohuby M, Korn M, Breitschopf K, Löhn M, Wohlfart P, Konkar A, Podeschwa M, Bärenz F, Pfenninger A, Schwahn U, Opatz T, Reimann M, Petry S, Tennagels N (2018) Acute and repeated treatment with 5-PAHSA or 9-PAHSA isomers does not improve glucose control in mice. Cell Metab 28:217–227

Plaisance EP, Lukasova M, Offermanns S, Zhang Y, Cao G, Judd RL (2009) Niacin stimulates adiponectin secretion through the GPR109A receptor. Am J Physiol Endocrinol Metab 296: E549–E558

Qu A, Shah YM, Manna SK, Gonzalez FJ (2012) Disruption of endothelial peroxisome proliferator-activated receptor γ accelerates diet-induced atherogenesis in LDL receptor-null mice. Arterioscler Thromb Vasc Biol 32:65–73

Ramms B, Gordts PLSM (2018) Apolipoprotein C-III in triglyceride-rich lipoprotein metabolism. Curr Opin Lipidol 29:171–179

Ranjbar R, Shafiee M, Hesari A, Ferns GA, Ghasemi F, Avan A (2019) The potential therapeutic use of renin-angiotensin system inhibitors in the treatment of inflammatory diseases. J Cell Physiol 234:2277–2295

Ruan CC, Kong LR, Chen XH, Ma Y, Pan XX, Zhang ZB, Gao PJ (2018) A2A receptor activation attenuates hypertensive cardiac remodeling via promoting Brown adipose tissue-derived FGF21. Cell Metab 28:476–489

Saremi A, Schwenke DC, Buchanan TA, Hodis HN, Mack WJ, Banerji M, Bray GA, Clement SC, Henry RR, Kitabchi AE, Mudaliar S, Ratner RE, Stentz FB, Musi N, Tripathy D, DeFronzo RA, Reaven PD (2013) Pioglitazone slows progression of atherosclerosis in prediabetes independent of changes in cardiovascular risk factors. Arterioscler Thromb Vasc Biol 33:393–399

Scheja L, Heeren J (2016) Metabolic interplay between white, beige, brown adipocytes and the liver. J Hepatol 64:1176–1186

Scheja L, Heeren J (2019) The endocrine function of adipose tissues in health and cardiometabolic disease. Nat Rev Endocrinol 15:507, manuscript in press

Schlein C, Talukdar S, Heine M, Fischer AW, Krott LM, Nilsson SK, Brenner MB, Heeren J, Scheja L (2016) FGF21 lowers plasma triglycerides by accelerating lipoprotein catabolism in white and brown adipose tissues. Cell Metab 23:441–453

Sidossis LS, Porter C, Saraf MK, Børsheim E, Radhakrishnan RS, Chao T, Ali A, Chondronikola M, Mlcak R, Finnerty CC, Hawkins HK, Toliver-Kinsky T, Herndon DN (2015) Browning of subcutaneous white adipose tissue in humans after severe adrenergic stress. Cell Metab 22:219–227

Singh AK, Aryal B, Chaube B, Rotllan N, Varela L, Horvath TL, Suárez Y, Fernández-Hernando C (2018) Brown adipose tissue derived ANGPTL4 controls glucose and lipid metabolism and regulates thermogenesis. Mol Metab 11:59–69

Skiba DS, Nosalski R, Mikolajczyk TP, Siedlinski M, Rios FJ, Montezano AC, Jawien J, Olszanecki R, Korbut R, Czesnikiewicz-Guzik M, Touyz RM, Guzik TJ (2017) Anti-atherosclerotic effect of the angiotensin 1-7 mimetic AVE0991 is mediated by inhibition of perivascular and plaque inflammation in early atherosclerosis. Br J Pharmacol 174:4055–4069

Stanford KI, Lynes MD, Takahashi H, Baer LA, Arts PJ, May FJ, Lehnig AC, Middelbeek RJW, Richard JJ, So K, Chen EY, Gao F, Narain NR, Distefano G, Shettigar VK, Hirshman MF, Ziolo MT, Kiebish MA, Tseng YH, Coen PM, Goodyear LJ (2018) 12,13-diHOME: an exercise-induced lipokine that increases skeletal muscle fatty acid uptake. Cell Metab 27:1111–1120

Stefan N, Kantartzis K, Celebi N, Staiger H, Machann J, Schick F, Cegan A, Elcnerova M, Schleicher E, Fritsche A, Häring HU (2010) Circulating palmitoleate strongly and independently predicts insulin sensitivity in humans. Diabetes Care 33:405–407

Stitziel NO, Stirrups KE, Masca NG, Erdmann J, Ferrario PG, König IR, Weeke PE, Webb TR, Auer PL, Schick UM, Lu Y, Zhang H, Dube MP, Goel A, Farrall M, Peloso GM, Won HH, Do R, van Iperen E, Kanoni S, Kruppa J, Mahajan A, Scott RA, Willenborg C, Braund PS, van Capelleveen JC, Doney AS, Donnelly LA, Asselta R, Merlini PA, Duga S, Marziliano N, Denny JC, Shaffer CM, El-Mokhtari NE, Franke A, Gottesman O, Heilmann S, Hengstenberg C, Hoffman P, Holmen OL, Hveem K, Jansson JH, Jöckel KH, Kessler T, Kriebel J, Laugwitz KL, Marouli E, Martinelli N, McCarthy MI, Van Zuydam NR, Meisinger C, Esko T, Mihailov E, Escher SA, Alver M, Moebus S, Morris AD, Müller-Nurasyid M, Nikpay M, Olivieri O, Lemieux Perreault LP, AlQarawi A, Robertson NR, Akinsanya KO, Reilly DF, Vogt TF, Yin W, Asselbergs FW, Kooperberg C, Jackson RD, Stahl E, Strauch K, Varga TV,

Waldenberger M, Zeng L, Kraja AT, Liu C, Ehret GB, Newton-Cheh C, Chasman DI, Chowdhury R, Ferrario M, Ford I, Jukema JW, Kee F, Kuulasmaa K, Nordestgaard BG, Perola M, Saleheen D, Sattar N, Surendran P, Tregouet D, Young R, Howson JM, Butterworth AS, Danesh J, Ardissino D, Bottinger EP, Erbel R, Franks PW, Girelli D, Hall AS, Hovingh GK, Kastrati A, Lieb W, Meitinger T, Kraus WE, Shah SH, McPherson R, Orho-Melander M, Melander O, Metspalu A, Palmer CN, Peters A, Rader D, Reilly MP, Loos RJ, Reiner AP, Roden DM, Tardif JC, Thompson JR, Wareham NJ, Watkins H, Willer CJ, Kathiresan S, Deloukas P, Samani NJ, Schunkert H (2016) Coding variation in ANGPTL4, LPL, and SVEP1 and the risk of coronary disease. N Engl J Med 374:1134–1144

Subramanian V, Golledge J, Ijaz T, Bruemmer D, Daugherty A (2010) Pioglitazone-induced reductions in atherosclerosis occur via smooth muscle cell-specific interaction with PPAR {gamma}. Circ Res 107:953–958

Sui W, Li H, Yang Y, Jing X, Xue F, Cheng J, Dong M, Zhang M, Pan H, Chen Y, Zhang Y, Zhou Q, Shi W, Wang X, Zhang H, Zhang C, Zhang Y, Cao Y (2019) Bladder drug mirabegron exacerbates atherosclerosis through activation of brown fat-mediated lipolysis. Proc Natl Acad Sci U S A 116:10937–10942

Superko HR, Zhao XQ, Hodis HN, Guyton JR (2017) Niacin and heart disease prevention: engraving its tombstone is a mistake. J Clin Lipidol 11:1309–1317

Talukdar S, Zhou Y, Li D, Rossulek M, Dong J, Somayaji V, Weng Y, Clark R, Lanba A, Owen BM, Brenner MB, Trimmer JK, Gropp KE, Chabot JR, Erion DM, Rolph TP, Goodwin B, Calle RA (2016) A long-acting FGF21 molecule, PF-05231023, decreases body weight and improves lipid profile in non-human Primates and type 2 diabetic subjects. Cell Metab 23:427–440

Taskinen MR, Packard CJ, Borén J (2019) Emerging evidence that apoC-III inhibitors provide novel options to reduce the residual CVD. Curr Atheroscler Rep 21:27

Thorp E, Kuriakose G, Shah YM, Gonzalez FJ, Tabas I (2007) Pioglitazone increases macrophage apoptosis and plaque necrosis in advanced atherosclerotic lesions of nondiabetic low-density lipoprotein receptor-null mice. Circulation 116:2182–2190

Tian Z, Miyata K, Tazume H, Sakaguchi H, Kadomatsu T, Horio E, Takahashi O, Komohara Y, Araki K, Hirata Y, Tabata M, Takanashi S, Takeya M, Hao H, Shimabukuro M, Sata M, Kawasuji M, Oike Y (2013) Perivascular adipose tissue-secreted angiopoietin-like protein 2 (Angptl2) accelerates neointimal hyperplasia after endovascular injury. J Mol Cell Cardiol 57:1–12

Tsutsumi K, Inoue Y, Shima A, Iwasaki K, Kawamura M, Murase T (1993) The novel compound NO-1886 increases lipoprotein lipase activity with resulting elevation of high density lipoprotein cholesterol, and long-term administration inhibits atherogenesis in the coronary arteries of rats with experimental atherosclerosis. J Clin Invest 92:411–417

van Marken Lichtenbelt WD, Vanhommerig JW, Smulders NM, Drossaerts JM, Kemerink GJ, Bouvy ND, Schrauwen P, Teule GJ (2009) Cold-activated brown adipose tissue in healthy men. N Engl J Med 360:1500–1508

van Wanrooij EJ, de Jager SC, van Es T, de Vos P, Birch HL, Owen DA, Watson RJ, Biessen EA, Chapman GA, van Berkel TJ, Kuiper J (2008) CXCR3 antagonist NBI-74330 attenuates atherosclerotic plaque formation in LDL receptor-deficient mice. Arterioscler Thromb Vasc Biol 28:251–257

Veillard NR, Kwak B, Pelli G, Mulhaupt F, James RW, Proudfoot AE, Mach F (2004) Antagonism of RANTES receptors reduces atherosclerotic plaque formation in mice. Circ Res 94:253–261

Veillard NR, Steffens S, Pelli G, Lu B, Kwak BR, Gerard C, Charo IF, Mach F (2005) Differential influence of chemokine receptors CCR2 and CXCR3 in development of atherosclerosis in vivo. Circulation 112:870–878

Villarroya F, Cereijo R, Villarroya J, Giralt M (2017) Brown adipose tissue as a secretory organ. Nat Rev Endocrinol 13:26–35

Wang GX, Zhao XY, Meng ZX, Kern M, Dietrich A, Chen Z, Cozacov Z, Zhou D, Okunade AL, Su X, Li S, Blüher M, Lin JD (2014) The brown fat-enriched secreted factor Nrg4 preserves metabolic homeostasis through attenuation of hepatic lipogenesis. Nat Med 20:1436–1443

Weng C, Shen Z, Li X, Jiang W, Peng L, Yuan H, Yang K, Wang J (2017) Effects of chemerin/ CMKLR1 in obesity-induced hypertension and potential mechanism. Am J Transl Res 9:3096–3104

Worthmann A, John C, Rühlemann MC, Baguhl M, Heinsen FA, Schaltenberg N, Heine M, Schlein C, Evangelakos I, Mineo C, Fischer M, Dandri M, Kremoser C, Scheja L, Franke A, Shaul PW, Heeren J (2017) Cold-induced conversion of cholesterol to bile acids in mice shapes the gut microbiome and promotes adaptive thermogenesis. Nat Med 23:839–849

Xiong W, Zhao X, Garcia-Barrio MT, Zhang J, Lin J, Chen YE, Jiang Z, Chang L (2017) MitoNEET in perivascular adipose tissue blunts atherosclerosis under mild cold condition in mice. Front Physiol 8:1032

Xue Y, Xu X, Zhang XQ, Farokhzad OC, Langer R (2016) Preventing diet-induced obesity in mice by adipose tissue transformation and angiogenesis using targeted nanoparticles. Proc Natl Acad Sci U S A 113:5552–5557

Yang ZH, Pryor M, Noguchi A, Sampson M, Johnson B, Pryor M, Donkor K, Amar M, Remaley AT (2019) Dietary palmitoleic acid attenuates atherosclerosis progression and hyperlipidemia in low-density lipoprotein receptor-deficient mice. Mol Nutr Food Res 63:e1900120

Yau H, Rivera K, Lomonaco R, Cusi K (2013) The future of thiazolidinedione therapy in the management of type 2 diabetes mellitus. Curr Diab Rep 13:329–341

Yore MM, Syed I, Moraes-Vieira PM, Zhang T, Herman MA, Homan EA, Patel RT, Lee J, Chen S, Peroni OD, Dhaneshwar AS, Hammarstedt A, Smith U, McGraw TE, Saghatelian A, Kahn BB (2014) Discovery of a class of endogenous mammalian lipids with anti-diabetic and anti-inflammatory effects. Cell 159:318–332

Young SG, Zechner R (2013) Biochemistry and pathophysiology of intravascular and intracellular lipolysis. Genes Dev 27:459–584

Zeman M, Vecka M, Perlík F, Staňková B, Hromádka R, Tvrzická E, Širc J, Hrib J, Žák A (2016) Pleiotropic effects of niacin: current possibilities for its clinical use. Acta Pharma 66:449–469

Zhang F, Hao G, Shao M, Nham K, An Y, Wang Q, Zhu Y, Kusminski CM, Hassan G, Gupta RK, Zhai Q, Sun X, Scherer PE, Oz OK (2018) An adipose tissue atlas: an image-guided identification of human-like BAT and beige depots in rodents. Cell Metab 27:252–262

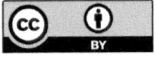

Microbiome and Cardiovascular Disease

Hilde Herrema, Max Nieuwdorp, and Albert K. Groen

Contents

1 Introduction 312
2 Gut and Oral Microbiome Communities: Potential Drivers of ASCVD? 313
   2.1 Other Microbiome Community Members 317
      2.1.1 Viruses and Bacteriophages 318
3 Microbiome-Derived Metabolites 319
   3.1 TMAO 320
   3.2 Imidazole-Propionate 320
   3.3 Short-Chain Fatty Acids 321
   3.4 Other Microbiome-Produced Metabolites Associated with ASCVD 322
4 Bile Acids 323
   4.1 Bile Acid Metabolism 323
   4.2 Regulation by Bile Acids 324
5 Summary and Future Perspectives 325
References 327

Abstract

Atherosclerotic cardiovascular disease (ASCVD) is a prime example of a systems disease. In the initial phase, apolipoprotein B-containing cholesterol-rich lipoproteins deposit excess cholesterol in macrophage-like cells that subsequently develop into foam cells. A multitude of systemic as well as

H. Herrema · M. Nieuwdorp
Departments of Internal and Experimental Vascular Medicine, Amsterdam University Medical Centers, Location AMC, Amsterdam, The Netherlands

A. K. Groen (✉)
Departments of Internal and Experimental Vascular Medicine, Amsterdam University Medical Centers, Location AMC, Amsterdam, The Netherlands

Department of Laboratory Medicine, University of Groningen, University Medical Center Groningen, Groningen, The Netherlands
e-mail: a.k.groen@amsterdamumc.nl

© The Author(s) 2020
A. von Eckardstein, C. J. Binder (eds.), *Prevention and Treatment of Atherosclerosis*,
Handbook of Experimental Pharmacology 270, https://doi.org/10.1007/164_2020_356

environmental factors are involved in further progression of atherosclerotic plaque formation. In recent years, both oral and gut microbiota have been proposed to play an important role in the process at different stages. Particularly bacteria from the oral cavity may easily reach the circulation and cause low-grade inflammation, a recognized risk factor for ASCVD. Gut-derived microbiota on the other hand can influence host metabolism on various levels. Next to translocation across the intestinal wall, these prokaryotes produce a great number of specific metabolites such as trimethylamine and short-chain fatty acids but can also metabolize endogenously formed bile acids and convert these into metabolites that may influence signal transduction pathways. In this overview, we critically discuss the novel developments in this rapidly emerging research field.

Keywords

ASCVD · Atherosclerosis · Bacteriophage · Bile acids · SCFA · TMAO

1   Introduction

Atherosclerotic cardiovascular diseases (ASCVD), including coronary heart disease and stroke, are still the main causes of death in the Western world. In the last decades, extensive research programs have attempted to unravel molecular mechanisms underlying these debilitating diseases. Substantial progress has been made particularly in identification of the causal role of low-density lipoprotein (Ference et al. 2017) and triglyceride-rich remnants (Nordestgaard 2016). Although the focal point in research is often directed to cholesterol-containing lipoproteins, the major predictive risk factor for ASCVD is age (Pencina et al. 2019). The vascular aging process that underlies ASCVD risk is a complex process in which lipoproteins and blood pressure interact with the vessel wall and a number of environmental factors exert a secondary influence. One of these factors, which has gained substantial interest in recent years, is the microbiome defined as all microorganisms that colonize the body. Although the vast majority of microbiome studies concentrate on the gut, the oral microbiome may play a significant role in the context of ASCVD development. In this overview, we will critically review recent literature that focuses on the role of the microbiome in ASCVD.

ASCVD is a prime example of a systems disease. The obligate substrate is deposition of cholesterol in the vessel wall. Once depot formation is initiated in the form of foam cells, a host of additional factors such as inflammatory processes further determine disease progression through a plethora of actions. Note that inflammatory processes may also control lipid levels in the blood, thereby exerting control on multiple steps in development of atherosclerosis. Until recently, most of the information about the importance of inflammation in ASCVD came from studies in animal models. The results of the CANTOS trial, which showed a beneficial effect on ASCVD events through antibody-mediated inhibition of interleukin-1β, have added critical insight in the role of inflammation in ASCVD development in humans (Ridker et al. 2017). Inflammation is an extremely complex process by itself, and it is therefore not surprising that novel inflammation-modulating factors pop up continuously as potential ASCVD influencers. Yet, the onset of the disease requires lipid disposition mediated primarily by apolipoprotein B (apoB)-containing lipoproteins. The dominant role of these lipoproteins was nicely exemplified by Mendelian randomization studies that make use of natural mutations in the genes encoding lipoproteins (reviewed in Holmes et al. 2017). This enabled studies into the effect of variations in circulating cholesterol carriers on ASCVD risk (Ference et al. 2017). In addition, LDL-C lowering trials using statins with or without ezetimibe or PCSK9 inhibitors have provided critical insight in the role of cholesterol carriers and ASCVD risk (Wright and Murphy 2016). Interestingly, there is linear relation between LDL-C levels and cardiovascular events in which zero disease risk was associated with circulating LDL-C levels of around 1 mM (Wright and Murphy 2016). This suggests that at this level, the risk of cardiovascular events is close to zero and no disposition of lipid in the vessel wall will occur. In the general population, however, the concentration of apoB-containing lipoproteins is much higher than 1 mM, and some degree of atherosclerotic plaques development is almost inevitable. Indeed in the 1960s of the last century, studies in young soldiers that died in the Korean and Vietnam wars demonstrated early signs of atherosclerotic plaque formation as early as 25 years of age in about 5% of the soldiers (Virmani et al. 1987). Fortunately, certainly at ages lower than 60 years, most atherosclerotic plaques are not symptomatic. A majority of current research initiatives therefore focuses on processes that induce vulnerability of the plaque to rupture, one of the main causes for acute coronary syndromes.

In short, lipid deposition in the vessel wall and complex inflammatory processes are critical for development of ASCVD. In addition, aging and environmental factors such as smoking and diet play an important role herein. More recently, both oral and gut microbiome have entered the spotlights. Before considering the role of the microbiome in ASCVD development in detail, we will first give an update on recent oral and gut microbiome literature and focus on host-microbiome interactions relevant for progression of ASCVD.

2 Gut and Oral Microbiome Communities: Potential Drivers of ASCVD?

The gut and oral microbiome are the first and second, respectively, largest and most complex communities of microorganisms in the human body and comprise bacteria, fungi, viruses, archaea, and protozoa. It is critical to point out that the vast majority of publications on the role of the gut and oral microbiome in human health and disease are heavily biased toward bacterial members of this community. The upcoming awareness of the critical role of other members of the microbiome to composition and function of the community – and thereby contribution to human metabolism – is likely to change this bias in the coming decade. We will first elaborate on the bacterial component of the (gut and oral) microbiome and their postulated role in ASCVD development. Mechanistically, both the gut and oral microbiome are currently considered to affect human metabolism and ASCVD by interaction with the host immune system (gut and oral) and by conversion of dietary components into hormone-like signals or biologically active metabolites (gut) (Fig. 1).

The gut microbiome (estimated number of species >1,000, 1.5–2 kg per person) is a critical component of digestion, maintenance of gut barrier function, and immunomodulation. The predominant bacterial phyla are *Bacteroidetes* and *Firmicutes*, with *Actinobacteria*, *Proteobacteria*, and *Verrucomicrobia* being less abundant (Shetty et al. 2017). Methanogens are dominant among the archaea (Paterson et al. 2017). The vast majority of gut bacteria are shared among individuals at higher taxonomic levels (phylum). However, interindividual variation at lower taxonomic levels (species, strain) is very high. Alterations at this level, in particular reduced number and diversity of bacterial genes, have been associated with metabolic diseases including ASCVD (reviewed in Aron-Wisnewsky and Clément 2016; Liu et al. 2019; Tilg et al. 2019).

ASCVD risk factors have been reported to associate with the gut microbiome; for example, *Clostridiales* and *Clostridium* spp. correlate negatively with C-reactive protein, an inflammatory marker (Karlsson et al. 2012). The gut microbiome of ASCVD patients has been associated with decreased abundance of gut commensals such as *Bacteroidetes* (incl. *Bacteroides* and *Prevotella*) compared to healthy controls (Emoto et al. 2016). A metagenome-wide association study (Jie et al. 2017) in fecal samples of ASCVD patients and healthy controls reproduced findings on the reduced abundance of *Bacteroidetes* in ASCVD patients and further reported that these patients had reduced abundance of presumably beneficial short-chain fatty acid-producing bacteria such as *Roseburia intestinalis* and *Faecalibacterium prausnitzii*. Conversely, the microbiome of ASCVD patients was enriched in species belonging to the *Enterobacteriaceae* family, which are oftentimes associated with gut microbiome dysbiosis and (metabolic) disease development. Interestingly, the relative abundance of bacteria typical for the oral cavity, in particular *Streptococcus* spp., was also higher in the gut microbiome of patients with ACVD compared to healthy controls.

With over 700 bacterial species, the oral cavity comprises the second largest and most diverse microbiome community after the gut in the human body. These species are located in a plethora of very complex niches including the hard surfaces of the teeth as well as the soft mucus linings of the mouth. The mouth is the major entrance point to the human body. Bacteria from the oral cavity, in particular those associated with oral infectious diseases and adapted to thrive in an inflammatory environment (e.g., caries (tooth decay) and periodontitis (gum disease)), have been associated with "off-site" effects on systemic diseases such as ASCVD (Hajishengallis 2015).

Although the number of studies that have associated differences in gut and oral microbiome composition with ASCVD is plentiful, it is important to point out that data on a causal role for the gut microbiome in ASCVD development in humans is more difficult to find. The strongest evidence for a causal role of the gut or oral microbiome in progression of ASCVD has been derived from animal studies,

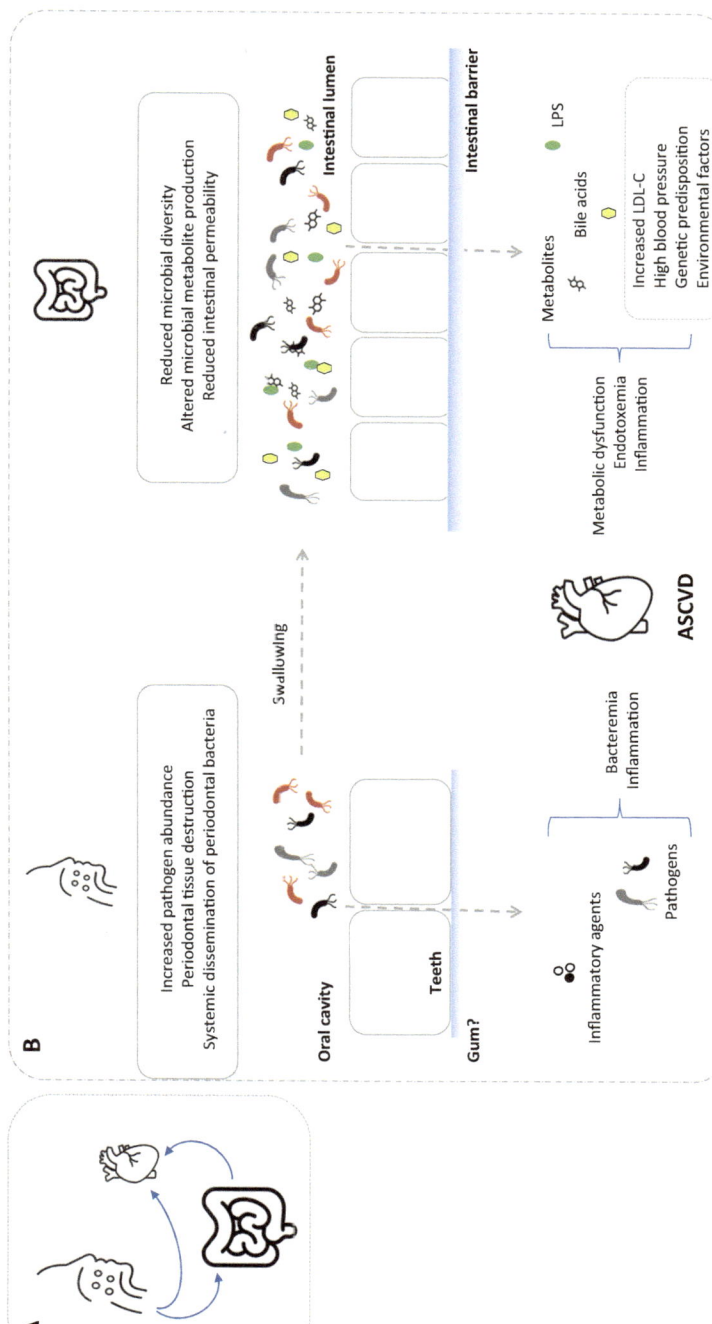

Fig. 1 Oral and gut microbiome have been implicated in the development of ASCVD (**a**). Increased pathogen abundance in the oral cavity, such as during periodontal disease, might reach the circulation and contribute to low-grade inflammation, a recognized risk factor for ASCVD. In addition, continuous swallowing of bacteria from the oral cavity has been suggested to alter gut microbiome composition, thereby contributing to ASCVD development (**b**). Please see text for details

Table 1 Overview of bacterial challenge studies carried out in germ-free mouse models

Mouse model	Diet + intervention(s)	Findings	Reference
Apoe−/− (gnotobiotic)	Chow, *Roseburia intestinalis* administration	Lesions and inflammation ↓in *R. intestinalis* vs control	Kasahara et al. (2018)
Apoe−/− (GF and CONV-R)	Chow, HFD, choline supplementation (both diets)	Chow: lesions and CH ↓ in CONV-R vs GF HFD: lesions and CH = in CONV-R vs GF Choline suppl: TMAO ↑, lesions = in CONV-R vs GF	Jonsson et al. (2018)
Apoe−/− (GF and CONV-R)	Chow	Lesions, LPS, and inflammation ↑ in CONV-R vs GF LDL-C ↓ in CONV-R vs GF	Kasahara et al. (2017)
Apoe−/− (GF by abx)	Chow without/with choline	Lesions, CH, and foam cells ↓ in choline-abx vs choline-no abx	Wang et al. (2011)
Apoe−/− (GF and CONV-R)	Chow without/with cholesterol	Chow without CH: lesions ↓ in CONV-R vs GF Chow with CH: lesions = in CONV-R vs GF	Stepankova et al. (2010)
Apoe−/− (GF and CONV-R)	HFD	Lesions = in CONV-R vs GF	Wright et al. (2000)

in particular mouse models (Table 1). Germ-free (sterile) apolipoprotein E-null (ApoE −/−) mice were shown to have increased atherosclerotic plaques compared to conventionally raised counterparts when fed a chow diet (Stepankova et al. 2010). These data were confirmed by Lindskog et al. but only with respect to the chow diet (Jonsson et al. 2018). Conversely, when germ-free ApoE −/− mice were fed a high-fat/high-cholesterol diet, the absence of microbiota increased atherogenesis, but the extent was still reduced compared to conventionally raised mice (Jonsson et al. 2018). However, there is some controversy around these data because Kasahara et al. reported decreased atherosclerosis in germ-free ApoE −/− mice on a chow diet (Kasahara et al. 2017). Since chow diets are not well characterized and composition differs from batch to batch, the apparent discrepancy may well be caused by subtle changes in the diet used in the different studies.

Convincing data for a causal role of the microbiota in ASCVD development came from fecal microbiota transplantation (FMT) studies showing that atherosclerosis was induced when FMT was carried out with feces derived from mice with proven atherosclerosis (Gregory et al. 2015). The question arises which factor is responsible for the atherosclerosis aggravating effect induced by the microbiome. Activation of inflammatory signaling pathways by the gut microbiome, or components thereof, has received a lot of attention in the past decade. This is exemplified by observations that transplantation of a pro-inflammatory microbiome into atherosclerosis-prone LDLR−/− mice accelerated phenotype development compared to LDLR−/− mice receiving a control microbiome (Brandsma et al. 2019). Translocation of lipopolysaccharide (LPS) across the intestinal wall into the blood seems a good mechanistic candidate. LPS is the major molecular component of the outer membrane of gram-negative bacteria, the most abundant bacteria in the gut (Raetz and Whitfield 2008). The lipid A component of LPS is a pathogen-associated molecular pattern, which activates Toll-like receptor 4 (TLR4) (Aderem and Underhill 1999). High-fat diet has been shown to increase gut permeability in mice. This may enhance the translocation of LPS into the circulation thereby inducing metabolic endotoxemia (Cani et al. 2007). In line, germ-free mice were demonstrated to be resistant to high-fat diet-induced insulin resistance and obesity (Rabot et al. 2010). Whether these results in mice can be translated to humans remains to be established.

Identification of atherosclerotic plaque-associated bacteria is suggestive of a direct role in plaque progression (Koren et al. 2011; Jonsson et al. 2017). Interestingly, many of these bacteria were also localized in the oral microbiome of patients with atherosclerosis. Indeed, a close association between periodontitis and ASCVD risk has been reported in a number of studies (Hajishengallis 2015). Gingival bleeding caused by periodontitis offers oral bacteria an easy entry into the circulation where they can attach to the atherosclerotic plaque. Whether they stay alive when bound to the plaque is not clear. As far as we are aware, no live bacteria have been cultured from plaques obtained during surgery. Yet, upon entry into the blood, the orally derived bacteria may be capable of activating endothelial cells, possibly leading to expression and secretion of metalloproteinases that in turn may decrease plaque stability. The activity of periodontitis has been shown to be reflected in systemic inflammation. This is important given the role of inflammation in the pathogenesis of ASCVD. Plasma levels of the inflammatory marker C-reactive protein (CRP) have been correlated with periodontitis status (Noack et al. 2005; Yoshii et al. 2009) as well as the pro-inflammatory cytokine IL-6 (Loos et al. 2005). These immune modulators may be either produced locally in the oral environment and subsequently secreted into the circulation or arise as a result of low-grade short-lived bacteremia (Torres De Heens et al. 2010). Given the high prevalence of periodontitis in the adult population, treatment of this disease may be an important modality to reduce the incidence of ASCVD (Lobo et al. 2019).

Summarizing these studies, it seems fair to conclude that activation of an inflammatory pathway is a reasonable way via which bacteria may promote progression of ASCVD. Whether the prokaryotes that enter the circulation via the oral cavity or gut play a role in affecting plaque stability has not yet been shown. In a study in mice, Jonsson et al. (2017) did not find differences in bacterial content between stable and labile plaques. However, activation of the inflammatory component of ASCVD may not be the only way by means of which the microbiota exert influence.

2.1 Other Microbiome Community Members

Although *bacteria* and *archaea* indeed account for >99% of microbiome mass (Shkoporov and Hill 2019), it should be realized, however, that both the oral and gut microbiome contain vast numbers of viruses, fungi, and – in most humans – protozoans. Although many of these less abundant community members have been linked to human disease (Hoffmann et al. 2013; Huseyin et al. 2017; Paterson et al. 2017; Laforest-Lapointe and Arrieta 2018), surprisingly little is known about trans-kingdom community-level interactions and the consequences thereof for human health. In order to deepen our understanding about the complexity of host-microbial interactions, it will be critical to address such interactions in the relevant ecosystem (e.g., the gut or oral cavity).

2.1.1 Viruses and Bacteriophages

Bacteriophages (phages), viruses of bacteria, are of particular interest because of their proven role in shaping microbial communities in many ecosystems (Fernández et al. 2018; Warwick-Dugdale et al. 2019). Furthermore, phages are abundantly present in the gut (estimated 1:1 ratio with bacteria), either as free phage or integrated into the bacterial genome as prophage (Reyes et al. 2012; Walk et al. 2016; Carding et al. 2017).

The many studies that have described a strong association of specific bacterial strains with ASCVD generally characterize the phylogenetic core, dynamics, and stability of the bacterial ecosystem by high-throughput 16S ribosomal RNA gene sequencing-based approaches. This precludes identification of integrated bacteriophage DNA in the bacterial DNA (see for recent reviews (Shetty et al. 2017; Hornung et al. 2018; Falony et al. 2019)). Increasingly accessible and affordable shotgun and long-read nanopore sequencing approaches together with rapidly emerging computational tools to unravel novel phage genomes are now rapidly solving part of the challenges phage researchers have faced in the past. These include the fact that the majority of gut bacteria (phage hosts) are strict anaerobes and thereby extremely difficult to culture. This has, until recent years, limited researchers to microscopic characterization of phages. The current collection of known gut phages therefore is a vast underrepresentation of the gut phageome. Interestingly, a healthy gut status in humans has been shown to mainly comprise integrated phages (Reyes et al. 2010; Minot et al. 2011), whereas cases of intestinal bowel disease have been associated with higher levels of free phages (Norman et al. 2015; Duerkop et al. 2018). Prophage integration has been shown to affect bacterial fitness and metabolic function in the gut (Duerkop et al. 2012; Hsu et al. 2019; Oh et al. 2019). Moreover, evidence for a direct role of phages in activation of the mammalian immune system, a critical element of ASCVD development, has recently been put forward (Gogokhia et al. 2019; Sweere et al. 2019). In line with long-standing observations that bacteriophages are able to pass the intestinal wall to enter the bloodstream, at least in experimental settings (Van Belleghem et al. 2019), these results support the urgency to carefully look into these viral members of the microbiome community in the gut and beyond. Implications for phages as modulators of (immune)metabolism are yet to be confirmed, but we predict this will be highly relevant for studies addressing the role of the microbiome in human ASCVD development.

3   Microbiome-Derived Metabolites

Gut bacteria are also considered to modulate human metabolism by production of small molecules including conversion of dietary components into hormone-like signals or biologically active metabolites (Fig. 2). It has been estimated that about 10% of the small molecules in the circulation are derived from the gut microbiome (Holmes et al. 2012). This estimate can very well be an underestimation because

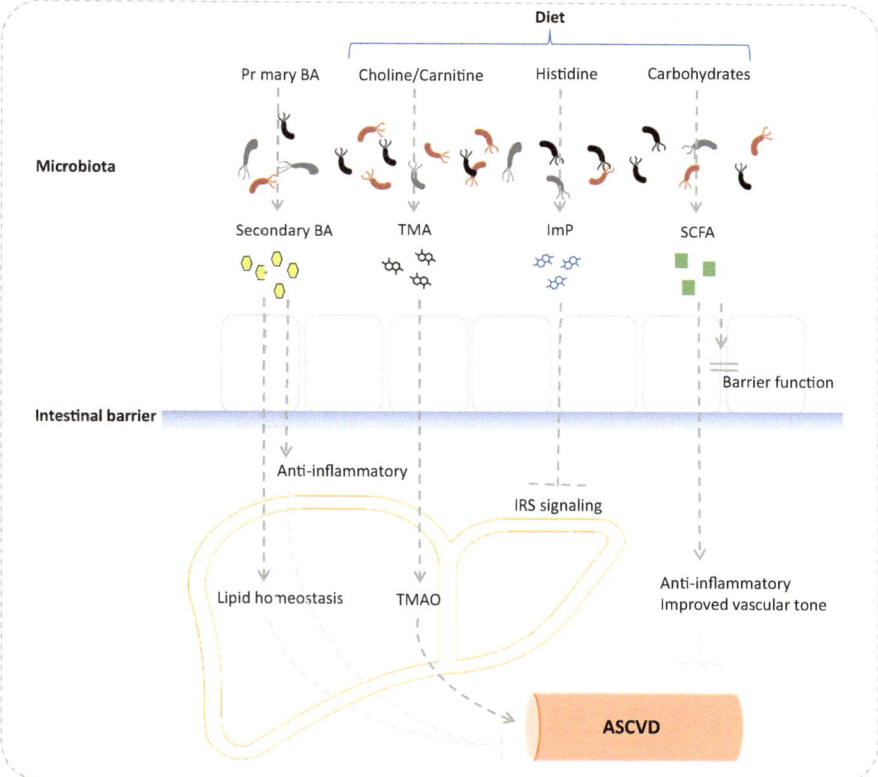

Fig. 2 Gut microbial metabolites have been implicated in ASCVD development. Primary bile acids are produced by the liver after which a small percentage is converted to secondary bile acids by colonic bacteria. Although evidence from human trials addressing if secondary bile acids might prevent ASCVD development is still warranted, secondary read outs associated with ASCVD (e.g., inflammation and LDL-C levels) have been reported to be reduced by bacteria capable of converting primary to secondary bile acids. TMA is produced by the microbiota from choline or carnitine precursors. In the liver, TMA is converted to TMAO which has been extensively linked to ASCVD development. ImP is a microbial metabolite of histidine. ImP directly inhibits insulin receptor-mediated signaling thereby leading to insulin resistance, a significant risk factor for the development of ASCVD. Whether ImP indeed affects ASCVD development is yet to be established. SCFA is a microbial fermentation product of complex carbohydrates. Many health benefits have been addressed to SCFA and include improved gut barrier function and reduced inflammation. Please see text for details

despite the major advances in development of metabolomics in the last decade, most circulating metabolites whether endogenous or microbial have not yet been identified.

3.1 TMAO

A wonderful example of how a bacterial metabolite can be identified to exert effect on ASCVD comes from the studies of the Hazen group in Cleveland Clinic (Zhu et al. 2017; Koeth et al. 2019; Wu et al. 2014). They demonstrated that nutrients such as choline and carnitine can be converted to trimethylamine (TMA) by gut bacteria that express TMA lyases. The gas TMA subsequently diffuses from the intestine into the circulation and is converted to trimethylamine N-oxide (TMAO) in the liver by the hepatic enzyme flavine monooxygenase 3 (FMO3) (Brown and Hazen 2015). TMAO activates atherosclerosis in mouse models, and TMAO plasma levels have been shown to correlate with incidence of cardiovascular disease in humans in a number of studies (Zhu et al. 2016, 2017). Several other studies, however, failed to show this correlation (Heianza et al. 2017; Kaysen et al. 2015; Mueller et al. 2015; Aldana-Hernández et al. 2019). Zhu et al. showed that TMAO may exert its action via influencing blood platelet hyperresponsiveness and thrombosis, which provides a mechanistic link between TMAO and cardiovascular risk (Zhu et al. 2016, 2017). Recently, Chen et al. showed that TMAO may induce ER stress (Chen et al. 2019). Unravelling the metabolic pathways involved in TMAO metabolism provides a beautiful example how the interaction between microbial activity and host metabolism can be elucidated. By developing specific inhibitors of TMA lyases, the Hazen group (Koh et al. 2018) may have produced the tools to treat patients at risk for ACSVD due to increased TMAO (Wang et al. 2015). In the original paper in which the Hazen group introduced the TMAO pathway, additional ASCVD-associated peaks in the MS spectra were observed (Wang et al. 2011). Characterization of these putative metabolites has not yet been published, but it seems justified to suggest that there is more to come.

3.2 Imidazole-Propionate

Metabolites produced by microbial metabolism of aromatic amino acids are good candidates. Recently the histidine derivative imidazole-propionate (ImP) has been linked to insulin resistance in humans. By detailed analysis of portal blood obtained from obese diabetic patients compared to "healthy" (nondiabetic) obese controls, the group was able to single out ImP as one of the compounds strongly increased in portal blood from the diabetics (Koh et al. 2018). The group of Backhed subsequently characterized the molecular mechanism of action in great detail (Koh et al. 2018). Extensive mechanistic studies in mice revealed that ImP impairs insulin signaling via p38 protein kinase. Identification of ImP is very recent, and its putative role in ASCVD has not been investigated yet. Since ASCVD is an almost inevitable comorbidity of diabetes, an aggravating effect of IMP on ASCVD may be expected to be published in the near future.

3.3   Short-Chain Fatty Acids

The short-chain fatty acids (SCFAs) butyrate, propionate, and acetate are produced from colonic fermentation of complex fibers by the gut microbiota. SCFAs are the main product of the digestive actions of the gut microbiota making them interesting candidates in the quest for microbial-derived metabolites influencing ASCVD. Lower levels of SCFA or SCFA-producing bacteria have been correlated with arterial stiffness, high blood pressure, and related end-organ damage (Pluznick 2013; Kim et al. 2018; Menni et al. 2018). Despite the abundant literature on diverse aspects of SCFA, metabolism insight in their impact on ASCVD in humans is limited to association studies. However, interesting effects have been observed in studies in animal models. A case in point is the recent study of Kasahara et al. in *Nature Microbiology* (Kasahara et al. 2018) that focused on the ameliorating action of butyrate on atherosclerotic plaque progression in ApoE −/− mice. Germ-free ApoE−/− mice were first colonized with a mixture of eight low butyrate-producing bacterial strains. Subsequently, mice were inoculated with the high butyrate-producing strain *Roseburia intestinalis* as well. This led to a significant reduction in atherosclerotic plaque size (compared to controls). Interestingly, butyrate, whether added to diet or produced by the bacteria, had no effect on plasma cholesterol or TMAO levels. The observed beneficial effect on plaque progression seemed mainly due to a tightening of gut barrier function which potentially reduces translocation of LPS in this animal model. This local effect of butyrate makes sense because this particular SCFA is almost completely metabolized by the colonic enterocytes. Besides this putative effect on gut barrier function, which clearly requires confirmation, SCFA have been implicated in modulation of inflammatory processes (Ohira et al. 2017). The G protein-coupled receptors GPR41 and GPR43 serve as SCFA receptors and have been shown to elicit intracellular signal transduction cascades mediated by mitogen-activated protein kinases (MAPKs) and protein kinase C (PKC) (den Besten et al. 2013). In addition, butyrate has been shown to inhibit histone deacetylases, thereby altering the acetylation state of histones and other proteins which may induce epigenetic changes in gene transcription (Vinolo et al. 2011). A direct effect of SCFAs on expression of COX1 and 2 and hence possibly on eicosanoid production, important regulators of inflammatory processes, has also been proposed (Nurmi et al. 2005; Al-Lahham et al. 2010).

Most studies aiming at increasing insight into the molecular mechanism via which SCFA exert influence on inflammatory processes derive from in vitro experiments with cultured cells or tissues (Vinolo et al. 2011). Butyrate and propionate have been shown to affect neutrophil function by increasing apoptosis via a caspase-dependent pathway (Aoyama et al. 2010). A problem with most in vitro studies is that supraphysiological concentrations are used to show the effects making translation to the human situation difficult. Furthermore, acetate, butyrate, and propionate sometimes exhibit contrasting effects (Cavaglieri et al. 2003) leading to controversy on their modes of action. It can, however, not be excluded that the SCFA concentration required to elicit an anti-inflammatory response varies with the type of inflammation (Al-Lahham et al. 2010).

Confirmation of the anti-inflammatory properties that are often associated with SCFA comes from animal experiments. In ApoE knockout mice, feeding with butyrate reduced atherosclerotic lesions and lowered macrophage migration accompanied by a decrease in pro-inflammatory cytokines (Aguilar et al. 2014). In mice treated intraperitoneally with acetate, inflammatory processes after kidney injuries were decreased leading to attenuation of the detrimental effects of inflammation on renal function (Andrade-Oliveira et al. 2015). Conversely, after systemic administration of supraphysiological doses of SCFA, renal tissue inflammation was increased due to dysregulation of T-cell response (Park et al. 2016). In another study in mice, SCFA receptors GPR41 and GPR43 were found to be required for an inflammatory response to bacterial infection and thus a protective pro-inflammatory response (Kim et al. 2013). In rodent models of colitis, oral acetate administration was shown to be protective (Masui et al. 2013).

As far as we are aware, no outcome trials have been carried out focusing on the effect of SCFA on ASCVD. However, a few human studies looked at the effect of SCFA on inflammatory aspects. A recent study investigated the effect of colonic infusions of SCFA, in concentrations found in the gut, on fasting levels of cytokines in overweight and obese subjects. The pro-inflammatory cytokine IL-1β decreased with a high acetate (60%) containing SCFA mixture compared to placebo and was significantly lower compared to a SCFA mixture containing high propionate (35%). Postprandial IL-1β levels as well as other pro-inflammatory cytokines including TNF-α, IL-6, and IL-8 did not change in the obese subjects neither in the fasting nor in the postprandial period (Canfora et al. 2017). In the study by van der Beek et al. (2016), a tendency for lower fasting plasma TNF-α concentrations was found after distal colonic acetate infusion with a 100 mmol/L yet not with a 180 mmol/L, as well as after proximal colonic acetate infusion.

3.4   Other Microbiome-Produced Metabolites Associated with ASCVD

A number of studies have appeared recently that aimed to identify bacteria as well as metabolites associated with different stages of cardiovascular disease (Wang et al. 2019; Würtz et al. 2015; Kurilshikov et al. 2019; Liu et al. 2019). Using a metagenomics approach, Kurilshikov et al. could link metabolic pathways encoded in the various bacteria to ASCVD risk but assessed risk directly in only one of the studied cohorts by measuring carotid IMT. In the other cohorts, a metabolic risk score was calculated from 33 established ASCVD biomarkers. An advantage of the metagenomics approach is that functional relations between

ASCVD risk and microbial pathway can be identified. This is important because many bacterial strains share metabolic pathways. ASCVD risk is associated strongly with pathways involved in amino acid metabolism (Newgard 2017). Metabolomics was investigated in this study using the NMR-based Nightingale platform which focuses mainly on lipoproteins, and the expected relations between ApoB-containing lipoproteins and ASCVD risk were observed. Using a multi-omics approach, in which state-of-the-art metabolomics was combined with 16S rRNA sequencing, a number of metabolic pathways and co-abundant bacterial groups were identified to associate with ASCVD severity (Liu et al. 2019). Although ASCVD severity was determined using coronary angiography, which enables accurate diagnosis of the extent of plaque formation, this limits the number patients that can be studied. By grouping bacteria by co-abundance, functional properties of these groups could be predicted linking ASCVD risk to taurine, sphingolipid, ceramide, and benzene metabolism. Identification of xenobiotics links environmental variables directly to microbiota and host metabolism which could lead in future studies to identification of molecular mechanisms.

4   Bile Acids

The most important endogenous molecules that undergo microbial modifications are the family of bile acids (BA).

4.1   Bile Acid Metabolism

These molecules are produced exclusively by the liver via two pathways that start separately but fuse after four steps to share most of the subsequent steps in the parts that produce the primary bile acid chenodeoxycholic acid (Kuipers et al. 2014). The so-called classic bile acid synthesis pathway starts with the conversion of cholesterol into 7-alpha-cholesterol catalyzed by the enzyme 7-alpha-hydroxylase and produce either cholic acid or chenodeoxycholic acid. In humans, this has been postulated to be the major pathway, but this hypothesis requires experimental validation. After synthesis is completed via a complex pathway consisting of enzymatic steps in the cellular cytosol as well as mitochondria, the molecules are conjugated in peroxisomes with either glycine or taurine (Russell 2003; Chiang and Ferrell 2019). In humans the ratio glycine/taurine is mostly around 3; rodents predominantly conjugate with taurine (Kuipers et al. 2014). Another substantial difference between rodents and humans is the fact that rodents convert the hydrophobic chenodeoxycholic acid into the very hydrophilic muricholic acids. This completely alters BA function and precludes direct translation of rodent data to humans (Kuipers et al. 2014).

In mice and man, BA are stored in the gallbladder and are expelled into the duodenum primarily after initiating intake of food (Behar 2013). The consensus is that sensors in the small intestine register arrival of fat and protein and activate gallbladder contraction through release of cholecystokinin, although also in the absence of food regular small contraction of the gallbladder must occur to maintain BA concentrations observed in the circulation (Sips et al. 2018). BA arriving in the terminal ileum are extremely efficiently absorbed via the sodium-dependent bile acid transporter (ASBT or SLC10A2) (Hagenbuch and Dawson 2004). Bile acids are highly toxic for bacteria which is probably an important reason why the small intestine is sparsely colonized relative to the colon. Depending on small intestinal motility and the bile salt hydrolase activity of the microbiota colonizing the small intestine, a small amount of bile acids enters the colon and is metabolized into a myriad of so-called secondary or more recently tertiary bile acids. The degree of metabolism strongly depends on the colonic microbiota composition of a given subject (Ridlon et al. 2006).

Secondary bile acids are hydrophobic and consequently highly toxic for bacteria; apparently bacteria that are able to dehydroxylate bile acids have evolved to create a toxic environment for their neighbors. Because of the fact that the secondary bile acids are hydrophobic, they can passively diffuse across the colonocyte cell membranes and enter the bloodstream. Whether this process is purely diffusion or whether transporters are also involved is not known. In humans, it is estimated that about 5% of the bile acid pool is not reabsorbed and is excreted via the feces. The variability may in part be caused by changes in absorptive capacity which might directly influence the risk on ASCVD. Note that although only 5% of the bile acids escapes the enterohepatic circulation, bile acid excretion is the major pathway for cholesterol export from the body, apart from neutral sterol excretion. Aging correlates negatively with bile acid synthesis (Einarsson et al. 1985); thus also cholesterol excretion via this route decreases with age pointing to a possible causal relation between BA excretion and ASCVD. The plasma concentration of taurocholate has been found to negatively correlate with longevity (Cheng et al. 2015). This could be due to increased absorptive capacity possibly increasing with age and also accounting for the decrease in synthesis, but this still has to be addressed experimentally. One report has described a negative correlation between bile acid synthesis rates and ASCVD events (Charach et al. 2018). Though highly interesting this study requires confirmation.

4.2   Regulation by Bile Acids

Besides the direct role of BA in cholesterol metabolism, they control diverse metabolic pathways via membrane and nuclear hormone receptors signaling. Particularly G-protein linked receptor TGR5 and the farnesoid X receptor (FXR) are important in this respect. Both receptors show a great preference for the more hydrophobic bile acids; hence microbial metabolism plays a major role in regulating BA control of metabolism.

The role of FXR in controlling progress of ASCVD is ambiguous. Hanniman et al. reported increased atherosclerosis development in FXR/ApoE double KO mice (Hanniman et al. 2005), whereas two other studies reported that loss of FXR in low-density lipoprotein receptor $-/-$ (LDLR) mice and ApoE$-/-$ mice reduced atherosclerotic lesion size (Guo et al. 2006; Zhang et al. 2006). Although differences in gut microbiota composition and sex of the mouse models used may play a role, the exact nature of these discrepancies is unclear. In contrast, FXR stimulation with the FXR agonists PX20606 and WAY-362450 did prevent atherosclerotic plaque formation in ApoE KO, LDLR $-/-$, or CETP transgene LDLR $-/-$ models (Hartman et al. 2009; Hambruch et al. 2012). Additionally, FXR stimulation modulates inflammatory responses, thereby reducing pro-inflammatory cytokine production. The first FDA-approved FXR agonist obeticholic acid (OCA) is currently tested in human trials (Neuschwander-Tetri et al. 2015). Unexpectedly, OCA induced an increase in LDL cholesterol and a concomitant decrease in HDL-C (Nevens et al. 2016). The underlying mechanism is not clear, and the effect on ASCVD has not yet been assessed; but the induced phenotype makes OCA a less attractive option to treat atherosclerosis in humans.

The other important BA receptor, TGR5, has a high affinity for secondary BA in particular lithocholate (Klindt et al. 2015). TGR5 stimulation activates thyroid hormone deiodinase 2 which converts inactive thyroxine (T4) into active 3,5,3′-triiodothyronine 12 (T3) and stimulates energy expenditure (Watanabe et al. 2006). Interestingly, TGR5 activation has immunosuppressive effects. TGR5 has been shown to reduce cytokine expression via inhibition of nuclear translocation of NF-κB (Pols et al. 2011; Yoneno et al. 2013). Furthermore, TGR5 activation with INT-777 inhibits the inflammasome, a major driver of the inflammatory component of ASCVD progression (Hao et al. 2017). In addition to its effects on immune cells, TGR5 also effects metabolism in endothelial cells (Keitel et al. 2007) where it may control nitric oxide (NO) production, through phosphorylation of endothelial nitric oxide synthase (eNOS) (Kida et al. 2013). The immunomodulatory functions of TGR5 make this receptor an interesting target to treat atherosclerosis, and because of its high affinity for lithocholic acid and deoxycholic acid, it may explain beneficial effects of the gut microbiota in ASCVD. So far, the effects of specific TGR5 agonists have only been studied in animal models; hence it is not clear whether the results can be translated to humans.

5 Summary and Future Perspectives

The etiology of ASCVD starts simple with disposition of lipids in the vessel wall but develops into an extremely complex myriad of aggravating and inhibiting factors when it progresses. Because so many factors are involved, it seems justified to assume that ASCVD develops in a unique way in any single patient. Up to now treatment of ASCVD mainly focuses on inhibiting the initiating factor, disposition of lipid in the vessel wall. Although perhaps successful in inhibiting progress of the disease, it does not induce regression of the plaques to a significant extent. Attempts to induce plaque regression have been very unsuccessful so far. Enhancing cholesterol efflux through increasing plasma HDL concentration has not worked probably by a lack of understanding of the molecular mechanism of cholesterol efflux in vivo.

The question arises whether influencing the composition of the microbiome can help. As discussed in this review, the bacterial component of the microbiome can influence the process of ASCVD development at many different stages. Particularly, the oral microbiome can easily invade a patient suffering from a very common periodontitis. This causes a systemic inflammatory response potentially aggravating atherosclerotic plaque progression.

Bacteria can initiate production of harmful molecules such as TMA or ImP that are likely to contribute to ASCVD development. Since many bacterial species are capable of TMA or ImP production, it is challenging to develop strategies to, e.g., eradicate these bacteria. Antibiotics treatment has been shown to reduce TMAO production in humans (Craciun and Balskus 2012) However, it is critical to point out that there are many objections to using antibiotics as means to intervene in microbiome-mediated cues to ASCVD development. These include significant consequences of antibiotic use for the gut microbial community, risk to develop antibiotic resistance, and the fact that antibiotics use has been associated with increased progression of ASCVD (Heianza et al. 2019).

Early initiatives aiming to specifically reduce production of TMA (instead of the bacterium) have shown promising results in lowering TMAO levels and ASCVD risk, at least in mice. Inhibition of the activity of TMA lyase, which hydrolyses choline to TMA, using the choline analog DMB reduced atherosclerosis burden in ApoE$-/-$ mice fed a choline-rich diet (Wang et al. 2015). More recently, it was shown that strategies aiming to inhibit phospholipase D, a bacterial enzyme that frees choline from phosphatidylcholine lipids, might be an interesting novel target to reduce choline-derived production of TMA (Chittim et al. 2019). More upstream in the cascade of microbial-metabolite production, it might be beneficial to develop strategies that aim to reduce intake of precursors of the presumably harmful metabolites. Although it is too early to tell if reduction of choline intake or alternative dietary strategies to reduce TMAO production will prevent ASCVD development (Washburn et al. 2019), these initiatives might provide feasible and economic solutions for reduction of these and other (e.g., ImP from histidine) microbiome-derived atherogenic metabolites. Important in this context is that humans usually have very low coherence to dietary interventions. In addition, high interindividual differences in response to dietary interventions (Walker et al. 2011; Cotillard et al. 2013; Kovatcheva-Datchary et al. 2015) make diet a challenging intervention to alter the microbiome and (markers of) ASCVD development.

The microbial modification of primary into secondary bile acids is in part facilitated by the bacterial enzyme bile salt hydrolase (BSH). BSH activity has been postulated to alter cholesterol accumulation, inflammation, and atherosclerosis development (Tremaroli and Bäckhed 2012), and BSH activity is present in a very wide range of bacteria (Joyce et al. 2014). A modified *E. coli* strain carrying the BSH gene was shown to enhance expression of genes involved in cholesterol efflux, immune homeostasis, and energy metabolism in mice (Joyce et al. 2014).

In line, a dedicated intervention study using BSH-active *Lactobacillus reuteri* in hypercholesterolemic humans showed that this probiotic effectively lowered LDL-C compared to placebo-treated subjects (Jones et al. 2012). Of interest in this context is that many probiotic strains are characterized by BSH activity (Begley et al. 2006). Whether or not the BSH activity underlies the beneficial effects of probiotic strain administration on parameters of ASCVD risk/health remains to be determined. Nevertheless, many probiotic strains have been associated with ASCVD health. *Bifidobacteria* and *Lactobacillus plantarum* have been associated with lowering of cholesterol (Tahri et al. 1996). Interestingly, *Lactobacillus plantarum* (Nguyen et al. 2007) and *Lactobacillus rhamnosus* (Qiu et al. 2018) were also reported to decrease TMAO and atherosclerosis development in mice prone to develop the disease. Likewise, in hypercholesterolemic humans, *Lactobacillus rhamnosus* was reported to reduce cholesterol levels (Costabile et al. 2017).

One can speculate that beneficial bacteria may produce molecules that halt or even induce regression of the process. As far as we know, studies to find these compounds have not been carried out. A good strategy may be to use modern machine learning methods to analyze the plasma of subjects with atherogenic plasma profile that do not show signs of ASCVD.

Acknowledgments MN is supported by a ZONMW-VIDI grant 2013 [016.146.327] and a Dutch Heart Foundation CVCN IN CONTROL Young Talent Grant 2013.

References

Aderem A, Underhill DM (1999) Mechanisms of phagocytosis in macrophages [in process citation]. Annu Rev Immunol 17:593

Aguilar EC, Leonel AJ, Teixeira LG et al (2014) Butyrate impairs atherogenesis by reducing plaque inflammation and vulnerability and decreasing NFκB activation. Nutr Metab Cardiovasc Dis 24:606–613. https://doi.org/10.1016/j.numecd.2014.01.002

Aldana-Hernández P, Leonard K-A, Zhao Y-Y et al (2019) Dietary choline or trimethylamine N-oxide supplementation does not influence atherosclerosis development in Ldlr−/− and Apoe−/− male mice. J Nutr 150:249–255. https://doi.org/10.1093/jn/nxz214

Al-Lahham SH, Peppelenbosch MP, Roelofsen H et al (2010) Biological effects of propionic acid in humans; metabolism, potential applications and underlying mechanisms. Biochim Biophys Acta 1801:1175–1183. https://doi.org/10.1016/j.bbalip.2010.07.007

Andrade-Oliveira V, Amano MT, Correa-Costa M et al (2015) Gut Bacteria products prevent AKI induced by ischemia-reperfusion. J Am Soc Nephrol 26:1877–1888. https://doi.org/10.1681/asn.2014030288

Aoyama M, Kotani J, Usami M (2010) Butyrate and propionate induced activated or non-activated neutrophil apoptosis via HDAC inhibitor activity but without activating GPR-41/GPR-43 pathways. Nutrition 26:653–661. https://doi.org/10.1016/j.nut.2009.07.006

Aron-Wisnewsky J, Clément K (2016) The gut microbiome, diet, and links to cardiometabolic and chronic disorders. Nat Rev Nephrol 12:169. https://doi.org/10.1038/nrneph.2015.191

Begley M, Hill C, Gahan CGM (2006) Bile salt hydrolase activity in probiotics. Appl Environ Microbiol 72:1729

Behar J (2013) Physiology and pathophysiology of the biliary tract: the gallbladder and sphincter of Oddi—a review. ISRN Physiol 2013:1. https://doi.org/10.1155/2013/837630

Brandsma E, Kloosterhuis NJ, Koster M et al (2019) A Proinflammatory gut microbiota increases systemic inflammation and accelerates atherosclerosis. Circ Res 124:94. https://doi.org/10.1161/CIRCRESAHA.118.313234

Brown JM, Hazen SL (2015) The gut microbial endocrine organ: bacterially derived signals driving Cardiometabolic diseases. Annu Rev Med 66:343. https://doi.org/10.1146/annurev-med-060513-093205

Canfora EE, van der Beek CM, Jocken JWE et al (2017) Colonic infusions of short-chain fatty acid mixtures promote energy metabolism in overweight/obese men: a randomized crossover trial. Sci Rep 7:2206. https://doi.org/10.1038/s41598-017-02546-x

Cani PD, Neyrinck AM, Fava F et al (2007) Selective increases of bifidobacteria in gut microflora improve high-fat-diet-induced diabetes in mice through a mechanism associated with endotoxaemia. Diabetologia 50:2374. https://doi.org/10.1007/s00125-007-0791-0

Carding SR, Davis N, Hoyles L (2017) Review article: the human intestinal virome in health and disease. Aliment Pharmacol Ther 46:800

Cavaglieri CR, Nishiyama A, Fernandes LC et al (2003) Differential effects of short-chain fatty acids on proliferation and production of pro- and anti-inflammatory cytokines by cultured lymphocytes. Life Sci 73:1683–1690

Charach G, Argov O, Geiger K et al (2018) Diminished bile acids excretion is a risk factor for coronary artery disease: 20-year follow up and long-term outcome. Ther Adv Gastroenterol 11. https://doi.org/10.1177/1756283X17743420

Chen S, Henderson A, Petriello MC et al (2019) Trimethylamine N-oxide binds and activates PERK to promote metabolic dysfunction. Cell Metab 30:1141. https://doi.org/10.1016/j.cmet.2019.08.021

Cheng S, Larson MG, McCabe EL et al (2015) Distinct metabolomic signatures are associated with longevity in humans. Nat Commun 6:6791. https://doi.org/10.1038/ncomms7791

Chiang JYL, Ferrell JM (2019) Bile acids as metabolic regulators and nutrient sensors. Annu Rev Nutr 39:175. https://doi.org/10.1146/annurev-nutr-082018-124344

Chittim CL, Martínez del Campo A, Balskus EP (2019) Gut bacterial phospholipase Ds support disease-associated metabolism by generating choline. Nat Microbiol 4:155. https://doi.org/10.1038/s41564-018-0294-4

Costabile A, Buttarazzi I, Kolida S et al (2017) An in vivo assessment of the cholesterol-lowering efficacy of lactobacillus plantarum ECGC 13110402 in normal to mildly hypercholesterolaemic adults. PLoS One 12:e0187964. https://doi.org/10.1371/journal.pone.0187964

Cotillard A, Kennedy SP, Kong LC et al (2013) Dietary intervention impact on gut microbial gene richness. Nature 500:585. https://doi.org/10.1038/nature12480

Craciun S, Balskus EP (2012) Microbial conversion of choline to trimethylamine requires a glycyl radical enzyme. Proc Natl Acad Sci U S A 109:21307. https://doi.org/10.1073/pnas.1215689109

den Besten G, van Eunen K, Groen AK et al (2013) The role of short-chain fatty acids in the interplay between diet, gut microbiota, and host energy metabolism. J Lipid Res 54:2325. https://doi.org/10.1194/jlr.r036012

Duerkop BA, Clements CV, Rollins D et al (2012) A composite bacteriophage alters colonization by an intestinal commensal bacterium. Proc Natl Acad Sci 109:17621. https://doi.org/10.1073/pnas.1206136109

Duerkop BA, Kleiner M, Paez-Espino D et al (2018) Murine colitis reveals a disease-associated bacteriophage community. Nat Microbiol 3:1023. https://doi.org/10.1038/s41564-018-0210-y

Einarsson K, Nilsell K, Leijd B, Angelin B (1985) Influence of age on secretion of cholesterol and synthesis of bile acids by the liver. N Engl J Med 313:277. https://doi.org/10.1056/nejm198508013130501

Emoto T, Yamashita T, Sasaki N et al (2016) Analysis of gut microbiota in coronary artery disease patients: a possible link between gut microbiota and coronary artery disease. J Atheroscler Thromb 23:908. https://doi.org/10.5551/jat.32672

Falony G, Vandeputte D, Caenepeel C et al (2019) The human microbiome in health and disease: hype or hope. Acta Clin Belgica 74:53. https://doi.org/10.1080/17843286.2019.1583782

Ference BA, Ginsberg HN, Graham I et al (2017) Low-density lipoproteins cause atherosclerotic cardiovascular disease. 1. Evidence from genetic, epidemiologic, and clinical studies. A consensus statement from the European Atherosclerosis Society Consensus Panel. Eur Heart J 38:2459–2472. https://doi.org/10.1093/eurheartj/ehx144

Fernández L, Rodríguez A, García P (2018) Phage or foe: an insight into the impact of viral predation on microbial communities. ISME J 12:1171

Gogokhia L, Buhrke K, Bell R et al (2019) Expansion of bacteriophages is linked to aggravated intestinal inflammation and colitis. Cell Host Microbe 25:285. https://doi.org/10.1016/j.chom.2019.01.008

Gregory JC, Buffa JA, Org E et al (2015) Transmission of atherosclerosis susceptibility with gut microbial transplantation. J Biol Chem 290:5647. https://doi.org/10.1074/jbc.M114.618249

Guo GL, Santamarina-Fojo S, Akiyama TE et al (2006) Effects of FXR in foam-cell formation and atherosclerosis development. Biochim Biophys Acta Mol Cell Biol Lipids 1761:1401. https://doi.org/10.1016/j.bbalip.2006.09.018

Hagenbuch B, Dawson P (2004) The sodium bile salt cotransport family SLC10. Pflugers Arch Eur J Physiol 447:566

Hajishengallis G (2015) Periodontitis: from microbial immune subversion to systemic inflammation. Nat Rev Immunol 15:30–44

Hambruch E, Miyazaki-Anzai S, Hahn U et al (2012) Synthetic farnesoid X receptor agonists induce high-density lipoprotein-mediated transhepatic cholesterol efflux in mice and monkeys and prevent atherosclerosis in cholesteryl ester transfer protein transgenic low-density lipoprotein receptor ($-/-$) mice. J Pharmacol Exp Ther 343:556. https://doi.org/10.1124/jpet.112.196519

Hanniman EA, Lambert G, McCarthy TC, Sinal CJ (2005) Loss of functional farnesoid X receptor increases atherosclerotic lesions in apolipoprotein E-deficient mice. J Lipid Res 46:2595. https://doi.org/10.1194/jlr.m500390-jlr200

Hao H, Cao L, Jiang C et al (2017) Farnesoid X receptor regulation of the NLRP3 Inflammasome underlies cholestasis-associated sepsis. Cell Metab 25:856. https://doi.org/10.1016/j.cmet.2017.03.007

Hartman HB, Gardell SJ, Petucci CJ et al (2009) Activation of farnesoid X receptor prevents atherosclerotic lesion formation in LDLR $-/-$ and apoE $-/-$ mice. J Lipid Res 50:1090. https://doi.org/10.1194/jlr.m800619-jlr200

Heianza Y, Ma W, Manson JAE et al (2017) Gut microbiota metabolites and risk of major adverse cardiovascular disease events and death: a systematic review and meta-analysis of prospective studies. J Am Heart Assoc 6:e004947

Heianza Y, Zheng Y, Ma W et al (2019) Duration and life-stage of antibiotic use and risk of cardiovascular events in women. Eur Heart J 40:3838. https://doi.org/10.1093/eurheartj/ehz231

Hoffmann C, Dollive S, Grunberg S et al (2013) Archaea and fungi of the human gut microbiome: correlations with diet and bacterial residents. PLoS One 8:e66019. https://doi.org/10.1371/journal.pone.0066019

Holmes E, Li JV, Marchesi JR, Nicholson JK (2012) Gut microbiota composition and activity in relation to host metabolic phenotype and disease risk. Cell Metab 16:559

Holmes MV, Ala-Korpela M, Smith GD (2017) Mendelian randomization in cardiometabolic disease: challenges in evaluating causality. Nat Rev Cardiol 14:577

Hornung B, Martins dos Santos VAP, Smidt H, Schaap PJ (2018) Studying microbial functionality within the gut ecosystem by systems biology. Genes Nutr 13:5

Hsu BB, Gibson TE, Yeliseyev V et al (2019) Dynamic modulation of the gut microbiota and Metabolome by bacteriophages in a mouse model. Cell Host Microbe 25:803. https://doi.org/10.1016/j.chom.2019.05.001

Huseyin CE, O'Toole PW, Cotter PD, Scanlan PD (2017) Forgotten fungi-the gut mycobiome in human health and disease. FEMS Microbiol Rev 41:479

Jie Z, Xia H, Zhong SL et al (2017) The gut microbiome in atherosclerotic cardiovascular disease. Nat Commun 8:845. https://doi.org/10.1038/s41467-017-00900-1

Jones ML, Martoni CJ, Parent M, Prakash S (2012) Cholesterol-lowering efficacy of a microencapsulated bile salt hydrolase-active Lactobacillus reuteri NCIMB 30242 yoghurt formulation in hypercholesterolaemic adults. Br J Nutr 107:1505. https://doi.org/10.1017/S0007114511004703

Jonsson A, Hållenius FF, Akrami R et al (2017) Bacterial profile in human atherosclerotic plaques. Atherosclerosis 263:177. https://doi.org/10.1016/j.atherosclerosis.2017.06.016

Jonsson AL, Caesar R, Akrami R et al (2018) Impact of gut microbiota and diet on the development of atherosclerosis in ApoE−/− mice. Arterioscler Thromb Vasc Biol 38:2318. https://doi.org/10.1161/ATVBAHA.118.311233

Joyce SA, MacSharry J, Casey PG et al (2014) Regulation of host weight gain and lipid metabolism by bacterial bile acid modification in the gut. Proc Natl Acad Sci U S A 111:7421–7426. https://doi.org/10.1073/pnas.1323599111

Karlsson FH, Fåk F, Nookaew I et al (2012) Symptomatic atherosclerosis is associated with an altered gut metagenome. Nat Commun 3:1245. https://doi.org/10.1038/ncomms2266

Kasahara K, Tanoue T, Yamashita T et al (2017) Commensal bacteria at the crossroad between cholesterol homeostasis and chronic inflammation in atherosclerosis. J Lipid Res 58:519. https://doi.org/10.1194/jlr.m072165

Kasahara K, Krautkramer KA, Org E et al (2018) Interactions between Roseburia intestinalis and diet modulate atherogenesis in a murine model. Nat Microbiol 3:1461. https://doi.org/10.1038/s41564-018-0272-x

Kaysen GA, Johansen KL, Chertow GM et al (2015) Associations of Trimethylamine N-oxide with nutritional and inflammatory biomarkers and cardiovascular outcomes in patients new to dialysis. J Ren Nutr 25:351. https://doi.org/10.1053/j.jrn.2015.02.006

Keitel V, Reinehr R, Gatsios P et al (2007) The G-protein coupled bile salt receptor TGR5 is expressed in liver sinusoidal endothelial cells. Hepatology 45:695. https://doi.org/10.1002/hep.21458

Kida T, Tsubosaka Y, Hori M et al (2013) Bile acid receptor tgr5 agonism induces no production and reduces monocyte adhesion in vascular endothelial cells. Arterioscler Thromb Vasc Biol 33:1663. https://doi.org/10.1161/ATVBAHA.113.301565

Kim MH, Kang SG, Park JH et al (2013) Short-chain fatty acids activate GPR41 and GPR43 on intestinal epithelial cells to promote inflammatory responses in mice. Gastroenterology 145:396–406.e10. https://doi.org/10.1053/j.gastro.2013.04.056

Kim S, Goel R, Kumar A et al (2018) Imbalance of gut microbiome and intestinal epithelial barrier dysfunction in patients with high blood pressure. Clin Sci 132:701. https://doi.org/10.1042/cs20180087

Klindt C, Deutschmann K, Reich M et al (2015) TGR5 knockout mice are highly susceptible to LCA induced liver damage. Z Gastroenterol 53. https://doi.org/10.1055/s-0035-1568049

Koeth RA, Lam-Galvez BR, Kirsop J et al (2019) L-Carnitine in omnivorous diets induces an atherogenic gut microbial pathway in humans. J Clin Invest 129:373. https://doi.org/10.1172/JCI94601

Koh A, Molinaro A, Ståhlman M et al (2018) Microbially produced imidazole propionate impairs insulin signaling through mTORC1. Cell 175:947. https://doi.org/10.1016/j.cell.2018.09.055

Koren O, Spor A, Felin J et al (2011) Human oral, gut, and plaque microbiota in patients with atherosclerosis. Proc Natl Acad Sci 108:4592. https://doi.org/10.1073/pnas.1011383107

Kovatcheva-Datchary P, Nilsson A, Akrami R et al (2015) Dietary fiber-induced improvement in glucose metabolism is associated with increased abundance of Prevotella. Cell Metab 22:971. https://doi.org/10.1016/j.cmet.2015.10.001

Kuipers F, Bloks VW, Groen AK (2014) Beyond intestinal soap – bile acids in metabolic control. Nat Rev Endocrinol 10:488

Kurilshikov A, van den Munckhof ICL, Chen L et al (2019) Gut microbial associations to plasma metabolites linked to cardiovascular phenotypes and risk. Circ Res 124:1808. https://doi.org/10.1161/CIRCRESAHA.118.314642

Laforest-Lapointe I, Arrieta M-C (2018) Microbial eukaryotes: a missing link in gut microbiome studies. mSystems 3:e00201. https://doi.org/10.1128/msystems.00201-17

Liu H, Chen X, Hu X et al (2019) Alterations in the gut microbiome and metabolism with coronary artery disease severity. Microbiome 7:68. https://doi.org/10.1186/s40168-019-0683-9

Lobo MG, Schmidt MM, Lopes RD et al (2019) Treating periodontal disease in patients with myocardial infarction: a randomized clinical trial. Eur J Intern Med 71:76. https://doi.org/10.1016/j.ejim.2019.08.012

Loos BG, Craandijk J, Hoek FJ et al (2005) Elevation of systemic markers related to cardiovascular diseases in the peripheral blood of periodontitis patients. J Periodontol 71:1528. https://doi.org/10.1902/jop.2000.71.10.1528

Masui R, Sasaki M, Funaki Y et al (2013) G protein-coupled receptor 43 moderates gut inflammation through cytokine regulation from mononuclear cells. Inflamm Bowel Dis 19:2848–2856. https://doi org/10.1097/01.MIB.0000435444.14860.ea

Menni C, Lin C, Cecelja M et al (2018) Gut microbial diversity is associated with lower arterial stiffness in women. Eur Heart J 39:2390. https://doi.org/10.1093/eurheartj/ehy226

Minot S, Sinha R, Chen J et al (2011) The human gut virome: inter-individual variation and dynamic response to diet. Genome Res 21:1616. https://doi.org/10.1101/gr.122705.111

Mueller DM, Allenspach M, Othman A et al (2015) Plasma levels of trimethylamine-N-oxide are confounded by impaired kidney function and poor metabolic control. Atherosclerosis 243:638. https://doi.org/10.1016/j.atherosclerosis.2015.10.091

Neuschwander-Tetri BA, Loomba R, Sanyal AJ et al (2015) Farnesoid X nuclear receptor ligand obeticholic acid for non-cirrhotic, non-alcoholic steatohepatitis (FLINT): a multicentre, randomised, placebo-controlled trial. Lancet 385:956. https://doi.org/10.1016/S0140-6736(14)61933-4

Nevens F, Andreone P, Mazzella G et al (2016) A placebo-controlled trial of Obeticholic acid in primary biliary cholangitis. N Engl J Med 375:631. https://doi.org/10.1056/nejmoa1509840

Newgard CB (2017) Metabolomics and metabolic diseases: where do we stand? Cell Metab 25:43–56

Nguyen TDT, Kang JH, Lee MS (2007) Characterization of Lactobacillus plantarum PH04, a potential probiotic bacterium with cholesterol-lowering effects. Int J Food Microbiol 113:358. https://doi.org/10.1016/j.ijfoodmicro.2006.08.015

Noack B, Genco RJ, Trevisan M et al (2005) Periodontal infections contribute to elevated systemic C-reactive protein level. J Periodontol 72:1221. https://doi.org/10.1902/jop.2000.72.9.1221

Nordestgaard BG (2016) Triglyceride-rich lipoproteins and atherosclerotic cardiovascular disease: new insights from epidemiology, genetics, and biology. Circ Res 118:547. https://doi.org/10.1161/CIRCRESAHA.115.306249

Norman JM, Handley SA, Baldridge MT et al (2015) Disease-specific alterations in the enteric virome in inflammatory bowel disease. Cell 160:447. https://doi.org/10.1016/j.cell.2015.01.002

Nurmi JT, Puolakkainen PA, Rautonen NE (2005) Bifidobacterium Lactis sp. 420 up-regulates cyclooxygenase (Cox)-1 and down-regulates Cox-2 gene expression in a Caco-2 cell culture model. Nutr Cancer 51:83–92. https://doi.org/10.1207/s15327914nc5101_12

Oh JH, Alexander LM, Pan M et al (2019) Dietary fructose and microbiota-derived short-chain fatty acids promote bacteriophage production in the gut symbiont lactobacillus reuteri. Cell Host Microbe 25:273. https://doi.org/10.1016/j.chom.2018.11.016

Ohira H, Tsutsui W, Fujioka Y (2017) Are short chain fatty acids in gut microbiota defensive players for inflammation and atherosclerosis? J Atheroscler Thromb 24:660. https://doi.org/10.5551/jat.rv17006

Park J, Goergen CJ, HogenEsch H, Kim CH (2016) Chronically elevated levels of short-chain fatty acids induce T cell-mediated ureteritis and hydronephrosis. J Immunol 196:2388–2400. https://doi.org/10.4049/jimmunol.1502046

Paterson MJ, Oh S, Underhill DM (2017) Host–microbe interactions: commensal fungi in the gut. Curr Opin Microbiol 40:131

Pencina MJ, Navar AM, Wojdyla D et al (2019) Quantifying importance of major risk factors for coronary heart disease. Circulation 139:1603. https://doi.org/10.1161/CIRCULATIONAHA.117.031855

Pluznick JL (2013) A novel SCFA receptor, the microbiota, and blood pressure regulation. Gut Microbes 5:202. https://doi.org/10.4161/gmic.27492

Pols TWH, Nomura M, Harach T et al (2011) TGR5 activation inhibits atherosclerosis by reducing macrophage inflammation and lipid loading. Cell Metab 14:747. https://doi.org/10.1016/j.cmet.2011.11.006

Qiu L, Tao X, Xiong H et al (2018) Lactobacillus plantarum ZDY04 exhibits a strain-specific property of lowering TMAO via the modulation of gut microbiota in mice. Food Funct 9:4299. https://doi.org/10.1039/c8fo00349a

Rabot S, Membrez M, Bruneau A et al (2010) Germ-free C57BL/6J mice are resistant to high-fat-diet-induced insulin resistance and have altered cholesterol metabolism. FASEB J 24:4948. https://doi.org/10.1096/fj.10-164921

Raetz CRH, Whitfield C (2008) Lipopolysaccharide endotoxins Christian. Annu Rev Biochem 71:635–700. https://doi.org/10.1146/annurev.biochem.71.110601.135414

Reyes A, Haynes M, Hanson N et al (2010) Viruses in the faecal microbiota of monozygotic twins and their mothers. Nature 466:334. https://doi.org/10.1038/nature09199

Reyes A, Semenkovich NP, Whiteson K et al (2012) Going viral: next-generation sequencing applied to phage populations in the human gut. Nat Rev Microbiol 10:607

Ridker PM, Everett BM, Thuren T et al (2017) Antiinflammatory therapy with canakinumab for atherosclerotic disease. N Engl J Med 377:1119. https://doi.org/10.1056/nejmoa1707914

Ridlon JM, Kang D-J, Hylemon PB (2006) Bile salt biotransformations by human intestinal bacteria. J Lipid Res 47:241. https://doi.org/10.1194/jlr.r500013-jlr200

Russell DW (2003) The enzymes, regulation, and genetics of bile acid synthesis. Annu Rev Biochem 72:137. https://doi.org/10.1146/annurev.biochem.72.121801.161712

Shetty SA, Hugenholtz F, Lahti L et al (2017) Intestinal microbiome landscaping: insight in community assemblage and implications for microbial modulation strategies. FEMS Microbiol Rev 41:182. https://doi.org/10.1093/femsre/fuw045

Shkoporov AN, Hill C (2019) Bacteriophages of the human gut: the "known unknown" of the microbiome. Cell Host Microbe 25:195

Sips FLP, Eggink HM, Hilbers PAJ et al (2018) In silico analysis identifies intestinal transit as a key determinant of systemic bile acid metabolism. Front Physiol 9:631. https://doi.org/10.3389/fphys.2018.00631

Stepankova R, Tonar Z, Bartova J et al (2010) Absence of microbiota (germ-free conditions) accelerates the atherosclerosis in ApoE-deficient mice fed standard low cholesterol diet. J Atheroscler Thromb 17:796. https://doi.org/10.5551/jat.3285

Sweere JM, van Belleghem JD, Ishak H et al (2019) Bacteriophage trigger antiviral immunity and prevent clearance of bacterial infection. Science 363:eaat9691. https://doi.org/10.1126/science.aat9691

Tahri K, Grill JP, Schneider F (1996) Bifidobacteria strain behavior toward cholesterol: coprecipitation with bile salts and assimilation. Curr Microbiol 33:187. https://doi.org/10.1007/s002849900098

Tilg H, Zmora N, Adolph TE, Elinav E (2019) The intestinal microbiota fuelling metabolic inflammation. Nat Rev Immunol 20:40. https://doi.org/10.1038/s41577-019-0198-4

Torres De Heens GL, Loos BG, van der Velden U (2010) Monozygotic twins are discordant for chronic periodontitis: clinical and bacteriological findings. J Clin Periodontol 37:120. https://doi.org/10.1111/j.1600-051X.2009.01511.x

Tremaroli V, Bäckhed F (2012) Functional interactions between the gut microbiota and host metabolism. Nature 489:242

van Belleghem JD, Dąbrowska K, Vaneechoutte M et al (2019) Interactions between bacteriophage, bacteria, and the mammalian immune system. Viruses 11:10

van der Beek CM, Canfora EE, Lenaerts K et al (2016) Distal, not proximal, colonic acetate infusions promote fat oxidation and improve metabolic markers in overweight/obese men. Clin Sci 130:2073–2082 https://doi.org/10.1042/cs20160263

Vinolo MAR, Rodrigues HG, Nachbar RT, Curi R (2011) Regulation of inflammation by short chain fatty acids. Nutrients 3:858–876. https://doi.org/10.3390/nu3100858

Virmani R, Robinowitz M, Geer JC et al (1987) Coronary artery atherosclerosis revisited in Korean war combat casualties. Arch Pathol Lab Med 111:972–976

Walk ST, de Vos WM, van der Oost J et al (2016) Healthy human gut phageome. Proc Natl Acad Sci 113:10400. https://doi.org/10.1073/pnas.1601060113

Walker AW, Ince J, Duncan SH et al (2011) Dominant and diet-responsive groups of bacteria within the human colonic microbiota. ISME J 5:220. https://doi.org/10.1038/ismej.2010.118

Wang Z, Klipfell E, Bennett BJ et al (2011) Gut flora metabolism of phosphatidylcholine promotes cardiovascular disease. Nature 472:57. https://doi.org/10.1038/nature09922

Wang Z, Roberts AB, Buffa JA et al (2015) Non-lethal inhibition of gut microbial Trimethylamine production for the treatment of atherosclerosis. Cell 163:1585. https://doi.org/10.1016/j.cell.2015.11.055

Wang Z, Zhu C, Nambi V et al (2019) Metabolomic pattern predicts incident coronary heart disease. Arterioscler Thromb Vasc Biol 39:1475. https://doi.org/10.1161/atvbaha.118.312236

Warwick-Dugdale J, Buchholz HH, Allen MJ, Temperton B (2019) Host-hijacking and planktonic piracy: how phages command the microbial high seas. Virol J 16:15

Washburn RL, Cox JE, Muhlestein JB et al (2019) Pilot study of novel intermittent fasting effects on metabolomic and trimethylamine N-oxide changes during 24-hour water-only fasting in the FEELGOOD trial. Nutrients 11:246. https://doi.org/10.3390/nu11020246

Watanabe M, Houten SM, Mataki C et al (2006) Bile acids induce energy expenditure by promoting intracellular thyroid hormone activation. Nature 439:484–489. https://doi.org/10.1038/nature04330

Wright RS, Murphy J (2016) PROVE-IT to IMPROVE-IT why LDL-C goals still matter in post-ACS patients. J Am Coll Cardiol 67:362–364

Wright SD, Burton C, Hernandez M et al (2000) Infectious agents are not necessary for murine atherogenesis. J Exp Med 191:1437. https://doi.org/10.1084/jem.191.8.1437

Wu J, Saleh MA, Kirabo A et al (2014) Changes in gut microbiota control metabolic endotoxemia-induced inflammation in high-fat diet-induced obesity and diabetes in mice. Diabetes 57:1470. https://doi.org/10.2337/db07-1403

Würtz P, Havulinna AS, Soininen P et al (2015) Metabolite profiling and cardiovascular event risk: a prospective study of 3 population-based cohorts. Circulation 131:774. https://doi.org/10.1161/CIRCULATIONAHA.114.013116

Yoneno K, Hisamatsu T, Shimamura K et al (2013) TGR5 signalling inhibits the production of pro-inflammatory cytokines by in vitro differentiated inflammatory and intestinal macrophages in Crohn's disease. Immunology 139:19. https://doi.org/10.1111/imm.12045

Yoshii S, Tsuboi S, Morita I et al (2009) Temporal association of elevated C-reactive protein and periodontal disease in men. J Periodontol 80:734. https://doi.org/10.1902/jop.2009.080537

Zhang Y, Wang X, Vales C et al (2006) FXR deficiency causes reduced atherosclerosis in Ldlr−/− mice. Arterioscler Thromb Vasc Biol 26:2316. https://doi.org/10.1161/01.ATV.0000235697. 35431.05

Zhu W, Gregory JC, Org E et al (2016) Gut microbial metabolite TMAO enhances platelet hyperreactivity and thrombosis risk. Cell 165:111. https://doi.org/10.1016/j.cell.2016.02.011

Zhu W, Wang Z, Tang WW, Hazen SL (2017) Gut microbe-generated TMAO from dietary choline is prothrombotic in subjects. Circulation 135:1671. https://doi.org/10.1186/s40945-017-0033-9.Using

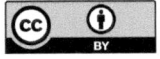

Smooth Muscle Cell-Proteoglycan-Lipoprotein Interactions as Drivers of Atherosclerosis

Sima Allahverdian, Carleena Ortega, and Gordon A. Francis

Contents

1   Introduction 336
2   Smooth Muscle Cell Phenotype Switch and Extracellular Matrix Production 336
3   Extracellular Matrix (ECM) 337
    3.1   Fibrillar Matrix 338
    3.2   Proteoglycans: Non-fibrillar Components of the ECM 339
4   Interactions Between SMCs and the ECM 342
5   SMC, ECM, and Lipoprotein Interactions in Diffuse Intimal Thickening (DIT) 343
6   SMC-ECM Interaction in Lipid Retention 344
    6.1   Deposition of Lipoproteins in the Artery Wall 344
    6.2   PG-Binding Sites in Lipoproteins 347
    6.3   The Variability of Interactions Between Lipoproteins and Proteoglycans 347
    6.4   Effects of Binding and Retention of Lipoproteins 348
7   Role of ECM Proteoglycans in Early Stages of Atherosclerosis Development in Animal
    Models 348
8   The Role of the ECM-SMC Interaction in Plaque Stability and Rupture 349
    8.1   Factors Involved in Plaque Instability 350
9   Therapeutic Targets and Interventions 351
10   Conclusion 352
References 352

Abstract

In humans, smooth muscle cells (SMCs) are the main cell type in the artery medial layer, in pre-atherosclerotic diffuse thickening of the intima, and in all stages of atherosclerotic lesion development. SMCs secrete the proteoglycans responsible for the initial binding and retention of atherogenic lipoproteins in the

S. Allahverdian · C. Ortega · G. A. Francis (✉)
Department of Medicine, Centre for Heart Lung Innovation, Providence Healthcare Research Institute, St. Paul's Hospital, University of British Columbia, Vancouver, BC, Canada
e-mail: gordon.francis@hli.ubc.ca

© The Author(s) 2020
A. von Eckardstein, C. J. Binder (eds.), *Prevention and Treatment of Atherosclerosis*, Handbook of Experimental Pharmacology 270, https://doi.org/10.1007/164_2020_364

artery intima, with this retention driving foam cell formation and subsequent stages of atherosclerosis. In this chapter we review current knowledge of the extracellular matrix generated by SMCs in medial and intimal arterial layers, their relationship to atherosclerotic lesion development and stabilization, how these findings correlate with mouse models of atherosclerosis, and potential therapies aimed at targeting the SMC matrix-lipoprotein interaction for atherosclerosis prevention.

Keywords

Atherosclerosis · Biglycan · Diffuse intimal thickening · Extracellular matrix · Lipoprotein retention · Proteoglycans · Response to retention · Smooth muscle · Smooth muscle cells

1 Introduction

Smooth muscle is the involuntary nonskeletal form of muscle cells, present in hollow organs such as the stomach, intestine, bladder and uterus, the respiratory tract, and arteries and veins of the circulatory system. Smooth muscle cells (SMCs) in the artery muscular or "medial" layer contract or relax to redistribute blood throughout the body and to regulate local blood pressure and blood vessel volume. In addition, in humans SMCs are the predominant cell type in the pre-atherosclerotic intima and all stages of atherosclerotic lesion development (Allahverdian et al. 2018). In the intimal layer, SMCs take on alternate phenotypes and roles including increased proliferation, increased production of matrix proteoglycans, uptake of lipoproteins and foam cell formation, loss of SMC markers and expression of macrophage markers, and stabilization of arteries against plaque rupture. In this chapter we review extracellular matrix (ECM) production by SMCs and its critical role in mediating the lipoprotein retention that drives atherosclerotic lesion development. We correlate these findings in humans with mouse models of atherosclerosis and how modification of the SMC-derived proteoglycan-lipoprotein interaction might be targeted as a means of preventing or treating atherosclerosis.

2 Smooth Muscle Cell Phenotype Switch and Extracellular Matrix Production

Vascular smooth muscle cells (SMCs), unlike skeletal and heart muscle cells, are highly plastic and show a spectrum of phenotypes in the medial and intimal artery layers, with contractile and synthetic being the extremes (Owens et al. 2004). SMCs switch their phenotypes depending on genetic preprogramming and local environmental signals including cytokines and mechanical forces. The majority of SMCs constituting the medial layer of healthy arteries exhibit a contractile phenotype with high levels of cytoplasmic contractile myofilaments, a low proliferation rate, and low protein synthesis. On the other end of the spectrum, intimal SMCs can exhibit either a contractile phenotype or a dedifferentiated, synthetic phenotype with reduced expression of contractile proteins and other differentiated SMC markers and high rates of proliferation and protein synthesis. The majority of SMCs in the intima are of synthetic phenotype. SMCs forming the fibrous cap over atheromas, however, retain SMC markers including α-SMA and show a more differentiated, contractile phenotype (Feil et al. 2014; Perisic Matic et al. 2016; Albarran-Juarez et al. 2016; Chappell et al. 2016). Although transdifferentiation of SMCs with partial or total loss of SMC markers and gain of some macrophage markers has been reported in both human and mouse atherosclerotic lesions, detailed studies have confirmed SMCs maintain their characteristics and do not function as macrophages (Feil et al. 2014; Allahverdian et al. 2014; Shankman et al. 2015; Vengrenyuk et al. 2015).

As the major cell type of the pre-atherosclerotic and atherosclerotic intima, the phenotypic characteristics and products generated by synthetic phenotype SMCs are key determinants of atherosclerotic lesion development (Nakashima et al. 2008). Some of these SMC products are components of the ECM (Wight 2018). ECM is a component of all tissues and organs including blood vessels that provides physical strength to the tissue and acts as a framework in which cells and other molecules are embedded and bound. In arteries, the composition of ECM varies in the intima, media, and adventitia, between healthy and atherosclerotic arteries, and with different stages of atherosclerosis. In particular, the marked increase in proteoglycan content of ECM in the pre-atherosclerotic diffuse intimal thickening (DIT) stage of intima development creates the conditions necessary for the initial retention of serum lipoproteins and initiation of foam cell and atherosclerotic lesion formation (Nakashima et al. 2008; Wight 2018).

3 Extracellular Matrix (ECM)

Extracellular matrix (ECM) is a non-cellular, well-organized, and highly dynamic three-dimensional network in which cells reside and function. ECM is comprised of both fibers and a non-fibrillar amorphous gelatinous material called ground substance. Fibrous protein components of ECM include collagens, elastin, fibronectin (FN), and laminins. The non-fibrillar substance consists of proteoglycans (including versican, perlecan, biglycan, and decorin), along with glycoproteins and hyaluronan. Proteoglycans consist of long chains of repeating disaccharides attached to a core protein, while glycoproteins are composed of short, highly branched chains of various monosaccharides with no repeating unit attached to a core protein (Fig. 1). Hyaluronan is a glycosaminoglycan molecule that has no protein core but forms a non-covalent complex with proteoglycans in the ECM.

ECM components interact with resident cells through their cell surface receptors and regulate their morphology as well as functions such as growth, migration, differentiation, and survival (Theocharis et al. 2016). The composition and structure of ECM varies from tissue to tissue, and alteration of this composition changes the overall structure of the tissue and the function and properties of the embedded cells. Moreover, growth factors, cytokines, and chemokines that bind to ECM molecules

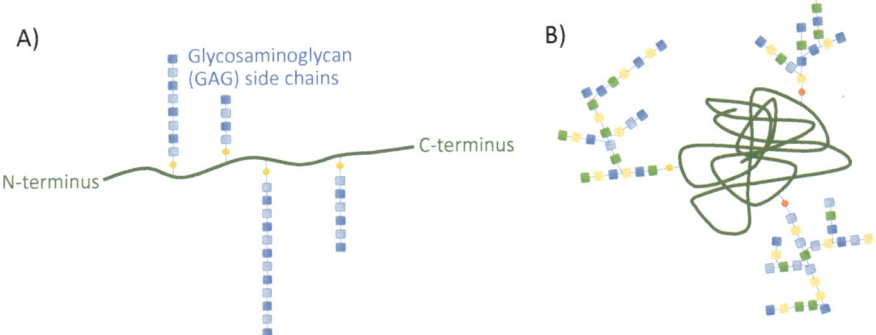

Fig. 1 Model structures of proteoglycans and glycoproteins. (**a**) Proteoglycans consist of a core protein (green line) with glycosaminoglycans (GAGs, blue beaded string), consisting of repeating disaccharide units of various lengths that are attached via O-glycosidic linkages (yellow circles) to the protein. Proteoglycans are distinguished by the size of their protein cores and by the number and type of GAGs attached to their protein cores. (**b**) Glycoproteins consist of a globular protein with a variety of monosaccharides (colored squares) covalently attached to the protein via O-glycosidic linkages (yellow circles) or N-glycosidic linkages (orange hexagon)

are released in response to different stimuli and modify local cellular function (Theocharis et al. 2016). All cell types synthesize and secrete ECM, with alteration of cellular properties due to physiological and pathologic conditions modulating the composition of ECM produced. In the following sections, we focus primarily on ECM produced by, and affecting the function of, arterial SMCs.

3.1   Fibrillar Matrix

Collagens, the most abundant protein in the human body and the major component of the ECM, have widespread distribution among tissues from bone and cartilage to vessel walls. Collagens are categorized into fibril-forming varieties including types I, II and III, present mainly in dermis, tendon, bone, and cartilage, and non-fibrillar collagens such as types IV and VIII, present in the basement membrane – the layer between the endothelium/epithelium and underlying cells – and fibril-associated forms including collagen types IX and XII, which do not form fibers themselves but are associated with collagen fibers (Theocharis et al. 2019). Collagens I and III are the main collagen forms in the medial and intimal layers of medium and large arteries and are the predominant collagens providing tensile strength to the vessel wall (Shekhonin et al. 1985; Frantz et al. 2010; Yue 2014). Collagens make up approximately 40% of all ECM in normal arteries, 10% of early atherosclerotic lesions, and 50% in advanced lesions (Wight 2018). Among the different subtypes, type I collagen is more highly expressed in SMC-rich fibrous caps compared to SMC-poor plaque shoulders. Collagen fibers are thus believed to play an important role in plaque stability (Rekhter 1999).

Elastin fibers are another major fibrillar component of ECM that provide recoil and elasticity to tissues undergoing repeated stretching, such as arteries. Elastic fibers constitute about 50% of the ECM in normal artery walls but only 20% of early and 10% of late atherosclerotic lesions (Wight 2018). Elastin is produced by assembly and crosslinking of its soluble precursor tropoelastin (Wise and Weiss 2009). Normal arteries contain mature crosslinked elastin fibers and negligible amounts of tropoelastin. Using atherosclerotic models, Phinikaridou et al. have shown that accumulation of tropoelastin is associated with plaque progression and instability. They also found that human endarterectomy specimens with ruptured plaques have higher tropoelastin content than stable plaques, suggesting this marker can be used as an indicator of plaque instability (Phinikaridou et al. 2018).

Fibronectin (FN) is another fibril-forming glycoprotein of the ECM. Fibronectin monomers are produced and secreted by cells to form FN fibers (Theocharis et al. 2016). The fibrillar form of FN is a homodimer with monomers linked at the cell surface by disulfide bonds. A soluble monomeric form of fibronectin is also present in plasma, which cells can utilize to assemble into fibers. Fibronectin fibers have binding sites for each other to form multimers. They can also bind to cell surface receptors such as integrins, as well as to collagens, heparin, and fibrin, and act as a bridge to make a network (Theocharis et al. 2016, 2019; Yue 2014). Fibronectin along with fibrinogen and vitronectin is the major component of the provisional matrix present in the intimal space during early stages of atherosclerosis. Fibronectin therefore plays an important role in initiation of the plaque but also later in formation of the fibrous cap to stabilize the plaque (Rohwedder et al. 2012; Finney et al. 2017).

The laminin family comprises 16 heterotrimeric glycoproteins (Theocharis et al. 2016). Each laminin fiber contains one α-, one β-, and one γ-chain in five, four, and three genetic variants, respectively. Laminins are a major component of the basement membrane underlying endothelial cells and surrounding SMCs in the intima. Laminin fibers of the basement membrane bind to each other to make a network to which cells adhere and interact with collagen IV to stabilize the overall structure. Interaction of laminin with collagen is mediated through bridging molecules like the proteoglycan perlecan. Laminin fibers interact with resident cells through multiple cell surface receptors including integrins to regulate cellular differentiation, adhesion, and migration (Theocharis et al. 2016, 2019).

3.2 Proteoglycans: Non-fibrillar Components of the ECM

Proteoglycans are complex macromolecules consisting of a core protein (e.g., versican; the entire proteoglycan molecule is named according to its core protein) to which one or more glycosaminoglycan molecules (GAGs) are covalently attached (Wight 2018) (Fig. 1). GAGs are linear negatively charged polysaccharides of varying length made up of repeating disaccharide units. There are six types of GAGs: chondroitin sulfate (CS), dermatan sulfate (DS), heparan sulfate (HS), heparin, keratan sulfate (KS), and hyaluronic acid (HA; also called hyaluronan). CS, DS, HS, and KS are linked to the different core proteins through O-glycosidic

Table 1 Summary of the various proteoglycans found in the arterial wall, their respective GAG chains, location, and their key role in atherogenesis and vascular homeostasis

Proteoglycan	Glycosaminoglycan (GAG)	Location	Role in atherogenesis and vascular homeostasis
Versican	CS	• Throughout the arterial wall • Enriched in areas with many SMCs (e.g., DIT, fibrous cap, and the edge of lipid cores)	• Provides a matrix that prepares SMC for proliferation and migration
Biglycan	CS, DS	• Abundant in DIT, plaque core, and fibrous cap	• Mediation of lipoprotein retention
Decorin	CS, DS	• Adventitia of normal and atherosclerotic arteries • Similar location as biglycan [e.g., deep (outer) intima in early atherosclerosis] but to a lesser extent • Enriched in the intima of atherosclerosis-resistant arteries	• May contribute to plaque stability
Perlecan	HS	• Basement membrane between endothelial cells and intimal SMCs (abundant in mice but not humans)	• In mice: permeability barrier and lipoprotein retention • In humans: unclear

linkage to make distinct PG families: CSPGs, DSPGs, HSPGs, and KSPGs. Binding of more than one type of GAG to a single core protein creates various PG subtypes. Hyaluronan is the only GAG that is synthesized at the cell membrane and not in the Golgi apparatus, and is only present in a protein-free form. Proteoglycans are abundant in the ECM and are also present on the cell surface and intracellularly. They interact with growth factors, cytokines, cell surface receptors, and other ECM molecules, through which they participate in multiple cellular functions including signaling, proliferation, migration, adhesion, differentiation, and apoptosis (Wight 2018; Theocharis et al. 2016; Yue 2014). Almost all cell types in the vessel wall can synthesize PGs, with SMCs being the major contributor. Proteoglycan content of the normal vessel wall is low, only 4% of total ECM, but it increases dramatically up to 50% in early atherosclerosis and 20% in late lesions (Wight 2018). There are more than 20 different PGs in blood vessels. As discussed below, the negative charge of PGs plays a critical role in the binding and retention of positively charged lipoproteins in the artery intima, a pivotal step in atherosclerotic lesion initiation. Key features of PGs involved in atherosclerotic lesion development are discussed here and summarized in Table 1.

3.2.1   Versican

Versican is a large aggregating CSPG (Wight 2018) that exists in at least four different isoforms, created by alternative splicing of mRNA from a single gene (V0–V3). These variants differ by the length of their core proteins and the number of GAGs attached. Versican forms complexes with hyaluronan, a long-chain GAG, to make high molecular weight aggregates. These aggregates provide a swelling pressure that resists tissue shrinkage and also a viscoelastic pericellular matrix that allows SMCs to change their shape to prepare them for proliferation and migration (Wight and Merrilees 2004). Immunostaining of the ECM of human coronary arteries showed the presence of versican in all layers of the artery wall but increased in areas of atherosclerotic arteries with high SMC content such as diffuse intimal thickening (DIT), fibrous cap, and the edge of the lipid core in advanced lesions (Gutierrez et al. 1997; Kolodgie et al. 2002). SMCs are the main source of versican, and its expression is upregulated by factors including platelet-derived growth factor (PDGF) and transforming growth factor-β1 (TGF-β1). Both PDGF and TGF-β1 increase the number of versican transcripts and elongation of CS chains in cultured SMCs (Schonherr et al. 1991).

3.2.2   Biglycan

The small leucine-rich proteoglycan (SLRP) family includes small core proteins (biglycan, decorin) containing a number of leucine-rich repeats (LRRs) that can have CS, DS, or KS side chains (Wight 2018). Biglycan, together with decorin, belongs to the same class of SLRPs due to their homologous genes and proteins and the presence of ten LRRs sandwiched between cysteine-rich regions (Gutierrez et al. 1997). The N-terminal domain of biglycan typically contains two CS/DS side chains (Iozzo 1999) or two DSPG chains (O'Brien et al. 1998; Gutierrez et al. 1997). Biglycan is the primary proteoglycan found in the intima of normal and atherosclerotic human arteries (Little et al. 2008) and is enriched in areas such as DIT (discussed further in Sect. 4), the plaque core, and fibrous cap (Gutierrez et al. 1997). The presence of growth factors such as PDGF and TGF-β1 transforms biglycan into "hyperelongated biglycan," which has more sulfate incorporated, conveying higher negative charge and longer GAG chains (Schonherr et al. 1993), and therefore increased binding capacity to low density lipoprotein (LDL) and other apolipoprotein B (apoB)-containing lipoproteins (Little et al. 2002). Biglycan concentrated in the deepest part of DIT colocalizes strongly with apoB in early and advancing fatty streaks and plays a critical role in mediating lipoprotein retention in the artery wall (outlined further in Sect. 4 below).

3.2.3   Decorin

Decorin is another member of the SLRP family (Iozzo 1999). Decorin's N-terminus has a single CS/DS chain (Wight 2018). Decorin is expressed in the adventitia of normal and atherosclerotic arteries (Gutierrez et al. 1997). Decorin is also found, although to a somewhat lesser extent than biglycan, in the deep (outer) intima of coronary arteries in early stages of atherosclerosis, suggesting it also has a role in lipoprotein retention. It is also often found in association with collagen fibers in atherosclerotic plaque and may have a role in plaque stability by increasing collagen fibrillogenesis (Wight 2018).

3.2.4   Perlecan

Perlecan, the most abundant HSPG in the mouse artery wall (Nakashima et al. 2008), is located in the basement membrane between the endothelial cells and intimal SMCs (Tran-Lundmark et al. 2008). Perlecan functions as a permeability barrier but also facilitates lipoprotein retention (Tran-Lundmark et al. 2008). Mice that were deficient in both HS-perlecan and apoE were shown to have higher flux but lower arterial retention of lipoproteins compared to apoE-single null mice (Tran-Lundmark et al. 2008). Human atherosclerotic lesions have low expression of perlecan, and the role of perlecan in development of human atherosclerosis is not clear.

4   Interactions Between SMCs and the ECM

In addition to SMCs being the primary source of proteoglycans and other ECM components in arteries, the composition and organization of ECM itself plays an important role in the regulation of SMC phenotype, i.e., the interaction between SMCs and ECM is *bidirectional*. Integrins, transmembrane receptors linking the intracellular SMC cytoskeleton to the ECM, play a critical role in this bidirectional signaling across the plasma membrane and regulation of SMC phenotype by ECM components (Finney et al. 2017; Adiguzel et al. 2009).

Fibrillar collagen I, a major component of ECM in the medial layer, induces a contractile and quiescent phenotype in human SMCs grown in culture, whereas monomeric (non-fibrillar) collagen type I, present in atherosclerotic plaque intima, enhances SMC proliferation, a characteristic feature of synthetic phenotype (Ichii et al. 2001; Koohestani et al. 2013; Yeh et al. 2012). This phenotypic shift was accompanied by alteration of gene expression in cultured human SMCs induced by polymerized compared to monomeric collagens (Ichii et al. 2001). Fibrillar collagen type I has also been shown to inhibit PDGF-induced proliferation and migration of SMCs (Raines et al. 2000). Collagen type IV and laminin, components of the basement membrane that surrounds arterial SMCs in the subendothelial space, induce a differentiated contractile phenotype in vascular SMCs grown in culture and diminish the synthetic phenotype induced by PDGF (Thyberg and Hultgardh-Nilsson 1994). In the same manner, integrins $\alpha1\beta1$ and $\alpha7\beta1$, which bind to collagen IV and laminin, respectively, are highly expressed in quiescent contractile SMCs and serve to maintain the spindle morphology and contractile phenotype of SMCs (Finney et al. 2017). Fibronectin, a major component of provisional matrix in the intima, induces both contractile and synthetic phenotype in vascular SMCs depending on the nature of integrins expressed by the local SMCs (Finney et al. 2017). Altogether various combinations of integrins expressed by SMCs and a variety of ECM components result in a complex SMC-ECM interaction that affects both SMC and ECM properties.

Smooth muscle cells also interact with non-fibrillar PG components of the ECM. Bingley et al. found that HSPGs extracted from rabbit aortae inhibit phenotypic change of the cultured SMCs and maintain them in a quiescent state (Bingley et al. 1998). Interestingly, they found that when applied in a periadventitial gel following injury of rabbit carotid artery, HSPGs inhibit neointima formation (Bingley et al. 1998). Different subtypes of versican have been shown to alter SMC phenotype differently (Wight et al. 2014). Hyaluronan, present in both early and advanced lesions (Krolikoski et al. 2019), enhances proliferation and migration of SMCs (Evanko et al. 1999) and when overexpressed in SMCs of apoE-deficient mice accelerates the progression of atherosclerosis (Chai et al. 2005).

5 SMC, ECM, and Lipoprotein Interactions in Diffuse Intimal Thickening (DIT)

Diffuse intimal thickening (DIT) is a layer of thickened intima composed of SMCs, elastin, and PGs. DIT is initiated in utero and is present in all humans in atherosclerosis-prone arteries such as the coronary arteries and abdominal aorta by the age of 2 years (Nakashima et al. 2008). DIT represents a pre-atherosclerotic stage that provides the "soil" for the initial deposition and retention of lipoproteins and subsequent stages of atherosclerosis (Nakashima et al. 2008; Dubland and Francis 2016). Versican and biglycan are the most abundant proteoglycans in this DIT layer of atherosclerosis-prone arteries, while the thin intimal layer of atherosclerosis-resistant arteries, such as the internal thoracic artery, is enriched in decorin (Merrilees et al. 2001).

Using immunohistochemical techniques, Nakashima et al. showed that biglycan is localized in the deeper region of DIT in human coronary arteries (Nakashima et al. 2007). Lipoproteins that diffuse in from the plasma are trapped and deposited in the deep intima in the early stages of atherosclerosis due to a charge-charge interaction between this proteoglycan and apolipoprotein B of the lipoproteins. In an in vitro model, overexpression of biglycan in rat vascular SMCs increased lipoprotein binding to matrix formed by the cultured cells, while expression of a GAG-deficient mutated biglycan blocked this binding and accumulation (O'Brien et al. 2004). This observation and colocalization of biglycan with apoB- and apoE-containing lipoproteins in both early and advanced human (Nakashima et al. 2007; O'Brien et al. 2004) and murine lesions (Kunjathoor et al. 2002) indicate the presence of biglycan is crucial for the initial and ongoing deposition of lipids in the artery wall.

Unlike biglycan, immunohistochemical studies show versican is predominantly localized in the superficial part of the thickened intima of coronary arteries (Merrilees et al. 2001). Although in vitro studies have shown versican is capable of binding to LDL and has a larger number of binding sites for LDL compared to biglycan (Camejo et al. 1988), it has not been detected in lipoprotein-rich areas of atherosclerotic lesions nor colocalized with apoE or apoB epitopes in either human or mouse atherosclerotic lesions (Wight and Merrilees 2004; Kunjathoor et al. 2002).

Decorin, like biglycan, is distributed in the deep intima although at lower levels and colocalizes with lipids with less intensity compared to biglycan (Nakashima et al. 2007; Otsuka et al. 2015). In vitro studies have shown decorin links LDL with collagen type I (Pentikainen et al. 1997), and in vivo studies have demonstrated colocalization of decorin with collagens and apoB in atherosclerotic lesions (Nakashima et al. 2007; Riessen et al. 1994). Moreover, overexpression of decorin in rat SMCs after balloon injury of the carotid arteries resulted in compact collagen-rich lesions with reduced intimal thickness (Fischer et al. 2000). These findings suggest that decorin has a primary role in collagen organization in atherogenesis and a secondary role in lipid retention.

Perlecan is a heparan sulfate proteoglycan and the most abundant PG in the mouse artery wall, present in basement membranes in the intima and media (Nakashima et al. 2008). Human atherosclerotic lesions express only low amounts of perlecan (Tran et al. 2007). Like biglycan in humans, perlecan is involved in lipid retention in mouse atherosclerosis (Kunjathoor et al. 2002). Vikramadithyan et al. have shown that heterozygous deficiency of perlecan in chow-fed apoE-deficient mice results in more than 70% reduction in early-stage atherosclerosis lesion size. However, these authors did not find any difference in lesion size in advanced atherosclerosis (Vikramadithyan et al. 2004). Tran-Lundmark et al. also showed more than 50% reduction in lesion size in HS-deficient perlecan apoE$^{-/-}$ mice compared to control apoE$^{-/-}$ mice (Tran-Lundmark et al. 2008).

The expression of key artery wall ECM components and their roles including lipoprotein binding and fibrous cap formation are indicated in Fig. 2.

6   SMC-ECM Interaction in Lipid Retention

The ability of SMC-generated PGs in the human arterial intima to bind atherogenic apoB-containing lipoproteins mediates what is considered to be the critical and rate-limiting step in atherogenesis, from which subsequent steps of atheroma development ensue. This is the so-called "response-to-retention" hypothesis of atherosclerosis (Williams and Tabas 1995). The interaction between atherogenic lipoproteins and PGs involves an ionic or electrostatic interaction between positively charged amino acids of aopB on lipoproteins and negatively charged sulfate groups on the PGs generated by SMCs (Camejo et al. 1998; Boren et al. 1998). The role of deposition of lipoproteins in the intimal space and specific interactions of SMC-ECM molecules and apolipoproteins that mediate retention of lipoproteins are outlined below.

6.1   Deposition of Lipoproteins in the Artery Wall

Movement of lipoproteins from the plasma to the intimal space involves transport across the vascular endothelium via transcytosis, a process that is independent of LDL receptor function (Simionescu and Simionescu 1991). In contrast to

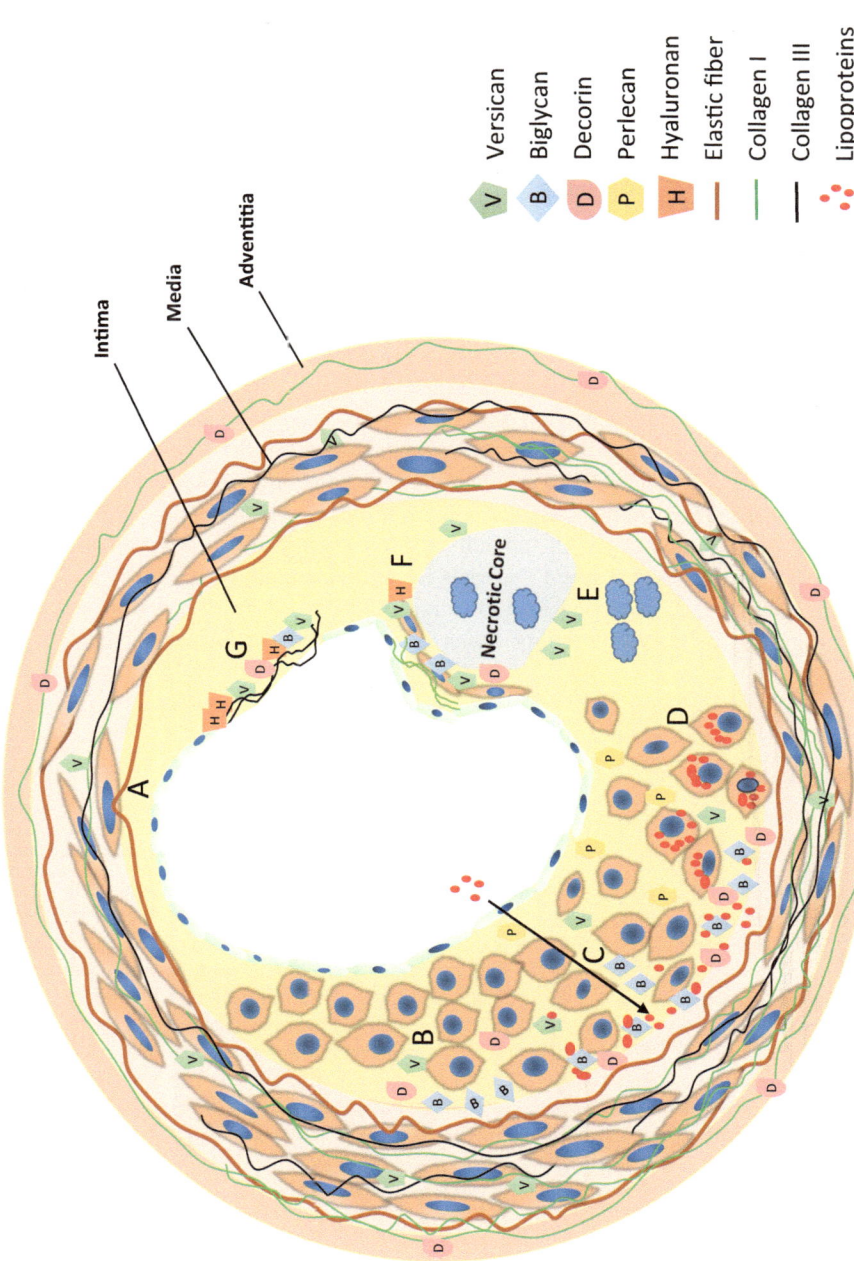

Fig. 2 Distribution of major ECM components in the normal artery wall and different stages of atherosclerosis. Composition of ECM varies in different layers of the artery wall and at different stages of atherosclerosis. (**a**) Collagen I and decorin in the adventitia, along with collagens I and III, elastic fibers, and versican

endocytosis and lysosomal degradation of lipoproteins mediated by the LDL receptor, endothelial transcytosis delivers lipoproteins including LDL and other apoB-
containing lipoproteins including very-low-density lipoproteins (VLDL), VLDL
remnants (intermediate-density lipoproteins), chylomicron remnants (Yang et al.
2018), and presumably lipoprotein (a) via endocytic uptake, intracellular transport,
and exocytosis into the ECM of the artery wall (Simionescu and Simionescu 1991;
Fung et al. 2018). Although transcytosis is the rate-limiting step in the movement of
LDL and other lipoproteins into the subendothelial layer, it does not equate to the
amount of LDL retained in the intimal space (Vasile et al. 1983). This was supported
by the in vivo observation that the rate of LDL entry into normal rabbit aorta
exceeded the rate of LDL accumulation (Carew et al. 1984). The retention of LDL
occurs more extensively in lesion-susceptible areas such as the aortic arch compared
with lesion-resistant arteries such as the descending thoracic aorta (Schwenke and
Carew 1988). The difference in LDL accumulation between atherosclerosis-
susceptible and atherosclerosis-resistant sites is also apparently independent of
LDL permeability, as an in vivo comparison of healthy and atherosclerosis-
susceptible arterial segments in rabbits showed they have similar LDL permeability
(Schwenke and Carew 1989). These findings indicate that retention of apoB-
containing lipoproteins, rather than the rate of transcytosis or endothelial permeability, is the rate-limiting factor in the amount of deposition of these lipoproteins in the
artery wall. These studies formed the basis for Williams and Tabas' "response-to-
retention" hypothesis, proposed in 1995, that highlighted the retention of apoB-
containing lipoproteins as the major driver of atherogenesis (Williams and Tabas
1995).

Fig. 2 (continued) in the medial layer make up the majority of ECM in normal arterial walls. (**b**)
Diffuse intimal thickening (DIT) is a thick layer of smooth muscle cells (SMCs) and proteoglycans
(PGs) present in atherosclerosis-prone arteries beginning from birth. Biglycan, decorin, and
versican secreted mainly by SMCs are the primary PGs in DIT, where biglycan and decorin are
located in the deep intima and versican mainly in the superficial intima. (**c**) ApoB-containing
lipoproteins that enter from the plasma via transcytosis through the endothelium are retained in
the deep intima in early atherosclerosis due to a charge-charge interaction between apoB and
glycosaminoglycan side chains of biglycan and decorin in the deep intima. (**d**) Trapped lipoproteins
are modified, aggregated, and taken up by surrounding SMCs and macrophages to make foam cells
(macrophages are omitted to emphasize the role of the ECM). Perlecan in mouse atheromas also
binds lipoproteins but does not participate in this retention in humans. (**e**) Apoptosis/necrosis of
foam cells leads to formation of a necrotic core in advanced atherosclerotic plaques, with versican
being prominent at the edge. (**f**) Stable plaques are defined by the presence of a thick fibrous cap
lying between the necrotic core and the luminal surface of the plaque. The fibrous caps consist of
more differentiated SMCs and are enriched in versican, biglycan, and collagen type I, with lesser
amounts of decorin and hyaluronan. (**g**) Unstable plaques with little or no fibrous cap show an
intense staining for hyaluronan, versican, and collagen type III at the site of erosion and weak
staining for biglycan and decorin

6.2   PG-Binding Sites in Lipoproteins

Lipoproteins delivered to the intima interact with the ECM via binding sites in their apolipoproteins (Usman et al. 2015). ApoB has been widely studied as the binding ligand of GAGs (Camejo et al. 1990; Srinivasan et al. 1988; Anber et al. 1997). Inhibition of the LDL-PG interaction by the presence of an anti-apoB antibody supports the observation that apoB is the binding site in lipoproteins (Sambandam et al. 1991). Modification of positively charged arginine and lysine residues in LDL abolished complex formation with CSPG, a GAG found in versican, biglycan, and decorin, indicating the importance of these amino acids in the apoB-PG interaction (Anber et al. 1997). The extent of apoB interaction with PGs is dependent on the degree of exposure of these positively charged residues in apoB (Camejo et al. 1990). The presence of hydropathic, hydroxyl-containing serine and threonine residues around positively charged lysine and arginine residues increases the hydrophilicity of these segments and enhances their ability to interact with PGs (Camejo et al. 1990). In addition, the hydrolysis of surface phospholipids on LDL by secretory phospholipase A2 results in smaller and denser LDL particles that have greater exposure of PG-binding apoB segments, accounting for the increased affinity of small dense LDL for biglycan and decorin when compared to native LDL (Sartipy et al. 1999).

Site B of apoB100, residues 3,359–3,369, has been proposed to be the principal site of binding with PGs (Boren et al. 1998). A single-point mutation in this region of apoB100 severely affects proteoglycan interactions, without affecting LDL receptor binding (Boren et al. 1998). Furthermore, Cardin and Weintraub identified the GAG-binding sequence of apoB100 to be either –X-B-B-X-B-X or –X-B-B-X-X-B-X where X is a hydropathic amino acid and B is either lysine or arginine (Cardin and Weintraub 1989). Chylomicron remnants, which are also atherogenic and deposit in the artery wall, contain the N-terminal 48% of apoB100 (apoB48) and therefore lack the GAG-binding Site B. GAG binding of apoB48 has been shown to be mediated by a lysine-rich cluster of amino acids in N-terminal residues 84–94, termed Site B-1b, exposed in this carboxyl-truncated form of apoB.

In addition to apoB, apoE and apoAI also colocalize with biglycan in human atherosclerotic plaques (O'Brien et al. 1998), but only apoE was found to have proteoglycan-binding domains (O'Brien et al. 1998; Olin et al. 2001). High-density lipoproteins (HDL) binding to GAGs appear to be limited to apoE-containing but not apoE-free HDL (Olin et al. 2001).

6.3   The Variability of Interactions Between Lipoproteins and Proteoglycans

Iverius initially demonstrated the interaction between GAGs and human plasma lipoproteins by equilibrating lipoproteins with a GAG-linked agarose gel, resulting in the interaction of LDL and VLDL, but not HDL, acetylated VLDL, or acetylated LDL, with heparin, DS, HS, and chondroitin-4-sulfate (Iverius 1972). Heparin and

CSPGs have the same binding site in apoB (Sambandam et al. 1991). The position of sulfation of GAGs was not found to be important; however increased sulfation, which confers higher negative charge, correlates with increased lipoprotein binding (Sambandam et al. 1991), confirming the electrostatic nature of the interaction between negatively charged GAGs and positively charged apoB-binding sites. The strength of the interaction between VLDL and LDL with different GAGs was heparin > DS > HS ~ C4-S (Iverius 1972). Contrary to this observation, Vijayagopal et al. observed greater affinity between LDL and CS than HSPG (Vijayagopal et al. 1983). This was supported by another publication that found CS/DSPG from bovine aorta was more potent than HS-PG in inducing complex formation with LDL and that the strongest complex formed is between LDL and CS/DSPG (Radhakrishnamurthy et al. 1990). Parallel with Iverius' observation, DSPG was determined to be more efficient in binding LDL than CSPG (Sambandam et al. 1991). The localization of lipoproteins in atherogenic plaques with biglycan and decorin (which may have DS side chains) as opposed to versican (a CSPG) aligns with this observation.

6.4 Effects of Binding and Retention of Lipoproteins

The retention of lipoproteins in the intima and their subsequent modification including oxidation and aggregation initiates a vicious cycle of further SMC proliferation and synthesis of elongated and more lipoprotein-attracting PGs that increase lipoprotein entrapment (Camejo et al. 1993; Chang et al. 2000). Macrophages infiltrating into the developing plaque secrete lipoprotein lipase, which can also act as a bridge between lipoproteins and PGs and thereby enhance lipoprotein retention. Macrophages also secrete inflammatory mediators that lead to further cell recruitment and plaque development (reviewed in Usman et al. 2015). The trapping of lipoproteins through interactions with PGs in the intima makes them a substrate for modifications including oxidation and aggregation. This converts the lipoproteins into ligands for scavenger receptors on macrophages and SMCs, leading to foam cell formation in both these cell types (Allahverdian et al. 2014; Wang et al. 2019). In this way, consistent with the response-to-retention theory of atherogenesis, SMC-dependent PG synthesis is the critical driver of subsequent stages of atherosclerotic lesion development.

7   Role of ECM Proteoglycans in Early Stages of Atherosclerosis Development in Animal Models

A key question, raised by the apparent pivotal importance of SMCs in producing the lipoprotein-binding PGs that drive lipoprotein retention and atherogenesis in humans, is how important this is in mice, the primary models used to study the determinants of atherosclerosis in man. Although small animals do not develop a pre-atherosclerotic SMC DIT layer like humans (Nakashima et al. 2008), several studies provide evidence that the initial binding of apoB-containing lipoproteins to subendothelial PGs in the artery wall is also a key step in atherogenesis in animal models of atherosclerosis. Perlecan and biglycan, but not versican, a major PG detected in human plaques, appear early in developing lesions in apoE$^{-/-}$ and LDLR$^{-/-}$ mice underneath the endothelium and in the absence of intimal thickening (Kunjathoor et al. 2002). The presence of these PGs around areas of extracellular lipid deposition suggests that they also contribute to lipoprotein retention in murine models of atherosclerosis. This supports the theory of PG-dependent lipoprotein retention, although these PGs are likely secreted by endothelial cells or activated macrophages rather than SMCs in the first stage of mouse atherosclerosis (Kinsella et al. 1997; Nugent et al. 2000; Chang et al. 2012). In intermediate and advanced lesions, PGs and lipoproteins are localized in SMC-rich areas of the mouse intima (Kunjathoor et al. 2002). In another study, Thompson et al. found that overexpression of biglycan by SMCs in LDLR$^{-/-}$ mice increases lipid retention and atherosclerosis development (Thompson et al. 2014). Moreover, apoE$^{-/-}$ mice heterozygous for deletion of perlecan have less atherosclerotic lesion area at early stages compared to apoE$^{-/-}$ mice with no deletion. This might be attributed partly to decreased lipoprotein retention in the perlecan$^{+/-}$ mice (Vikramadithyan et al. 2004). In another study, Skalen et al. used transgenic mice expressing recombinant LDL with proteoglycan binding site-defective apoB and showed those mice develop significantly less atherosclerosis compared to mice expressing wild-type control LDL (Skalen et al. 2002). These studies demonstrate a key role for PGs for initial subendothelial lipid retention at early stages of mouse atherosclerosis and a likely role for SMC-derived PGs in later stages of murine models of this disease.

8 The Role of the ECM-SMC Interaction in Plaque Stability and Rupture

Stable plaque is defined by the presence of a thick fibrous cap lying between the necrotic core and luminal surface of the plaque. It consists of SMCs embedded in a collagen-proteoglycan matrix with varying degrees of macrophage and lymphocyte infiltration and has a critical role in maintaining integrity of the plaque. Unstable plaques are prone to erosion and rupture that leads to platelet adhesion and luminal thrombus formation, the most common cause of acute coronary syndromes and sudden cardiac death (Allahverdian et al. 2018). Plaque rupture involves breakage of a large lipid/necrotic core with large luminal thrombus, thin fibrous cap, and a dense infiltration of inflammatory cells (Kolodgie et al. 2004).

Extracellular matrix components of atherosclerotic lesions have a key role in maintaining stability of plaques and accumulate in topographically distinct patterns in different plaque types. Kolodgie et al. found that the fibrous caps of stable lesions show increased amounts of versican, biglycan, and collagen type I staining and significantly less decorin and hyaluronan (Kolodgie et al. 2002). With SMCs being the main producer of collagen and PGs in the fibrous matrix (Pietila and Nikkari 1983), it is not surprising that the number of SMCs in fibrous caps is directly correlated with plaque stability (Allahverdian et al. 2018). One study found collagen VIII deficiency in apoE$^{-/-}$ mice resulted in thinning of the fibrous cap, which suggests that this collagen plays an important role in protecting the plaque from rupture (Lopes et al. 2013).

Eroded plaques show an intense staining for hyaluronan, versican, and collagen type III at the plaque/thrombus interface and weak staining for biglycan and decorin. Cell surface receptor for hyaluronan, CD44, has been shown to be expressed by a subset of SMCs at the plaque/thrombus interface in erosions (Kolodgie et al. 2002) and mediates adhesion of platelets to hyaluronan (Day 1999). Exposure of versican-hyaluronan to flowing blood at the de-endothelialized surface of the eroded plaque promotes platelet attachment and may play an important role in the development of thrombosis via a CD44-dependent mechanism (Koshiishi et al. 1994).

Fibrous caps owe their strength and resistance to rupture to their collagen fiber content and therefore the content and synthetic capacity of collagen-producing SMCs (Doran et al. 2008; Libby 2008). Thinned fibrous cap areas contain very few SMCs with little to absent staining for PGs or hyaluronan and scattered strands of collagen type I (Kolodgie et al. 2002). Factors that alter the abundance or function of SMCs thereby alter ECM production by SMCs and plaque stability.

8.1 Factors Involved in Plaque Instability

Pro-inflammatory cytokines have been shown to reduce the number of intimal SMCs, thereby compromising ECM production (Geng et al. 1997; Kockx and Knaapen 2000). Various cytokines and growth factors, normally present in athero-sclerotic plaques, also either stimulate or suppress collagen synthesis by vascular SMCs (Amento et al. 1991). Moreover, reduction of SMC density in plaque and the fibrous cap as a result of apoptosis results in diminished ECM production and may lead to plaque instability. von der Thusen et al. found that induction of vascular SMC apoptosis by overexpression of p53 in the fibrous cap of carotid plaques of apoE$^{-/-}$ mice results in reduction of cell density, cap thinning, and plaque destabilization (von der Thusen et al. 2002). Low endothelial shear stress (ESS) has been shown to induce SMC apoptosis (Qi et al. 2008) and therefore indirectly affect collagen content of atherosclerotic plaques. Frontini et al. found that lipid loading of human vascular SMCs impairs their ability to assemble fibrillar collagen and fibronectin (Frontini et al. 2009), which may contribute to reducing plaque stability. Others found that enhancement of cholesterol efflux preserves the assembly of fibrillar collagen and fibronectin by SMCs (Beyea et al. 2012).

An imbalance between synthesis and degradation of ECM leads to thinning of the fibrous cap and plaque rupture. Members of the matrix metalloproteinases (MMP) and tissue inhibitor of metalloproteinase (TIMP) families can alter the quantity and composition of ECM and affect plaque stability (Newby et al. 2009). Although macrophages are the main source of MMPs in atherosclerosis (Shah et al. 1995), secretion of different MMPs by SMCs also plays an important role in cap thinning and plaque destabilization. Members of the MMP family with collagenase activity, including MMP-1, MMP-8, MMP-13, and the activator of MMP collagenases, MMP-14, weaken the plaque by degrading collagen fibers (Libby 2008; Deguchi et al. 2005). The concentration, production, and expression of MMP-9 (Loftus et al. 2000), MMP-1, and MMP-13 (Sukhova et al. 1999) are significantly higher in unstable compare to stable carotid plaques.

Low endothelial shear stress (ESS) has also been shown to play an important role in plaque instability. In an ex vivo model of porcine carotid atherosclerosis, low ESS resulted in an increase in MMP expression (Gambillara et al. 2005). Low ESS is also associated with a diminished SMC and collagen content, a high MMP expression and activity, and a marked thinning of the fibrous cap in mouse carotid and porcine coronary plaques (Cheng et al. 2006; Koskinas et al. 2013).

9   Therapeutic Targets and Interventions

The critical role of SMC-dependent PG synthesis and lipoprotein retention in subsequent atherosclerosis development makes the PG-lipoprotein interaction a potentially profound and novel point of therapeutic intervention to prevent ischemic vascular disease. Vazquez and colleagues introduced the chP3R99 monoclonal antibody (mAb) against ECM GAGs as a potential therapeutic for atherosclerosis in 2012 (Soto et al. 2012). The mAb binds to sulfated GAGs such as heparin, HS, and DS and had the strongest affinity for CS in aorta (Soto et al. 2012). It prevented 70% of LDL-CS complex formation and abolished 80% of LDL oxidation in vitro (Soto et al. 2012). The mAb also demonstrated the capacity to (1) prevent foam cell formation by the inhibition of LDL retention and oxidation in the arteries of rats; (2) decrease the intima-media ratio, a measure of DIT formation; and (3) decrease macrophage infiltration in the aorta of New Zealand white rabbits (Soto et al. 2012). Thereafter, they delivered the mAb chP3R99 via subcutaneous injections to apoE$^{-/-}$ mice fed a high-fat and high-cholesterol diet and determined that the vaccination stimulated an immune response against various sulfated GAGs via the induction of a secondary anti-idiotype response (Ab2) that mirrors GAG antigenic determinants (Brito et al. 2012). The Ab2 gave rise to synthesis of anti-idiotype antibodies (Ab3) that have a specificity homologous to that of Ab1 (Brito et al. 2012). Further research using chP3R99 in the same mouse model established the chP3R99-LALA variant restricted the progression of atherosclerosis in apoE$^{-/-}$ mice by preventing initial CS-LDL complex formation (Delgado-Roche et al. 2015). Both the efficiency of the chP3R99-LALA mAb in initiating the anti-idiotype cascade and anti-atherogenic benefits were dose-dependent in apoE$^{-/-}$ mice but were independent of the sex and age of the mice (Sarduy et al. 2017). The mAb was also shown to decrease inflammation and halt lesion development of advanced stages of atherosclerosis in male apoE$^{-/-}$ mice (Brito et al. 2017). These findings strongly confirm the relevance of the "response-to-retention" hypothesis of atherogenesis and provide the exciting possibility of developing an immunization that could block the PG-lipoprotein interaction lifelong as a novel means of preventing atherosclerosis.

10   Conclusion

Smooth muscle cells (SMCs) are the most abundant cell type in the healthy human artery wall as well as the pre-atherosclerotic and atherosclerotic intimal layer. The ECM components secreted by SMCs are critical factors in maintaining normal arterial architecture and stability but also in predicting propensity to atherosclerosis. In particular, the secretion of PGs by intimal SMCs promotes the initial and ongoing binding and retention of atherogenic lipoproteins in the artery wall. This retention of lipoproteins is necessary for further development of atherosclerosis, apparently in mice as well as in humans, making the proteoglycan-lipoprotein interaction a novel and exciting potential point of intervention for the future treatment and prevention of atherosclerosis.

Acknowledgments   This work is supported by a Heart and Stroke Foundation Grant-In-Aid to GAF.

References

Adiguzel E, Ahmad PJ, Franco C, Bendeck MP (2009) Collagens in the progression and complications of atherosclerosis. Vasc Med 14(1):73–89

Albarran-Juarez J, Kaur H, Grimm M, Offermanns S, Wettschureck N (2016) Lineage tracing of cells involved in atherosclerosis. Atherosclerosis 251:445–453

Allahverdian S, Chehroudi AC, McManus BM, Abraham T, Francis GA (2014) Contribution of intimal smooth muscle cells to cholesterol accumulation and macrophage-like cells in human atherosclerosis. Circulation 129(15):1551–1559

Allahverdian S, Chaabane C, Boukais K, Francis GA, Bochaton-Piallat ML (2018) Smooth muscle cell fate and plasticity in atherosclerosis. Cardiovasc Res 114(4):540–550

Amento EP, Ehsani N, Palmer H, Libby P (1991) Cytokines and growth factors positively and negatively regulate interstitial collagen gene expression in human vascular smooth muscle cells. Arterioscler Thromb 11(5):1223–1230

Anber V, Millar JS, McConnell M, Shepherd J, Packard CJ (1997) Interaction of very-low-density, intermediate-density, and low-density lipoproteins with human arterial wall proteoglycans. Arterioscler Thromb Vasc Biol 17(11):2507–2514

Beyea MM, Reaume S, Sawyez CG, Edwards JY, O'Neil C, Hegele RA et al (2012) The oxysterol 24(s),25-epoxycholesterol attenuates human smooth muscle-derived foam cell formation via reduced low-density lipoprotein uptake and enhanced cholesterol efflux. J Am Heart Assoc 1(3): e000810

Bingley JA, Hayward IP, Campbell JH, Campbell GR (1998) Arterial heparan sulfate proteoglycans inhibit vascular smooth muscle cell proliferation and phenotype change in vitro and neointimal formation in vivo. J Vasc Surg 28(2):308–318

Boren J, Olin K, Lee I, Chait A, Wight TN, Innerarity TL (1998) Identification of the principal proteoglycan-binding site in LDL. A single-point mutation in apo-B100 severely affects proteoglycan interaction without affecting LDL receptor binding. J Clin Invest 101 (12):2658–2664

Brito V, Mellal K, Portelance SG, Perez A, Soto Y (2012) deBlois D, et al. induction of anti-anti-idiotype antibodies against sulfated glycosaminoglycans reduces atherosclerosis in apolipoprotein E-deficient mice. Arterioscler Thromb Vasc Biol 32(12):2847–2854

Brito V, Mellal K, Zoccal KF, Soto Y, Menard L, Sarduy R et al (2017) Atheroregressive potential of the treatment with a chimeric monoclonal antibody against sulfated glycosaminoglycans on pre-existing lesions in apolipoprotein E-deficient mice. Front Pharmacol 8:782

Camejo G, Olofsson SO, Lopez F, Carlsson P, Bondjers G (1988) Identification of Apo B-100 segments mediating the interaction of low density lipoproteins with arterial proteoglycans. Arteriosclerosis 8(4):368–377

Camejo G, Rosengren B, Olson U, Lopez F, Olofson SO, Westerlund C et al (1990) Molecular basis of the association of arterial proteoglycans with low density lipoproteins: its effect on the structure of the lipoprotein particle. Eur Heart J 11(Suppl E):164–173

Camejo G, Fager G, Rosengren B, Hurt-Camejo E, Bondjers G (1993) Binding of low density lipoproteins by proteoglycans synthesized by proliferating and quiescent human arterial smooth muscle cells. J Biol Chem 268(19):14131–14137

Camejo G, Hurt-Camejo E, Wiklund O, Bondjers G (1998) Association of apo B lipoproteins with arterial proteoglycans: pathological significance and molecular basis. Atherosclerosis 139 (2):205–222

Cardin AD, Weintraub HJ (1989) Molecular modeling of protein-glycosaminoglycan interactions. Arteriosclerosis 9(1):21–32

Carew TE, Pittman RC, Marchand ER, Steinberg D (1984) Measurement in vivo of irreversible degradation of low density lipoprotein in the rabbit aorta. Predominance of intimal degradation. Arteriosclerosis 4(3):214–224

Chai S, Chai Q, Danielsen CC, Hjorth P, Nyengaard JR, Ledet T et al (2005) Overexpression of hyaluronan in the tunica media promotes the development of atherosclerosis. Circ Res 96 (5):583–591

Chang MY, Potter-Perigo S, Tsoi C, Chait A, Wight TN (2000) Oxidized low density lipoproteins regulate synthesis of monkey aortic smooth muscle cell proteoglycans that have enhanced native low density lipoprotein binding properties. J Biol Chem 275(7):4766–4773

Chang MY, Chan CK, Braun KR, Green PS, O'Brien KD, Chait A et al (2012) Monocyte-to-macrophage differentiation: synthesis and secretion of a complex extracellular matrix. J Biol Chem 287(17):14122–14135

Chappell J, Harman JL, Narasimhan VM, Yu H, Foote K, Simons BD et al (2016) Extensive proliferation of a subset of differentiated, yet plastic, medial vascular smooth muscle cells contributes to neointimal formation in mouse injury and atherosclerosis models. Circ Res 119 (12):1313–1323

Cheng C, Tempel D, van Haperen R, van der Baan A, Grosveld F, Daemen MJ et al (2006) Atherosclerotic lesion size and vulnerability are determined by patterns of fluid shear stress. Circulation 113(23):2744–2753

Day AJ (1999) The structure and regulation of hyaluronan-binding proteins. Biochem Soc Trans 27 (2):115–121

Deguchi JO, Aikawa E, Libby P, Vachon JR, Inada M, Krane SM et al (2005) Matrix metalloproteinase-13/collagenase-3 deletion promotes collagen accumulation and organization in mouse atherosclerotic plaques. Circulation 112(17):2708–2715

Delgado-Roche L, Brito V, Acosta E, Perez A, Fernandez JR, Hernandez-Matos Y et al (2015) Arresting progressive atherosclerosis by immunization with an anti-glycosaminoglycan monoclonal antibody in apolipoprotein E-deficient mice. Free Radic Biol Med 89:557–566

Doran AC, Meller N, McNamara CA (2008) Role of smooth muscle cells in the initiation and early progression of atherosclerosis. Arterioscler Thromb Vasc Biol 28(5):812–819

Dubland JA, Francis GA (2016) So much cholesterol: the unrecognized importance of smooth muscle cells in atherosclerotic foam cell formation. Curr Opin Lipidol 27(2):155–161

Evanko SP, Angello JC, Wight TN (1999) Formation of hyaluronan- and versican-rich pericellular matrix is required for proliferation and migration of vascular smooth muscle cells. Arterioscler Thromb Vasc Biol 19(4):1004–1013

Feil S, Fehrenbacher B, Lukowski R, Essmann F, Schulze-Osthoff K, Schaller M et al (2014) Transdifferentiation of vascular smooth muscle cells to macrophage-like cells during atherogenesis. Circ Res 115(7):662–667

Finney AC, Stokes KY, Pattillo CB, Orr AW (2017) Integrin signaling in atherosclerosis. Cell Mol Life Sci 74(12):2263–2282

Fischer JW, Kinsella MG, Clowes MM, Lara S, Clowes AW, Wight TN (2000) Local expression of bovine decorin by cell-mediated gene transfer reduces neointimal formation after balloon injury in rats. Circ Res 86(6):676–683

Frantz C, Stewart KM, Weaver VM (2010) The extracellular matrix at a glance. J Cell Sci 123 (Pt 24):4195–4200

Frontini MJ, O'Neil C, Sawyez C, Chan BM, Huff MW, Pickering JG (2009) Lipid incorporation inhibits Src-dependent assembly of fibronectin and type I collagen by vascular smooth muscle cells. Circ Res 104(7):832–841

Fung KYY, Fairn GD, Lee WL (2018) Transcellular vesicular transport in epithelial and endothelial cells: challenges and opportunities. Traffic 19(1):5–18

Gambillara V, Montorzi G, Haziza-Pigeon C, Stergiopulos N, Silacci P (2005) Arterial wall response to ex vivo exposure to oscillatory shear stress. J Vasc Res 42(6):535–544

Geng YJ, Henderson LE, Levesque EB, Muszynski M, Libby P (1997) Fas is expressed in human atherosclerotic intima and promotes apoptosis of cytokine-primed human vascular smooth muscle cells. Arterioscler Thromb Vasc Biol 17(10):2200–2208

Gutierrez P, O'Brien KD, Ferguson M, Nikkari ST, Alpers CE, Wight TN (1997) Differences in the distribution of versican, decorin, and biglycan in atherosclerotic human coronary arteries. Cardiovasc Pathol 6(5):271–278

Ichii T, Koyama H, Tanaka S, Kim S, Shioi A, Okuno Y et al (2001) Fibrillar collagen specifically regulates human vascular smooth muscle cell genes involved in cellular responses and the pericellular matrix environment. Circ Res 88(5):460–467

Iozzo RV (1999) The biology of the small leucine-rich proteoglycans. Functional network of interactive proteins. J Biol Chem 274(27):18843–18846

Iverius PH (1972) The interaction between human plasma lipoproteins and connective tissue glycosaminoglycans. J Biol Chem 247(8):2607–2613

Kinsella MG, Tsoi CK, Jarvelainen HT, Wight TN (1997) Selective expression and processing of biglycan during migration of bovine aortic endothelial cells. The role of endogenous basic fibroblast growth factor. J Biol Chem 272(1):318–325

Kockx MM, Knaapen MW (2000) The role of apoptosis in vascular disease. J Pathol 190 (3):267–280

Kolodgie FD, Burke AP, Farb A, Weber DK, Kutys R, Wight TN et al (2002) Differential accumulation of proteoglycans and hyaluronan in culprit lesions: insights into plaque erosion. Arterioscler Thromb Vasc Biol 22(10):1642–1648

Kolodgie FD, Burke AP, Wight TN, Virmani R (2004) The accumulation of specific types of proteoglycans in eroded plaques: a role in coronary thrombosis in the absence of rupture. Curr Opin Lipidol 15(5):575–582

Koohestani F, Braundmeier AG, Mahdian A, Seo J, Bi J, Nowak RA (2013) Extracellular matrix collagen alters cell proliferation and cell cycle progression of human uterine leiomyoma smooth muscle cells. PLoS One 8(9):e75844

Koshiishi I, Shizari M, Underhill CB (1994) CD44 can mediate the adhesion of platelets to hyaluronan. Blood 84(2):390–396

Koskinas KC, Sukhova GK, Baker AB, Papafaklis MI, Chatzizisis YS, Coskun AU et al (2013) Thin-capped atheromata with reduced collagen content in pigs develop in coronary arterial regions exposed to persistently low endothelial shear stress. Arterioscler Thromb Vasc Biol 33 (7):1494–1504

Krolikoski M, Monslow J, Pure E et al (2019) Matrix Biol 78-79:201–218

Kunjathoor VV, Chiu DS O'Brien KD, LeBoeuf RC (2002) Accumulation of biglycan and perlecan, but not versican, in lesions of murine models of atherosclerosis. Arterioscler Thromb Vasc Biol 22(3):462–468

Libby P (2008) The molecular mechanisms of the thrombotic complications of atherosclerosis. J Intern Med 263(5):517–527

Little PJ, Tannock L, Olin KL, Chait A, Wight TN (2002) Proteoglycans synthesized by arterial smooth muscle cells in the presence of transforming growth factor-beta1 exhibit increased binding to LDLs. Arterioscler Thromb Vasc Biol 22(1):55–60

Little PJ, Osman N, O'Brien KD (2008) Hyperelongated biglycan: the surreptitious initiator of atherosclerosis. Curr Opin Lipidol 19(5):448–454

Loftus IM, Naylor AR, Goodall S, Crowther M, Jones L, Bell PR et al (2000) Increased matrix metalloproteinase-9 activity in unstable carotid plaques. A potential role in acute plaque disruption. Stroke 31(1):40–47

Lopes J, Adiguzel E, Gu S, Liu SL, Hou G, Heximer S et al (2013) Type VIII collagen mediates vessel wall remodeling after arterial injury and fibrous cap formation in atherosclerosis. Am J Pathol 182(6):2241–2253

Merrilees MJ, Beaumont B, Scott LJ (2001) Comparison of deposits of versican, biglycan and decorin in saphenous vein and internal thoracic, radial and coronary arteries: correlation to patency. Coron Artery Dis 12(1):7–16

Nakashima Y, Fujii H, Sumiyoshi S, Wight TN, Sueishi K (2007) Early human atherosclerosis: accumulation of lipid and proteoglycans in intimal thickenings followed by macrophage infiltration. Arterioscler Thromb Vasc Biol 27(5):1159–1165

Nakashima Y, Wight TN, Sueishi K (2008) Early atherosclerosis in humans: role of diffuse intimal thickening and extracellular matrix proteoglycans. Cardiovasc Res 79(1):14–23

Newby AC, George SJ, Ismail Y, Johnson JL, Sala-Newby GB, Thomas AC (2009) Vulnerable atherosclerotic plaque metalloproteinases and foam cell phenotypes. Thromb Haemost 101 (6):1006–1011

Nugent MA, Nugent HM, Iozzo RV, Sanchack K, Edelman ER (2000) Perlecan is required to inhibit thrombosis after deep vascular injury and contributes to endothelial cell-mediated inhibition of intimal hyperplasia. Proc Natl Acad Sci U S A 97(12):6722–6727

O'Brien KD, Olin KL, Alpers CE, Chiu W, Ferguson M, Hudkins K et al (1998) Comparison of apolipoprotein and proteoglycan deposits in human coronary atherosclerotic plaques: colocalization of biglycan with apolipoproteins. Circulation 98(6):519–527

O'Brien KD, Lewis K, Fischer JW, Johnson P, Hwang JY, Knopp EA et al (2004) Smooth muscle cell biglycan overexpression results in increased lipoprotein retention on extracellular matrix: implications for the retention of lipoproteins in atherosclerosis. Atherosclerosis 177(1):29–35

Olin KL, Potter-Perigo S, Barrett PH, Wight TN, Chait A (2001) Biglycan, a vascular proteoglycan, binds differently to HDL2 and HDL3: role of apoE. Arterioscler Thromb Vasc Biol 21 (1):129–135

Otsuka F, Kramer MC, Woudstra P, Yahagi K, Ladich E, Finn AV et al (2015) Natural progression of atherosclerosis from pathologic intimal thickening to late fibroatheroma in human coronary arteries: a pathology study. Atherosclerosis 241(2):772–782

Owens GK, Kumar MS, Wamhoff BR (2004) Molecular regulation of vascular smooth muscle cell differentiation in development and disease. Physiol Rev 84(3):767–801

Pentikainen MO, Oorni K, Lassila R, Kovanen PT (1997) The proteoglycan decorin links low density lipoproteins with collagen type I. J Biol Chem 272(12):7633–7638

Perisic Matic L, Rykaczewska U, Razuvaev A, Sabater-Lleal M, Lengquist M, Miller CL et al (2016) Phenotypic modulation of smooth muscle cells in atherosclerosis is associated with downregulation of LMOD1, SYNPO2, PDLIM7, PLN, and SYNM. Arterioscler Thromb Vasc Biol 36(9):1947–1961

Phinikaridou A, Lacerda S, Lavin B, Andia ME, Smith A, Saha P et al (2018) Tropoelastin: a novel marker for plaque progression and instability. Circ Cardiovasc Imaging 11(8):e007303

Pietila K, Nikkari T (1983) Role of the arterial smooth muscle cell in the pathogenesis of atherosclerosis. Med Biol 61(1):31–44

Qi YX, Qu MJ, Long DK, Liu B, Yao QP, Chien S et al (2008) Rho-GDP dissociation inhibitor alpha downregulated by low shear stress promotes vascular smooth muscle cell migration and apoptosis: a proteomic analysis. Cardiovasc Res 80(1):114–122

Radhakrishnamurthy B, Srinivasan SR, Vijayagopal P, Berenson GS (1990) Arterial wall proteoglycans--biological properties related to pathogenesis of atherosclerosis. Eur Heart J 11 (Suppl E):148–157

Raines EW, Koyama H, Carragher NO (2000) The extracellular matrix dynamically regulates smooth muscle cell responsiveness to PDGF. Ann N Y Acad Sci 902:39–51; discussion-2

Rekhter MD (1999) Collagen synthesis in atherosclerosis: too much and not enough. Cardiovasc Res 41(2):376–384

Riessen R, Isner JM, Blessing E, Loushin C, Nikol S, Wight TN (1994) Regional differences in the distribution of the proteoglycans biglycan and decorin in the extracellular matrix of atherosclerotic and restenotic human coronary arteries. Am J Pathol 144(5):962–974

Rohwedder I, Montanez E, Beckmann K, Bengtsson E, Duner P, Nilsson J et al (2012) Plasma fibronectin deficiency impedes atherosclerosis progression and fibrous cap formation. EMBO Mol Med 4(7):564–576

Sambandam T, Baker JR, Christner JE, Ekborg SL (1991) Specificity of the low density lipoprotein-glycosaminoglycan interaction. Arterioscler Thromb 11(3):561–568

Sarduy R, Brito V, Castillo A, Soto Y, Grinan T, Marleau S et al (2017) Dose-dependent induction of an idiotypic cascade by anti-glycosaminoglycan monoclonal antibody in apoE(−/−) mice: association with atheroprotection. Front Immunol 8:232

Sartipy P, Camejo G, Svensson L, Hurt-Camejo E (1999) Phospholipase A(2) modification of low density lipoproteins forms small high density particles with increased affinity for proteoglycans and glycosaminoglycans. J Biol Chem 274(36):25913–25920

Schonherr E, Jarvelainen HT, Sandell LJ, Wight TN (1991) Effects of platelet-derived growth factor and transforming growth factor-beta 1 on the synthesis of a large versican-like chondroitin sulfate proteoglycan by arterial smooth muscle cells. J Biol Chem 266(26):17640–17647

Schonherr E, Jarvelainen HT, Kinsella MG, Sandell LJ, Wight TN (1993) Platelet-derived growth factor and transforming growth factor-beta 1 differentially affect the synthesis of biglycan and decorin by monkey arterial smooth muscle cells. Arterioscler Thromb 13(7):1026–1036

Schwenke DC, Carew TE (1988) Quantification in vivo of increased LDL content and rate of LDL degradation in normal rabbit aorta occurring at sites susceptible to early atherosclerotic lesions. Circ Res 62(4):699–710

Schwenke DC, Carew TE (1989) Initiation of atherosclerotic lesions in cholesterol-fed rabbits. II. Selective retention of LDL vs. selective increases in LDL permeability in susceptible sites of arteries. Arteriosclerosis 9(6):908–918

Shah PK, Falk E, Badimon JJ, Fernandez-Ortiz A, Mailhac A, Villareal-Levy G et al (1995) Human monocyte-derived macrophages induce collagen breakdown in fibrous caps of atherosclerotic plaques. Potential role of matrix-degrading metalloproteinases and implications for plaque rupture. Circulation 92(6):1565–1569

Shankman LS, Gomez D, Cherepanova OA, Salmon M, Alencar GF, Haskins RM et al (2015) KLF4-dependent phenotypic modulation of smooth muscle cells has a key role in atherosclerotic plaque pathogenesis. Nat Med 21(6):628–637

Shekhonin BV, Domogatsky SP, Muzykantov VR, Idelson GL, Rukosuev VS (1985) Distribution of type I, III, IV and V collagen in normal and atherosclerotic human arterial wall: immunomorphological characteristics. Coll Relat Res 5(4):355–368

Simionescu N, Simionescu M (1991) Cellular interactions of lipoproteins with the vascular endothelium: endocytosis and transcytosis. Target Diagn Ther 5:45–95

Skalen K, Gustafsson M, Rydberg EK, Hulten LM, Wiklund O, Innerarity TL et al (2002) Subendothelial retention of atherogenic lipoproteins in early atherosclerosis. Nature 417 (6890):750–754

Soto Y, Acosta E, Delgado L, Perez A, Falcon V, Becquer MA et al (2012) Antiatherosclerotic effect of an antibody that binds to extracellular matrix glycosaminoglycans. Arterioscler Thromb Vasc Biol 32(3):595–604

Srinivasan SR, Vijayagopal P, Eberle K, Dalferes ER Jr, Radhakrishnamurthy B, Berenson GS (1988) Low density lipoprotein binding affinity of arterial wall isomeric chondroitin sulfate proteoglycans. Atherosclerosis 72(1):1–9

Sukhova GK, Schonbeck U, Rabkin E, Schoen FJ, Poole AR, Billinghurst RC et al (1999) Evidence for increased collagenolysis by interstitial collagenases-1 and -3 in vulnerable human atheromatous plaques. Circulation 99(19):2503–2509

Theocharis AD, Skandalis SS, Gialeli C, Karamanos NK (2016) Extracellular matrix structure. Adv Drug Deliv Rev 97:4–27

Theocharis AD, Manou D, Karamanos NK (2019) The extracellular matrix as a multitasking player in disease. FEBS J 286(15):2830–2869

Thompson JC, Tang T, Wilson PG, Yoder MH, Tannock LR (2014) Increased atherosclerosis in mice with increased vascular biglycan content. Atherosclerosis 235(1):71–75

Thyberg J, Hultgardh-Nilsson A (1994) Fibronectin and the basement membrane components laminin and collagen type IV influence the phenotypic properties of subcultured rat aortic smooth muscle cells differently. Cell Tissue Res 276(2):263–271

Tran PK, Agardh HE, Tran-Lundmark K, Ekstrand J, Roy J, Henderson B et al (2007) Reduced perlecan expression and accumulation in human carotid atherosclerotic lesions. Atherosclerosis 190(2):264–270

Tran-Lundmark K, Tran PK, Paulsson-Berne G, Friden V, Soininen R, Tryggvason K et al (2008) Heparan sulfate in perlecan promotes mouse atherosclerosis: roles in lipid permeability, lipid retention, and smooth muscle cell proliferation. Circ Res 103(1):43–52

Usman A, Ribatti D, Sadat U, Gillard JH (2015) From lipid retention to immune-mediate inflammation and associated angiogenesis in the pathogenesis of atherosclerosis. J Atheroscler Thromb 22(8):739–749

Vasile E, Simionescu M, Simionescu N (1983) Visualization of the binding, endocytosis, and transcytosis of low-density lipoprotein in the arterial endothelium in situ. J Cell Biol 96 (6):1677–1689

Vengrenyuk Y, Nishi H, Long X, Ouimet M, Savji N, Martinez FO et al (2015) Cholesterol loading reprograms the microRNA-143/145-myocardin axis to convert aortic smooth muscle cells to a dysfunctional macrophage-like phenotype. Arterioscler Thromb Vasc Biol 35(3):535–546

Vijayagopal P, Srinivasan SR, Radhakrishnamurthy B, Berenson GS (1983) Hemostatic properties and serum lipoprotein binding of a heparan sulfate proteoglycan from bovine aorta. Biochim Biophys Acta 758(1):70–83

Vikramadithyan RK, Kako Y, Chen G, Hu Y, Arikawa-Hirasawa E, Yamada Y et al (2004) Atherosclerosis in perlecan heterozygous mice. J Lipid Res 45(10):1806–1812

von der Thusen JH, van Vlijmen BJ, Hoeben RC, Kockx MM, Havekes LM, van Berkel TJ et al (2002) Induction of atherosclerotic plaque rupture in apolipoprotein E−/− mice after adenovirus-mediated transfer of p53. Circulation 105(17):2064–2070

Wang Y, Dubland JA, Allahverdian S, Asonye E, Sahin B, Jaw JE et al (2019) Smooth muscle cells contribute the majority of foam cells in ApoE (apolipoprotein E)-deficient mouse atherosclerosis. Arterioscler Thromb Vasc Biol 39(5):876–887

Wight TN (2018) A role for proteoglycans in vascular disease. Matrix Biol 71-72:396–420

Wight TN, Merrilees MJ (2004) Proteoglycans in atherosclerosis and restenosis: key roles for versican. Circ Res 94(9):1158–1167

Wight TN, Kinsella MG, Evanko SP, Potter-Perigo S, Merrilees MJ (2014) Versican and the regulation of cell phenotype in disease. Biochim Biophys Acta 1840(8):2441–2451

Williams KJ, Tabas I (1995) The response-to-retention hypothesis of early atherogenesis. Arterioscler Thromb Vasc Biol 15(5):551–561

Wise SG, Weiss AS (2009) Tropoelastin. Int J Biochem Cell Biol 41(3):494–497

Yang H, Zhang N, Okoro EU, Guo Z (2018) Transport of apolipoprotein B-containing lipoproteins through endothelial cells is associated with apolipoprotein e-carrying HDL-like particle formation. Int J Mol Sci 19(11):3593

Yeh YT, Lee CI, Lim SH, Chen LJ, Wang WL, Chuang YJ et al (2012) Convergence of physical and chemical signaling in the modulation of vascular smooth muscle cell cycle and proliferation by fibrillar collagen-regulated P66Shc. Biomaterials 33(28):6728–6738

Yue B (2014) Biology of the extracellular matrix: an overview. J Glaucoma 23(8 Suppl 1):S20–S23

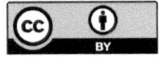

Anti-inflammatory and Immunomodulatory Therapies in Atherosclerosis

Justine Deroissart, Florentina Porsch, Thomas Koller, and Christoph J. Binder

Contents

1 Introduction 360
2 Targeting Innate Immune Responses 362
   2.1 Targeting the NLRP3 Inflammasome 362
      2.1.1 Targeting the IL-1 Signaling Pathway 365
      2.1.2 NLRP3 Inhibitors 366
   2.2 Targeting TNF and Interleukins 367
      2.2.1 Tumor Necrosis Factor (TNF) 367
      2.2.2 IL-6 369
   2.3 Targeting Chronic Inflammation Using Broad Anti-inflammatory Drugs 370
      2.3.1 Methotrexate 370
      2.3.2 Low-Dose Colchicine 372
   2.4 Targeting Chemokine Signaling 374
      2.4.1 Targeting the CCR5 Axis 374
      2.4.2 Targeting the CCR2 Axis 375
3 Modulation of the Adaptive Immune Response 376
   3.1 Strategies Targeting the Homeostatic Balance Between Regulatory and Effector T
      Cells 377
      3.1.1 Low-Dose IL-2 Therapy 378
      3.1.2 Alternative Means to Expand Regulatory T Cells 379
   3.2 Strategies Targeting B Cells and Humoral Immunity 379
      3.2.1 Anti-CD20 Mediated B Cell Depletion (Rituximab) 380
      3.2.2 Other B Cell Depleting Antibodies 382
      3.2.3 B Cell Depletion via Targeting of the BAFF/APRIL System 382
      3.2.4 IgE Neutralization (Omalizumab) 382
   3.3 Strategies Targeting the Interaction Between T Cells and Antigen-Presenting
      Cells 383
      3.3.1 Targeting Co-stimulatory Pathways 383
      3.3.2 Immunization Against LDL-Related Antigens 385
      3.3.3 Tolerogenic Vaccination 386
      3.3.4 Immunization Against Pathogen-Derived Antigens 386

J. Deroissart · F. Porsch · T. Koller · C. J. Binder (✉)
Department of Laboratory Medicine, Medical University of Vienna, Vienna, Austria
e-mail: christoph.binder@meduniwien.ac.at

© The Author(s) 2021
A. von Eckardstein, C. J. Binder (eds.), *Prevention and Treatment of Atherosclerosis*,
Handbook of Experimental Pharmacology 270, https://doi.org/10.1007/164_2021_505

4 Conclusion 387
References 388

Abstract

Hypercholesterolemia is a major risk factor in atherosclerosis development and lipid-lowering drugs (i.e., statins) remain the treatment of choice. Despite effective reduction of LDL cholesterol in patients, a residual cardiovascular risk persists in some individuals, highlighting the need for further therapeutic intervention. Recently, the CANTOS trial paved the way toward the development of specific therapies targeting inflammation, a key feature in atherosclerosis progression. The pre-existence of multiple drugs modulating both innate and adaptive immune responses has significantly accelerated the number of translational studies applying these drugs to atherosclerosis. Additional preclinical research has led to the discovery of new therapeutic targets, offering promising perspectives for the treatment and prevention of atherosclerosis. Currently, both drugs with selective targeting and broad unspecific anti-inflammatory effects have been tested. In this chapter, we aim to give an overview of current advances in immunomodulatory treatment approaches for atherosclerotic cardiovascular diseases.

Keywords

Adaptive immunity · Anti-inflammatory therapy · Atherosclerosis ·
Cardiovascular diseases · Immunotherapy · Inflammation · Innate immunity

1   Introduction

Atherosclerosis is a lipid-driven disease that is characterized by the formation of plaques in the subendothelial space of arteries. Therefore, lipid-lowering drugs such as statins are considered the treatment of choice as their reduction of circulating low-density lipoprotein (LDL) can prevent plaque formation and progression in patients (Ference et al. 2017; Borén et al. 2020). A crucial step in disease initiation involves the retention of LDL and other ApoB-carrying lipoproteins within the vascular wall due to their ability to bind intimal proteoglycans. Subsequent enzymatic and non-enzymatic modifications of these lipoprotein particles result in the formation of damage-associated molecular patterns (DAMPs) that trigger an inflammatory response. This includes the activation of endothelial cells by oxidized phospholipids and other lipid species. In response, the endothelium secretes chemoattractant cytokines like monocyte chemoattractant protein-1 (MCP-1), growth factors (macrophage colony-stimulating factor (MCSF), granulocyte-macrophage colony-stimulating factor (GMCSF)) and upregulates the expression of genes coding for adhesion molecules (VCAM-1 and ICAM-1), allowing the recruitment and differentiation of inflammatory monocytes. Monocytes recruited into the intima become lesional macrophages, which take up oxidized LDL and aggregated LDL via scavenger receptors (CD36, SR-A), ultimately leading to foam cell formation – a rate-limiting step that greatly contributes to the development and progression of atherosclerotic plaques (Borén et al. 2020). Excess accumulation of modified lipoproteins, formation of foam cells, subsequent macrophage cell death, and impaired clearance of these apoptotic cells, all contribute to chronic inflammation in the vascular wall (Borén et al. 2020; Libby 2021). Studies over the past 20 years have focused on the chronic inflammatory nature of atherosclerosis and have demonstrated the detrimental role of inflammation in its pathophysiology. This work led to the consideration of markers of inflammation such as IL-6 and high-sensitivity C-reactive protein (hsCRP) as biomarker for risk stratification of cardiovascular patients (Ridker et al. 2000a, b, 2009). According to this concept, patients with signs of inflammation (i.e., elevated levels of hsCRP or IL-6) are considered at higher risk of experiencing a cardiovascular event during their lifetime compared to individuals without residual inflammation. Additionally, both innate and adaptive immunity have been found to play a crucial role in the initiation, progression, and rupture of atherosclerotic plaques (Gisterå and Hansson 2017; Wolf and Ley 2019; Libby 2021). Since the importance of the immune system in atherosclerotic plaque development is becoming increasingly clear, novel treatments that target both innate and adaptive immunity have been developed with the aim to complement already established lipid-lowering therapies (Bäck et al. 2019). This chapter aims to introduce the reader to these novel anti-inflammatory and immunomodulatory treatments, which range from small molecule drugs to antibodies and vaccination strategies.

To optimally target the inflammatory component of atherosclerosis, one needs to understand the chronic inflammatory nature of this specific process. Chronic inflammation is typically the consequence of a non-resolving inflammation due to an impaired clearance and persistent presence of the inciting trigger combined with a hampered removal of freshly recruited inflammatory cells (Tabas and Glass 2013). In atherosclerosis the main triggers of inflammation are sterile DAMPs that result from the pathological accumulation of lipids in the vascular wall. Therefore, optimal strategies targeting chronic inflammation are either directed toward limiting the generation and activity of disease-specific DAMPs or the inflammatory response they incite. Other strategies aim at dampening inflammation or enhancing the resolution processes. Clearly, the more targeted anti-inflammatory treatments are to a specific pathophysiology, the lower the risk of adverse effects such as a reduction of the host's capacity to fight infections. Thus, careful assessment of the risks and benefits of each anti-inflammatory strategy is needed during the development of these treatments. Modulating both the innate and adaptive responses offers promising possibilities to limit chronic inflammation in the vascular wall.

2 Targeting Innate Immune Responses

2.1 Targeting the NLRP3 Inflammasome

Accumulating evidence shows that the nucleotide-binding oligomerization domain, leucine-rich repeat-containing receptor (NLR) family pyrin domain-containing 3 (NLRP3) inflammasome plays a central role in plaque formation, growth, and stability. Its activation is typically necessary for the secretion of proinflammatory cytokines, such as IL-1β and IL-18, which in turn activate the innate immune system. Ligation of both pattern recognition receptors (PRRs) and tumor necrosis factor receptor (TNFR) can activate the NF-κB pathway, which promotes the transcription of proinflammatory cytokines like tumor necrosis factor-α (TNF-α) and interleukin IL-6 while also initiating the priming of the NLRP3 inflammasome. The latter involves the production of cytosolic NLRP3 protein as well as the inactive form of IL-1 family cytokines: pro-IL-1β and pro-IL-18 (Kelley et al. 2019). Although several PRRs can trigger the formation of inflammasomes, such as NACHT, LRR, and PYD domains-containing protein 1 (NLRP1), NLR family CARD domain-containing protein 4 (NLRC4), and absent in melanoma 2 (AIM2), the NLRP3 inflammasome displays unique activation properties. A large variety of pathogen-associated molecular patterns (PAMPs) (microbial, viral, fungal molecules) and DAMPs (urate crystals) can activate NLRP3. In the context of atherosclerosis, cholesterol crystals (Duewell et al. 2010) have been suggested as key DAMPs driving NLRP3 activation. Importantly, NLRP3 also senses perturbations of cellular homeostasis such as lysosome rupture, ion channel disturbances (K+ efflux), and mitochondrial stress resulting from various stimuli (Kelley et al. 2019). In its activated form, NLRP3 can recruit the apoptosis-associated speck-like protein which contains a caspase recruitment domain (ASC) and the inactivated form of caspase-1 (pro-caspase-1). The proximity of pro-caspase 1 proteins within the complex leads to caspase-1 activation, which proceeds to the proteolytic activation of pro-IL-1β, pro-IL-18, and the propyroptotic factor gasdermin D (GSDMD) involved in pyroptosis, a lytic cell death necessary for cytokine release.

With respect to atherogenesis, important insights came from studies by Duewell and colleagues, who showed that lipid accumulation in the vessel wall leads to the formation of cholesterol crystals which are taken up by macrophages where they activate the NLRP3 inflammasome (Rajamaki et al. 2010; Duewell et al. 2010). In parallel, many studies have investigated the role of NLRP3-derived cytokines (i.e., the IL-1 cytokine family: mainly IL-1β, IL-1α, IL-18, and IL-1R antagonist (IL-1Ra)), as well as proteins involved in NLRP3 activation (ASC, caspase-1) in murine atherosclerosis using transgenic mice. Targeting IL-1 signaling using recombinant IL-1Ra, which competes with IL-1α and IL-1β for binding of IL-1 receptors, in Apoe$^{-/-}$ mice prone to atherosclerosis, resulted in reduced fatty streak formation. This indicates an important role of IL-1Ra in the suppression of lesion development during the early phase of the disease (Elhage et al. 1998; Isoda et al. 2004; Merhi-Soussi et al. 2005). Similarly, overexpression of IL-1Ra in Ldlr$^{-/-}$ mice, fed a high-cholesterol/high-fat diet (containing cholate) for 10 weeks led to a reduction of

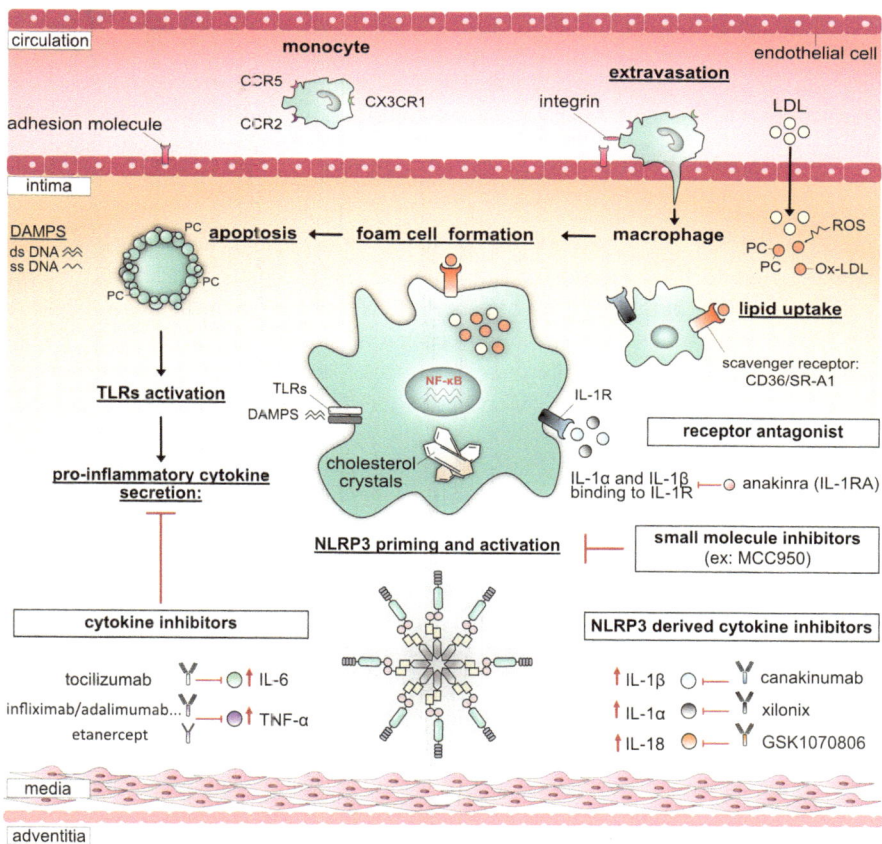

Fig. 1 Therapies targeting innate immune responses in atherosclerosis. Proinflammatory cytokines such as IL-6, TNF, IL-1, and IL-18 actively modulate atherosclerosis development. Therefore, several strategies aim at reducing their levels in circulation. The NLRP3 inflammasome greatly contributes to the secretion of such cytokines and several therapeutic approaches have been developed to prevent its deleterious effects. Drugs targeting NLRP3 are of three types: monoclonal antibodies targeting NLRP3 products (i.e., IL1-α-Xilonix, IL1-β-Canakinumab, IL-18-GSK1070806), recombinant proteins (i.e., IL-1-receptor antagonist-Anakinra), and NLRP3 direct inhibitors (i.e., MCC950). While some of these therapies were assessed in large clinical trials (i.e., Canakinumab), others remained inconclusive due to the low number of patients involved in the study (i.e., Xilonix), or were not investigated in humans yet. The potential benefit of such therapies still requires to be evaluated in robust clinical trials

atherosclerotic lesion area (Devlin et al. 2002). Taken together, these studies suggest that targeting the NLRP3 inflammasome using small molecule inhibitors or targeting NLRP3 products represents promising therapeutic targets for cardiovascular diseases (Fig. 1).

Regarding NLRP3 products, the two IL-1 isoforms (IL-1α and IL-1β) share molecular similarities but are produced by different cellular sources and seem to display different release mechanisms. The release of IL-1α can be inflammasome-dependent or independent, according to the nature of the activating stimulus (Groß et al. 2012). In contrast to IL-1β, the precursor form of IL-1α is active and acts as an alarmin. IL-1α is constitutively expressed as a membrane-bound protein on the surface of various cell types including non-immune cells like epithelial cells. When cells expressing IL-1α undergo cell death, IL-1α is released and acts as an alarmin, inducing IL-1β production and contributing to local inflammation. Additionally, IL-1α can be produced by macrophages, in an inflammasome-independent manner (Freigang et al. 2013). IL-1β on the other hand is mainly produced by hematopoietic cells like dendritic cells, monocytes, and macrophages with its activation requiring (in the majority of cases) the NLRP3 inflammasome. Importantly, IL-1β has been detected in human atherosclerotic plaques and its circulating levels correlate with the severity of coronary atherosclerosis (Galea et al. 1996; Dewberry et al. 2000). Despite these discrepancies, the two IL-1 isoforms share similar downstream effector functions as they both signal via the IL-1 receptor family (IL-1R). Mechanistically, IL-1 signaling impacts various cell types within the atherosclerotic lesion, affecting plaque size and stability. It also contributes to the activation status of endothelial cells, which express adhesion molecules (VCAM-1 and ICAM-1) for the recruitment of leukocytes (Wang et al. 1995). Furthermore, IL-1β induces MCP-1 secretion, which promotes monocyte recruitment and is strongly associated with cardiovascular risk (Jun et al. 2009).

The importance of IL-1α has only recently been appreciated. A small study carried out in coronary artery disease (CAD) patients and healthy control subjects showed higher expression of IL-1α in peripheral blood mononuclear cells (PBMC) of CAD patients (Wæhre et al. 2004). Additionally, IL-1α has been described as the key driver of the senescence-associated secretory phenotype (SASP) of vascular SMCs that can promote vascular inflammation (Clarke et al. 2010; Gardner et al. 2015). Another study carried out by S. Freigang and colleagues also suggests that IL-1α greatly contributes to vascular inflammation in atherosclerosis. Reconstitution of cholesterol fed Ldlr$^{-/-}$ mice with bone marrow from IL-1b–/–, IL-1a–/– and wild-type mice resulted in dramatically reduced atherosclerosis in IL-1α-deficient chimeras but not IL-1β-deficient or wild-type chimeras (Freigang et al. 2013). Similarly, D. Gomez et al showed that antibody-mediated inhibition of IL-1β in Apoe$^{-/-}$ mice with established atherosclerosis failed to decrease lesion size but resulted in adverse plaque remodeling (Gomez et al. 2018). In contrast, other studies suggest beneficial effects of IL-1β targeting in murine atherosclerosis (Kirii et al. 2003; Bhaskar et al. 2011).

Thus, IL-1α and IL-1β may affect plaque formation at different time points in lesion development (Kirii et al. 2003; Duewell et al. 2010; Bhaskar et al. 2011; Gomez et al. 2018; Vromman et al. 2019). While IL-1α appears to be important for the early phase of atherosclerosis, IL-1β seems to be more involved in the progression of established plaques (Vromman et al. 2019). Additionally, Vromman et al. showed that the anatomical location of plaques matters in the response to therapies targeting IL-1 signaling. For example, neutralization of IL-1α or both isoforms using either an anti-IL1α and/or an anti-IL-1β monoclonal antibody reduces the lesion area in aortic roots but not in the brachiocephalic arteries in Apoe $^{-/-}$ mice. Moreover, compensatory outward remodeling was more impaired in the brachiocephalic artery compared to the aortic roots during early atherosclerosis.

In summary, the NLRP3 inflammasome and inflammasome-derived cytokines represent attractive points for therapeutic intervention in cardiovascular diseases. Careful design of preclinical studies will allow better dissection of the mechanistic and physiological aspects of IL-1 inhibition and improvement of the development of new therapies.

2.1.1 Targeting the IL-1 Signaling Pathway

Anti-IL-1 β (Canakinumab)

The recent CANTOS (Canakinumab. Anti-Inflammatory Thrombosis Outcome Study) trial has made a profound impact on the field of atherosclerotic cardiovascular disease. It showed for the first time in a large phase 3 clinical trial that therapeutic targeting of inflammation provides a clinical benefit to patients with stable atherosclerosis. The goal of the study was to evaluate the effect of canakinumab, a monoclonal antibody targeting IL-1β, on adverse cardiac events in patients with a history of MI and elevated hsCRP (hsCRP ≥ 2 mg/L). 10,061 patients, most of whom were on statin therapy, received either placebo or canakinumab at three different doses: 50 mg, 150 mg, or 300 mg, every 3 months. The best results were obtained with the intermediate dose (150 mg) which led to a 15% reduction in the primary endpoint of nonfatal MI, nonfatal stroke, or cardiovascular death. However, as IL-1β is also a crucial cytokine in the host immune response against bacterial infection, its inhibition also significantly increased the number of fatal infections (Ridker et al. 2017). Despite these non-negligible side effects, this study clearly demonstrates a beneficial effect of inhibiting IL-1β signaling.

To better predict positive outcomes of canakinumab therapy in patients, an additional analysis of the CANTOS trial was conducted (Ridker et al. 2018b). Within the canakinumab treated group, patients with hsCRP levels <2 mg/L following treatment had a 25% reduction in major adverse cardiovascular events while no significant benefits were observed in patients with levels ≥ 2 mg/L. Importantly, cardiovascular mortality and all-cause mortality were both reduced by 31% in patients with hsCRP levels <2 mg/L. This was not the case in patients with levels ≥ 2 mg/L where no benefits were shown. This analysis clearly documented the need to assess the successful impact on inflammation to optimally appreciate the protective effect of this intervention.

Another analysis published by the CANTOS group indicates that targeting IL-1β alone may not sufficiently alleviate CVD risk, as both IL-6 and IL-18 levels remain predictors of future cardiovascular events in patients receiving anti-IL-1β treatment. Briefly, in patients treated with canakinumab, the risk of major adverse cardiac events (MACE) increased by 15% and 42% for each tertile increase in IL-18 and IL-6 levels, respectively. This suggests a residual inflammatory component that needs to be considered for further cardiovascular risk reduction. Drugs targeting the IL-6 cytokine are currently tested in clinical trials and might benefit patients with sustained elevated IL-6 levels by preventing recurrent CVD events (Biasucci et al. 2020; Ridker et al. 2020).

IL-1 Receptor Antagonist (Anakinra)

Anakinra is an antagonist of the IL-1 receptor, blocking the action of both IL-1α and IL-1β isoforms. Since 2001, it has been used as a treatment in patients with rheumatoid arthritis (RA), who are also known to be at high risk of cardiovascular disease (Nurmohamed 2009; Avina-Zubieta et al. 2012; Primdahl et al. 2013). Anakinra was assessed in small clinical trials in patients with myocardial infarction: The "Virginia Commonwealth University-Anakinra Remodeling Trial 1-2-3" (VCU ART1-2-3) and the "Markers of inflammation in non-ST elevation acute coronary syndromes"(MRC ILA-HEART) study (Abbate et al. 2010, 2013, 2020; Morton et al. 2015). In VCU ART, this type of interleukin-1 blockade significantly reduced the systemic inflammatory response with a strong reduction of hsCRP levels in patients with ST-Elevation Myocardial Infarction (STEMI) as well as decreasing the incidence of heart failure. In the MRC ILA-Heart trial, a reduction of IL-6 and hsCRP levels was also observed in non-STEMI (NSTEMI) patients who received Anakinra daily for 2 weeks. However, by day 30, the hsCRP levels in patients treated with Anakinra were significantly higher than in the placebo group, and an unexpected increase of late recurrent ischemic events was observed. Interestingly, a recent study carried out by the Interleukin-1 Genetics Consortium supports the hypothesis that long-term IL-1 inhibition may be associated with an increase in cardiovascular events. In this study, individuals who carried four IL-1Ra raising alleles were found to have an increased odds ratio for coronary heart disease (1.15) compared to those carrying no IL-1Ra raising alleles. Additionally, the concentration of proatherogenic lipids, including LDL cholesterol, increased with each extra allele present (Freitag et al. 2015). However, the VCU-ART study showed no effect on recurrent ischemic events, while there was an increase of MACE upon Anakinra treatment after 1 year in the MRC ILA-Heart trial.

In summary, the relationship between IL-1 targeting and clinical outcomes seems more complex than originally thought. Currently attempted therapeutic strategies include targeting IL-1β (Canakinumab) or both IL-1α and IL-1β with the human recombinant IL-1RA (Anakinra). Further understanding of the distinct roles of the different IL-1 isoforms would enhance our understanding of clinical trial data (CANTOS, VCU ART-1/2/3, MRC ILA-HEART) and improve future trial design.

2.1.2   NLRP3 Inhibitors

Despite the importance of the NLRP3 inflammasome in many inflammatory diseases, there is currently no approved inflammasome inhibitor for the treatment or prevention of atherosclerosis. Nevertheless, many small molecule compounds targeting the NLRP3 inflammasome have been developed, with promising results. Importantly, both canonical and non-canonical NLRP3 activation pathways can be targeted.

MCC950

MCC950 is a small molecule inhibitor of the NLRP3 pathway, with a mechanism which is yet to be fully understood (Coll et al. 2015). Nevertheless, it was found to reduce atherosclerotic lesion formation in Apoe$^{-/-}$ mice. This was associated with decreased expression of the adhesion molecules ICAM-1 and VCAM-1, as well as reduced macrophage infiltration within plaques and no change in necrotic core size (Van Der Heijden et al. 2017). This early data suggests that MCC950 represents an interesting candidate to target NLRP3 induced inflammation in atherosclerosis.

Tranilast

Tranilast, which was originally used to treat allergy, was shown to inhibit NLRP3 by facilitating its ubiquitination and impairing ASC oligomerization (Huang et al. 2018; Chen et al. 2020). The effect of Tranilast on atherosclerosis was assessed in Watanabe heritable hyperlipidemic rabbits and resulted in decreased atherosclerosis upon treatment (Matsumura et al. 1999). Recently, another study carried out in mice showed that Tranilast decreased the initiation and progression of atherosclerosis in both Ldlr$^{-/-}$ and Apoe$^{-/-}$ prone atherosclerotic mice (Chen et al. 2020). Thus, pharmacologic manipulation of NLRP3 ubiquitination offers a new strategy for protection against atherosclerosis.

Despite encouraging results from animal models, many questions remain to be answered concerning the safety of NLRP3 inhibitors. It will be critical to further examine how these compounds affect the activity of other inflammasomes and how the host immune response is affected in the long run. The initiation of new clinical trials evaluating the benefit of NLRP3 inhibitors in the context of cardiovascular diseases will also depend on these factors.

2.2 Targeting TNF and Interleukins

2.2.1 Tumor Necrosis Factor (TNF)

Tumor necrosis factor (TNF) is a proinflammatory cytokine with a broad spectrum of functions and targets. It controls inflammatory responses by regulating leukocyte activation, maturation, and cytokine/chemokine release. TNF secretion can be triggered by the recognition of PAMPs and DAMPs, but also by cytokines and interferon such as IL-1, GM-CSF, TGF-β, TNF-α itself (autocrine loop), and IFN-γ (Zelová and Hošek 2013). It is mainly produced by macrophages and T cells, but many other cell types, including non-immune cells such as endothelial cells and smooth muscle cells (SMCs), can also secrete TNF. Importantly, TNF seems to be highly expressed in human atherosclerotic plaques (Rus et al. 1991; Canault et al. 2006). Ohta et al showed that TNF enhances the expression of ICAM-1, VCAM-1, and MCP-1 in endothelial cells, favoring monocyte recruitment into the vascular wall. Additionally, an increase of scavenger receptor A dependent uptake of oxidized LDL by macrophages has been described, as well as decreased IL-1β and INF-γ mRNA expression, which together strongly support a deleterious role of TNF in murine atherosclerosis (Ohta et al. 2005; Xiao et al. 2009). Interestingly, recent studies suggest that TNF might also be involved in the regulation of the NLRP3 inflammasome (Sode et al. 2014; Bauernfeind et al. 2016; McGeough et al. 2017).

TNF is a central mediator of the inflammatory response and its signaling mechanism is well described. Many biological agents interfering with TNF signaling have been developed and tested in clinical trials in the context of inflammatory diseases associated with high cardiovascular risk, such as rheumatoid arthritis (RA), psoriatic arthritis, and Crohn's disease. For example, treatment with TNF blockers (infliximab or etanercept) in RA is associated with a lower incidence of cardiovascular events (Jacobsson et al. 2005). Two meta-analyses also confirmed that RA patients treated with anti-TNF therapy have a lower risk of cardiovascular events in comparison with patients treated with disease-modifying antirheumatic drugs (DMARDs) (Barnabe et al. 2011; Roubille et al. 2015). Currently, five different anti-TNF drugs are approved for clinical use, which include soluble TNF-receptor (etanercept) and TNF monoclonal antibodies (adalimumab, infliximab, golimumab, and certolizumab pegol). The evidence for their use in atherosclerotic cardiovascular disease will be discussed below.

Adalimumab

While adalimumab has been used as a safe therapy in a myriad of inflammatory diseases (Burmester et al. 2020), no large-scale trial regarding its effect on atherosclerotic cardiovascular disease exists. A small study in RA patients showed that treatment with adalimumab improves endothelial-dependent vasodilatation (Gonzalez-Juanatey et al. 2006), findings which were confirmed in a second study by the same authors. In this latter study, a comparison of baseline and post-treatment (12 months) carotid artery wall thickness (intima-media) measurement in RA patients showed no statistical difference (Gonzalez-Juanatey et al. 2012). Nevertheless, these observations suggest that adalimumab may improve the state of subclinical atherosclerosis in RA patients. Improvement of endothelial cell function was also observed in a study involving 14 psoriatic patients (Avgerinou et al. 2011). After 12 weeks of adalimumab treatment, no significant change on hsCRP level compared to baseline was observed, but ICAM-1 expression was decreased and the flow-mediated dilation (FMD), used as a marker of endothelial dysfunction, was improved. A larger study (NCT01722214) included 107 psoriatic patients randomized to receive either adalimumab for 52 weeks or placebo for 16 weeks followed by adalimumab for 36 weeks (per-protocol setting). At 16 weeks, the adalimumab treatment group had no difference in vascular inflammation compared to the placebo control group. At the 52-week time point, there was no difference observed in the ascending aorta with adalimumab, but a modest increase in vascular inflammation in carotids was described (Bissonnette et al. 2017). Thus, in lieu of a large clinical trial, the effect of adalimumab in ASCVD remains unclear.

Golimumab

Golimumab is a fully-humanized monoclonal anti-TNF antibody approved for the treatment of RA, ankylosing spondylitis (AS), psoriatic arthritis, and ulcerative colitis. Golimumab has a greater affinity for the soluble (sTNF) vs. the transmembrane form (mTNF). While no data exist regarding the therapeutic benefit of golimumab in atherosclerosis, a pilot study in patients with ASCVD provided encouraging results (Tam et al. 2014). This randomized, double-blind, placebo-controlled trial aimed to assess the efficacy of Golimumab in preventing atherosclerosis progression and arterial stiffness in AS patients. A total of 20 patients received 50 mg of Golimumab monthly, with 21 receiving placebo treatment, for 1 year. After 6 months, no significant change in vascular parameters (i.e. aortic stiffness, carotid intima/media thickness) was observed between the two groups. However, a significant progression of the mean intima-media thickness (IMT) was only seen in the placebo group and not in the golimumab group. Maximum IMT, pulse wave velocity (PWV), and augmentation index (Aix) remained unchanged (paired t-test analysis). Nevertheless, no significant difference concerning vascular parameters was demonstrated between the two groups after 1 year of treatment. Further large-scale studies are needed to fully validate the potential effects seen in this study.

In addition to these findings in AS patients, TNF inhibitors were found to improve the overall pathologic profile of RA and psoriasis patients at high cardiovascular risk. Therapeutic targeting of TNF has shown benefit in the prevention of atherosclerosis in RA (Del Porto et al. 2007), which might also be the case in psoriasis (Sattar et al. 2007). Interestingly, a recent meta-analysis that includes 7,697 coronary artery disease (CAD) patients and 9,655 control patients has investigated the association of *TNF* gene polymorphisms and CAD susceptibility (Huang et al. 2020). The authors concluded that there was no association of *TNF* 308G/A, 857C/T, 863C/A, and 1031 T polymorphisms with CAD susceptibility. However, the *TNF* 238G/A genotype showed a significant association with higher CAD susceptibility in the subgroup of Europeans and North Asians, which suggests a direct role of TNF in CAD. Additionally, several studies described an adverse effect of TNF inhibitors on lipid profiles and described an increase of total cholesterol and triglycerides levels (Curtis et al. 2012; Hassan et al. 2016). In summary, further large-scale studies are required to evaluate the potential benefits of anti-TNF agents.

2.2.2 IL-6

Interleukin-6 (IL-6) is a pleiotropic cytokine involved in different arms of the immune system. It can result in both pro- and anti-inflammatory outcomes which can be explained by the different signaling pathways engaged: the classical pathway, the trans-signaling pathway, and the blockade pathway. The classical pathway occurs in a few cell types such as T cells, hepatocytes, and monocytes. It involves the IL-6 receptor (IL-6R) and glycoprotein 130 (gp130), a signal transducer sub-unit of the IL-6 receptor. In the trans-signaling pathway, the mechanism involves the signal transducer gp130 as well as soluble IL-6 receptor (sIL-6R). In contrast to the classical pathway, trans-signaling can occur in any cell type expressing a membrane-bound gp130 protein. In this scenario, sIL-6 binds to sIL-6R and forms a complex that can activate signaling through gp130 resulting in a greater magnitude of proinflammatory state. IL-6 signaling can also be blocked via the soluble form of gp130 which acts as a natural inhibitor of trans-signaling by binding sIL-6/IL-6R complex (Jostock et al. 2001).

Despite inconclusive data from experimental models (Elhage et al. 2001; Song and Schindler 2004; Schieffer et al. 2004; Schuett et al. 2012), shreds of evidence from translational studies identify IL-6 as a key regulator of atherogenesis. Expression of IL-6 was detected in human atherosclerotic plaques (Seino et al. 1994; Rus et al. 1996; Schieffer et al. 2000). Several studies found that high levels of IL-6 are associated with increased cardiovascular risk in human (Mendall et al. 1997; Ridker et al. 2000b; Fisman et al. 2006; Zakai et al. 2007; Danesh et al. 2008; Lefkou et al. 2010). Among them, a study from J. Danesh and colleagues, who compared serial measurements of serum IL-6 between patients with a history of coronary heart disease and controls. Results showed that long-term exposure to circulating IL-6 was associated with an increased risk of coronary artery disease (Danesh et al. 2008). However, follow-up studies of the CANTOS trial showed that patients with elevated IL-6 levels after canakinumab treatment have no significant benefit as opposed to patients with lower IL-6 levels (Ridker et al. 2018a, 2020).

Collectively, these studies and the studies based on the CANTOS trial suggest an important role of IL-6 in cardiovascular diseases. Targeting the IL-6 axis may be crucial to reduce the residual inflammation responsible for the increased risk of cardiovascular events.

Several clinical trials tested the therapeutic benefit of targeting the IL-6 axis using Tocilizumab (Table 1). However, higher-powered studies are required to better evaluate the safety and efficiency of current IL-6 targeting agents, and appreciate their benefit in preventing atherosclerosis.

2.3   Targeting Chronic Inflammation Using Broad Anti-inflammatory Drugs

Given the importance of inflammation in atherosclerosis, the usage of broad anti-inflammatory drugs could potentially reduce the risk of atherosclerotic events. Well known for their anti-inflammatory properties, methotrexate and colchicine are widely used as main treatments in inflammatory diseases with a high risk of CVD, notably RA, psoriasis, and other rheumatologic disorders (Saag et al. 2008; Singh et al. 2012). The repurposing of these two drugs as a therapeutic approach against atherosclerosis was evaluated in several clinical trials discussed below.

2.3.1   Methotrexate

Treatment with low-dose methotrexate (LD-MTX) reduces the levels of circulating CRP, IL-6, TNF-alpha and cardiovascular events in RA patients (Choi et al. 2002; Wessels et al. 2008; Westlake et al. 2010; Roubille et al. 2015). An important feature of LD-MTX is its ability to increase adenosine production and stimulate the adenosine A_{2A} receptor, which has been shown to promote the expression of several proteins involved in reverse cholesterol transport, thus potentially reducing foam cell formation (Reiss et al. 2008). The potential benefit of LD-MTX in the treatment of atherosclerosis was recently assessed in the cardiovascular inflammation reduction trial (CIRT) which is discussed below.

Table 1 Tocilizumab therapy and consequences on CVD risk factors

Drug	Target	Approval	Cohort	Trial design	Effect	References
Tocilizumab	IL-6R	RA patients	RA patients	Non-randomized pilot study	• Improved endothelial function and aortic stiffness ↑CRP level Modification of total cholesterol levels	Protogerou et al. (2011)
			RA patients	Non-randomized pilot study	• Side effect on lipid profile: consequences on cardiovascular risk were not assessed	Strang et al. (2013)
			RA patients	Randomized, double-blind placebo-controlled	• Side effect on lipid profile: consequences on cardiovascular risk were not assessed	McInnes et al. (2015)
			Non-ST-elevation myocardial infarction (NSTEMI) patients	Randomized, double-blind placebo-controlled	↑ Inflammation and primary percutaneous coronary intervention related to high-sensitivity troponin T release ↑CRP level	Kleveland et al. (2016)

Cardiovascular Inflammation Reduction Trial (CIRT)

The CIRT trial was performed in parallel with the CANTOS trial and aimed to determine if LD-MTX could reduce cardiovascular events in patients with stable atherosclerosis and high cardiovascular risk (Everett et al. 2013). The double-blind trial included 4,786 patients with a history of myocardial infarction or multivessel coronary disease, as well as either type 2 diabetes or metabolic syndrome. Patients were randomized and treated with either LD-MTX (2,391) or placebo (2,395). The final primary endpoint was a composite of nonfatal myocardial infarction, nonfatal stroke, cardiovascular death, and hospitalization for unstable angina that led to urgent revascularization. After a median follow-up of 2.3 years, the primary endpoint occurred in 201 patients in the methotrexate group and 207 patients in the placebo group (HR 0.96, 95% CI 0.79–1.16). Also, treatment with LD-MTX did not reduce plasma levels of CRP, IL-1β, IL-6, TNF-α. No significant difference between the two groups for any component of the primary endpoint was found.

Considering the success of the CANTOS trial and the beneficial effect seen with LD-MTX in RA patients, the CIRT trial results are disappointing. While CANTOS targeted a specific and well-defined pathway, the CIRT trial used a drug with a large spectrum of anti-inflammatory effects with molecular consequences which are not yet understood. Besides the different mechanisms of action, an additional explanation for the discrepant results between CIRT and CANTOS may be differences in the study design of the two studies. Patients recruited to the CIRT trial had a lower residual inflammatory profile (median baseline CRP: 1.6 mg/L) compared to patients from the CANTOS trial, where patient recruitment was based on hsCRP levels ≥ 2 mg/L as a marker of high residual inflammation (median baseline CRP: 4.2 mg/L). In support of this explanation, treatment of RA patients with LD-MTX led to a reduction of hsCRP (Westlake et al. 2010) and decreased cardiovascular risk.

These data demonstrate that the design of future clinical trials needs to consider inclusion criteria that target individuals with a high inflammatory profile.

2.3.2 Low-Dose Colchicine

Colchicine is an inexpensive anti-inflammatory drug used in patients with gout, familial Mediterranean fever, and pericarditis. By preventing microtubule assembly, colchicine can disrupt inflammasome activation, microtubule-based inflammatory cell chemotaxis, phagocytosis, and other host immune mechanisms. The first benefit of colchicine in ischemic heart disease (IHD) has been observed in familial Mediterranean fever patients (Langevitz et al. 2001). Patients diagnosed with FMF show a sustained inflammatory response which puts them at a higher risk of suffering a heart attack in comparison with the general population. Langevitz and colleagues showed that treatment with colchicine lowered the risk of IHD in FMF patients compared to untreated patients with other inflammatory conditions and similar rates of risk factors. Also, patients taking colchicine achieved a frequency of IHD comparable to the general population. To assess the potential benefit of colchicine in atherosclerosis, several clinical trials such as the low-dose colchicine trial (LoDoCo), or more recently the colchicine cardiovascular outcomes trial (COLCOT), have been carried out and will be discussed below.

LoDoCo-MI and LoDoCo-1/2 Trials

In 2007, a small pilot study had demonstrated the potential of low-dose colchicine to reduce hsCRP levels, independently of lowering cholesterol (Atorvastatin), in patients with stable coronary artery disease (Nidorf and Thompson 2007). However, in the randomized and placebo-controlled LoDoCo (Low-Dose Colchicine)-MI study (237 patients), colchicine at 0.5 mg/day for 30 days failed to reduce hsCRP levels ($\leq$ 2 mg/L) in patients with recent MI (Hennessy et al. 2019).

Subsequently, the LoDoCo (Low-Dose Colchicine) trial was designed as a prospective study to assess the efficiency and safety of long-term low-dose colchicine usage in patients with stable coronary disease. 532 patients on lipid-lowering medication and antithrombotic therapy were randomized and treated with a daily dose of colchicine (0.5 mg/mL) or no colchicine. After a median follow-up of 3 years, the primary outcome (acute coronary syndrome, out-of-hospital cardiac arrest, or non-cardioembolic ischemic stroke) had occurred in 5.3% of patients in the low-dose colchicine group, as opposed to 16% in the non-treated group (Nidorf et al. 2013). To validate the observations from the LoDoCo study, a large-scale study (LoDoCo 2) involving 5,522 patients was conducted. LoDoCo 2 confirmed the significant treatment benefit of low-dose colchicine in reducing CVD risk in patients with stable coronary disease. The primary endpoint was a composite of cardiovascular death, spontaneous (non-procedural) myocardial infarction, ischemic stroke, or ischemia-driven coronary revascularization. The secondary endpoint was a composite of cardiovascular death, spontaneous MI, or ischemic stroke. Primary endpoints occurred in 6.8% of patients in the low-dose colchicine group as opposed to 9.6% in the placebo-treated group, and secondary endpoints occurred in 4.2% in the colchicine group and 5.7% in the placebo group. However, an increase in death from non-cardiovascular diseases was observed in the colchicine treated group, which further justifies the need for more targeted therapies that limit undesirable side effects (Nidorf et al. 2019, 2020; Pradhan 2021).

COLCOT Trial

Another recent double-blind randomized placebo-controlled colchicine intervention study, named COLCOT (colchicine cardiovascular outcomes trial), aimed to assess the benefit of colchicine in patients with a recent acute MI (Tardif et al. 2019). In total, 4,745 patients were divided into two groups that were given oral colchicine at 0.5 mg/day or a placebo. The primary efficacy endpoint was a composite of death from cardiovascular causes, myocardial infarction, stroke, urgent hospitalization for angina leading to coronary revascularization, or resuscitated cardiac arrest. At a median of 23 months, the primary composite endpoint had occurred in 5.5% of the treatment group and 7.1% in the placebo group (hazard ratio, 0.77). Remarkably, the hazard ratio for stroke (HR = 0.26) and hospitalization for angina (HR = 0.50) indicate an important benefit in the colchicine treated group for these two particular primary endpoints. Overall, colchicine showed a good safety and tolerability profile despite a slight but significant increase in pneumonia occurrence (0.9%) in the colchicine group compared to the placebo group (0.4%). There were no differences in peripheral blood counts and CRP levels among the treated group compared to the placebo. Recent follow-up analysis suggests that the main benefit of colchicine therapy occurs when treatment is initiated in the first 3 days post-MI (Bouabdallaoui et al. 2020).

Additionally, the repurposed usage of low-dose colchicine has shown multiple benefits for the treatment of stable coronary artery diseases. A recent pilot study carried out in 80 patients with recent acute coronary syndrome suggests that low-dose colchicine uptake on a regular basis can efficiently stabilize plaques on top of optimal medical therapy (Vaidya et al. 2018). Further upcoming data from large-scale trials such as CLEAR-Synergy (4,000 patients with ST-elevation myocardial infarction undergoing percutaneous coronary intervention (NCT03048825)) will help to validate its efficiency and tolerability in coronary diseases.

2.4   Targeting Chemokine Signaling

Considerable work has been carried out on the identification of inflammatory mediators that actively participate in the progression of atherosclerosis which has increased the number of potential new therapeutic targets. Among them, chemokines were identified as key players in leukocyte recruitment/adhesion and activation as well as promotion of local inflammation in arteries. The contribution of chemokines to plaque formation/destabilization and thrombus formation has been extensively reviewed elsewhere (Zernecke and Weber 2014).

Despite the proven relevance of specific chemokines in atherogenesis, the clinical evaluation of drugs targeting specific chemokines or chemokine pairings has not progressed much. This is mainly due to the complexity of the "working network" within which chemokines operate and their critical role in fundamental host defense.

Several chemokines and their receptors such as CCL5/CCR5 (including heterodimeric interactions), CCL2/CCR2, CX3CL1/CX3CR1 are an active part of disease progression (Combadière et al. 2008). Drugs targeting those axes were developed in the context of other diseases like human immunodeficiency virus infections and facilitate the establishment of new clinical studies involving patients with cardiovascular diseases. Currently, drugs used to disrupt chemokine–receptor interactions rely on four main strategies: the modification of the chemokine N-terminal domain, the synthesis of small molecules used as a receptor antagonist, the usage of specific antibodies targeting chemokines, and other drugs interfering with chemokines' heterodimeric interactions. Here, we will focus on promising chemokine targeting therapies with available clinical data in the context of atherosclerosis.

2.4.1   Targeting the CCR5 Axis

Expression of CCL5 and CCR5 has been identified in atherosclerotic plaques more than 15 years ago (Wilcox et al. 1994; Pattison et al. 1996; Veillard et al. 2004). Atheroprotective effects resulting from the perturbation of CCR5/RANTES (Regulated on Activation, Normal T cell Expressed and Secreted) interactions were described in several mouse studies. The genetic inactivation of CCR5 in chow or high-fat diet-fed Apoe$^{-/-}$ mice was shown to be protective in advanced atherosclerosis, but not in the early phase of the disease. The atheroprotective effect was associated with a decrease of macrophage numbers in plaques and reduced levels of circulating IL-6. The plaque quality was also affected by an increased content of SMCs, promoting plaque stabilization (Kuziel et al. 2003; Braunersreuther et al. 2007; Quinones et al. 2007). Moreover, a natural variant of *CCR5* (CCR5Δ32 polymorphism) which reduces the cell surface expression of CCR5, is associated with a reduced risk of coronary artery diseases and MI (Szalai et al. 2001; González et al. 2001). Thus, the CCR5 pathway appears to be an interesting potential target for antiatherosclerotic therapy.

Maraviroc

The CCR5 inhibitor maraviroc is one of the few small molecules targeting a chemokine/receptor interaction approved by the US Food and Drug Administration and the European Medicines Agency as a preventive treatment for HIV (2007). HIV-associated inflammation increases HIV patients' risk of cardiovascular disease (Shah et al. 2018), which suggests a potential role of maraviroc in modulating the atherogenic risk of these patients. This was confirmed preclinically as the treatment of atherosclerosis-prone Apoe$^{-/-}$ mice with maraviroc has been found to reduce atherosclerotic lesion development (Cipriani et al. 2013).

A recent pilot study in HIV patients showed that maraviroc treatment decreases carotid intima-media thickness, reflecting potential anti-atherogenic effects (Francisci et al. 2019). Additionally, an anti-human CCR5 monoclonal antibody (HGS004-Human Genome Sciences), tested in a clinical trial in HIV patients, showed a good safety profile and could be an interesting candidate for atherosclerosis therapy (Lalezari et al. 2008). Finally, a phase 4 clinical trial evaluating the efficacy of maraviroc in modulating atherosclerosis in HIV patients has been completed (NCT03402815) and results are forthcoming. This data will provide crucial information regarding the future of CCR5 axis targeting therapy in atherosclerosis.

2.4.2 Targeting the CCR2 Axis

Many pieces of evidence from experimental models demonstrate the proatherogenic role of CCR2 and its ligand CCL2/MCP-1 (Monocyte chemoattractant protein 1) (França et al. 2017). Notably, CCR2 signaling can promote monocyte recruitment to atherosclerotic lesions and foam cell formation (Boring et al. 1998; Bobryshev 2006). A recent discovery by Winter et al showed that the recruitment of myeloid cells within atherosclerotic lesions is subject to circadian regulation (Winter et al. 2018). This establishes a new concept of chrono-pharmacology-based therapy for the treatment of atherosclerosis, which is particularly relevant for the usage of CCR2 antagonists given their role in the promotion of monocyte recruitment (Winter et al. 2018).

MNL1202

In an effort to develop a specific antagonist of CCR2, a humanized antibody MNL1202 has been generated and tested in a phase 2 clinical trial in patients at risk for CVD (with at least 2 risk factors for atherosclerotic CVD, hsCRP level >3 mg/L, and receiving or not receiving lipid-lowering drugs). The direct blocking of CCR2 with MLN1202 was well tolerated and significantly reduced hsCRP levels in the antibody-treated group compared to the placebo-treated group (Gilbert et al. 2011). Thus MLN1202 appears to be a promising candidate to target atherosclerosis-associated inflammation.

Despite encouraging preclinical results, few molecules targeting chemokines and their receptors have been approved for clinical use yet. The fundamental role of chemokine signaling during both innate and adaptive immune response suggests that its targeting likely critically impairs the host immune response. For example, treatment with the CCL5 variant Met-RANTES or deficiency in CCL5 delays viral clearance by macrophages and impairs T-cell function (Makino et al. 2002). In this regard, the specific targeting of chemokine heteromerization represents a good alternative as it poses fewer risks of immunological side effects than chemokine antagonists. Up to now, 11 heteromeric chemokine pairs have been reported (Koenen and Weber 2010), expanding the therapeutic possibilities. Importantly, preclinical studies are carried out in a pathogen-free context, which is not representative of human pathogen exposure. Thus, future studies must assess the risk of long-term exposure to such chemokine targeting therapies. The complexity of the chemokine network, the lack of data concerning the toxicity of their targeting agents, and the availability of other, safer therapeutic approaches have drastically slowed down the translation of chemokine targeted therapies to human cardiovascular disease. Future studies should include a parallel assessment of risks and benefits provided by molecules targeting chemokine interactions to better appreciate the net effect on patients with cardiovascular diseases.

3   Modulation of the Adaptive Immune Response

Adaptive immunity plays a key role in driving and modulating the pathogenesis of atherosclerosis (Sage et al. 2018; ; Wolf and Ley 2019; Libby 2021). The adaptive branch of immunity consists primarily of T and B cells, both of which have the capacity to induce immune responses that are specifically targeted to disease-associated antigens. Adaptive immunity therefore represents an attractive therapeutic target as its modulation could allow for a more specific response, potentially reducing the risks of weakened host defenses associated with broad anti-inflammatory therapies (Fig. 2).

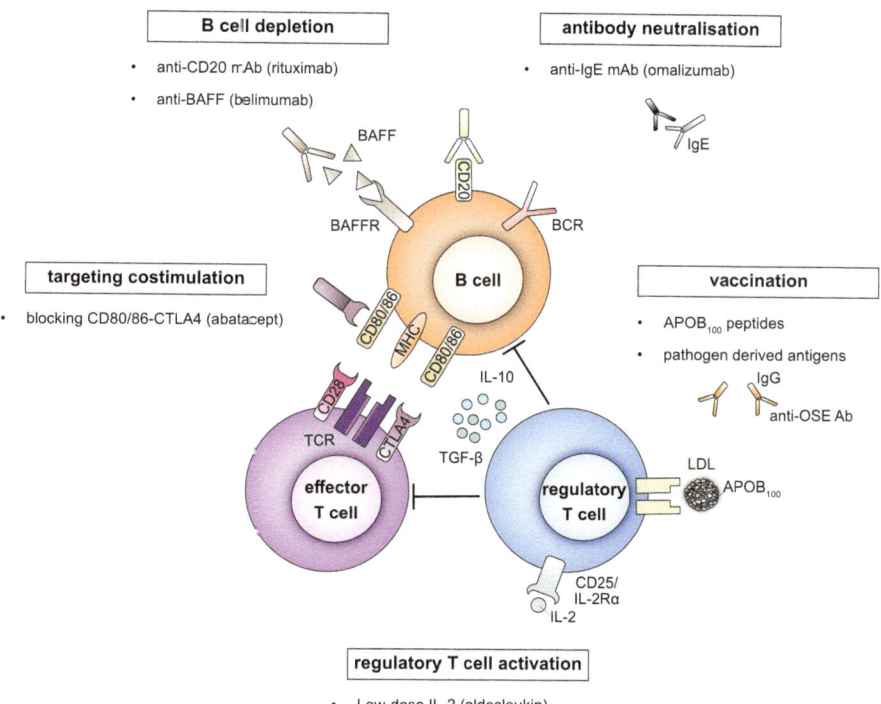

Fig. 2 Targeting adaptive immune responses in atherosclerosis. Regulatory T cells (T_{regs}) play a protective role in atherosclerosis via their immunosuppressive capacities such as the secretion of IL10 and TGFβ. They can suppress the activity of proatherogenic effector T cells such as TH1 cells. T_{reg} numbers can be increased in a non-specific manner via the use of low-dose IL2 or in an antigen-specific manner by immunization with ApoB100-derived peptides. Furthermore, blocking effector T cell activation by inhibiting the interaction between co-stimulatory CD80/CD86 on antigen-presenting cells such as B cells and CD28 on T cells has been shown to reduce atherosclerosis in mice. B2 cells and many of their effector functions including some proatherogenic antibody isotypes such as IgE have been shown to promote atherogenesis. Thus, B cell depleting antibodies such as anti-CD20 or anti-BAFF antibodies have been shown to protect mice from atherosclerosis. Additionally, the depletion of proatherogenic antibodies such as IgE may have beneficial effects. On the other hand, immunization with modified LDL has been shown to induce protective antibody responses (both IgG and IgM) against oxidation-specific epitopes (OSE) that ameliorate atherosclerosis in preclinical studies

3.1 Strategies Targeting the Homeostatic Balance Between Regulatory and Effector T Cells

Although no therapies targeting T cells are currently in clinical use for the treatment and prevention of cardiovascular disease, some therapeutic approaches have shown promise in preclinical models and are being evaluated in clinical trials. In atherosclerosis-prone mice, regulatory T cells (T_{regs}) have been shown to be beneficial both in the progression and regression of atherosclerosis (Ait-Oufella et al. 2006; Mor et al.

2007; Klingenberg et al. 2013; Sharma et al. 2020). In contrast, many effector T cells are thought to be proatherogenic, particularly IFNγ-secreting T helper 1 (Th1) (Saigusa et al. 2020; Buono et al. 2005). In humans, cardiovascular disease is associated with an imbalance in T_{reg} and effector T cells, where T_{regs} are decreased in patients with acute coronary syndrome and low numbers are associated with increased rates of acute coronary events (Mor et al. 2006; Han et al. 2007; Cheng et al. 2008; Ammirati et al. 2010; Wigren et al. 2012).

Therefore, the aim of T cell-targeted therapeutic approaches in atherosclerosis is to change the homeostatic balance of different T cell subsets by expanding atheroprotective, immunosuppressive T_{regs} while suppressing putatively proatherogenic effector T cell populations (Foks et al. 2015). This could be achieved on the one hand by the stimulation of non-specific T_{regs} by targeting pathways such as interleukin-2 (IL-2). On the other hand, specific T_{regs} can be expanded with the use of tolerogenic vaccines against atherosclerosis-relevant antigens.

3.1.1 Low-Dose IL-2 Therapy

Interleukin-2 is a cytokine that plays a key role in the regulation of T cell activity and survival. Although IL-2 has the ability to regulate all T cells, it appears to be particularly important in the development and survival of T_{regs} (Boyman and Sprent 2012). The activation threshold for T_{regs} is lower than for other effector T cells (Yu et al. 2009), which may explain the somewhat paradoxical effect of IL-2 therapy. While high-dose IL-2 therapy is thought to promote effector immunity, low-dose IL-2 stimulates immunosuppressive T_{regs} (Klatzmann and Abbas 2015). A potential added benefit of this therapy could be the IL-2 mediated expansion of innate lymphoid cells 2 (ILC2) (Van Gool et al. 2014). ILC2 cells represent a rare subset of immune cells that likely exert atheroprotective functions via the secretion of type-2 cytokines such as IL-5 and IL-13 (Binder et al. 2004; Cardilo-Reis et al. 2012; Newland et al. 2017). Preclinical studies have shown that administration of recombinant IL-2 complexed with monoclonal antibodies against IL-2 increases the levels of T_{regs} and reduces atherosclerotic plaque burden in mice (Foks et al. 2011; Dinh et al. 2012; Proto et al. 2018).

The IL-2 analogue aldesleukin is currently approved for the treatment of advanced renal cell carcinoma and metastatic melanoma. In cardiovascular disease, low-dose IL-2 therapy is being evaluated in clinical trials with the aim to increase T_{reg} numbers, thereby limiting post-ischemic inflammatory responses and promoting myocardial healing in the setting of ischemic heart disease and acute coronary syndrome. The low-dose Interleukin-2 in patients with stable ischemic heart disease and acute coronary syndromes (LILACS) study is a randomized, placebo-controlled, double-blind phase I/IIa clinical trial that aims to assess the safety and tolerability of escalating doses of recombinant IL2, as well as its ability to alter T_{reg}, effector T cell and other immune cell populations (NCT03113773; expected completion date 06/2021; Zhao et al. 2018). Preliminary results indicate the treatment is well tolerated and induces robust increases in T_{regs} without affecting effector T cells. Interestingly, a dose-dependent reduction in B cells was also seen, which may have further beneficial effects on atherosclerosis (Zhao et al. 2020a). The subsequent low-dose IL-2 for the Reduction of Vascular Inflammation In Acute Coronary Syndromes (IVORY) phase II trial will assess changes in vascular inflammation in patients with acute coronary syndromes (NCT04241601; expected completion date 01/2024; Zhao et al. 2020b).

One limitation of low-dose IL-2 therapy are potential off-target effects, which include mild increases in NK cells and eosinophils (Zhao et al. 2020a). Furthermore, initially protective T_{regs} may undergo a phenotypic switch toward a proinflammatory T_H1-like phenotype with progressing disease in mice (Li et al. 2016; Butcher et al. 2016; Wolf et al. 2020). It remains to be addressed whether this switch can occur in humans.

3.1.2   Alternative Means to Expand Regulatory T Cells

Alternative options to harness the immunosuppressive capacity of T_{regs} is by ex vivo expansion of T_{regs}, where autologous naïve Tregs are isolated from the blood and expanded in vivo using a cytokine cocktail or antigenic stimuli. The adoptive transfer of T_{regs} has been tested in humans in the setting of transplantation (Trzonkowski et al. 2009; Brunstein et al. 2011; Di Ianni et al. 2011; Mathew et al. 2018) and type 1 diabetes (Marek-Trzonkowska et al. 2014), but not cardiovascular disease. Another way to expand T_{regs} is using tolerogenic non-FcR binding anti-CD3 antibodies such as teplizumab, which have shown promise in clinical trials for the treatment and prevention of type 1 diabetes (Herold et al. 2013, 2019). However, the effect of anti-CD3 on atherosclerosis has so far only been addressed in preclinical murine studies alone (Steffens et al. 2006; Kita et al. 2014) or in combination with IL-2 complex (Kasahara et al. 2014), where it was associated with reduced atherosclerosis progression or increased T_{reg}-dependent plaque regression.

3.2   Strategies Targeting B Cells and Humoral Immunity

B cells play a well-established role in the pathogenesis of atherosclerosis, with different B cell subsets having distinct effects on the pathogenesis of atherosclerosis (Sage et al.). B cells exert their function primarily via the generation of humoral immunity in the form of highly specific antibodies, but they also have the capacity to act as antigen-presenting cells to T cells and to secrete cytokines. The most abundant B cell type, follicular B2 cells, as well as B cell-derived germinal center B cells that arise upon interaction with follicular T helper cells, are generally considered proatherogenic (Clement et al. 2015; Tay et al. 2018; Centa et al. 2019; Bagchi-Chakraborty et al. 2019). In contrast, marginal zone B2 cells may protect from atherosclerosis by suppressing T follicular helper cells (Nus et al. 2017) and potentially via the secretion of atheroprotective IgM (Grasset et al. 2015). B1 cells, which can be further subdivided into B1a and B1b cells, represent an innate-like B cell type that can secrete germline-encoded natural antibodies that are typically of the IgM class in a T cell-independent manner. Their atheroprotective function, which is dependent on their ability to secrete IgM, is well-established in mice (Lewis et al. 2009; Kyaw et al. 2012; Rosenfeld et al. 2015; Gruber et al. 2016; Tsiantoulas et al.

2017). Other minor B cell subsets include B1 cell derived innate response activator (IRA) B cells that can promote atherosclerosis via the secretion of GM-CSF and the subsequent induction of Th1-differentiation (Hilgendorf et al. 2014) and IL-10-secreting B regulatory cells (Bregs), whose role in atherosclerosis remains controversial (Strom et al. 2015; Sage et al. 2015; Douna et al. 2019).

Although most evidence on the role of B cells in atherosclerosis stems from preclinical studies, B cells also appear to be key players in human cardiovascular disease. Patients suffering from autoimmune diseases such as systemic lupus erythematosus (SLE) and rheumatoid arthritis have an increased risk of cardiovascular disease independently of other risk factors (Hollan et al. 2013). A genome wide association study (GWAS) and transcriptome analysis of the Framingham Heart Study cohort recently revealed genes associated with B cell activation and differentiation to be the most deregulated genes between patients with and without coronary heart disease, suggesting a key function for B cells in modulating atherosclerosis (Huan et al. 2013). B cells are present in the vascular wall of human atherosclerotic plaques (Hamze et al. 2013; Kortelainen and Porvari 2014), where they may undergo antigen-driven clonal expansion ((Burioni et al. 2009). However, it is currently not clear how findings from murine B cell subsets and their functions in cardiovascular disease translate to human B cells. For example, although B1 cells are a well-described atheroprotective subset in mice, the nature and existence of the human equivalent of murine B1 cells remain controversial (Griffin et al. 2011; Upadhye et al. 2020). McNamara and colleagues have recently found a subset of CXCR4-expressing B1 cells that correlated with the levels of IgM directed against MDA-LDL and that inversely correlated with plaque volume and stenosis (Upadhye et al. 2019). Furthermore, increased levels of CD86-expressing CD19+ B cells were found to associate with an increased risk of stroke, while CD40-expressing CD19+ B cells showed a negative association (Mantani et al. 2014).

Overall, the aim of B cell-targeted therapy is to reduce the proatherogenic effects of follicular B2 cells, ideally while preserving atheroprotective IgM-secreting B1 cells (Porsch and Binder 2019). Currently, B cell depletion therapy is primarily used in the treatment of B cell malignancies and in the treatment of autoimmune diseases. An alternative therapeutic target is humoral immunity. On the one hand, putatively proatherogenic antibody classes such as IgE may be neutralized. On the other hand, passive and active immunization strategies may be harnessed to specifically target atherosclerosis-associated antigens such as oxidation-specific epitopes.

3.2.1 Anti-CD20 Mediated B Cell Depletion (Rituximab)

Given the strong evidence for a proatherogenic role of follicular B2 cells, the major B cell type in the body, some high-risk patients may benefit from their depletion. Indeed, preclinical studies suggest that anti-CD20 mediated B cell depletion could ameliorate the development of several cardiovascular pathologies including atherosclerosis (Ait-Oufella et al. 2010; Kyaw et al. 2010), myocardial infarction (Zouggari et al. 2013), myocardial infarction-accelerated atherosclerosis (Kyaw et al. 2021), abdominal aortic aneurysm (Schaheen et al. 2016), and hypertension (Chan et al. 2015).

In mice, anti-CD20 treatment preferentially depletes B2 cells, while preserving atheroprotective B1 cells (Hamaguchi et al. 2005). In line with that, anti-CD20 treatment of Ldlr$^{-/-}$ and Apoe$^{-/-}$ mice potently decreases B2 cell numbers and IgG levels and induces significant reductions in atherosclerosis (Ait-Oufella et al. 2010; Kyaw et al. 2010). In the context of acute myocardial infarction, Zouggari et al. could show that anti-CD20 mediated B2 cell depletion was associated with reduced inflammation and CCL7-mediated monocyte mobilization while improving cardiac function, reducing infarct size and fibrosis (Zouggari et al. 2013). Furthermore, anti-CD20 mediated B2 cell depletion significantly reduced myocardial infarction-accelerated atherosclerosis (Kyaw et al. 2021).

Rituximab is a CD20-targeted monoclonal antibody that has been approved for the treatment of some B cell malignancies (NHL, CLL) and autoimmune diseases (rheumatoid arthritis, granulomatosis with polyangiitis, pemphigus vulgaris) for more than two decades. Given its long clinical use, there is increasing evidence on its effect on cardiovascular parameters. Although a recent meta-analysis could not show an effect on short-term cardiovascular adverse events in randomized placebo-controlled trials involving rituximab, long-term follow-up data is lacking (Morris-Rosenfeld et al. 2014). Similarly, a study assessing the effects of biologic and conventional disease-modifying antirheumatic drugs on incident cardiovascular disease in rheumatoid arthritis patients with a mean follow-up of 4 years could find no beneficial effects of rituximab on cardiovascular risk, although the number of patients on rituximab in this study was relatively low (Ozen et al. 2020). However, several small human studies could show reductions in carotid intima-media thickness (Kerekes et al. 2009; Benucci et al. 2013; Novikova et al. 2016), improved flow-mediated dilation (Kerekes et al. 2009; Benucci et al. 2013; Hsue et al. 2014) and decreased arterial thickness (Provan et al. 2015) in patients receiving rituximab.

The Rituximab in patients with acute ST-elevation myocardial infarction (RITA-MI) trial was a prospective, open-label, single-arm phase I/IIa trial testing a single intravenous injection of rituximab in patients with STEMI within 48 h of symptom onset with a 6-month follow-up. Preliminary data suggests the treatment is well tolerated at all doses tested and resulted in a rapid, robust reduction of circulating B cells by a mean 96.3% that persisted throughout the follow-up period in a dose-dependent manner. Interestingly, immunoglobulin levels were not affected at that point. Additionally, clinical cardiac parameters including ejection fraction and (cardiac) biomarkers such as C-reactive protein (CRP) and B-type natriuretic peptide (BNP) were improved at follow-up (NCT03072199; Zhao et al. 2021). A subsequent phase IIb trial, RITA-MI 2, will be carried out in the form of a placebo-controlled randomized trial, which will allow further assessment of whether anti-CD20-mediated B cell depletion provides clinical benefits compared to placebo treatment (Zhao et al. 2021). The ICFEr-RITU2 trial is another phase II clinical trial assessing the safety of rituximab and the effect of rituximab on cardiac fibrotic remodeling in patients with chronic heart failure with reduced ejection fraction (HFrEF; NCT03332888; Sánchez-Trujillo et al. 2019). Furthermore, the risk of atherosclerotic cardiovascular disease was reduced in patients receiving rituximab following kidney transplantation (Kim et al. 2019), further supporting the potential of anti-CD20 mediated B cell depletion in the treatment of cardiovascular disease.

3.2.2   Other B Cell Depleting Antibodies

In addition to rituximab, there are emerging targets on B cells such as CD19 (inebilizumab, blinatumomab) and CD22 (inotuzumab ozogamicin) that are being targeted to deplete B cells in cancer and autoimmune disease (Hofmann et al. 2018). However, these receptors are also expressed on B1 cells, and may thus interfere with atheroprotective B cell effects. Additionally, there are therapies targeting receptors expressed on antibody-secreting plasma cells such as CD38 (daratumumab) and SLAMF7 (elotuzumab), which are used in the treatment of multiple myeloma (Radocha et al. 2021). However, the effect of such B cell depleting agents on cardiovascular disease has not been assessed directly.

3.2.3   B Cell Depletion via Targeting of the BAFF/APRIL System

An alternative means to deplete B cells is via the targeting of the B cell activating factor (BAFF)/A Proliferation-Inducing Ligand (APRIL) system, which is made up of soluble mediators that are required for B cell survival. BAFF appears to be particularly important in the survival of B2 cells (Rauch et al. 2009). In preclinical studies, BAFFR deficiency and anti-BAFFR mAb administration have been shown to robustly and selectively deplete B2 cells, thus decreasing atherosclerotic lesion formation (Kyaw et al. 2012; Sage et al. 2012) and improving recovery from myocardial infarction (Zouggari et al. 2013). However, there is also evidence that BAFF may promote Breg differentiation (Yang et al. 2010) and that BAFF overexpression might protect from atherosclerosis (Jackson et al. 2016). BAFF may also exert atheroprotective functions via inhibition of TLR9-IRF7-dependent proinflammatory signaling in macrophages. Indeed, BAFF neutralization promoted lesion formation in atherosclerosis-prone mice and increased lesional CXCL10 content, suggesting potential adverse effects of BAFF-targeted therapies (Tsiantoulas et al. 2018). Belimumab is a BAFF-targeting antibody that is approved for the treatment of SLE, which robustly depletes B cells, plasma cells, and immunoglobulins. So far, the effect of belimumab on cardiovascular disease has not been assessed in human patients.

3.2.4   IgE Neutralization (Omalizumab)

The primary effector function of B cells is the generation of humoral immunity in the form of antigen-specific antibodies. There is ample epidemiological and preclinical experimental evidence suggesting an important role for humoral immunity and different antibody classes in atherosclerosis (Khamis et al. 2016; Sage et al. 2017; Tay et al. 2018; Centa et al. 2019; van den Berg et al. 2019). IgE is a class-switched, typically follicular B cell-derived antibody class that is associated with allergic responses. It can trigger proinflammatory responses via interaction with FcεRI receptors on mast cells, basophils, macrophages, and vascular cells (Wu and Zarrin 2014). Plasma IgE levels correlate with coronary heart disease in humans (Kounis and Hahalis 2016). Interestingly, patients suffering from asthma are also at increased risk for cardiovascular disease (Tattersall et al. 2015). Preclinical studies suggest a proatherogenic role for IgE in Apoe$^{-/-}$ and Ldlr$^{-/-}$ mice (Wang et al. 2011; Wezel et al. 2015; Tsiantoulas et al. 2017; Zhang et al. 2020). Antibody-mediated IgE neutralization was found to reduce atherosclerotic lesion formation in Ldlr$^{-/-}$ mice in the context of secreted IgM deficiency (Tsiantoulas et al. 2017).

Omalizumab is an IgE-neutralizing antibody that interferes with the interaction of IgE and its receptors, resulting in the reduction of IgE levels. It is approved for the treatment of severe asthma and chronic idiopathic urticaria. Although a clinical trial suggested potential cardiovascular side effects of omalizumab treatment, this clinical trial was biased by the dramatically increased cardiovascular disease burden at baseline in the patients receiving omalizumab (Iribarren et al. 2017a). A subsequent pooled analysis of randomized, double-blind placebo-controlled trials involving omalizumab did not show an increased cardiovascular risk (Iribarren et al. 2017b) Therefore, the effect of IgE neutralization on cardiovascular disease remains to be evaluated in a clinical trial setting.

3.3 Strategies Targeting the Interaction Between T Cells and Antigen-Presenting Cells

Efficient T cell activation is crucially dependent on the engagement of co-stimulatory pathways. It has been hypothesized that T cells require two signals in order to become fully activated, one being antigen-presentation via MHC-molecules, the other being co-stimulation by receptors expressed on the surface of antigen-presenting cells such as dendritic cells, macrophages, and B cells. Inhibition of such co-stimulatory pathways may therefore interfere with the activation, proliferation, and differentiation of T cells, which may have beneficial effects on atherosclerosis. In contrast, targeting co-inhibitory pathways with the use of immune checkpoint inhibitors in cancer therapy may enhance T cell activity, which could have detrimental effects on cardiovascular disease.

3.3.1 Targeting Co-stimulatory Pathways

Abatacept
CD80 (B7-1) and CD86 (B7-2) are expressed on activated antigen-presenting cells, where they can interact with both the co-stimulatory CD28 receptor and the inhibitory CTLA4 receptor on T cells (Sharpe and Freeman 2002).

Abatacept is a recombinant biologic consisting of the Ig-domain of CTLA4 and a human IgG1 Fc region. It binds CD80/CD86 with high affinity, thus blocking the interaction of CD80/CD86 with the co-stimulatory CD28 receptor and activation of T cells. Preclinical studies suggest a primarily proatherogenic role for CD80/CD86. However, CD80/CD86 may also be required for the efficient induction of T$_{regs}$ (Ait-Oufella et al. 2006). However, abatacept was shown to reduce atherosclerosis in different murine models of atherosclerosis (Ma et al. 2013; Ewing et al. 2013).

Abatacept is currently clinically approved for the treatment of rheumatoid, juvenile idiopathic, and psoriatic arthritis, while the highly similar belatacept is used in patients receiving kidney transplants. Some clinical trials suggest slightly reduced cardiovascular disease risk in patients receiving abatacept compared to TNF inhibitors (Zhang et al. 2016; Kang et al. 2018; Jin et al. 2018; Hsieh et al. 2020).

CD40-CD40L

Another important co-stimulatory signal is provided by the CD40-CD40L interaction, a member of the tumor necrosis factor receptor (TNFR) family. Targeting this pathway reduced atherosclerosis in mice (Lutgens et al. 2000, 2010; Schönbeck et al. 2000), but not in others (Zirlik et al. 2007). Additionally, CD40-signaling intermediates, the so-called TNF-receptor associated factors (TRAFs), have been targeted successfully by a small molecule inhibitor in mouse models (Lutgens et al. 2010; Chatzigeorgiou et al. 2014). Importantly, no immunosuppressive side effects were observed with this inhibitor (Seijkens et al. 2018) and a newly developed delivery system, linking a TRAF6 inhibitor to a HDL particle, was found to be safe in non-human primates (Lameijer et al. 2018). Based on these initial findings, further assessment of CD40-TRAF inhibition needs to be carried out to verify its role in human atherosclerosis. While CD40-CD40L targeting therapeutics have not been approved for clinical use yet, several antagonistic antibodies are currently being evaluated in clinical trials for the treatment of inflammatory conditions (Karnell et al. 2019).

Co-inhibitory Pathways

Recent years have seen the emergence of cancer immunotherapy and the widespread use of immune checkpoint inhibitors. Immune checkpoint inhibitors are used clinically with the aim to enhance anti-tumor immunity by T cells. Many of these drugs target pathways that have been described to play a proatherogenic role. Given the prominent role of effector T cells and these immunomodulatory pathways in cardiovascular disease, such T cell-simulating therapy is expected to have detrimental effects on atherosclerosis (Simons et al. 2019). Importantly, a recent study by Drobni et al. could demonstrate a threefold increased risk for cardiovascular events and more than threefold increased aortic plaque volumes in patients receiving immune checkpoint inhibitor therapy (Drobni et al. 2020). Additionally, atherosclerotic mice which underwent short-term check point inhibition therapy developed a more vulnerable, proinflammatory atherosclerotic phenotype due to an access of effector T cells, endothelial activation, and increased CD8+ T cell recruitment (Poels et al. 2020). This study highlights the importance of cardiovascular risk awareness in cancer patients receiving checkpoint inhibitor immunotherapy.

Vaccination Strategies

Vaccines represent an attractive future therapeutic avenue, as they may provide a durable, antigen-specific approach, thus limiting adverse effects on the host immune response. However, vaccination approaches remain challenging, as they require the targeting of specific self-antigens that may trigger unwanted autoimmune responses.

Unlike traditional vaccines that aim at enhancing the activity of the adaptive immune system against pathogens, the idea behind immunization strategies against atherosclerosis is either to induce immunological tolerance or to neutralize atherosclerosis-specific antigens without inducing a considerable inflammatory response. Additionally, passive immunization strategies offer the opportunity to directly administer antibodies that may modulate inflammatory and metabolic pathogenic mechanisms in atherosclerosis, although their effect is transient.

3.3.2   Immunization Against LDL-Related Antigens

LDL and particularly its modified forms represent well-established immunogenic epitopes that have previously been shown to play a role in atherosclerosis and to be recognized by various components of the immune system. LDL can undergo oxidative modifications that result in the formation of a variety of lipid peroxidation-derived oxidation-specific epitopes (OSE), including phosphorylcholine (PC)-containing oxidized phospholipids and malondialdehyde (MDA), which are highly immunogenic and trigger inflammation in the vascular wall. Notably, OSE are targeted by specific circulating antibodies that have been shown to neutralize their proinflammatory activities. Thus, several experimental studies have addressed the effect of immunization with modified LDL or parts of its main lipoprotein component, Apolipoprotein B (ApoB).

Palinski and colleagues were able to show that immunization with malondialdehyde (MDA)-modified LDL reduced atherogenesis in LDLR-deficient rabbits (Palinski et al. 1995), which was further confirmed by several groups using modified LDL in rabbits (Ameli et al. 1996; Nilsson et al. 1997; Asgary et al. 2007) and mice (George et al. 1998; Freigang et al. 1998; Zhou et al. 2001; Binder et al. 2004; Van Puijvelde et al. 2006). Specific advanced MDA adducts have been shown to be particularly immunogenic, which may further impact the effect of vaccination on atherogenesis (Gonen et al. 2014).

Although the mechanisms responsible for the atheroprotective effects observed in these studies have not been fully elucidated, several pathways play a role, including the induction of neutralizing antibodies that interfere with the proinflammatory effects of these OSE. However, even though several preclinical studies have shown a prominent induction of humoral immunity upon immunization (George et al. 1998; Freigang et al. 1998; Zhou et al. 2001; Binder et al. 2004) and the inverse association between plaque size and antibody levels against OSEs (Zhou et al. 2001), it is currently not clear how these findings translate to the clinic.

Passive immunization via administration of antibodies against OSE has shown promise in preclinical models (Schiopu et al. 2004, 2007; Poulsen et al. 2016). The phase II GLACIER trial failed to show reduced vascular inflammation following administration of a recombinant IgG1 antibody against MDA-modified ApoB100 (Lehrer-Graiwer et al. 2015). However, the relatively short follow-up period, the use of FDG-PET instead of coronary artery assessments, and the patient selection criteria may have been a limitation of this study. Given the proposed atheroprotective role of IgM against oxidation-specific epitopes, it will be interesting to assess the effect of passive administration of IgM antibodies (or single chain and other class switch variants thereof) on human atherosclerosis in the future. One attractive candidate is the IgM antibody E06, which binds the phosphocholine (PC) headgroup of oxidized phospholipids (oxPLs), thus blocking the proinflammatory properties of oxPL and the uptake of oxLDL by macrophages (Shaw et al. 2000; Que et al. 2018).

3.3.3 Tolerogenic Vaccination

Another proposed atheroprotective mechanism is tolerization, which is associated with the induction of immunosuppressive T_{regs} that may limit inflammation via IL10, TGFβ and the suppression of T effector functions. Several preclinical studies found the reduction in atherosclerotic lesion formation upon administration of modified LDL or ApoB100-derived peptides to be associated with significant increases in T_{reg} numbers (Fredrikson et al. 2008; Wigren et al. 2011; Herbin et al. 2012).

In addition to lipid-derived antigens, peptide-based vaccination strategies based on ApoB100-derived peptides, many of which are recognized by autoantibodies from sera of patients with coronary heart disease, have also shown promise in preclinical studies (Fredrikson et al. 2003). Administration of several ApoB100 peptides, including P210, P45, P74, (Fredrikson et al. 2003, 2005, 2008; Dunér et al. 2021), P2 (Chyu et al. 2005), P3 (Tse et al. 2013), P18 (Kimura et al. 2018), P265 and P295 (Gisterå et al. 2017), has been shown to reduce lesion formation in murine atherosclerosis

However, several challenges remain before the clinical implementation of inflammation-restraining tolerogenic T cell vaccine is possible. Given that the interaction of TCRs with their cognate peptide is dependent on the efficient presentation on MHC type II molecules, HLA types need to be matched. The necessity for HLA matching has resulted in tetramer-based approaches to allow the identification of antigen-specific T cell populations (Kimura et al. 2017, 2018). The considerable heterogeneity of the human HLA locus and the need to adapt peptides to individual HLA types present a major challenge in the design of T-cell based peptide vaccines. Furthermore, the efficient induction of tolerance critically depends on dose, choice of adjuvant, and the route of administration (Van Puijvelde et al. 2006, 2007; Klingenberg et al. 2010; Czerkinsky and Holmgren 2012).

3.3.4 Immunization Against Pathogen-Derived Antigens

Some studies suggest that vaccination against common diseases such as influenza and pneumonia can reduce cardiovascular risk (Ren et al. 2015; Barnes et al. 2015). A double-blind randomized placebo-controlled clinical trial (Influenza Vaccination After Myocardial Infarction, IAMI; NCT02831608) is currently underway to assess the effect of influenza vaccination on cardiovascular outcomes in patients with preexisting cardiovascular disease (Fröbert et al. 2017). While it cannot be excluded that inflammation associated with infections may affect the plaque, the potential beneficial effect of pneumococcal vaccination may be due to its ability to induce antibodies that react with the oxidation-specific epitope, PC (Binder et al. 2003; Caligiuri et al. 2007). Initial studies have evaluated the consequences of the molecular mimicry between oxidized LDL and the CPS of pneumococci and demonstrated that immunization of $Ldlr^{-/-}$ mice with pneumococcal extracts induced PC-specific

IgM and reduced lesion formation (Binder et al. 2003). A similar effect has been observed when Apoe$^{-/-}$ mice were immunized with PC-conjugated KLH (Caligiuri et al. 2007).

These studies suggested the possibility that existing pneumococcal vaccines could be repurposed to trigger anti-atherogenic immunity in humans. However, PC is not a major antigenic component of pneumococcal vaccines due to poor immunogenicity, and several studies indicated that unlike natural infections vaccination with existing vaccines does not trigger robust anti-OxLDL antibody titers. Small-scale clinical trials of the 13-valent conjugated pneumococcal vaccine Prevnar-13 did not find an induction of antibodies against oxLDL or phosphorylcholine in a small cohort of patients with metabolic diseases (Grievink et al. 2020; Shiri-Sverdlov et al. 2021), which may be due to the fact that PC is only a minimal constituent of Prevnar-13. The AUSPICE trial to assess the effect of the pneumococcal polysaccharide vaccine Pneumovax 23 on antibody levels against oxidation-specific epitopes and several cardiovascular disease markers in 4725 patients is currently underway (ACTRN12615000536561; Ren et al. 2016).

Heat shock proteins (HSPs) represent a group of highly conserved stress-associated proteins that can act as autoantigens either due to cross-reactivity against microbial-derived HSPs or following their expression during endothelial injury (Wick et al. 2014). Preclinical studies show that administration of microbial HSPs or HSP-related peptides protects mice from atherosclerosis (Maron et al. 2002; Van Puijvelde et al. 2007; Jing et al. 2011; Klingenberg et al. 2012; Grundtman et al. 2015). The atheroprotective mechanism may involve induction of cross-reactive antibodies against MDA-LDL (Kyrklund et al. 2020) or tolerogenic activation of T_{regs} (Van Puijvelde et al. 2007).

4 Conclusion

The immune system represents a versatile and essential part of human homeostasis which harbors great potential for the treatment and prevention of atherosclerosis. While the identification of relevant therapeutic targets remains challenging, it has greatly improved over the last decade as various anti-inflammatory and immuno-modulatory approaches have been studied. These range from modulation of the innate immune system by interfering with cytokines and their production, chemokines and general inflammation, to the adaptive immune system where B cells, T cells, their interaction and their potential in immunization are utilized. While these approaches have proven promising in multiple preclinical studies, with some translation into human trials, a wider application and breakthrough into the clinic is yet to occur. One factor which slows the translation of preclinical findings into the clinic is the immune system's essential role in fighting infections. Unspecific modulation or downregulation of the immune system can lead to unwanted side effects such as increased infections. It is thus important to conduct further research in order to harvest the positive potential while minimizing side effects. Research into potential biomarkers such as hsCRP and IL-6 – but with even greater specificity for the atherogenic disease process – represents an important step toward solving this issue, as they allow the identification of patients who are most likely benefiting from immunomodulatory treatment. Moreover, highly specific biomarkers would also be needed to monitor a successful response to anti-inflammatory or immunomodulatory treatments. Additionally, further research into the immune system's role in human atherosclerosis, combined with large-scale clinical trials will pave the way for immunomodulatory treatments to become a realistic addition to standard atherosclerosis therapies.

References

Abbate A, Kontos MC, Grizzard JD et al (2010) Interleukin-1 blockade with Anakinra to prevent adverse cardiac remodeling after acute myocardial infarction (Virginia Commonwealth University Anakinra remodeling trial [VCU-ART] pilot study). AJC 105:1371–1377. https://doi.org/10.1016/j.amjcard.2009.12.059

Abbate A, Van Tassell BW, Biondi-Zoccai G et al (2013) Effects of interleukin-1 blockade with anakinra on adverse cardiac remodeling and heart failure after acute myocardial infarction [from the Virginia commonwealth university-anakinra remodeling trial (2) (vcu-art 2) pilot study]. Am J Cardiol 111:1394–1400. https://doi.org/10.1016/j.amjcard.2013.01.287

Abbate A, Trankle CR, Buckley LF et al (2020) Interleukin-1 blockade inhibits the acute inflammatory response in patients with ST-segment-elevation myocardial infarction. J Am Heart Assoc 9:e014941. https://doi.org/10.1161/JAHA.119.014941

Ait-Oufella H, Salomon BL, Potteaux S et al (2006) Natural regulatory T cells control the development of atherosclerosis in mice. Nat Med 12:178–180. https://doi.org/10.1038/nm1343

Ait-Oufella H, Herbin O, Bouaziz J-D et al (2010) B cell depletion reduces the development of atherosclerosis in mice. J Exp Med 207:1579–1587. https://doi.org/10.1084/jem.20100155

Ameli S, Hultgårdh-Nilsson A, Regnström J et al (1996) Effect of immunization with homologous LDL and oxidized LDL on early atherosclerosis in hypercholesterolemic rabbits. Arterioscler Thromb Vasc Biol 16:1074–1079. https://doi.org/10.1161/01.ATV.16.8.1074

Ammirati E, Cianflone D, Banfi M et al (2010) Circulating CD4+CD25hiCD127lo regulatory T-cell levels do not reflect the extent or severity of carotid and coronary atherosclerosis. Arterioscler Thromb Vasc Biol 30:1832–1841. https://doi.org/10.1161/ATVBAHA.110.206813

Asgary S, Saberi SA, Azampanah S (2007) Effect of immunization against ox-LDL with two different antigens on formation and development of atherosclerosis. Lipids Health Dis 6:32. https://doi.org/10.1186/1476-511X-6-32

Avgerinou G, Tousoulis D, Siasos G et al (2011) Anti-tumor necrosis factor alpha treatment with adalimumab improves significantly endothelial function and decreases inflammatory process in patients with chronic psoriasis. Int J Cardiol 151:382–383. https://doi.org/10.1016/j.ijcard.2011.06.112

Avina-Zubieta JA, Thomas J, Sadatsafavi M et al (2012) Risk of incident cardiovascular events in patients with rheumatoid arthritis: a meta-analysis of observational studies. Ann Rheum Dis 71:1524–1529. https://doi.org/10.1136/annrheumdis-2011-200726

Bäck M, Yurdagul A, Tabas I et al (2019) Inflammation and its resolution in atherosclerosis: mediators and therapeutic opportunities. Nat Rev Cardiol 16:389–406

Bagchi-Chakraborty J, Francis A, Bray T et al (2019) B cell Fcγ receptor IIb modulates atherosclerosis in male and female mice by controlling adaptive germinal center and innate B1-cell responses. Arterioscler Thromb Vasc Biol 39:1379. https://doi.org/10.1161/ATVBAHA.118.312272

Barnabe C, Martin B-J, Ghali WA (2011) Systematic review and meta-analysis: anti-tumor necrosis factor α therapy and cardiovascular events in rheumatoid arthritis. Arthritis Care Res (Hoboken) 63:522–529. https://doi.org/10.1002/acr.20371

Barnes M, Heywood AE, Mahimbo A et al (2015) Acute myocardial infarction and influenza: a meta-analysis of case-control studies. Heart 101:1738–1747. https://doi.org/10.1136/heartjnl-2015-307691

Bauernfeind F, Niepmann S, Knolle PA, Hornung V (2016) Aging-associated TNF production primes Inflammasome activation and NLRP3-related metabolic disturbances. J Immunol 197:2900–2908. https://doi.org/10.4049/jimmunol.1501336

Benucci M, Saviola G, Manfredi M et al (2013) Factors correlated with improvement of endothelial dysfunction during rituximab therapy in patients with rheumatoid arthritis. Biol Theory 7:69–75. https://doi.org/10.2147/BTT.S39182

Bhaskar V, Yin J, Mirza AM et al (2011) Monoclonal antibodies targeting IL-1 beta reduce biomarkers of atherosclerosis in vitro and inhibit atherosclerotic plaque formation in apolipoprotein E-deficient mice. Atherosclerosis 216:313–320. https://doi.org/10.1016/j.atherosclerosis.2011.02.026

Biasucci LM, Pedicino D, Liuzzo G (2020) Promises and challenges of targeting inflammation to treat cardiovascular disease: the post-CANTOS era. Eur Heart J 41:2164–2167. https://doi.org/10.1093/eurheartj/ehz586

Binder CJ, Hörkkö S, Dewan A et al (2003) Pneumococcal vaccination decreases atherosclerotic lesion formation: molecular mimicry between Streptococcus pneumoniae and oxidized LDL. Nat Med 9:736–743. https://doi.org/10.1038/nm876

Binder CJ, Hartvigsen K, Chang M-K et al (2004) IL-5 links adaptive and natural immunity specific for epitopes of oxidized LDL and protects from atherosclerosis. J Clin Invest 114:427–437. https://doi.org/10.1172/JCI20479

Bissonnette R, Harel F, Krueger JG et al (2017) TNF-alpha; antagonist and vascular inflammation in patients with psoriasis vulgaris: a randomized placebo-controlled study. J Invest Dermatol 137:1638. https://doi.org/10.1016/j.jid.2017.02.977

Bobryshev YV (2006) Monocyte recruitment and foam cell formation in atherosclerosis. Micron 37:208–222

Borén J, John Chapman M, Krauss RM et al (2020) Low-density lipoproteins cause atherosclerotic cardiovascular disease: pathophysiological, genetic, and therapeutic insights: a consensus statement from the European atherosclerosis society consensus panel. Eur Heart J 41:2313–2330

Boring L, Gosling J, Cleary M, Charo IF (1998) Decreased lesion formation in CCR2(−/−) mice reveals a role for chemokines in the initiation of atherosclerosis. Nature 394:894–897. https://doi.org/10.1038/29788

Bouabdallaoui N, Tardif JC, Waters DD et al (2020) Time-to-treatment initiation of colchicine and cardiovascular outcomes after myocardial infarction in the colchicine cardiovascular outcomes trial (COLCOT). Eur Heart J 41:4092–4099. https://doi.org/10.1093/eurheartj/ehaa659

Boyman O, Sprent J (2012) The role of interleukin-2 during homeostasis and activation of the immune system. Nat Rev Immunol 12:180–190

Braunersreuther V, Zernecke A, Arnaud C et al (2007) Ccr5 but not Ccr1 deficiency reduces development of diet-induced atherosclerosis in mice. Arterioscler Thromb Vasc Biol 27:373–379. https://doi.org/10.1161/01.ATV.0000253886.44609.ae

Brunstein CG, Miller JS, Cao Q et al (2011) Infusion of ex vivo expanded T regulatory cells in adults transplanted with umbilical cord blood: safety profile and detection kinetics. Blood 117:1061–1070. https://doi.org/10.1182/blood-2010-07-293795

Buono C, Binder CJ, Stavrakis G et al (2005) T-bet deficiency reduces atherosclerosis and alters plaque antigen-specific immune responses. Arterioscler Thromb Vasc Biol 39(7):1379–1389

Burioni R, Canducci F, Saita D et al (2009) Antigen-driven evolution of B lymphocytes in coronary atherosclerotic plaques. J Immunol 183:2537–2544. https://doi.org/10.4049/jimmunol.0901076

Burmester GR, Gordon KB, Rosenbaum JT et al (2020) Long-term safety of adalimumab in 29,967 adult patients from global clinical trials across multiple indications: an updated analysis. Adv Ther 37:364–380. https://doi.org/10.1007/s12325-019-01145-8

Butcher MJ, Filipowicz AR, Waseem TC et al (2016) Atherosclerosis-driven Treg plasticity results in formation of a dysfunctional subset of plastic IFNγ+ Th1/Tregs. Circ Res 119:1190–1203. https://doi.org/10.1161/CIRCRESAHA.116.309764

Caligiuri G, Khallou-Laschet J, Vandaele M et al (2007) Phosphorylcholine-targeting immunization reduces atherosclerosis. J Am Coll Cardiol 50:540–546. https://doi.org/10.1016/J.JACC.2006.11.054

Canault M, Peiretti F, Kopp F et al (2006) The TNF alpha converting enzyme (TACE/ADAM17) is expressed in the atherosclerotic lesions of apolipoprotein E-deficient mice: possible contribution to elevated plasma levels of soluble TNF alpha receptors. Atherosclerosis 187:82–91. https://doi.org/10.1016/j.atherosclerosis.2005.08.031

Cardilo-Reis L, Gruber S, Schreier SM et al (2012) Interleukin-13 protects from atherosclerosis and modulates plaque composition by skewing the macrophage phenotype. EMBO Mol Med 4:1072–1086. https://doi.org/10.1002/emmm.201201374

Centa M, Jin H, Hofste L et al (2019) Germinal center-derived antibodies promote atherosclerosis plaque size and stability. Circulation 139:2466. https://doi.org/10.1161/CIRCULATIONAHA.118.038534

Chan CT, Sobey CG, Lieu M et al (2015) Obligatory role for B cells in the development of angiotensin II-dependent hypertension. Hypertension 66:1023–1033. https://doi.org/10.1161/HYPERTENSIONAHA.115.05779

Chatzigeorgiou A, Seijkens T, Zarzycka B et al (2014) Blocking CD40-TRAF6 signaling is a therapeutic target in obesity-associated insulin resistance. Proc Natl Acad Sci U S A 111:2686–2691. https://doi.org/10.1073/pnas.1400419111

Chen S, Wang Y, Pan Y et al (2020) Novel role for Tranilast in regulating NLRP3 ubiquitination, vascular inflammation, and atherosclerosis. J Am Heart Assoc 9:e015513. https://doi.org/10.1161/JAHA.119.015513

Cheng X, Yu X, Ding Y et al (2008) The Th17/Treg imbalance in patients with acute coronary syndrome. Clin Immunol 127:89–97. https://doi.org/10.1016/J.CLIM.2008.01.009

Choi HK, Hernán MA, Seeger JD et al (2002) Methotrexate and mortality in patients with rheumatoid arthritis: a prospective study. Lancet 359:1173–1177. https://doi.org/10.1016/S0140-6736(02)08213-2

Chyu KY, Zhao X, Reyes OS et al (2005) Immunization using an Apo B-100 related epitope reduces atherosclerosis and plaque inflammation in hypercholesterolemic apo E (−/−) mice. Biochem Biophys Res Commun 338:1982–1989. https://doi.org/10.1016/j.bbrc.2005.10.141

Cipriani S, Francisci D, Mencarelli A et al (2013) Efficacy of the CCR5 antagonist maraviroc in reducing early, ritonavir-induced atherogenesis and advanced plaque progression in mice. Circulation 127:2114–2124. https://doi.org/10.1161/CIRCULATIONAHA.113.001278

Clarke MCH, Talib S, Figg NL, Bennett MR (2010) Vascular smooth muscle cell apoptosis induces interleukin-1-directed inflammation: effects of hyperlipidemia-mediated inhibition of phagocytosis. Circ Res 106:363–372. https://doi.org/10.1161/CIRCRESAHA.109.208389

Clement M, Guedj K, Andreata F et al (2015) Control of the T follicular helper–germinal center B-cell Axis by CD8 + regulatory T cells limits atherosclerosis and tertiary lymphoid organ development. Circulation 131:560–570. https://doi.org/10.1161/CIRCULATIONAHA.114.010988

Coll RC, Robertson AAB, Chae JJ et al (2015) A small-molecule inhibitor of the NLRP3 inflammasome for the treatment of inflammatory diseases. Nat Med 21:248–257. https://doi.org/10.1038/nm.3806

Combadière C, Potteaux S, Rodero M et al (2008) Combined inhibition of CCL2, CX3CR1, and CCR5 abrogates Ly6Chi and Ly6Clo monocytosis and almost abolishes atherosclerosis in hypercholesterolemic mice. Circulation 117:1649–1657. https://doi.org/10.1161/CIRCULATIONAHA.107.745091

Curtis JR, John A, Baser O (2012) Dyslipidemia and changes in lipid profiles associated with rheumatoid arthritis and initiation of anti-tumor necrosis factor therapy. Arthritis Care Res 64:1282–1291. https://doi.org/10.1002/acr.21693

Czerkinsky C, Holmgren J (2012) Mucosal delivery routes for optimal immunization: targeting immunity to the right tissues. Curr Top Microbiol Immunol 354:1–18

Danesh J, Kaptoge S, Mann AG et al (2008) Long-term interleukin-6 levels and subsequent risk of coronary heart disease: two new prospective studies and a systematic review. PLoS Med 5:0600–0610. https://doi.org/10.1371/journal.pmed.0050078

Del Porto F, Laganà B, Lai S et al (2007) Response to anti-tumour necrosis factor alpha blockade is associated with reduction of carotid intima-media thickness in patients with active rheumatoid arthritis. Rheumatology 46:1111–1115. https://doi.org/10.1093/rheumatology/kem089

Devlin CM, Kuriakose G, Hirsch E, Tabas I (2002) Genetic alterations of IL-1 receptor antagonist in mice affect plasma cholesterol level and foam cell lesion size. Proc Natl Acad Sci U S A 99:6280–6285. https://doi.org/10.1073/pnas.092324399

Dewberry R, Holden H, Crossman D, Francis S (2000) Interleukin-1 receptor antagonist expression in human endothelial cells and atherosclerosis. Arterioscler Thromb Vasc Biol 20:2394–2400. https://doi.org/10.1161/01.ATV.20.11.2394

Di Ianni M, Falzetti F, Carotti A et al (2011) Tregs prevent GVHD and promote immune reconstitution in HLA-haploidentical transplantation. Blood 117:3921–3928. https://doi.org/10.1182/blood-2010-10-311894

Dinh TN, Kyaw TS, Kanellakis P et al (2012) Cytokine therapy with interleukin-2/anti-interleukin-2 monoclonal antibody complexes expands CD4+CD25+Foxp3+ regulatory T cells and attenuates development and progression of atherosclerosis. Circulation 126:1256–1266. https://doi.org/10.1161/CIRCULATIONAHA.112.099044

Douna H, Amersfoort J, Schaftenaar FH et al (2019) Bidirectional effects of IL-10+ regulatory B cells in Ldlr−/− mice. Atherosclerosis 280:118–125. https://doi.org/10.1016/J.ATHEROSCLEROSIS.2018.11.019

Drobni ZD, Alvi RM, Taron J et al (2020) Association between immune checkpoint inhibitors with cardiovascular events and atherosclerotic plaque. Circulation 142:2299–2311. https://doi.org/10.1161/CIRCULATIONAHA.120.049981

Duewell P, Kono H, Rayner KJ et al (2010) NLRP3 inflammasomes are required for atherogenesis and activated by cholesterol crystals. Nature 464:1357–1361. https://doi.org/10.1038/nature08938

Dunér P, Mattisson IY, Fogelstrand P et al (2021) Antibodies against apo B100 peptide 210 inhibit atherosclerosis in apoE−/− mice. Sci Rep 11:9022. https://doi.org/10.1038/s41598-021-88430-1

Elhage R, Maret A, Pieraggi MT et al (1998) Differential effects of interleukin-1 receptor antagonist and tumor necrosis factor binding protein on fatty-streak formation in apolipoprotein E-deficient mice. Circulation 97:242–244. https://doi.org/10.1161/01.CIR.97.3.242

Elhage R, Clamens S, Besnard S et al (2001) Involvement of interleukin-6 in atherosclerosis but not in the prevention of fatty streak formation by 17β-estradiol in apolipoprotein E-deficient mice. Atherosclerosis 156:315–320. https://doi.org/10.1016/S0021-9150(00)00682-1

Everett BM, Pradhan AD, Solomon DH et al (2013) Rationale and design of the cardiovascular inflammation reduction trial: a test of the inflammatory hypothesis of atherothrombosis. Am Heart J 166:199–207. https://doi.org/10.1016/j.ahj.2013.03.018

Ewing MM, Karper JC, Abdul S et al (2013) T-cell co-stimulation by CD28–CD80/86 and its negative regulator CTLA-4 strongly influence accelerated atherosclerosis development. Int J Cardiol 168:1965–1974. https://doi.org/10.1016/J.IJCARD.2012.12.085

Ference BA, Ginsberg HN, Graham I et al (2017) Low-density lipoproteins cause atherosclerotic cardiovascular disease. 1. Evidence from genetic, epidemiologic, and clinical studies. A consensus statement from the European Atherosclerosis Society Consensus Panel. Eur Heart J 38:2459–2472. https://doi.org/10.1093/eurheartj/ehx144

Fisman EZ, Benderly M, Esper RJ et al (2006) Interleukin-6 and the risk of future cardiovascular events in patients with angina pectoris and/or healed myocardial infarction. Am J Cardiol 98:14–18. https://doi.org/10.1016/j.amjcard.2006.01.045

Foks AC, Frodermann V, ter Borg M et al (2011) Differential effects of regulatory T cells on the initiation and regression of atherosclerosis. Atherosclerosis 218:53–60. https://doi.org/10.1016/j.atherosclerosis.2011.04.029

Foks AC, Lichtman AH, Kuiper J (2015) Treating atherosclerosis with regulatory T cells. Arterioscler Thromb Vasc Biol 35:280–287. https://doi.org/10.1161/ATVBAHA.114.303568

França CN, Izar MCO, Hortêncio MNS et al (2017) Monocyte subtypes and the CCR2 chemokine receptor in cardiovascular disease. Clin Sci 131:1215–1224

Francisci D, Pirro M, Schiaroli E et al (2019) Maraviroc intensification modulates atherosclerotic progression in HIV-suppressed patients at high cardiovascular risk. A randomized, crossover pilot study. Open Forum Infect Dis 6:1–7. https://doi.org/10.1093/ofid/ofz112

Fredrikson GN, Söderberg I, Lindholm M et al (2003) Inhibition of atherosclerosis in ApoE-null mice by immunization with ApoB-100 peptide sequences. Arterioscler Thromb Vasc Biol 23:879–884. https://doi.org/10.1161/01.ATV.0000067937.93716.DB

Fredrikson GN, Andersson L, Söderberg I et al (2005) Atheroprotective immunization with MDA-modified apo B-100 peptide sequences is associated with activation of Th2 specific antibody expression. Autoimmunity 38:171–179. https://doi.org/10.1080/08916930500050525

Fredrikson GN, Björkbacka H, Söderberg I et al (2008) Treatment with apo B peptide vaccines inhibits atherosclerosis in human apo B-100 transgenic mice without inducing an increase in peptide-specific antibodies. J Intern Med 264:563–570. https://doi.org/10.1111/j.1365-2796.2008.01995.x

Freigang S, Hörkkö S, Miller E et al (1998) Immunization of LDL receptor–deficient mice with homologous malondialdehyde-modified and native LDL reduces progression of atherosclerosis by mechanisms other than induction of high titers of antibodies to oxidative neoepitopes. Arterioscler Thromb Vasc Biol 18:1972–1982. https://doi.org/10.1161/01.ATV.18.12.1972

Freigang S, Ampenberger F, Weiss A et al (2013) Fatty acid-induced mitochondrial uncoupling elicits inflammasome-independent IL-1α and sterile vascular inflammation in atherosclerosis. Nat Immunol 14:1045–1053. https://doi.org/10.1038/ni.2704

Freitag D, Butterworth AS, Willeit P et al (2015) Cardiometabolic effects of genetic upregulation of the interleukin 1 receptor antagonist: a Mendelian randomisation analysis. Lancet Diabetes Endocrinol 3:243–253. https://doi.org/10.1016/S2213-8587(15)00034-0

Fröbert O, Götberg M, Angerås O et al (2017) Design and rationale for the influenza vaccination after myocardial infarction (IAMI) trial. A registry-based randomized clinical trial. Am Heart J 189:94–102. https://doi.org/10.1016/j.ahj.2017.04.003

Galea J, Armstrong J, Gadsdon P et al (1996) Interleukin-1β in coronary arteries of patients with ischemic heart disease. Arterioscler Thromb Vasc Biol 16:1000–1006. https://doi.org/10.1161/01.ATV.16.8.1000

Gardner SE, Humphry M, Bennett MR, Clarke MCH (2015) Senescent vascular smooth muscle cells drive inflammation through an interleukin-1α-dependent senescence-associated secretory phenotype. Arterioscler Thromb Vasc Biol 35:1963–1974. https://doi.org/10.1161/ATVBAHA.115.305896

George J, Afek A, Gilburd B et al (1998) Hyperimmunization of apo-E-deficient mice with homologous malondialdehyde low-density lipoprotein suppresses early atherogenesis. Atherosclerosis 138:147–152. https://doi.org/10.1016/S0021-9150(98)00015-X

Gilbert J, Lekstrom-Himes J, Donaldson D et al (2011) Effect of CC chemokine receptor 2 CCR2 blockade on serum C-reactive protein in individuals at atherosclerotic risk and with a single nucleotide polymorphism of the monocyte chemoattractant protein-1 promoter region. Am J Cardiol 107:906–911. https://doi.org/10.1016/j.amjcard.2010.11.005

Gisterå A, Hansson GK (2017) The immunology of atherosclerosis. Nat Rev Nephrol 13:368–380

Gisterå A, Hermansson A, Strodthoff D et al (2017) Vaccination against T-cell epitopes of native ApoB100 reduces vascular inflammation and disease in a humanized mouse model of atherosclerosis. J Intern Med 281:383–397. https://doi.org/10.1111/joim.12589

Gomez D, Baylis RA, Durgin BG et al (2018) Interleukin-1β has atheroprotective effects in advanced atherosclerotic lesions of mice. Nat Med 24:1418–1429. https://doi.org/10.1038/s41591-018-0124-5

Gonen A, Hansen LF, Turner WW et al (2014) Atheroprotective immunization with malondialdehyde-modified LDL is hapten specific and dependent on advanced MDA adducts: implications for development of an atheroprotective vaccine. J Lipid Res 55:2137–2155. https://doi.org/10.1194/jlr.M053256

González P, Alvarez R, Batalla A et al (2001) Genetic variation at the chemokine receptors CCR5/CCR2 in myocardial infarction. Genes Immun 2:191–195. https://doi.org/10.1038/sj.gene.6363760

Gonzalez-Juanatey C, Llorca J, Sanchez Andrade A et al (2006) Short-term adalimumab therapy improves endothelial function in patients with rheumatoid arthritis refractory to infliximab. Clin Exp Rheumatol 24(3):3C9–312

Gonzalez-Juanatey C, Vazquez-Rodriguez TR, Miranda-Filloy JA et al (2012) Anti-TNF-alpha-adalimumab therapy is associated with persistent improvement of endothelial function without progression of carotid intima-media wall thickness in patients with rheumatoid arthritis refractory to conventional therapy. Mediators Inflamm 2012:674265. https://doi.org/10.1155/2012/674265

Grasset EK, Duhlin A, Agardh HE et al (2015) Sterile inflammation in the spleen during atherosclerosis provides oxidation-specific epitopes that induce a protective B-cell response. Proc Natl Acad Sci 112(16):E2030–E2038. https://doi.org/10.1073/pnas.1421227112

Grievink HW, Gal P, Ozsvar Kozma M et al (2020) The effect of a 13-valent conjugate pneumococcal vaccine on circulating antibodies against oxidized LDL and phosphorylcholine in man, a randomized placebo-controlled clinical trial. Biology (Basel) 9:1–10. https://doi.org/10.3390/biology9110345

Griffin DO, Holodick NE, Rothstein TL (2011) Human B1 cells in umbilical cord and adult peripheral blood express the novel phenotype CD20+ CD27+ CD43+ CD70. J Exp Med 208:67–80. https://doi.org/10.1084/jem.20101499

Groß O, Yazdi AS, Thomas CJ et al (2012) Inflammasome activators induce interleukin-1α secretion via distinct pathways with differential requirement for the protease function of Caspase-1. Immunity 36:388–400. https://doi.org/10.1016/j.immuni.2012.01.018

Gruber S, Hendrikx T, Tsiantoulas D et al (2016) sialic acid-binding immunoglobulin-like lectin G promotes atherosclerosis and liver inflammation by suppressing the protective functions of B-1 cells. Cell Rep 14:2348–2361. https://doi.org/10.1016/j.celrep.2016.02.027

Grundtman C, Jakic B, Buszko M et al (2015) Mycobacterial heat shock protein 65 (mbHSP65)-induced atherosclerosis: preventive oral tolerization and definition of atheroprotective and atherogenic mbHSP65 peptides. Atherosclerosis 242:303–310. https://doi.org/10.1016/j.atherosclerosis.2015.06.044

Hamaguchi Y, Uchida J, Cain DW et al (2005) The peritoneal cavity provides a protective niche for B1 and conventional B lymphocytes during anti-CD20 immunotherapy in mice. J Immunol 174:4389–4399. https://doi org/10.4049/JIMMUNOL.174.7.4389

Hamze M, Desmetz C, Berthe ML et al (2013) Characterization of resident B cells of vascular walls in human atherosclerotic patients. J Immunol 191:3006–3016. https://doi.org/10.4049/jimmunol.1202870

Han S, Liu P, Zhang W et al (2007) The opposite-direction modulation of CD4+CD25+ Tregs and T helper 1 cells in acute coronary syndromes. Clin Immunol 124:90–97. https://doi.org/10.1016/J.CLIM.2007.03.546

Hassan S, Milman U, Feld J et al (2016) Effects of anti-TNF-α treatment on lipid profile in rheumatic diseases: an analytical cohort study. Arthritis Res Ther 18:261. https://doi.org/10.1186/s13075-016-1148-1

Hennessy T, Soh L, Bowman M et al (2019) The low dose colchicine after myocardial infarction (LoDoCo-MI) study: a pilot randomized placebo controlled trial of colchicine following acute myocardial infarction. Am Heart J 215:62–69. https://doi.org/10.1016/j.ahj.2019.06.003

Herbin O, Ait-Oufella H, Yu W et al (2012) Regulatory T-cell response to apolipoprotein B100–derived peptides reduces the development and progression of atherosclerosis in mice. Arterioscler Thromb Vasc Biol 32:605–612. https://doi.org/10.1161/ATVBAHA.111.242800

Herold KC, Gitelman SE, Willi SM et al (2013) Teplizumab treatment may improve C-peptide responses in participants with type 1 diabetes after the new-onset period: a randomised controlled trial. Diabetologia 56:391–400. https://doi.org/10.1007/s00125-012-2753-4

Herold KC, Bundy BN, Long SA et al (2019) An anti-CD3 antibody, teplizumab, in relatives at risk for type 1 diabetes. N Engl J Med 381:603–613. https://doi.org/10.1056/nejmoa1902226

Hilgendorf I, Theurl I, Gerhardt LMS et al (2014) Innate response activator B cells aggravate atherosclerosis by stimulating T Helper-1 adaptive Immunity. Clinical perspective. Circulation 129:1677–1687. https://doi.org/10.1161/CIRCULATIONAHA.113.006381

Hofmann K, Clauder AK, Manz RA (2018) Targeting B cells and plasma cells in autoimmune diseases. Front Immunol 9:835

Hollan I, Meroni PL, Ahearn JM et al (2013) Cardiovascular disease in autoimmune rheumatic diseases. Autoimmun Rev 12:1004–1015

Hsieh MJ, Lee CH, Tsai ML et al (2020) Biologic agents reduce cardiovascular events in rheumatoid arthritis not responsive to tumour necrosis factor inhibitors: a national cohort study. Can J Cardiol 36:1739–1746. https://doi.org/10.1016/j.cjca.2020.01.003

Hsue PY, Scherzer R, Grunfeld C et al (2014) Depletion of B-cells with rituximab improves endothelial function and reduces inflammation among individuals with rheumatoid arthritis. J Am Heart Assoc 3. https://doi.org/10.1161/JAHA.114.001267

Huan T, Zhang B, Wang Z et al (2013) A systems biology framework identifies molecular underpinnings of coronary heart disease. Arterioscler Thromb Vasc Biol 33:1427. https://doi.org/10.1161/ATVBAHA.112.300112

Huang Y, Jiang H, Chen Y et al (2018) Tranilast directly targets <scp>NLRP</scp> 3 to treat inflammasome-driven diseases. EMBO Mol Med 10(4):e8689. https://doi.org/10.15252/emmm.201708689

Huang R, Zhao SR, Li Y et al (2020) Association of tumor necrosis factor-α gene polymorphisms and coronary artery disease susceptibility: a systematic review and meta-analysis. BMC Med Genet 21:29. https://doi.org/10.1186/s12881-020-0952-2

Iribarren C, Rahmaoui A, Long AA et al (2017a) Cardiovascular and cerebrovascular events among patients receiving omalizumab: results from EXCELS, a prospective cohort study in moderate to severe asthma. J Allergy Clin Immunol 139:1489–1495. https://doi.org/10.1016/j.jaci.2016.07.038

Iribarren C, Rothman KJ, Bradley MS et al (2017b) Cardiovascular and cerebrovascular events among patients receiving omalizumab: pooled analysis of patient-level data from 25 randomized, double-blind, placebo-controlled clinical trials. J Allergy Clin Immunol 139:1678–1680. https://doi.org/10.1016/j.jaci.2016.12.953

Isoda K, Sawada S, Ishigami N et al (2004) Lack of interleukin-1 receptor antagonist modulates plaque composition in apolipoprotein E-deficient mice. Arterioscler Thromb Vasc Biol 24:1068–1073. https://doi.org/10.1161/01.ATV.0000127025.48140.a3

Jackson SW, Scharping NE, Jacobs HM et al (2016) Cutting edge: BAFF overexpression reduces atherosclerosis via TACI-dependent B cell activation. J Immunol 197:4529–4534. https://doi.org/10.4049/jimmunol.1601198

Jacobsson LTH, Turesson C, Gülfe A et al (2005) Treatment with tumor necrosis factor blockers is associated with a lower incidence of first cardiovascular events in patients with rheumatoid arthritis. J Rheumatol 32:1213–1218

Jin Y, Kang EH, Brill G et al (2018) Cardiovascular (CV) risk after initiation of abatacept versus TNF inhibitors in rheumatoid arthritis patients with and without baseline CV disease. J Rheumatol 45:1240–1248. https://doi.org/10.3899/jrheum.170926

Jing H, Yong L, Haiyan L et al (2011) Oral administration of Lactococcus lactis delivered heat shock protein 65 attenuates atherosclerosis in low-density lipoprotein receptor-deficient mice. Vaccine 29:4102–4109. https://doi.org/10.1016/j.vaccine.2011.03.105

Jostock T, Müllberg J, Özbek S et al (2001) Soluble gp130 is the natural inhibitor of soluble interleukin-6 receptor transsignaling responses. Eur J Biochem 268:160–167. https://doi.org/10.1046/j.1432-1327.2001.01867.x

Jun HL, Hee JU, Park JW et al (2009) Interleukin-1β promotes the expression of monocyte chemoattractant protein-1 in human aorta smooth muscle cells via multiple signaling pathways. Exp Mol Med 41:757–764. https://doi.org/10.3858/emm.2009.41.10.082

Kang EH, Jin Y, Brill G et al (2018) Comparative cardiovascular risk of abatacept and tumor necrosis factor inhibitors in patients with rheumatoid arthritis with and without diabetes mellitus: a multidatabase cohort study. J Am Heart Assoc 7:e007393. https://doi.org/10.1161/JAHA.117.007393

Karnell JL, Rieder SA, Ettinger R, Kolbeck R (2019) Targeting the CD40-CD40L pathway in autoimmune diseases: humoral immunity and beyond. Adv Drug Deliv Rev 141:92–103

Kasahara K, Sasaki N, Yamashita T et al (2014) CD3 antibody and IL-2 complex combination therapy inhibits atherosclerosis by augmenting a regulatory immune response. J Am Heart Assoc 3. https://doi.org/10.1161/JAHA.113.000719

Kelley N, Jeltema D, Duan Y, He Y (2019) The NLRP3 inflammasome: an overview of mechanisms of activation and regulation. Int J Mol Sci 20:3328

Kerekes G, Soltész P, Dér H et al (2009) Effects of rituximab treatment on endothelial dysfunction, carotid atherosclerosis, and lipid profile in rheumatoid arthritis. Clin Rheumatol 28:705–710. https://doi.org/10.1007/s10067-009-1095-1

Khamis RY, Hughes AD, Caga-anan M et al (2016) EBioMedicine high serum immunoglobulin G and M levels predict freedom from adverse cardiovascular events in hypertension : a nested case-control substudy of the Anglo-Scandinavian cardiac outcomes trial. EBioMedicine 9:372–380. https://doi.org/10.1016/j.ebiom.2016.06.012

Kim DG, Lee J, Seo WJ et al (2019) Rituximab protects against development of atherosclerotic cardiovascular disease after kidney transplantation: a propensity-matched study. Sci Rep 9:1–8. https://doi.org/10.1038/s41598-019-52942-8

Kimura T, Tse K, McArdle S et al (2017) Atheroprotective vaccination with MHC-II-restricted ApoB peptides induces peritoneal IL-10-producing CD4 T cells. Am J Physiol Circ Physiol 312:H781–H790. https://doi.org/10.1152/ajpheart.00798.2016

Kimura T, Kobiyama K, Winkels H et al (2018) Regulatory CD4+ T cells recognize major histocompatibility complex class II molecule-restricted peptide epitopes of apolipoprotein B. Circulation 138:1130–1143. https://doi.org/10.1161/CIRCULATIONAHA.117.031420

Kirii H, Niwa T, Yamada Y et al (2003) Lack of interleukin-1beta decreases the severity of atherosclerosis in ApoE-deficient mice. Arterioscler Thromb Vasc Biol 23:656–660. https://doi.org/10.1161/01.ATV.0000064374.15232.C3

Kita T, Yamashita T, Sasaki N et al (2014) Regression of atherosclerosis with anti-CD3 antibody via augmenting a regulatory T-cell response in mice. Cardiovasc Res 102:107–117. https://doi.org/10.1093/cvr/cvu002

Klatzmann D, Abbas AK (2015) The promise of low-dose interleukin-2 therapy for autoimmune and inflammatory diseases. Nat Rev Immunol 15:283–294. https://doi.org/10.1038/nri3823

Kleveland O, Kunszt G, Bratlie M et al (2016) Effect of a single dose of the interleukin-6 receptor antagonist tocilizumab on inflammation and troponin T release in patients with non-ST-elevation myocardial infarction: a double-blind, randomized, placebo-controlled phase 2 trial. Eur Heart J 37:2406–2413. https://doi.org/10.1093/eurheartj/ehw171

Klingenberg R, Lebens M, Hermansson A et al (2010) Intranasal immunization with an apolipoprotein B-100 fusion protein induces antigen-specific regulatory T cells and reduces atherosclerosis. Arterioscler Thromb Vasc Biol 30:946–952. https://doi.org/10.1161/ATVBAHA.109.202671

Klingenberg R, Ketelhuth DFJ, Strodthoff D et al (2012) Subcutaneous immunization with heat shock protein-65 reduces atherosclerosis in Apoe −/− mice. Immunobiology 217:540–547. https://doi.org/10.1016/j.imbio.2011.06.006

Klingenberg R, Gerdes N, Badeau RM et al (2013) Depletion of FOXP3+ regulatory T cells promotes hypercholesterolemia and atherosclerosis. J Clin Invest 123:1323–1334. https://doi.org/10.1172/JCI63891

Koenen RR, Weber C (2010) Therapeutic targeting of chemokine interactions in atherosclerosis. Nat Rev Drug Discov 9:141–153. https://doi.org/10.1038/nrd3048

Kortelainen ML, Porvari K (2014) Adventitial macrophage and lymphocyte accumulation accompanying early stages of human coronary atherogenesis. Cardiovasc Pathol 23:193–197. https://doi.org/10.1016/j.carpath.2014.03.001

Kounis NG, Hahalis G (2016) Serum IgE levels in coronary artery disease. Atherosclerosis 251:498–500. https://doi.org/10.1016/j.atherosclerosis.2016.05.045

Kuziel WA, Dawson TC, Quinones M et al (2003) CCR5 deficiency is not protective in the early stages of atherogenesis in apoE knockout mice. Atherosclerosis 167:25–32. https://doi.org/10.1016/S0021-9150(02)00382-9

Kyaw T, Tay C, Khan A et al (2010) Conventional B2 B cell depletion ameliorates whereas its adoptive transfer aggravates atherosclerosis. J Immunol 185:4410–4419. https://doi.org/10.4049/jimmunol.1000033

Kyaw T, Tay C, Hosseini H et al (2012) Depletion of B2 but not B1a B cells in BAFF receptor-deficient ApoE−/− mice attenuates atherosclerosis by potently ameliorating arterial inflammation. PLoS One 7:e29371. https://doi.org/10.1371/journal.pone.0029371

Kyaw T, Loveland P, Kanellakis P et al (2021) Alarmin-activated B cells accelerate murine atherosclerosis after myocardial infarction via plasma cell-immunoglobulin-dependent mechanisms. Eur Heart J 42:938–947. https://doi.org/10.1093/eurheartj/ehaa995

Kyrklund M, Bildo M, Akhi R et al (2020) Humoral immune response to heat shock protein 60 of Aggregatibacter actinomycetemcomitans and cross-reactivity with malondialdehyde acetaldehyde-modified LDL. PLoS One 15:e0230682. https://doi.org/10.1371/journal.pone.0230682

Lalezari J, Yadavalli GK, Para M et al (2008) Safety, pharmacokinetics, and antiviral activity of HGS004, a novel fully human IgG4 monoclonal antibody against CCR5, in HIV-1–infected patients. J Infect Dis 197:721–727. https://doi.org/10.1086/527327

Lameijer M, Binderup T, Van Leent MMT et al (2018) Efficacy and safety assessment of a TRAF6-targeted nanoimmunotherapy in atherosclerotic mice and non-human primates. Nat Biomed Eng 2:279–292. https://doi.org/10.1038/s41551-018-0221-2

Langevitz P, Livneh A, Neumann L et al (2001) Prevalence of ischemic heart disease in patients with familial Mediterranean fever. Isr Med Assoc J 3:9–12

Lefkou E, Fragakis N, Ioannidou E et al (2010) Increased levels of proinflammatory cytokines in children with family history of coronary artery disease. Clin Cardiol 33:E6. https://doi.org/10.1002/clc.20434

Lehrer-Graiwer J, Singh P, Abdelbaky A et al (2015) FDG-PET imaging for oxidized LDL in stable atherosclerotic disease: a phase II study of safety, tolerability, and anti-inflammatory activity. JACC Cardiovasc Imaging 8:493–494. https://doi.org/10.1016/J.JCMG.2014.06.021

Lewis MJ, Malik TH, Ehrenstein MR et al (2009) Immunoglobulin M is required for protection against atherosclerosis in low-density lipoprotein receptor-deficient mice. Circulation 120:417–426. https://doi.org/10.1161/CIRCULATIONAHA.109.868158

Li J, McArdle S, Gholami A et al (2016) CCR5+T-bet+FoxP3+ effector CD4 T cells drive atherosclerosis. Circ Res 118:1540–1552. https://doi.org/10.1161/CIRCRESAHA.116.308648

Libby P (2021) The changing landscape of atherosclerosis. Nature 592:524–533. https://doi.org/10.1038/s41586-021-03392-8

Lutgens E, Cleutjens KBJM, Heeneman S et al (2000) Both early and delayed anti-CD40L antibody treatment induces a stable plaque phenotype. Proc Natl Acad Sci U S A 97:7464–7469. https://doi.org/10.1073/pnas.97.13.7464

Lutgens E, Lievens D, Beckers L et al (2010) Deficient CD40-TRAF6 signaling in leukocytes prevents atherosclerosis by skewing the immune response toward an antiinflammatory profile. J Exp Med 207:391–404. https://doi.org/10.1084/jem.20091293

Ma K, Lv S, Liu B et al (2013) CTLA4-IgG ameliorates homocysteine-accelerated atherosclerosis by inhibiting T-cell overactivation in apoE−/− mice. Cardiovasc Res 97:349–359. https://doi.org/10.1093/cvr/cvs330

Makino Y, Cook DN, Smithies O et al (2002) Impaired T cell function in RANTES-deficient mice. Clin Immunol 102:302–309. https://doi.org/10.1006/clim.2001.5178

Mantani PT, Ljungcrantz I, Andersson L et al (2014) Circulating CD40+ and CD86+ B cell subsets demonstrate opposing associations with risk of stroke. Arterioscler Thromb Vasc Biol 34:211–218. https://doi.org/10.1161/ATVBAHA.113.302667

Marek-Trzonkowska N, Myśliwiec M, Dobyszuk A et al (2014) Therapy of type 1 diabetes with CD4+CD25highCD127-regulatory T cells prolongs survival of pancreatic islets - results of one year follow-up. Clin Immunol 153:23–30. https://doi.org/10.1016/j.clim.2014.03.016

Maron R, Sukhova G, Faria AM et al (2002) Mucosal administration of heat shock protein-65 decreases atherosclerosis and inflammation in aortic arch of low-density lipoprotein receptor-deficient mice. Circulation 106:1708–1715. https://doi.org/10.1161/01.CIR.0000029750.99462.30

Mathew JM, H-Voss J, LeFever A et al (2018) A phase i clinical trial with ex vivo expanded recipient regulatory t cells in living donor kidney transplants. Sci Rep 8:7428. https://doi.org/10.1038/s41598-018-25574-7

Matsumura T, Kugiyama K, Sugiyama S et al (1999) Suppression of atherosclerotic development in Watanabe heritable hyperlipidemic rabbits treated with an oral antiallergic drug, tranilast. Circulation 99:919–924. https://doi.org/10.1161/01.CIR.99.7.919

McGeough MD, Wree A, Inzaugarat ME et al (2017) TNF regulates transcription of NLRP3 inflammasome components and inflammatory molecules in cryopyrinopathies. J Clin Invest 127:4488–4497. https://doi.org/10.1172/JCI90699

McInnes IB, Thompson L, Giles JT et al (2015) Effect of interleukin-6 receptor blockade on surrogates of vascular risk in rheumatoid arthritis: MEASURE, a randomised, placebo-controlled study. Ann Rheum Dis 74:694–702. https://doi.org/10.1136/annrheumdis-2013-204345

Mendall MA, Patel P, Asante M et al (1997) Relation of serum cytokine concentrations to cardiovascular risk factors and coronary heart disease. Heart 78:273–277. https://doi.org/10.1136/hrt.78.3.273

Merhi-Soussi F, Kwak BR, Magne D et al (2005) Interleukin-1 plays a major role in vascular inflammation and atherosclerosis in male apolipoprotein E-knockout mice. Cardiovasc Res 66:583–593. https://doi.org/10.1016/j.cardiores.2005.01.008

Mor A, Luboshits G, Planer D et al (2006) Altered status of CD4+CD25+ regulatory T cells in patients with acute coronary syndromes. Eur Heart J 27:2530–2537. https://doi.org/10.1093/eurheartj/ehl222

Mor A, Planer D, Luboshits G et al (2007) Role of naturally occurring CD4+CD25+ regulatory T cells in experimental atherosclerosis. Arterioscler Thromb Vasc Biol 27:893–900. https://doi.org/10.1161/01.ATV.0000259365.31469.89

Morris-Rosenfeld S, Lipinski MJ, McNamara CA (2014) Understanding the role of B cells in atherosclerosis: potential clinical implications. Expert Rev Clin Immunol 10:77–89. https://doi.org/10.1586/1744666X.2014.857602

Morton AC, Rothman AMK, Greenwood JP et al (2015) The effect of interleukin-1 receptor antagonist therapy on markers of inflammation in non-ST elevation acute coronary syndromes: the MRC-ILA heart study. Eur Heart J 36:377–384. https://doi.org/10.1093/eurheartj/ehu272

Newland SA, Mohanta S, Clément M et al (2017) Type-2 innate lymphoid cells control the development of atherosclerosis in mice. Nat Commun 8:15781. https://doi.org/10.1038/ncomms15781

Nidorf M, Thompson PL (2007) Effect of colchicine (0.5 mg twice daily) on high-sensitivity C-reactive protein independent of aspirin and atorvastatin in patients with stable coronary artery disease. Am J Cardiol 99:805–807. https://doi.org/10.1016/j.amjcard.2006.10.039

Nidorf SM, Eikelboom JW, Budgeon CA, Thompson PL (2013) Low-dose colchicine for secondary prevention of cardiovascular disease. J Am Coll Cardiol 61:404–410. https://doi.org/10.1016/j.jacc.2012.10.027

Nidorf SM, Fiolet ATL, Eikelboom JW et al (2019) The effect of low-dose colchicine in patients with stable coronary artery disease: the LoDoCo2 trial rationale, design, and baseline characteristics. Am Heart J 218:46–56. https://doi.org/10.1016/j.ahj.2019.09.011

Nidorf SM, Fiolet ATL, Mosterd A et al (2020) Colchicine in patients with chronic coronary disease. N Engl J Med 383:1838–1847. https://doi.org/10.1056/NEJMoa2021372

Nilsson J, Calara F, Regnstrom J et al (1997) Immunization with homologous oxidized low density lipoprotein reduces neointimal formation after balloon injury in hypercholesterolemic rabbits. J Am Coll Cardiol 30:1886–1891. https://doi.org/10.1016/S0735-1097(97)00366-5

Novikova DS, Popkova TV, Lukina GV et al (2016) The effects of rituximab on lipids, arterial stiffness and carotid intima-media thickness in rheumatoid arthritis. J Korean Med Sci 31:202–207. https://doi.org/10.3346/jkms.2016.31.2.202

Nurmohamed MT (2009) Cardiovascular risk in rheumatoid arthritis. Autoimmun Rev 8:663–667

Nus M, Sage AP, Lu Y et al (2017) Marginal zone B cells control the response of follicular helper T cells to a high-cholesterol diet. Nat Med 23:601. https://doi.org/10.1038/nm.4315

Ohta H, Wada H, Niwa T et al (2005) Disruption of tumor necrosis factor-α gene diminishes the development of atherosclerosis in ApoE-deficient mice. Atherosclerosis 180:11–17. https://doi.org/10.1016/j.atherosclerosis.2004.11.016

Ozen G, Pedro S, Michaud K (2020) The risk of cardiovascular events associated with disease-modifying antirheumatic drugs in rheumatoid arthritis. J Rheumatol 48(5):648–655. https://doi.org/10.3899/jrheum.200265

Palinski W, Miller E, Witztum JL (1995) Immunization of low density lipoprotein (LDL) receptor-deficient rabbits with homologous malondialdehyde-modified LDL reduces atherogenesis. Proc Natl Acad Sci USA 92:821–825. https://doi.org/10.1073/PNAS.92.3.821

Pattison JM, Nelson PJ, Huie P et al (1996) RANTES chemokine expression in transplant-associated accelerated atherosclerosis. J Heart Lung Transplant 15:1194–1199

Poels K, van Leent MMT, Reiche ME et al (2020) Antibody-mediated inhibition of CTLA4 aggravates atherosclerotic plaque inflammation and progression in hyperlipidemic mice. Cell 9:1987. https://doi.org/10.3390/cells9091987

Porsch F, Binder CJ (2019) Impact of B-cell–targeted therapies on cardiovascular disease. Arterioscler Thromb Vasc Biol 39:1705–1714. https://doi.org/10.1161/ATVBAHA.119.311996

Poulsen CB, Al-Mashhadi AL, Von Wachenfeldt K et al (2016) Treatment with a human recombinant monoclonal IgG antibody against oxidized LDL in atherosclerosis-prone pigs reduces cathepsin S in coronary lesions. Int J Cardiol 215:506–515. https://doi.org/10.1016/j.ijcard.2016.03.222

Pradhan AD (2021) Time to commence or time out for colchicine in secondary prevention of cardiovascular disease? Eur Heart J. https://doi.org/10.1093/eurheartj/ehab210

Primdahl J, Clausen J, Hørslev-Petersen K (2013) Results from systematic screening for cardiovascular risk in outpatients with rheumatoid arthritis in accordance with the EULAR recommendations. Ann Rheum Dis 72:1771–1776. https://doi.org/10.1136/annrheumdis-2013-203688

Proto JD, Doran AC, Gusarova G et al (2018) Regulatory T cells promote macrophage efferocytosis during inflammation resolution. Immunity 49:666–677. https://doi.org/10.1016/J.IMMUNI.2018.07.015

Protogerou AD, Zampeli E, Fragiadaki K et al (2011) A pilot study of endothelial dysfunction and aortic stiffness after interleukin-6 receptor inhibition in rheumatoid arthritis. Atherosclerosis 219:734–736. https://doi.org/10.1016/j.atherosclerosis.2011.09.015

Provan SA, Berg IJ, Hammer HB et al (2015) The impact of newer biological disease modifying anti-rheumatic drugs on cardiovascular risk factors: a 12-month longitudinal study in rheumatoid arthritis patients treated with rituximab, abatacept and tociliziumab. PLoS One 10: e0130709. https://doi.org/10.1371/journal.pone.0130709

Que X, Hung MY, Yeang C et al (2018) Oxidized phospholipids are proinflammatory and proatherogenic in hypercholesterolaemic mice. Nature 558:301–306. https://doi.org/10.1038/s41586-018-0198-8

Quinones MP, Martinez HG Jimenez F et al (2007) CC chemokine receptor 5 influences late-stage atherosclerosis. Atherosclerosis 195:e92–e103. https://doi.org/10.1016/j.atherosclerosis.2007.03.026

Radocha J, van de Donk NWCJ, Weisel K (2021) Monoclonal antibodies and antibody drug conjugates in multiple myeloma. Cancers (Basel) 13

Rajamaki K, Lappalainen J, Oorni K et al (2010) Cholesterol crystals activate the NLRP3 inflammasome in human macrophages: a novel link between cholesterol metabolism and inflammation. PLoS One 5:7. https://doi.org/10.1371/journal.pone.0011765

Rauch M, Tussiwand R, Bosco N, Rolink AG (2009) Crucial role for BAFF-BAFF-R signaling in the survival and maintenance of mature B cells. PLoS One 4:e5456. https://doi.org/10.1371/journal.pone.0005456

Reiss AB, Carsons SE, Anwar K et al (2008) Atheroprotective effects of methotrexate on reverse cholesterol transport proteins and foam cell transformation in human THP-1 monocyte/macrophages. Arthritis Rheum 58:3675–3683. https://doi.org/10.1002/art.24040

Ren S, Newby D, Li SC et al (2015) Effect of the adult pneumococcal polysaccharide vaccine on cardiovascular disease: a systematic review and meta-analysis. Open Hear 2:e000247. https://doi.org/10.1136/openhrt-2015-000247

Ren S, Hure A, Peel R et al (2016) Rationale and design of a randomized controlled trial of pneumococcal polysaccharide vaccine for prevention of cardiovascular events: the Australian study for the prevention through immunization of cardiovascular events (AUSPICE). Am Heart J 177:58–65. https://doi.org/10.1016/j.ahj.2016.04.003

Ridker PM, Hennekens CH, Buring JE, Rifai N (2000a) C-reactive protein and other markers of inflammation in the prediction of cardiovascular disease in women. N Engl J Med 342:836–843. https://doi.org/10.1056/NEJM200003233421202

Ridker PM, Rifai N, Stampfer MJ, Hennekens CH (2000b) Plasma concentration of interleukin-6 and the risk of future myocardial infarction among apparently healthy men. Circulation 101:1767–1772. https://doi.org/10.1161/01.CIR.101.15.1767

Ridker PM, Danielson E, Fonseca FA et al (2009) Reduction in C-reactive protein and LDL cholesterol and cardiovascular event rates after initiation of rosuvastatin: a prospective study of the JUPITER trial. Lancet 373:1175–1182. https://doi.org/10.1016/S0140-6736(09)60447-5

Ridker PM, Everett BM, Thuren T et al (2017) Antiinflammatory therapy with canakinumab for atherosclerotic disease. N Engl J Med 377:1119–1131. https://doi.org/10.1056/NEJMoa1707914

Ridker PM, Libby P, MacFadyen JG et al (2018a) Modulation of the interleukin-6 signalling pathway and incidence rates of atherosclerotic events and all-cause mortality: analyses from the Canakinumab anti-inflammatory thrombosis outcomes study (CANTOS). Eur Heart J 39:3499–3507. https://doi.org/10.1093/eurheartj/ehy310

Ridker PM, MacFadyen JG, Everett BM et al (2018b) Relationship of C-reactive protein reduction to cardiovascular event reduction following treatment with canakinumab: a secondary analysis from the CANTOS randomised controlled trial. Lancet 391:319–328. https://doi.org/10.1016/S0140-6736(17)32814-3

Ridker PM, MacFadyen JG, Thuren T, Libby P (2020) Residual inflammatory risk associated with interleukin-18 and interleukin-6 after successful interleukin-1b inhibition with canakinumab: further rationale for the development of targeted anti-cytokine therapies for the treatment of atherothrombosis. Eur Heart J 41:2153–2163. https://doi.org/10.1093/eurheartj/ehz542

Rosenfeld SM, Perry HM, Gonen A et al (2015) B-1b cells secrete atheroprotective IgM and attenuate atherosclerosis. Circ Res 117

Roubille C, Richer V, Starnino T et al (2015) The effects of tumour necrosis factor inhibitors, methotrexate, non-steroidal anti-inflammatory drugs and corticosteroids on cardiovascular events in rheumatoid arthritis, psoriasis and psoriatic arthritis: a systematic review and meta-analysis. Ann Rheum Dis 74:480–489

Rus FG, Niculescu F, Vlaicu R (1991) Tumor necrosis factor-alpha in human arterial wall with atherosclerosis. Atherosclerosis 89:247–254. https://doi.org/10.1016/0021-9150(91)90066-C

Rus HG, Vlaicu R, Niculescu F (1996) Interleukin-6 and interleukin-8 protein and gene expression in human arterial atherosclerotic wall. Atherosclerosis 127:263–271. https://doi.org/10.1016/S0021-9150(96)05968-0

Saag KG, Gim GT, Patkar NM et al (2008) American College of Rheumatology 2008 recommendations for the use of nonbiologic and biologic disease-modifying antirheumatic drugs in rheumatoid arthritis. Arthritis Care Res 59:762–784

Sage AP, Tsiantoulas D, Baker L et al (2012) BAFF receptor deficiency reduces the development of atherosclerosis in mice--brief report. Arterioscler Thromb Vasc Biol 32:1573–1576. https://doi.org/10.1161/ATVBAHA.111.244731

Sage AP, Nus M, Baker LL et al (2015) Regulatory B cell-specific interleukin-10 is dispensable for atherosclerosis development in mice. Arterioscler Thromb Vasc Biol 35:1770–1773. https://doi.org/10.1161/ATVBAHA.115.305568

Sage AP, Nus M, Bagchi Chakraborty J et al (2017) X-box binding protein-1 dependent plasma cell responses limit the development of atherosclerosis. Circ Res 121:270–281. https://doi.org/10.1161/CIRCRESAHA.117.310884

Sage AP, Tsiantoulas D, Binder CJ, Mallat Z (2018) The role of B cells in atherosclerosis. Nat Rev Cardiol 16(3):180–196. https://doi.org/10.1038/s41569-018-0106-9

Saigusa R, Winkels H, Ley KT (2020) Cell subsets and functions in atherosclerosis. Nat Rev Cardiol 17:387. https://doi.org/10.1038/s41569-020-0352-5

Sánchez-Trujillo L, Jerjes-Sanchez C, Rodriguez D et al (2019) Phase II clinical trial testing the safety of a humanised monoclonal antibody anti-CD20 in patients with heart failure with reduced ejection fraction, ICFEr-RITU2: study protocol. BMJ Open 9:e022826. https://doi.org/10.1136/bmjopen-2018-022826

Sattar N, Crompton P, Cherry L et al (2007) Effects of tumor necrosis factor blockade on cardiovascular risk factors in psoriatic arthritis: a double-blind, placebo-controlled study. Arthritis Rheum 56:831–839. https://doi.org/10.1002/art.22447

Schaheen B, Downs EA, Serbulea V et al (2016) B-cell depletion promotes aortic infiltration of immunosuppressive cells and is protective of experimental aortic aneurysm. Arterioscler Thromb Vasc Biol 36:2191–2202. https://doi.org/10.1161/ATVBAHA.116.307559

Schieffer B, Schieffer E, Hilfiker-Kleiner D et al (2000) Expression of angiotensin II and interleukin 6 in human coronary atherosclerotic plaques. Circulation 101:1372–1378. https://doi.org/10.1161/01.CIR.101.12.1372

Schieffer B, Selle T, Hilfiker A et al (2004) Impact of interleukin-6 on plaque development and morphology in experimental atherosclerosis. Circulation 110:3493–3500. https://doi.org/10.1161/01.CIR.0000148135.08582.97

Schiopu A, Bengtsson J, Söderberg I et al (2004) Recombinant human antibodies against aldehyde-modified apolipoprotein B-100 peptide sequences inhibit atherosclerosis. Circulation 110:2047–2052. https://doi.org/10.1161/01.CIR.0000143162.56057.B5

Schiopu A, Frendéus B, Jansson B et al (2007) Recombinant antibodies to an oxidized low-density lipoprotein epitope induce rapid regression of atherosclerosis in Apobec-1−/−/low-density lipoprotein receptor−/−mice. J Am Coll Cardiol 50:2313–2318. https://doi.org/10.1016/J.JACC.2007.07.081

Schönbeck U, Sukhova GK, Shimizu K et al (2000) Inhibition of CD40 signaling limits evolution of established atherosclerosis in mice. Proc Natl Acad Sci U S A 97:7458–7463. https://doi.org/10.1073/pnas.97.13.7458

Schuett H, Oestreich R, Waetzig GH et al (2012) Transsignaling of interleukin-6 crucially contributes to atherosclerosis in mice. Arterioscler Thromb Vasc Biol 32:281–290. https://doi.org/10.1161/ATVBAHA.111.229435

Seijkens TTP, van Tiel CM, Kusters PJH et al (2018) Targeting CD40-induced TRAF6 signaling in macrophages reduces atherosclerosis. J Am Coll Cardiol 71:527–542. https://doi.org/10.1016/j.jacc.2017.11.055

Seino Y, Ikeda U, Ikeda M et al (1994) Interleukin 6 gene transcripts are expressed in human atherosclerotic lesions. Cytokine 6:87–91. https://doi.org/10.1016/1043-4666(94)90013-2

Shah ASV, Stelzle D, Ken Lee K et al (2018) Global burden of atherosclerotic cardiovascular disease in people living with HIV systematic review and meta-analysis. Circulation 138:1100–1112

Sharma M, Schlegel MP, Afonso MS et al (2020) Regulatory T cells license macrophage pro-resolving functions during atherosclerosis regression. Circ Res 127:335–353. https://doi.org/10.1161/CIRCRESAHA.119.316461

Sharpe AH, Freeman GJ (2002) The B7-CD28 superfamily. Nat Rev Immunol 2:116–126

Shaw PX, Hörkkö S, Chang MK et al (2000) Natural antibodies with the T15 idiotype may act in atherosclerosis, apoptotic clearance, and protective immunity. J Clin Invest 105:1731–1740. https://doi.org/10.1172/JCI8472

Shiri-Sverdlov R, Dos Reis IM, Oligschlaeger Y et al (2021) The influence of a conjugated pneumococcal vaccination on plasma antibody levels against oxidized low-density lipoprotein in metabolic disease patients: a single-arm pilot clinical trial. Antioxidants 10:1–12. https://doi.org/10.3390/antiox10010129

Simons KH, de Jong A, Jukema JW et al (2019) T cell co-stimulation and co-inhibition in cardiovascular disease: a double-edged sword. Nat Rev Cardiol 2019:1–19. https://doi.org/10.1038/s41569-019-0164-7

Singh JA, Furst DE, Bharat A et al (2012) 2012 update of the 2008 American college of rheumatology recommendations for the use of disease-modifying antirheumatic drugs and biologic agents in the treatment of rheumatoid arthritis. Arthritis Care Res 64:625–639. https://doi.org/10.1002/acr.21641

Sode J, Vogel U, Bank S et al (2014) Anti-TNF treatment response in rheumatoid arthritis patients is associated with genetic variation in the NLRP3-inflammasome. PLoS One 9:e100361. https://doi.org/10.1371/journal.pcne.0100361

Song L, Schindler C (2004) IL-6 and the acute phase response in murine atherosclerosis. Atherosclerosis 177:43–51. https://doi.org/10.1016/j.atherosclerosis.2004.06.018

Steffens S, Burger F, Pelli G et al (2006) Short-term treatment with anti-CD3 antibody reduces the development and progression of atherosclerosis in mice. Circulation 114:1977–1984. https://doi.org/10.1161/CIRCULATIONAHA.106.627430

Strang AC, Bisoendial RJ, Kootte RS et al (2013) Pro-atherogenic lipid changes and decreased hepatic LDL receptor expression by tocilizumab in rheumatoid arthritis. Atherosclerosis 229:174–181. https://doi.org/10.1016/j.atherosclerosis.2013.04.031

Strom AC, Cross AJ, Cole JE et al (2015) B regulatory cells are increased in hypercholesterolaemic mice and protect from lesion development via IL-10. Thromb Haemost 114:835–847. https://doi.org/10.1160/TH14-12-1084

Szalai C, Duba J, Prohászka Z et al (2001) Involvement of polymorphisms in the chemokine system in the susceptibility for coronary artery disease (CAD). Coincidence of elevated Lp (a) and MCP-1-2518 G/G genotype in CAD patients. Atherosclerosis 158:233–239. https://doi.org/10.1016/S0021-9150(01)00423-3

Tabas I, Glass CK (2013) Anti-inflammatory therapy in chronic disease: challenges and opportunities. Science 339:166–172

Tam LS, Shang Q, Kun EW et al (2014) The effects of golimumab on subclinical atherosclerosis and arterial stiffness in ankylosing spondylitis-a randomized, placebo-controlled pilot trial. Rheumatol (United Kingdom) 53:1065–1074. https://doi.org/10.1093/rheumatology/ket469

Tardif JC, Kouz S, Waters DD et al (2019) Efficacy and safety of low-dose colchicine after myocardial infarction. N Engl J Med 381:2497–2505. https://doi.org/10.1056/NEJMoa1912388

Tattersall MC, Guo M, Korcarz CE et al (2015) Asthma predicts cardiovascular disease events: the multi-ethnic study of atherosclerosis. Arterioscler Thromb Vasc Biol 35:1520–1525. https://doi.org/10.1161/ATVBAHA.115.305452

Tay C, Liu Y-H, Kanellakis P et al (2018) Follicular B cells promote atherosclerosis via T cell–mediated differentiation into plasma cells and secreting pathogenic immunoglobulin G. Arterioscler Thromb Vasc Biol 38:5. https://doi.org/10.1161/ATVBAHA.117.310678

Trzonkowski P, Bieniaszewska M, Juścińska J et al (2009) First-in-man clinical results of the treatment of patients with graft versus host disease with human ex vivo expanded CD4+CD25+-CD127- T regulatory cells. Clin Immunol 133:22–26. https://doi.org/10.1016/j.clim.2009.06.001

Tse K, Gonen A, Sidney J et al (2013) Atheroprotective vaccination with MHC-II restricted peptides from ApoB-100. Front Immunol 4:493. https://doi.org/10.3389/fimmu.2013.00493

Tsiantoulas D, Bot I, Ozsvar-Kozma M et al (2017) Increased plasma IgE accelerate atherosclerosis in secreted IgM deficiency. Circ Res 120:78–84. https://doi.org/10.1161/CIRCRESAHA.116.309606

Tsiantoulas D, Sage AP, Göderle L et al (2018) B cell–activating factor neutralization aggravates atherosclerosis. Circulation 138:2263–2273. https://doi.org/10.1161/CIRCULATIONAHA.117.032790

Upadhye A, Srikakulapu P, Gonen A et al (2019) Diversification and CXCR4-dependent establishment of the bone marrow B-1a cell Pool governs atheroprotective IgM production linked to human coronary atherosclerosis. Circ Res 125:e55–e70. https://doi.org/10.1161/CIRCRESAHA.119.315786

Upadhye A, Sturek JM, McNamara CA (2020) 2019 Russell Ross memorial lecture in vascular biology. Arterioscler Thromb Vasc Biol 40:309–322. https://doi.org/10.1161/ATVBAHA.119.313064

Vaidya K, Arnott C, Martínez GJ et al (2018) Colchicine therapy and plaque stabilization in patients with acute coronary syndrome: a CT coronary angiography study. JACC Cardiovasc Imaging 11:305–316. https://doi.org/10.1016/j.jcmg.2017.08.013

van den Berg VJ, Vroegindewey MM, Kardys I et al (2019) Anti-oxidized LDL antibodies and coronary artery disease: a systematic review. Antioxidants 8:10

Van Der Heijden T, Kritikou E, Venema W et al (2017) NLRP3 Inflammasome inhibition by MCC950 reduces atherosclerotic lesion development in apolipoprotein E-deficient mice-brief report. Arterioscler Thromb Vasc Biol 37:1457–1461. https://doi.org/10.1161/ATVBAHA.117.309575

Van Gool F, Molofsky AB, Morar MM et al (2014) Interleukin-5-producing group 2 innate lymphoid cells control eosinophilia induced by interleukin-2 therapy. Blood 124:3572–3576. https://doi.org/10.1182/blood-2014-07-587493

Van Puijvelde GHM, Hauer AD, De Vos P et al (2006) Induction of oral tolerance to oxidized low-density lipoprotein ameliorates atherosclerosis. Circulation 114:1968–1976. https://doi.org/10.1161/CIRCULATIONAHA.106.615609

Van Puijvelde GHM, Van Es T, Van Wanrooij EJA et al (2007) Induction of oral tolerance to HSP60 or an HSP60-peptide activates t cell regulation and reduces atherosclerosis. Arterioscler Thromb Vasc Biol 27:2677–2683. https://doi.org/10.1161/ATVBAHA.107.151274

Veillard NR, Kwak B, Pelli G et al (2004) Antagonism of RANTES receptors reduces atherosclerotic plaque formation in mice. Circ Res 94:253–261. https://doi.org/10.1161/01.RES.0000109793.17591.4E

Vromman A, Ruvkun V, Shvartz E et al (2019) Stage-dependent differential effects of interleukin-1 isoforms on experimental atherosclerosis. Eur Heart J 40:2482–2491. https://doi.org/10.1093/eurheartj/ehz008

Wæhre T, Yndestad A, Smith C et al (2004) Increased expression of interleukin-1 in coronary artery disease with downregulatory effects of HMG-CoA reductase inhibitors. Circulation 109:1966–1972. https://doi.org/10.1161/01.CIR.0000125700.33637.B1

Wang X, Feuerstein GZ, Gu JL et al (1995) Interleukin-1β induces expression of adhesion molecules in human vascular smooth muscle cells and enhances adhesion of leukocytes to smooth muscle cells. Atherosclerosis 115:89–98. https://doi.org/10.1016/0021-9150(94)05503-B

Wang J, Cheng X, Xiang M-X et al (2011) IgE stimulates human and mouse arterial cell apoptosis and cytokine expression and promotes atherogenesis in Apoe−/− mice. J Clin Invest 121:3564–3577. https://doi.org/10.1172/JCI46028

Wessels JAM, Huizinga TWJ, Guchelaar HJ (2008) Recent insights in the pharmacological actions of methotrexate in the treatment of rheumatoid arthritis. Rheumatology 47:249–255

Westlake SL, Colebatch AN, Baird J et al (2010) The effect of methotrexate on cardiovascular disease in patients with rheumatoid arthritis: a systematic literature review. Rheumatology 49:295–307. https://doi.org/10.1093/rheumatology/kep366

Wezel A, Lagraauw HM, van der Velden D et al (2015) Mast cells mediate neutrophil recruitment during atherosclerotic plaque progression. Atherosclerosis 241:289–296. https://doi.org/10.1016/j.atherosclerosis.2015.05.028

Wick G, Jakic B, Buszko M et al (2014) The role of heat shock proteins in atherosclerosis. Nat Rev Cardiol 11:516–529

Wigren M, Kolbus D, Dunér P et al (2011) Evidence for a role of regulatory T cells in mediating the atheroprotective effect of apolipoprotein B peptide vaccine. J Intern Med 269:546–556. https://doi.org/10.1111/j.1365-2796.2010.02311.x

Wigren M, Björkbacka H, Andersson L et al (2012) Low levels of circulating CD4+FoxP3+ T cells are associated with an increased risk for development of myocardial infarction but not for stroke. Arterioscler Thromb Vasc Biol 32:2000–2004. https://doi.org/10.1161/ATVBAHA.112.251579

Wilcox JN, Nelken NA, Coughlin SR et al (1994) Local expression of inflammatory cytokines in human atherosclerotic plaques. J Atheroscler Thromb 1:S10–S13. https://doi.org/10.5551/jat1994.1.Supplemment1_S10

Winter C, Silvestre-Roig C, Ortega-Gomez A et al (2018) Chrono-pharmacological targeting of the CCL2-CCR2 Axis ameliorates atherosclerosis. Cell Metab 28:175–182. https://doi.org/10.1016/j.cmet.2018.05.002

Wolf D, Ley K (2019) Immunity and inflammation in atherosclerosis. Circ Res 124:315–327

Wolf D, Gerhardt T, Winkels H et al (2020) Pathogenic autoimmunity in atherosclerosis evolves from initially protective apolipoprotein B $_{100}$ −reactive CD4 $^+$ T-regulatory cells. Circulation 142:1279–1293. https://doi.org/10.1161/CIRCULATIONAHA.119.042863

Wu LC, Zarrin AA (2014) The production and regulation of IgE by the immune system. Nat Rev Immunol 14:247–259

Xiao N, Yin M, Zhang L et al (2009) Tumor necrosis factor-alpha deficiency retards early fatty-streak lesion by influencing the expression of inflammatory factors in apoE-null mice. Mol Genet Metab 96:239–244. https://doi.org/10.1016/j.ymgme.2008.11.166

Yang M, Sun L, Wang S et al (2010) Novel function of B cell-activating factor in the induction of IL-10-producing regulatory B cells. J Immunol 184:3321–3325. https://doi.org/10.4049/jimmunol.0902551

Yu A, Zhu L, Altman NH, Malek TR (2009) A low Interleukin-2 receptor signaling threshold supports the development and homeostasis of T regulatory cells. Immunity 30:204–217. https://doi.org/10.1016/j.immuni.2008.11.014

Zakai NA, Katz R, Jenny NS et al (2007) Inflammation and hemostasis biomarkers and cardiovascular risk in the elderly: the cardiovascular health study. J Thromb Haemost 5:1128–1135. https://doi.org/10.1111/j.1538-7836.2007.02528.x

Zelová H, Hošek J (2013) TNF-α signalling and inflammation: interactions between old acquaintances. Inflamm Res 62:641–651

Zernecke A, Weber C (2014) Chemokines in atherosclerosis: proceedings resumed. Arterioscler Thromb Vasc Biol 34:742–750. https://doi.org/10.1161/ATVBAHA.113.301655

Zhang J, Xie F, Yun H et al (2016) Comparative effects of biologics on cardiovascular risk among older patients with rheumatoid arthritis. Ann Rheum Dis 75:1813–1818. https://doi.org/10.1136/annrheumdis-2015-207870

Zhang X, Li J, Luo S et al (2020) IgE contributes to atherosclerosis and obesity by affecting macrophage polarization, macrophage protein network, and foam cell formation. Arterioscler Thromb Vasc Biol 40:597–610. https://doi.org/10.1161/ATVBAHA.119.313744

Zhao TX, Kostapanos M, Griffiths C et al (2018) Low-dose interleukin-2 in patients with stable ischaemic heart disease and acute coronary syndromes (LILACS): protocol and study rationale for a randomised, double-blind, placebo-controlled, phase I/II clinical trial. BMJ Open 8: e022452. https://doi.org/10.1136/bmjopen-2018-022452

Zhao T, Sriranjan R, Lu Y et al (2020a) Low dose interleukin-2 in patients with stable ischaemic heart disease and acute coronary syndrome (LILACS). Eur Heart J 41:2. https://doi.org/10.1093/ehjci/ehaa946.1735

Zhao TX, Newland SA, Mallat Z (2020b) 2019 ATVB plenary lecture: Interleukin-2 therapy in cardiovascular disease: the potential to regulate innate and adaptive immunity. Arterioscler Thromb Vasc Biol 40:853–864. https://doi.org/10.1161/ATVBAHA.119.312287

Zhao TX, Ur-Rahman MA, Sage AP et al (2021) Rituximab in patients with acute ST-elevation myocardial infarction (RITA-MI): an experimental medicine safety study. Cardiovasc Res. https://doi.org/10.1093/cvr/cvab113

Zhou X, Caligiuri G, Hamsten A et al (2001) LDL immunization induces T-cell–dependent antibody formation and protection against atherosclerosis. Arterioscler Thromb Vasc Biol 21:108–114. https://doi.org/10.1161/01.ATV.21.1.108

Zirlik A, Maier C, Gerdes N et al (2007) CD40 ligand mediates inflammation independently of CD40 by interaction with Mac-1. Circulation 115:1571–1580. https://doi.org/10.1161/CIRCULATIONAHA.106.683201

Zouggari Y, Ait-Oufella H, Bonnin P et al (2013) B lymphocytes trigger monocyte mobilization and impair heart function after acute myocardial infarction. Nat Med 19:1273–1280. https://doi.org/10.1038/nm.3284

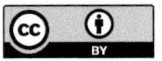

Neutrophil Extracellular Traps in Atherosclerosis and Thrombosis

Thomas M. Hofbauer, Anna S. Ondracek, and Irene M. Lang

Contents

1 Introduction 406
2 Neutrophils and Neutrophil Extracellular Traps 407
3 NETs in Venous Thrombosis 409
4 NETs in Atherosclerosis and Arterial Thrombosis 410
    4.1 Atherosclerosis 410
    4.2 Arterial Thrombosis 411
5 Neutrophil Extracellular Traps as a Therapeutic Target 413
    5.1 PAD-4 Inhibitors: Cl-Amidine 413
    5.2 Deoxyribonuclease 414
    5.3 Heparin 414
6 Summary 415
References 416

Abstract

Despite effective therapeutic and preventive strategies, atherosclerosis and its complications still represent a substantial health burden. Leukocytes and inflammatory mechanisms are increasingly recognized as drivers of atherosclerosis. Neutrophil granulocytes within the circulation were recently shown to undergo neutrophil extracellular trap (NET) formation, linking innate immunity with acute complications of atherosclerosis. In this chapter, we summarize mechanisms of NET formation, evidence for their involvement in atherosclerosis and thrombosis, and potential therapeutic regimens specifically targeting NET components.

Thomas M. Hofbauer and Anna S. Ondracek contributed equally to this work.

T. M. Hofbauer · A. S. Ondracek · I. M. Lang (✉)
Department of Cardiology, Internal Medicine II, Medical University of Vienna, Vienna, Austria
e-mail: irene.lang@meduniwien.ac.at

© The Author(s) 2020
A. von Eckardstein, C. J. Binder (eds.), *Prevention and Treatment of Atherosclerosis*,
Handbook of Experimental Pharmacology 270, https://doi.org/10.1007/164_2020_409

405

Keywords

Atherosclerosis · Cl-amidine · Deoxyribonuclease · Heparin · Myocardial
infarction · Neutrophil extracellular traps · Neutrophils · Thrombosis

Abbreviations

AAA	Abdominal aortic aneurysm
citH3	Citrullinated histone H3
DNase	Deoxyribonuclease
dsDNA	Double-stranded DNA
DVT	Deep vein thrombosis
ET	Extracellular traps
HIT	Heparin-induced thrombocytopenia
IL	Interleukin
MI	Myocardial infarction
MPO	Myeloperoxidase
NE	Neutrophil elastase
NETs	Neutrophil extracellular traps
PAD	Peripheral artery disease
PAD-4	Peptidylarginine deiminase 4
PE	Pulmonary embolism
PMA	Phorbol myristate acetate
ROS	Reactive oxygen species
tPA	Tissue plasminogen activator
VTE	Venous thromboembolism

1   Introduction

Atherosclerosis accounts for a substantial global disease burden. In recent decades, significant progress in understanding atherosclerosis was made. The identification of modifiable risk factors (Catapano et al. 2016), e.g. arterial hypertension or hyper-cholesterolemia, and the advent of percutaneous primary coronary intervention for treating acute complications of atherosclerosis like acute myocardial infarction (MI) (Beran et al. 2002) have led to a further reduction in incidence, cardiovascular morbidity, and markedly improved prognosis (Herrington et al. 2016). Still, due to the growing global population, the absolute number of deaths attributed to athero-sclerotic disease is rising (Barquera et al. 2015) and increasing the need for novel therapies.

Besides traditional risk factors, inflammation and leukocytes are increasingly recognized as contributors to vascular disease and its complications. Pathomechanisms are manifold, with T cells (Bullenkamp et al. 2016), B cells

(Sage et al. 2019), dendritic cells (Gil-Pulido and Zernecke 2017), monocytes, and macrophages (Moroni et al. 2019) being implicated. Recently, neutrophils were suggested to significantly promote atherosclerosis (Doring et al. 2015), particularly its acute vascular syndromes (Mangold et al. 2015). Upon activation, neutrophils are able to undergo drastic morphological changes, leading to cellular disintegration and release of intracellular content into the extracellular space, in a process called neutrophil extracellular trap (NET) formation (Brinkmann et al. 2004). Besides atherosclerosis (Doring et al. 2017), NETs have emerged as important drivers of disease (Papayannopoulos 2018), including auto-immunity, sepsis, and cancer.

In this chapter, we aim to give a broad overview of the role of vascular NETs in atherosclerotic disease and its specific manifestations. Finally, we discuss potential therapeutic regimens targeting NETs and their components.

2 Neutrophils and Neutrophil Extracellular Traps

Under physiological conditions, neutrophil granulocytes comprise approximately 60% of total leukocytes in humans (Bainton et al. 1971). Neutrophils have a rather short lifespan and are released from the bone marrow into the circulation (Ley et al. 2018). Neutrophils are crucial fighters of the innate immune system, being the first cell population recruited to sites of inflammation and injury (Distelmaier et al. 2014). Neutrophils are critical for host defense (Wang and Arase 2014).

Their abundance and cellular properties enable them to effectively fight pathogens by phagocytosis, degranulation, or cytokine secretion (Witko-Sarsat et al. 2000). Neutrophils are equipped with numerous types of granules (Cowland and Borregaard 2016) containing catalytic enzymes, such as myeloperoxidase (MPO) and serine proteases. Upon phagocytosis of pathogens, neutrophils can fuse their granules with phagolysosomes, resulting in intracellular degradation of pathogens. Alternatively, neutrophils can release their granular content into the extracellular space (Cowland and Borregaard 2016).

Another effector mechanism of neutrophils was identified only 15 years ago, although first evidence had already emerged in 1996: It was reported that phorbol myristate acetate (PMA) could rapidly induce cell death of neutrophils. Thereby, neutrophils underwent substantial morphological changes different from apoptosis or necrosis, including signs of nuclear decondensation (Takei et al. 1996). Extending this finding, the group of Arturo Zychlinsky demonstrated that not only PMA, but also lipopolysaccharide (LPS) or interleukin (IL)-8 led to the appearance of extracellular structures described as fragile fibers of decondensed DNA covered in histones and granule proteins. Gram-positive as well as gram-negative bacteria could be ensnared by these NETs, and presence of neutrophil elastase (NE) or MPO promoted degradation of important bacterial virulence factors (Brinkmann et al. 2004).

Using live-cell imaging, NET formation was found to be an active process, different from apoptosis and necrosis. After stimulation, isolated neutrophils first flattened, forming intracellular vacuoles, followed by loss of the nuclear lobular shape and further expanding in the cytoplasm. In this stage, neutrophils were still viable, containing the vital dye calcein blue but were not positive for Annexin V. This was reversed upon ultimate rupture of the plasma membrane. Furthermore, and in contrast to apoptosis, chromatin was decondensed. Intracellular membranes were fragmented, enabling mixing of nuclear, granular, and cytoplasmic components, which was not a feature of necrosis (Fuchs et al. 2007).

An important pre-requisite for NET formation is the presence of reactive oxygen species (ROS) (Fuchs et al. 2007; Hakkim et al. 2011). Inhibiting ROS production diminished NET formation, and neutrophils isolated from chronic granulomatous disease patients carrying mutations in the phagocyte NADPH oxidase did not produce NETs in response to PMA. However, when hydrogen peroxide was added to the system, the ability to form NETs was restored. These experiments indicated that NETosis is dependent on assembly and activation of the NADPH oxidase (Fuchs et al. 2007) and can be triggered by protein kinase C signaling via the raf-MEK-ERK pathway (Hakkim et al. 2011).

ROS serve as substrate for MPO, but presence of both is an essential stimulus for activation of NE (Metzler et al. 2014). Upon nuclear translocation, NE degrades core histones, facilitating decondensation of chromatin in synergy with histone citrullination by the calcium-dependent enzyme peptidyl arginine deiminase 4 (PAD-4) (Wang et al. 2004). Subsequent disintegration of intracellular membranes enables adsorption of granular proteases and antimicrobials onto chromatin. Rupture of the outer cell membrane finally leads to expulsion of cellular meshwork resulting in formation of NETs (Remijsen et al. 2011). Many of these released NET-associated proteins were shown to be degraded by neutrophil proteases in vitro, probably reducing their capacity to act as autoantigens in vivo (de Bont et al. 2020).

Since their discovery, pathways of NET formation are under thorough debate. Numerous triggers were reported; however, key events essential for NETosis could hardly be connected by signaling molecules to describe defined intracellular cascades. Even the absolute necessity of PAD-4 activity for NET formation is in question. Knockout or inhibition of PAD-4 was, on the one hand, reported to disrupt mouse and human NET formation (Lewis et al. 2015; Li et al. 2010; Martinod et al. 2013) while, on the other hand, other groups still observed NETs in response to the same stimuli independent of PAD-4 activity (Claushuis et al. 2018; Kenny et al. 2017). These conflicting data highlight the problems regarding different methods and also different interpretations of results. Nevertheless, citrullinated histone H3 (citH3) is still considered the most specific marker for NET formation. Differentiation between "vital" and "suicidal" NETosis even questions terminology itself by indicating that NET formation does not have to result in immediate cell death (Desai et al. 2016; Madhusoodanan 2017). Despite uncertainty regarding NET formation, it is increasingly recognized that presence of NETs fundamentally influences disease, including atherosclerosis and thrombosis.

Recently, the exclusivity of extracellular trap (ET) formation to neutrophils came into debate. Among granulocytes, mast cells (Campillo-Navarro et al. 2017) and eosinophils (Mukherjee et al. 2018) were reported capable of forming ETs. Another group even found monocytes to release ETs containing myeloperoxidase and citH3

(Granger et al. 2017). Furthermore, evidence implicated macrophages to equally expel their intracellular content in a process of ET formation (Doster et al. 2018). However, the significance of these non-neutrophil-associated ETs so far remains incompletely understood.

3   NETs in Venous Thrombosis

Deep vein thrombosis (DVT) and its major complications are prevalent in Europe and associated with high morbidity and mortality. Virchow's triad (Kumar et al. 2010) serves as an excellent framework for understanding risk factors of thrombosis, which are hypercoagulability, vascular dysfunction, and stasis. Recently, however, it was proposed to extend this triad to a tetrad, taking into account the paramount influence of the immune system and its dysregulation on thrombosis (Kapoor et al. 2018). In a rat model of inferior vena cava ligation, pro-inflammatory neutrophils were observed in emerging thrombi and vein walls (Wakefield et al. 1995). In humans, the pro-inflammatory markers interleukin (IL)-6 and C-reactive protein in plasma were increased in DVT and gradually declined after disease onset (Roumen-Klappe et al. 2002), while C-reactive protein predicted post-thrombotic syndrome (Roumen-Klappe et al. 2009).

The potential role of NETs in venous thrombosis was indicated by a flow chamber experiment, where NETs provided a fibrous scaffold for fibrin, von Willebrand factor (vWF) and platelets. NETs were then observed in thrombi of baboons subjected to experimental DVT (Fuchs et al. 2010). In a mouse model of DVT, large amounts of DNA were observed in thrombi, forming NET-like structures (von Bruhl et al. 2012). These observations were complemented by another group showing that fresh parts of thrombi were rich in the NET-specific marker citH3, which co-localized with vWF (Brill et al. 2012).

The first observation of NETs in human venous thrombosis was presented in a case report of a patient suffering from microscopic polyangiitis and DVT: both in kidney and thrombus samples, NETs were abundantly present (Nakazawa et al. 2012). Characterizing thrombi based on histological methods, DNA webs and citH3 were concentrated in organizing sections of thrombi, but not in already organized parts (Savchenko et al. 2014). Extending these findings, plasma DNA levels were found increased, diagnosing DVT with a sensitivity of 81%. Also, thrombus DNA positively correlated with D-dimer, vWF activity, the clinical Wells score, and neutrophil-derived MPO (Diaz et al. 2013). Similar results were obtained with concentrations of nucleosomes, which were elevated in DVT patients and positively correlated with neutrophil activation (van Montfoort et al. 2013).

Venous thromboembolism, mainly presenting as pulmonary embolism (PE), is a major complication of DVT (Di Nisio et al. 2016). Levels of nuclear DNA were shown to be elevated in PE (Arnalich et al. 2013) and independently predictive of mortality (Jimenez-Alcazar et al. 2018). In chronic thromboembolic pulmonary hypertension, a long-term sequela of PE (Lang 2004) characterized by the apposition of non-resolving, organized clots (Galie et al. 2016), neutrophils were shown to be hyperresponsive (Rose et al. 2003) and present in superficial areas of thrombi (Quarck et al. 2015), while soluble NET surrogates were increased compared to healthy controls (Aldabbous et al. 2016).

4   NETs in Atherosclerosis and Arterial Thrombosis

4.1   Atherosclerosis

First evidence for the importance of neutrophils in human atherosclerosis arose indirectly, when increased MPO levels predicted risk of coronary artery disease independently of traditional risk factors (Zhang et al. 2001). High numbers of circulating neutrophils as important source of MPO were linked to both formation and severity of atherosclerotic lesions (Huang et al. 2001) and chronic stable angina pectoris (Avanzas et al. 2004). Direct assessment of human atherosclerotic lesions revealed presence of MPO (Daugherty et al. 1994) and neutrophils (Tavora et al. 2009) producing pro-inflammatory IL-8 (Marino et al. 2015). The extent of neutrophil infiltration was associated with a pro-inflammatory state and rupture-prone lesions (Ionita et al. 2010). Furthermore, levels of the NET surrogate markers dsDNA and chromatin were independently associated with the severity of coronary atherosclerosis and occurrence of adverse cardiovascular events (Borissoff et al. 2013).

Experimental models to identify mechanistic pathways of atherosclerosis typically rely on mice deficient for Apo E or low-density lipoprotein receptor, which are fed with a high-fat diet to develop atherosclerotic lesions. This led to the identification of a plethora of contributors underlying lesion formation and progression and confirmed a significant role for neutrophils in plaque development.

MPO-positive neutrophils were predominantly found in lesional caps of plaques (van Leeuwen et al. 2008) and plaque regions with already high inflammatory activity outnumbering present macrophages (Rotzius et al. 2010). Depletion of neutrophils was shown to attenuate lesion formation (Zernecke et al. 2008); however, protective effects were only apparent if depletion was performed within the first weeks, confining the effect of neutrophil activity to early stages of plaque development (Drechsler et al. 2010).

In *Apo E* knockout mice, neutrophils adhered to the luminal site of carotid atherosclerotic lesions and released DNA, indicative of NET formation, an interpretation which was supported by visualization of NETs in human endarterectomy samples (Megens et al. 2012). Presence of NETs was further verified in atherosclerotic lesions of mice in conjunction with an increase of the pro-inflammatory markers IL-1α, IL-1β, and IL-6 (Warnatsch et al. 2015). NETs, via histones, induced lytic cell death of smooth muscle cells in atherosclerotic lesions, leading to decreased plaque stability (Silvestre-Roig et al. 2019).

Recently, atherosclerotic lesions were classified into rupture-prone or erosion-prone phenotypes (Quillard et al. 2017). A growing body of evidence suggests that pathomechanisms are profoundly different in these two entities. Rupture-prone lesions typically contain many macrophages, harbor large lipid pools but have low interstitial collagen and few smooth muscle cells covered by thin fibrous caps. Disruption of fibrous caps makes up about two thirds of coronary events (Prati et al. 2013; Virmani et al. 2000). Conversely, eroded plaques typically present with a thick or even intact fibrous cap with a discontinuous endothelial layer (Libby 2017). Neutrophil infiltration appears to be critical for erosion as shown by an optical coherence tomography study to distinguish between plaque rupture and erosion in acute coronary syndrome. Of 25 included patients, seven exhibited erosion, and levels of systemic MPO were strikingly increased compared to patients with plaque rupture (Ferrante et al. 2010). Characterization of human endarterectomy samples demonstrated that presence of NETs was positively correlated with endothelial cell apoptosis, a hallmark feature of eroded plaques. Yet, the extent of NET burden was not different in both lesion types, emphasizing the power of neutrophil effector function (Quillard et al. 2015).

4.2 Arterial Thrombosis

The role of NETs in arterial thrombosis was mostly studied in two major conditions, acute myocardial infarction and ischemic stroke.

4.2.1 Acute Myocardial Infarction

Apart from atherosclerosis itself, neutrophils are critically involved in myocardial infarction, an acute manifestation of stable disease. Naruko et al. discovered that neutrophils were abundantly present in both ruptured and eroded plaques of patients who have died from MI (Naruko et al. 2002). The emergence of catheter-based thrombus aspiration in MI (Beran et al. 2002) made a detailed examination of thrombi in a high number of patients possible, and enabled a new view on atherosclerosis outside of autopsy specimens. This provided crucial insights into pathomechanisms underlying coronary thrombosis. Analyses revealed that leukocytes are a major component of fresh thrombi (Rittersma et al. 2005). The majority of thrombus leukocytes were neutrophils which co-localized with large quantities of endothelin-1 (Adlbrecht et al. 2007), a potent vasoconstrictor and pro-inflammatory mediator associated with left ventricular dysfunction after MI (Taylor et al. 2004). Neutrophil accumulation at the culprit site was associated with a local increase in pro-thrombotic complement factors and infarct size (Distelmaier et al. 2009). This was corroborated by the observation that thrombus neutrophil count was associated with impaired coronary microcirculation and reduced left ventricular function at six-month follow-up (Arakawa et al. 2009).

Ultimately, the presence of NETs was demonstrated in culprit site thrombi (de Boer et al. 2013). NETs were decorated with pro-inflammatory interleukin-17, which drives neutrophil accumulation (Liao et al. 2012) and is suggested to be important in the pathogenesis of MI (Mora-Ruiz et al. 2019). NETs in culprit site thrombi were confirmed by another group, which demonstrated NET formation to be induced by high mobility group box 1, an important danger-associated molecular pattern (Maugeri et al. 2014). In comparison with venous thrombi, NET burden was significantly higher in coronary thrombi and positively correlated with infarct size (Mangold et al. 2015). Recently, levels of dsDNA measured one day after MI were also associated with microvascular obstruction, myocardial salvage index, and left ventricular ejection fraction at four months (Helseth et al. 2019). Furthermore, neutrophils isolated from the culprit lesion site were more prone to undergo NETosis ex vivo in comparison with neutrophils harvested from a non-infarct related coronary artery (Stakos et al. 2015). The same group also found NETs to be decorated with tissue factor, an important mediator of coagulation. NETs were also shown to contribute to myocardial fibrosis by leading to increased activation and differentiation of fibrocytes at the culprit site (Hofbauer et al. 2019).

Circadian rhythms and neutrophil aging were recently proposed to modulate neutrophil migratory properties into tissues with substantial influence on vascular health and thrombo-inflammatory reactions in ischemia reperfusion (Adrover et al. 2019; Steffens et al. 2017).

4.2.2 Acute Ischemic Stroke

NETs were also shown to be associated with acute ischemic stroke. Concentrations of plasma DNA identified patients at risk of death at follow-up (Rainer et al. 2003), while nucleosomes were correlated with neurological dysfunction and infarction volume (Geiger et al. 2006). Another group demonstrated that DNA was increased after stroke (Tsai et al. 2011). Correspondingly, immunohistological analysis of thrombectomy samples revealed large numbers of neutrophils positive for citH3 (Laridan et al. 2017). NET burden in ischemic stroke thrombi retrieved via endovascular therapy was associated with the complexity of intervention, measured as duration of procedure and number of required wire passes (Ducroux et al. 2018). With respect to prognosis and outcome, soluble NET markers were associated with a higher NIHSS score, an indicator of stroke severity. Increased all-cause mortality was reported in patients with citH3 levels ranging in the upper quartile (Valles et al. 2017). Mechanistically, a mouse model of cerebral artery ischemia/reperfusion revealed significant exacerbation of brain injury after infusion of exogenous histones, highlighting the cytotoxic properties of NET components and their devastating influence on vascular tissues (De Meyer et al. 2012).

4.2.3 Other Conditions Associated with Arterial Thrombosis

In other diseases associated with arterial thrombosis, most evidence is available in *abdominal aortic aneurysm* (AAA). AAA, characterized by vessel dilation and formation of multilayered intraluminal thrombi (Delbosc et al. 2011), is increasingly being recognized as an inflammatory condition (Piechota-Polanczyk et al. 2015). Neutrophils appear to be crucial, as their depletion using a specific, cytotoxic antibody resulted in drastically reduced AAA formation (Eliason et al. 2005). NETs were shown to be abundantly present in the luminal part of human AAA thrombi and adventitia, and to be induced by periodontal pathogens (Delbosc et al. 2011) associated with AAA progression (Nakano et al. 2011). Finally, NETs co-localized with IL-1β in AAA thrombi (Meher et al. 2018), a pro-inflammatory mediator that drives AAA (Johnston et al. 2013) and NET (Keshari et al. 2012) formation.

In other pathologies associated with arterial thrombosis, evidence for the influence of NETs is scarce. *Peripheral artery disease* thrombi contain NETs to a similar extent as coronary and stroke thrombi (Farkas et al. 2019). Comparing plasma samples of DVT and PAD patients, neutrophil elastase alpha1 anti-trypsin complex, a specific marker for NETs, was increased in PAD (Kremers et al. 2019). Increased NET markers were also observed in *thrombotic microangiopathies* like thrombotic thrombocytopenic purpura or hemolytic uremic syndrome, with plasma levels being reflective of disease activity (Fuchs et al. 2012).

5 Neutrophil Extracellular Traps as a Therapeutic Target

Given their importance in the pathogenesis of atherosclerotic vascular disease, there is an interest in finding therapeutic compounds to inhibit NETs and block their detrimental effects. Several pathways have been suggested, targeting various NET components.

5.1 PAD-4 Inhibitors: Cl-Amidine

Since activation of PAD-4 is regarded critical for efficient uncoiling of chromatin in NETosis (Wang et al. 2009), inhibition of this key enzyme was suggested as a potential therapeutic regimen. Initially, synthetic PAD-4 inhibitors such as Cl-amidine were envisioned for treatment of rheumatoid arthritis (Kearney et al. 2005; Luo et al. 2006), a disease exacerbated by PAD-mediated excessive formation of citrullinated proteins that promote auto-immunity (Turunen et al. 2016). As Cl-amidine was characterized to irreversibly block PAD4, it critically interferes with NET formation (Wang et al. 2009). Cl-amidine was shown to attenuate disease severity in mouse models of sepsis (Biron et al. 2017), collagen-induced arthritis (Willis et al. 2011) and systemic lupus erythematosus, where it decreased NET formation and reduced deposition of inflammatory immunoglobulin and complement factors in the kidney (Knight et al. 2013). Daily subcutaneous treatment of ApoE knockout mice with Cl-amidine could alleviate atherosclerotic lesions under high-fat diet, while accumulation of neutrophils and macrophages into lesions was reduced (Knight et al. 2014). Thrombus formation induced by photochemical injury of the carotid artery could be significantly delayed by pre-treatment with Cl-amidine (Knight et al. 2013). It was demonstrated that Cl-amidine treatment reduces infarct size in a mouse model of coronary artery ligation and was associated with improved cardiac function (Novotny et al. 2018). In a model of ischemic stroke, administration of Cl-amidine prevented thrombotic occlusions (Pena-Martinez et al. 2019). These observations emphasize a certain dependency of NETosis on enzymatic PAD4 activity despite conflicting results and render pharmaceutical PAD-4 inhibition, a potentially promising target for treatment of human atherosclerotic and thrombotic disease.

5.2   Deoxyribonuclease

Deoxyribonuclease (DNase) degrades NETs by hydrolysis of the DNA backbone (Fuchs et al. 2010). Two isoforms of different cellular origins target DNA strands in vivo. DNase 1, secreted by the non-hematopoietic compartment, preferentially degrades protein-free DNA, while leukocyte-derived DNase 1 like 3 (DNase 1L3) cleaves DNA:protein complexes (Napirei et al. 2009). Adequate DNase activity was suggested to be crucial for a homeostatic balance between NET formation and degradation. Indeed, neutrophilic mice deficient in both plasmatic DNases developed severe disseminated thrombosis. However, reconstitution with or presence of just one functional DNase type was sufficient to protect mice from vascular occlusion (Jimenez-Alcazar et al. 2017). Targeting chromatin and NETs by DNase 1 was shown to be beneficial in experimental DVT (Brill et al. 2012; von Bruhl et al. 2012) and ischemic injury, including intestinal ischemia (Boettcher et al. 2017a), testicular torsion (Boettcher et al. 2017b), and ischemic stroke (Pena-Martinez et al. 2019).

In atherosclerotic mice, injection of DNase reduced lesion size and attenuated lesional NET burden as well as pro-inflammatory cytokines (Warnatsch et al. 2015). Furthermore, DNase 1 was used in rodent models of cardiac ischemia. Although one study reports reduction of neutrophil infiltration by DNase 1 alone in a model of ischemia/reperfusion, the authors could only show improved cardiac function by co-administration of tissue plasminogen activator (tPA) (Ge et al. 2015). In contrast, DNase 1 treatment improved cardiac function in mice after coronary artery ligation, without any reduction in neutrophil infiltration to the ischemic myocardium (Vogel et al. 2015). These apparently contradictory results may be due to variations in methodology of ligation, duration of ischemia, and timing of DNase application. In vitro, DNase 1 was shown to accelerate tPA-mediated thrombolysis of human coronary (Mangold et al. 2015) and cerebral (Laridan et al. 2017) thrombi in comparison with tPA alone. Importantly, in MI patients, low DNase activity was associated with increased infarct size (Mangold et al. 2015).

Considering the mounting evidence on the benefits of DNase application in different well-established disease models, these data raise the possibility of DNase 1 treatment of patients in neutrophil-driven disease settings in which NET formation plays a pathogenic role.

5.3   Heparin

Due to their anticoagulant properties, unfractionated heparin and low molecular weight heparins are long recognized therapeutic cornerstones for deep vein thrombosis (Mazzolai et al. 2018) and MI (Neumann et al. 2019). Given the inflammatory component of thrombotic diseases, it is intriguing that heparins have a variety of anti-inflammatory effects (Mulloy et al. 2016; Rao et al. 2010) which seem to be unrelated to their anticoagulant activity (Rao et al. 2010). In a model of acute inflammation, diminished accumulation of neutrophils was at least in part ascribed to the ability of heparin oligosaccharides to block L- and P-selectin (Nelson et al.

1993). Likewise, CD11b-dependent adhesion could be attenuated by interaction with heparin (Salas et al. 2000; Wang et al. 2002). Furthermore, heparins can not only limit NET formation itself as shown by treatment in vitro and in vivo (Manfredi et al. 2017), but can also target existing NETs in various ways: heparin was shown to inhibit enzymatic activity of neutrophil elastase and Cathepsin G (Fryer et al. 1997), two major enzymes present in NETs (Folco et al. 2018). Binding and displacement of histones by heparin promotes NETs disassembly, limiting their pro-thrombotic properties in vitro (Fuchs et al. 2010) and in vivo (von Bruhl et al. 2012). At the same time, excessive release of histones during cell death and NETosis was suggested to counteract the anti-thrombotic function of heparin, potentially explaining non-responsiveness to heparin (Longstaff et al. 2016).

These observations stimulated the development of heparinoids that lack anticoagulant properties while keeping their anti-inflammatory effects (Rao et al. 2010). Indeed, sevuparin, a low-anticoagulant heparin analog, inhibited NE and histone H4, proteins associated with NETs (Rasmuson et al. 2019). In another study, non-anticoagulant heparin prevented histone-mediated cytotoxicity and improved survival in a murine sepsis model (Wildhagen et al. 2014). Thus, it might be a crucial therapeutic add-on to reduce NET burden without increasing risk of bleeding complications.

6 Summary

A summary of the content of this chapter is provided in the central Fig. 1. Taken together, NETs are important for the initiation and progression of thrombosis in the setting of atherosclerosis, including VTE, MI, and stroke. For these reasons, NETs

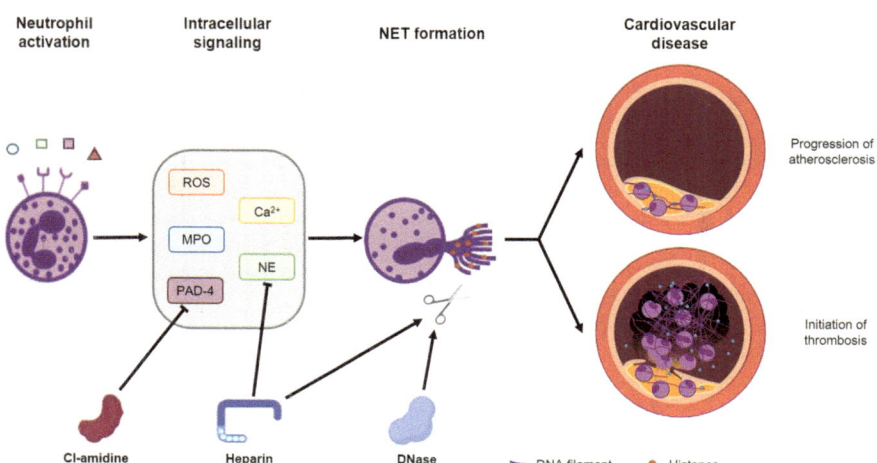

Fig. 1 The central figure summarizes mechanisms of NET formation, its pathways and consequences in atherosclerosis and thrombosis. The figure was constructed using Biorender and Microsoft PowerPoint

have emerged as potential targets for treatment. Despite promising in vitro and experimental in vivo data, adequately powered clinical trials are required to assess clinical benefits and safety of anti-NETotic regimens.

References

Adlbrecht C, Bonderman D, Plass C, Jakowitsch J, Beran G, Sperker W, Siostrzonek P, Glogar D, Maurer G, Lang IM (2007) Active endothelin is an important vasoconstrictor in acute coronary thrombi. Thromb Haemost 97:642–649

Adrover JM, Del Fresno C, Crainiciuc G, Cuartero MI, Casanova-Acebes M, Weiss LA, Huerga-Encabo H, Silvestre-Roig C, Rossaint J, Cossio I, Lechuga-Vieco AV, Garcia-Prieto J, Gomez-Parrizas M, Quintana JA, Ballesteros I, Martin-Salamanca S, Aroca-Crevillen A, Chong SZ, Evrard M, Balabanian K, Lopez J, Bidzhekov K, Bachelerie F, Abad-Santos F, Munoz-Calleja-C, Zarbock A, Soehnlein O, Weber C, Ng LG, Lopez-Rodriguez C, Sancho D, Moro MA, Ibanez B, Hidalgo A (2019) A neutrophil timer coordinates immune defense and vascular protection. Immunity 50:390–402.e10. https://doi.org/10.1016/j.immuni.2019.01.002

Aldabbous L, Abdul-Salam V, McKinnon T, Duluc L, Pepke-Zaba J, Southwood M, Ainscough AJ, Hadinnapola C, Wilkins MR, Toshner M, Wojciak-Stothard B (2016) Neutrophil extracellular traps promote angiogenesis: evidence from vascular pathology in pulmonary hypertension. Arterioscler Thromb Vasc Biol 36:2078–2087. https://doi.org/10.1161/atvbaha.116.307634

Arakawa K, Yasuda S, Hao H, Kataoka Y, Morii I, Kasahara Y, Kawamura A, Ishibashi-Ueda H, Miyazaki S (2009) Significant association between neutrophil aggregation in aspirated thrombus and myocardial damage in patients with ST-segment elevation acute myocardial infarction. Circ J 73:139–144

Arnalich F, Maldifassi MC, Ciria E, Codoceo R, Renart J, Fernandez-Capitan C, Herruzo R, Garcia-Rio F, Lopez-Collazo E, Montiel C (2013) Plasma levels of mitochondrial and nuclear DNA in patients with massive pulmonary embolism in the emergency department: a prospective cohort study. Crit Care 17:R90. https://doi.org/10.1186/cc12735

Avanzas P, Arroyo-Espliguero R, Cosin-Sales J, Quiles J, Zouridakis E, Kaski JC (2004) Multiple complex stenoses, high neutrophil count and C-reactive protein levels in patients with chronic stable angina. Atherosclerosis 175:151–157. https://doi.org/10.1016/j.atherosclerosis.2004.03.013

Bainton DF, Ullyot JL, Farquhar MG (1971) The development of neutrophilic polymorphonuclear leukocytes in human bone marrow. J Exp Med 134:907–934

Barquera S, Pedroza-Tobias A, Medina C, Hernandez-Barrera L, Bibbins-Domingo K, Lozano R, Moran AE (2015) Global overview of the epidemiology of atherosclerotic cardiovascular disease. Arch Med Res 46:328–338. https://doi.org/10.1016/j.arcmed.2015.06.006

Beran G, Lang I, Schreiber W, Denk S, Stefenelli T, Syeda B, Maurer G, Glogar D, Siostrzonek P (2002) Intracoronary thrombectomy with the X-sizer catheter system improves epicardial flow and accelerates ST-segment resolution in patients with acute coronary syndrome: a prospective, randomized, controlled study. Circulation 105:2355–2360

Biron BM, Chung CS, O'Brien XM, Chen Y, Reichner JS, Ayala A (2017) Cl-amidine prevents histone 3 citrullination and neutrophil extracellular trap formation, and improves survival in a murine sepsis model. J Innate Immun 9:22–32. https://doi.org/10.1159/000448808

Boettcher M, Eschenburg G, Mietzsch S, Jimenez-Alcazar M, Klinke M, Vincent D, Tiemann B, Bergholz R, Reinshagen K, Fuchs TA (2017a) Therapeutic targeting of extracellular DNA improves the outcome of intestinal ischemic reperfusion injury in neonatal rats. Sci Rep 7:15377. https://doi.org/10.1038/s41598-017-15807-6

Boettcher M, Meier D, Jimenez-Alcazar M, Eschenburg G, Mietzsch S, Vincent D, Klinke M, Trochimiuk M, Appl B, Tiemann B, Bergholz R, Reinshagen K, Fuchs TA (2017b) Degradation of extracellular DNA by DNase1 significantly reduces testicular damage after testicular torsion in rats. Urology 109:223.e1–223.e7. https://doi.org/10.1016/j.urology.2017.07.031

Borissoff JI, Joosen IA, Versteylen MO, Brill A, Fuchs TA, Savchenko AS, Gallant M, Martinod K, Ten Cate H, Hofstra L, Crijns HJ, Wagner DD, Kietselaer B (2013) Elevated levels of circulating DNA and chromatin are independently associated with severe coronary atherosclerosis and a prothrombotic state. Arterioscler Thromb Vasc Biol 33:2032–2040. https://doi.org/10.1161/atvbaha.113.301627

Brill A, Fuchs TA, Savchenko AS, Thomas GM, Martinod K, De Meyer SF, Bhandari AA, Wagner DD (2012) Neutrophil extracellular traps promote deep vein thrombosis in mice. J Thromb Haemost 10:136–144. https://doi.org/10.1111/j.1538-7836.2011.04544.x

Brinkmann V, Reichard U, Goosmann C, Fauler B, Uhlemann Y, Weiss DS, Weinrauch Y, Zychlinsky A (2004) Neutrophil extracellular traps kill bacteria. Science 303:1532–1535. https://doi.org/10.1126/science.1092385

Bullenkamp J, Dinkla S, Kaski JC, Dumitriu IE (2016) Targeting T cells to treat atherosclerosis: odyssey from bench to bedside. Eur Heart J Cardiovasc Pharmacother 2:194–199. https://doi.org/10.1093/ehjcvp/pvw001

Campillo-Navarro M, Leyva-Paredes K, Donis-Maturano L, Gonzalez-Jimenez M, Paredes-Vivas Y, Cerbulo-Vazquez A, Serafin-Lopez J, Garcia-Perez B, Ullrich SE, Flores-Romo L, Perez-Tapia SM, Estrada-Parra S, Estrada-Garcia I, Chacon-Salinas R (2017) Listeria monocytogenes induces mast cell extracellular traps. Immunobiology 222:432–439. https://doi.org/10.1016/j.imbio.2016.08.006

Catapano AL, Graham I, De Backer G, Wiklund O, Chapman MJ, Drexel H, Hoes AW, Jennings CS, Landmesser U, Pedersen TR, Reiner Z, Riccardi G, Taskinen MR, Tokgozoglu L, Verschuren WMM, Vlachopoulos C, Wood DA, Zamorano JL, Cooney MT (2016) 2016 ESC/EAS guidelines for the management of dyslipidaemias. Eur Heart J 37:2999–3058. https://doi.org/10.1093/eurheartj/ehw272

Claushuis TAM, van der Donk LEH, Luitse AL, van Veen HA, van der Wel NN, van Vught LA, Roelofs J, de Boer OJ, Lankelma JM, Boon L, de Vos AF, van 't Veer C, van der Poll T (2018) Role of peptidylarginine deiminase 4 in neutrophil extracellular trap formation and host defense during Klebsiella pneumoniae-induced pneumonia-derived sepsis. J Immunol 201:1241–1252. https://doi.org/10.4049/jimmunol.1800314

Cowland JB, Borregaard N (2016) Granulopoiesis and granules of human neutrophils. Immunol Rev 273:11–28. https://doi.org/10.1111/imr.12440

Daugherty A, Dunn JL, Rateri DL, Heinecke JW (1994) Myeloperoxidase, a catalyst for lipoprotein oxidation, is expressed in human atherosclerotic lesions. J Clin Invest 94:437–444. https://doi.org/10.1172/jci117342

de Boer OJ, Li X, Teeling P, Mackaay C, Ploegmakers HJ, van der Loos CM, Daemen MJ, de Winter RJ, van der Wal AC (2013) Neutrophils, neutrophil extracellular traps and interleukin-17 associate with the organisation of thrombi in acute myocardial infarction. Thromb Haemost 109:290–297. https://doi.org/10.1160/th12-06-0425

de Bont CM, Eerden N, Boelens WC, Pruijn GJM (2020) Neutrophil proteases degrade autoepitopes of NET-associated proteins. Clin Exp Immunol 199:1–8. https://doi.org/10.1111/cei.13392

De Meyer SF, Suidan GL, Fuchs TA, Monestier M, Wagner DD (2012) Extracellular chromatin is an important mediator of ischemic stroke in mice. Arterioscler Thromb Vasc Biol 32:1884–1891. https://doi.org/10.1161/atvbaha.112.250993

Delbosc S, Alsac JM, Journe C, Louedec L, Castier Y, Bonnaure-Mallet M, Ruimy R, Rossignol P, Bouchard P, Michel JB, Meilhac O (2011) Porphyromonas gingivalis participates in pathogenesis of human abdominal aortic aneurysm by neutrophil activation. Proof of concept in rats. PLoS One 6:e18679. https://doi.org/10.1371/journal.pone.0018679

Desai J, Mulay SR, Nakazawa D, Anders HJ (2016) Matters of life and death. How neutrophils die or survive along NET release and is "NETosis" = necroptosis? Cell Mol Life Sci 73:2211–2219. https://doi.org/10.1007/s00018-016-2195-0

Di Nisio M, van Es N, Buller HR (2016) Deep vein thrombosis and pulmonary embolism. Lancet 388:3060–3073. https://doi.org/10.1016/s0140-6736(16)30514-1

Diaz JA, Fuchs TA, Jackson TO, Kremer Hovinga JA, Lammle B, Henke PK, Myers DD Jr, Wagner DD, Wakefield TW (2013) Plasma DNA is elevated in patients with deep vein thrombosis. J Vasc Surg Venous Lymphat Disord:1. https://doi.org/10.1016/j.jvsv.2012.12.002

Distelmaier K, Adlbrecht C, Jakowitsch J, Winkler S, Dunkler D, Gerner C, Wagner O, Lang IM, Kubicek M (2009) Local complement activation triggers neutrophil recruitment to the site of thrombus formation in acute myocardial infarction. Thromb Haemost 102:564–572. https://doi.org/10.1160/th09-02-0103

Distelmaier K, Winter MP, Dragschitz F, Redwan B, Mangold A, Gleiss A, Perkmann T, Maurer G, Adlbrecht C, Lang IM (2014) Prognostic value of culprit site neutrophils in acute coronary syndrome. Eur J Clin Investig 44:257–265. https://doi.org/10.1111/eci.12228

Doring Y, Drechsler M, Soehnlein O, Weber C (2015) Neutrophils in atherosclerosis: from mice to man. Arterioscler Thromb Vasc Biol 35:288–295. https://doi.org/10.1161/atvbaha.114.303564

Doring Y, Soehnlein O, Weber C (2017) Neutrophil extracellular traps in atherosclerosis and atherothrombosis. Circ Res 120:736–743. https://doi.org/10.1161/circresaha.116.309692

Doster RS, Rogers LM, Gaddy JA, Aronoff DM (2018) Macrophage extracellular traps: a scoping review. J Innate Immun 10:3–13. https://doi.org/10.1159/000480373

Drechsler M, Megens RT, van Zandvoort M, Weber C, Soehnlein O (2010) Hyperlipidemia-triggered neutrophilia promotes early atherosclerosis. Circulation 122:1837–1845. https://doi.org/10.1161/circulationaha.110.961714

Ducroux C, Di Meglio L, Loyau S, Delbosc S, Boisseau W, Deschildre C, Ben Maacha M, Blanc R, Redjem H, Ciccio G, Smajda S, Fahed R, Michel JB, Piotin M, Salomon L, Mazighi M, Ho-Tin-Noe B, Desilles JP (2018) Thrombus neutrophil extracellular traps content impair tPA-induced thrombolysis in acute ischemic stroke. Stroke 49:754–757. https://doi.org/10.1161/strokeaha.117.019896

Eliason JL, Hannawa KK, Ailawadi G, Sinha I, Ford JW, Deogracias MP, Roelofs KJ, Woodrum DT, Ennis TL, Henke PK, Stanley JC, Thompson RW, Upchurch GR Jr (2005) Neutrophil depletion inhibits experimental abdominal aortic aneurysm formation. Circulation 112:232–240. https://doi.org/10.1161/circulationaha.104.517391

Farkas AZ, Farkas VJ, Gubucz I, Szabo L, Balint K, Tenekedjiev K, Nagy AI, Sotonyi P, Hidi L, Nagy Z, Szikora I, Merkely B, Kolev K (2019) Neutrophil extracellular traps in thrombi retrieved during interventional treatment of ischemic arterial diseases. Thromb Res 175:46–52. https://doi.org/10.1016/j.thromres.2019.01.006

Ferrante G, Nakano M, Prati F, Niccoli G, Mallus MT, Ramazzotti V, Montone RA, Kolodgie FD, Virmani R, Crea F (2010) High levels of systemic myeloperoxidase are associated with coronary plaque erosion in patients with acute coronary syndromes: a clinicopathological study. Circulation 122:2505–2513. https://doi.org/10.1161/circulationaha.110.955302

Folco EJ, Mawson TL, Vromman A, Bernardes-Souza B, Franck G, Persson O, Nakamura M, Newton G, Luscinskas FW, Libby P (2018) Neutrophil extracellular traps induce endothelial cell activation and tissue factor production through interleukin-1alpha and cathepsin G. Arterioscler Thromb Vasc Biol 38:1901–1912. https://doi.org/10.1161/atvbaha.118.311150

Fryer A, Huang YC, Rao G, Jacoby D, Mancilla E, Whorton R, Piantadosi CA, Kennedy T, Hoidal J (1997) Selective O-desulfation produces nonanticoagulant heparin that retains pharmacological activity in the lung. J Pharmacol Exp Ther 282:208–219

Fuchs TA, Abed U, Goosmann C, Hurwitz R, Schulze I, Wahn V, Weinrauch Y, Brinkmann V, Zychlinsky A (2007) Novel cell death program leads to neutrophil extracellular traps. J Cell Biol 176:231–241. https://doi.org/10.1083/jcb.200606027

Fuchs TA, Brill A, Duerschmied D, Schatzberg D, Monestier M, Myers DD Jr, Wrobleski SK, Wakefield TW, Hartwig JH, Wagner DD (2010) Extracellular DNA traps promote thrombosis. Proc Natl Acad Sci U S A 107:15880–15885. https://doi.org/10.1073/pnas.1005743107

Fuchs TA, Kremer Hovinga JA, Schatzberg D, Wagner DD, Lammle B (2012) Circulating DNA and myeloperoxidase indicate disease activity in patients with thrombotic microangiopathies. Blood 120:1157–1164. https://doi.org/10.1182/blood-2012-02-412197

Galie N, Humbert M, Vachiery JL, Gibbs S, Lang I, Torbicki A, Simonneau G, Peacock A, Vonk Noordegraaf A, Beghetti M, Ghofrani A, Gomez Sanchez MA, Hansmann G, Klepetko W, Lancellotti P, Matucci M, McDonagh T, Pierard LA, Trindade PT, Zompatori M, Hoeper M (2016) 2015 ESC/ERS guidelines for the diagnosis and treatment of pulmonary hypertension: the Joint Task Force for the Diagnosis and Treatment of Pulmonary Hypertension of the European Society of Cardiology (ESC) and the European Respiratory Society (ERS): Endorsed by: Association for European Paediatric and Congenital Cardiology (AEPC), International Society for Heart and Lung Transplantation (ISHLT). Eur Heart J 37:67–119. https://doi.org/10.1093/eurheartj/ehv317

Ge L, Zhou X, Ji WJ, Lu RY, Zhang Y, Zhang YD, Ma YQ, Zhao JH, Li YM (2015) Neutrophil extracellular traps in ischemia-reperfusion injury-induced myocardial no-reflow: therapeutic potential of DNase-based reperfusion strategy. Am J Physiol Heart Circ Physiol 308:H500–H509. https://doi.org/10.1152/ajpheart.00381.2014

Geiger S, Holdenrieder S, Stieber P, Hamann GF, Bruening R, Ma J, Nagel D, Seidel D (2006) Nucleosomes in serum of patients with early cerebral stroke. Cerebrovasc Dis 21:32–37. https://doi.org/10.1159/000089591

Gil-Pulido J, Zernecke A (2017) Antigen-presenting dendritic cells in atherosclerosis. Eur J Pharmacol 816:25–31. https://doi.org/10.1016/j.ejphar.2017.08.016

Granger V, Faille D, Marani V, Noel B, Gallais Y, Szely N, Flament H, Pallardy M, Chollet-Martin S, de Chaisemartin L (2017) Human blood monocytes are able to form extracellular traps. J Leukoc Biol 102:775–781. https://doi.org/10.1189/jlb.3MA0916-411R

Hakkim A, Fuchs TA, Martinez NE, Hess S, Prinz H, Zychlinsky A, Waldmann H (2011) Activation of the Raf-MEK-ERK pathway is required for neutrophil extracellular trap formation. Nat Chem Biol 7:75–77. https://doi.org/10.1038/nchembio.496

Helseth R, Shetelig C, Andersen GO, Langseth MS, Limalanathan S, Opstad TB, Arnesen H, Hoffmann P, Eritsland J, Seljeflot I (2019) Neutrophil extracellular trap components associate with infarct size, ventricular function, and clinical outcome in STEMI. Mediat Inflamm 2019:7816491. https://doi.org/10.1155/2019/7816491

Herrington W, Lacey B, Sherliker P, Armitage J, Lewington S (2016) Epidemiology of atherosclerosis and the potential to reduce the global burden of atherothrombotic disease. Circ Res 118:535–546. https://doi.org/10.1161/circresaha.115.307611

Hofbauer TM, Mangold A, Scherz T, Seidl V, Panzenbock A, Ondracek AS, Muller J, Schneider M, Binder T, Hell L, Lang IM (2019) Neutrophil extracellular traps and fibrocytes in ST-segment elevation myocardial infarction. Basic Res Cardiol 114:33. https://doi.org/10.1007/s00395-019-0740-3

Huang ZS, Jeng JS, Wang CH, Yip PK, Wu TH, Lee TK (2001) Correlations between peripheral differential leukocyte counts and carotid atherosclerosis in non-smokers. Atherosclerosis 158:431–436

Ionita MG, van den Borne P, Catanzariti LM, Moll FL, de Vries JP, Pasterkamp G, Vink A, de Kleijn DP (2010) High neutrophil numbers in human carotid atherosclerotic plaques are associated with characteristics of rupture-prone lesions. Arterioscler Thromb Vasc Biol 30:1842–1848. https://doi.org/10.1161/atvbaha.110.209296

Jimenez-Alcazar M, Rangaswamy C, Panda R, Bitterling J, Simsek YJ, Long AT, Bilyy R, Krenn V, Renne C, Renne T, Kluge S, Panzer U, Mizuta R, Mannherz HG, Kitamura D, Herrmann M, Napirei M, Fuchs TA (2017) Host DNases prevent vascular occlusion by neutrophil extracellular traps. Science 358:1202–1206. https://doi.org/10.1126/science.aam8897

Jimenez-Alcazar M, Limacher A, Panda R, Mean M, Bitterling J, Peine S, Renne T, Beer JH, Aujesky D, Lammle B, Fuchs TA (2018) Circulating extracellular DNA is an independent predictor of mortality in elderly patients with venous thromboembolism. PLoS One 13: e0191150. https://doi.org/10.1371/journal.pone.0191150

Johnston WF, Salmon M, Su G, Lu G, Stone ML, Zhao Y, Owens GK, Upchurch GR Jr, Ailawadi G (2013) Genetic and pharmacologic disruption of interleukin-1beta signaling inhibits experimental aortic aneurysm formation. Arterioscler Thromb Vasc Biol 33:294–304. https://doi.org/10.1161/atvbaha.112.300432

Kapoor S, Opneja A, Nayak L (2018) The role of neutrophils in thrombosis. Thromb Res 170:87–96. https://doi.org/10.1016/j.thromres.2018.08.005

Kearney PL, Bhatia M, Jones NG, Yuan L, Glascock MC, Catchings KL, Yamada M, Thompson PR (2005) Kinetic characterization of protein arginine deiminase 4: a transcriptional corepressor implicated in the onset and progression of rheumatoid arthritis. Biochemistry 44:10570–10582. https://doi.org/10.1021/bi050292m

Kenny EF, Herzig A, Kruger R, Muth A, Mondal S, Thompson PR, Brinkmann V, Bernuth HV, Zychlinsky A (2017) Diverse stimuli engage different neutrophil extracellular trap pathways. elife 6. https://doi.org/10.7554/eLife.24437

Keshari RS, Jyoti A, Dubey M, Kothari N, Kohli M, Bogra J, Barthwal MK, Dikshit M (2012) Cytokines induced neutrophil extracellular traps formation: implication for the inflammatory disease condition. PLoS One 7:e48111. https://doi.org/10.1371/journal.pone.0048111

Knight JS, Zhao W, Luo W, Subramanian V, O'Dell AA, Yalavarthi S, Hodgin JB, Eitzman DT, Thompson PR, Kaplan MJ (2013) Peptidylarginine deiminase inhibition is immunomodulatory and vasculoprotective in murine lupus. J Clin Invest 123:2981–2993. https://doi.org/10.1172/jci67390

Knight JS, Luo W, O'Dell AA, Yalavarthi S, Zhao W, Subramanian V, Guo C, Grenn RC, Thompson PR, Eitzman DT, Kaplan MJ (2014) Peptidylarginine deiminase inhibition reduces vascular damage and modulates innate immune responses in murine models of atherosclerosis. Circ Res 114:947–956. https://doi.org/10.1161/circresaha.114.303312

Kremers BMM, Birocchi S, van Oerle R, Zeerleder S, Spronk HMH, Mees BME, Luken BM, Ten Cate H, Ten Cate-Hoek AJ (2019) Searching for a common thrombo-inflammatory basis in patients with deep vein thrombosis or peripheral artery disease. Front Cardiovasc Med 6:33. https://doi.org/10.3389/fcvm.2019.00033

Kumar DR, Hanlin E, Glurich I, Mazza JJ, Yale SH (2010) Virchow's contribution to the understanding of thrombosis and cellular biology. Clin Med Res 8:168–172. https://doi.org/10.3121/cmr.2009.866

Lang IM (2004) Chronic thromboembolic pulmonary hypertension--not so rare after all. N Engl J Med 350:2236–2238. https://doi.org/10.1056/NEJMp048088

Laridan E, Denorme F, Desender L, Francois O, Andersson T, Deckmyn H, Vanhoorelbeke K, De Meyer SF (2017) Neutrophil extracellular traps in ischemic stroke thrombi. Ann Neurol 82:223–232. https://doi.org/10.1002/ana.24993

Lewis HD, Liddle J, Coote JE, Atkinson SJ, Barker MD, Bax BD, Bicker KL, Bingham RP, Campbell M, Chen YH, Chung CW, Craggs PD, Davis RP, Eberhard D, Joberty G, Lind KE, Locke K, Maller C, Martinod K, Patten C, Polyakova O, Rise CE, Rudiger M, Sheppard RJ, Slade DJ, Thomas P, Thorpe J, Yao G, Drewes G, Wagner DD, Thompson PR, Prinjha RK, Wilson DM (2015) Inhibition of PAD4 activity is sufficient to disrupt mouse and human NET formation. Nat Chem Biol 11:189–191. https://doi.org/10.1038/nchembio.1735

Ley K, Hoffman HM, Kubes P, Cassatella MA, Zychlinsky A, Hedrick CC, Catz SD (2018) Neutrophils: new insights and open questions. Sci Immunol 3. https://doi.org/10.1126/sciimmunol.aat4579

Li P, Li M, Lindberg MR, Kennett MJ, Xiong N, Wang Y (2010) PAD4 is essential for antibacterial innate immunity mediated by neutrophil extracellular traps. J Exp Med 207:1853–1862. https://doi.org/10.1084/jem.20100239

Liao YH, Xia N, Zhou SF, Tang TT, Yan XX, Lv BJ, Nie SF, Wang J, Iwakura Y, Xiao H, Yuan J, Jevallee H, Wei F, Shi GP, Cheng X (2012) Interleukin-17A contributes to myocardial ischemia/reperfusion injury by regulating cardiomyocyte apoptosis and neutrophil infiltration. J Am Coll Cardiol 59:420–429. https://doi.org/10.1016/j.jacc.2011.10.863

Libby P (2017) Superficial erosion and the precision management of acute coronary syndromes: not one-size-fits-all. Eur Heart J 38:801–803. https://doi.org/10.1093/eurheartj/ehw599

Longstaff C, Hogwood J, Gray E, Komorowicz E, Varju I, Varga Z, Kolev K (2016) Neutralisation of the anti-coagulant effects of heparin by histones in blood plasma and purified systems. Thromb Haemost 115:591–599. https://doi.org/10.1160/th15-03-0214

Luo Y, Knuckley B, Lee YH, Stallcup MR, Thompson PR (2006) A fluoroacetamidine-based inactivator of protein arginine deiminase 4: design, synthesis, and in vitro and in vivo evaluation. J Am Chem Soc 128:1092–1093. https://doi.org/10.1021/ja0576233

Madhusoodanan J (2017) Core concept: role player or cellular rubbish? Biologists debate the function of neutrophil extracellular traps. Proc Natl Acad Sci U S A 114:13309–13311. https://doi.org/10.1073/pnas.1719978115

Manfredi AA, Rovere-Querini P, D'Angelo A, Maugeri N (2017) Low molecular weight heparins prevent the induction of autophagy of activated neutrophils and the formation of neutrophil extracellular traps. Pharmacol Res 123:146–156. https://doi.org/10.1016/j.phrs.2016.08.008

Mangold A, Alias S, Scherz T, Hofbauer T, Jakowitsch J, Panzenbock A, Simon D, Laimer D, Bangert C, Kammerlander A, Mascherbauer J, Winter MP, Distelmaier K, Adlbrecht C, Preissner KT, Lang IM (2015) Coronary neutrophil extracellular trap burden and deoxyribonuclease activity in ST-elevation acute coronary syndrome are predictors of ST-segment resolution and infarct size. Circ Res 116:1182–1192. https://doi.org/10.1161/circresaha.116.304944

Marino F, Tozzi M, Schembri L, Ferraro S, Tarallo A, Scanzano A, Legnaro M, Castelli P, Cosentino M (2015) Production of IL-8, VEGF and elastase by circulating and intraplaque neutrophils in patients with carotid atherosclerosis. PLoS One 10:e0124565. https://doi.org/10.1371/journal.pone.0124565

Martinod K, Demers M, Fuchs TA, Wong SL, Brill A, Gallant M, Hu J, Wang Y, Wagner DD (2013) Neutrophil histone modification by peptidylarginine deiminase 4 is critical for deep vein thrombosis in mice. Proc Natl Acad Sci U S A 110:8674–8679. https://doi.org/10.1073/pnas.1301059110

Maugeri N, Campana L, Gavina M, Covino C, De Metrio M, Panciroli C, Maiuri L, Maseri A, D'Angelo A, Bianchi ME, Rovere-Querini P, Manfredi AA (2014) Activated platelets present high mobility group box 1 to neutrophils, inducing autophagy and promoting the extrusion of neutrophil extracellular traps. J Thromb Haemost 12:2074–2088. https://doi.org/10.1111/jth.12710

Mazzolai L, Aboyans V, Ageno W, Agnelli G, Alatri A, Bauersachs R, Brekelmans MPA, Buller HR, Elias A, Farge D, Konstantinides S, Palareti G, Prandoni P, Righini M, Torbicki A, Vlachopoulos C, Brodmann M (2018) Diagnosis and management of acute deep vein thrombosis: a joint consensus document from the European Society of Cardiology working groups of aorta and peripheral vascular diseases and pulmonary circulation and right ventricular function. Eur Heart J 39:4208–4218 https://doi.org/10.1093/eurheartj/ehx003

Megens RT, Vijayan S, Lievens D, Doring Y, van Zandvoort MA, Grommes J, Weber C, Soehnlein O (2012) Presence of luminal neutrophil extracellular traps in atherosclerosis. Thromb Haemost 107:597–598. https://doi.org/10.1160/th11-09-0650

Meher AK, Spinosa M, Davis JP, Pope N, Laubach VE, Su G, Serbulea V, Leitinger N, Ailawadi G, Upchurch GR Jr (2018) Novel role of IL (Interleukin)-1beta in neutrophil extracellular trap formation and abdominal aortic aneurysms. Arterioscler Thromb Vasc Biol 38:843–853. https://doi.org/10.1161/atvbaha.117.309897

Metzler KD, Goosmann C, Lubojemska A, Zychlinsky A, Papayannopoulos V (2014) A myeloperoxidase-containing complex regulates neutrophil elastase release and actin dynamics during NETosis. Cell Rep 8:883–896. https://doi.org/10.1016/j.celrep.2014.06.044

Mora-Ruiz MD, Blanco-Favela F, Chavez Rueda AK, Legorreta-Haquet MV, Chavez-Sanchez L (2019) Role of interleukin-17 in acute myocardial infarction. Mol Immunol 107:71–78. https://doi.org/10.1016/j.molimm.2019.01.008

Moroni F, Ammirati E, Norata GD, Magnoni M, Camici PG (2019) The role of monocytes and macrophages in human atherosclerosis, plaque neoangiogenesis, and atherothrombosis. Mediat Inflamm 2019:7434376. https://doi.org/10.1155/2019/7434376

Mukherjee M, Lacy P, Ueki S (2018) Eosinophil extracellular traps and inflammatory pathologies-untangling the web! Front Immunol 9:2763. https://doi.org/10.3389/fimmu.2018.02763

Mulloy B, Hogwood J, Gray E, Lever R, Page CP (2016) Pharmacology of heparin and related drugs. Pharmacol Rev 68:76–141. https://doi.org/10.1124/pr.115.011247

Nakano K, Wada K, Nomura R, Nemoto H, Inaba H, Kojima A, Naka S, Hokamura K, Mukai T, Nakajima A, Umemura K, Kamisaki Y, Yoshioka H, Taniguchi K, Amano A, Ooshima T (2011) Characterization of aortic aneurysms in cardiovascular disease patients harboring Porphyromonas gingivalis. Oral Dis 17:370–378. https://doi.org/10.1111/j.1601-0825.2010.01759.x

Nakazawa D, Tomaru U, Yamamoto C, Jodo S, Ishizu A (2012) Abundant neutrophil extracellular traps in thrombus of patient with microscopic polyangiitis. Front Immunol 3:333. https://doi.org/10.3389/fimmu.2012.00333

Napirei M, Ludwig S, Mezrhab J, Klockl T, Mannherz HG (2009) Murine serum nucleases--contrasting effects of plasmin and heparin on the activities of DNase1 and DNase1-like 3 (DNase1l3). FEBS J 276:1059–1073. https://doi.org/10.1111/j.1742-4658.2008.06849.x

Naruko T, Ueda M, Haze K, van der Wal AC, van der Loos CM, Itoh A, Komatsu R, Ikura Y, Ogami M, Shimada Y, Ehara S, Yoshiyama M, Takeuchi K, Yoshikawa J, Becker AE (2002) Neutrophil infiltration of culprit lesions in acute coronary syndromes. Circulation 106:2894–2900

Nelson RM, Cecconi O, Roberts WG, Aruffo A, Linhardt RJ, Bevilacqua MP (1993) Heparin oligosaccharides bind L- and P-selectin and inhibit acute inflammation. Blood 82:3253–3258

Neumann FJ, Sousa-Uva M, Ahlsson A, Alfonso F, Banning AP, Benedetto U, Byrne RA, Collet JP, Falk V, Head SJ, Juni P, Kastrati A, Koller A, Kristensen SD, Niebauer J, Richter DJ, Seferovic PM, Sibbing D, Stefanini GG, Windecker S, Yadav R, Zembala MO (2019) 2018 ESC/EACTS guidelines on myocardial revascularization. Eur Heart J 40:87–165. https://doi.org/10.1093/eurheartj/ehy394

Novotny J, Chandraratne S, Weinberger T, Philippi V, Stark K, Ehrlich A, Pircher J, Konrad I, Oberdieck P, Titova A, Hoti Q, Schubert I, Legate KR, Urtz N, Lorenz M, Pelisek J, Massberg S, von Bruhl ML, Schulz C (2018) Histological comparison of arterial thrombi in mice and men and the influence of Cl-amidine on thrombus formation. PLoS One 13:e0190728. https://doi.org/10.1371/journal.pone.0190728

Papayannopoulos V (2018) Neutrophil extracellular traps in immunity and disease. Nat Rev Immunol 18:134–147. https://doi.org/10.1038/nri.2017.105

Pena-Martinez C, Duran-Laforet V, Garcia-Culebras A, Ostos F, Hernandez-Jimenez M, Bravo-Ferrer I, Perez-Ruiz A, Ballenilla F, Diaz-Guzman J, Pradillo JM, Lizasoain I, Moro MA (2019) Pharmacological modulation of neutrophil extracellular traps reverses thrombotic stroke tPA (tissue-type plasminogen activator) resistance. Stroke 50:3228–3237. https://doi.org/10.1161/strokeaha.119.026848

Piechota-Polanczyk A, Jozkowicz A, Nowak W, Eilenberg W, Neumayer C, Malinski T, Huk I, Brostjan C (2015) The abdominal aortic aneurysm and intraluminal thrombus: current concepts of development and treatment. Front Cardiovasc Med 2:19. https://doi.org/10.3389/fcvm.2015.00019

Prati F, Uemura S, Souteyrand G, Virmani R, Motreff P, Di Vito L, Biondi-Zoccai G, Halperin J, Fuster V, Ozaki Y, Narula J (2013) OCT-based diagnosis and management of STEMI associated with intact fibrous cap. JACC Cardiovasc Imaging 6:283–287. https://doi.org/10.1016/j.jcmg.2012.12.007

Quarck R, Wynants M, Verbeken E, Meyns B, Delcroix M (2015) Contribution of inflammation and impaired angiogenesis to the pathobiology of chronic thromboembolic pulmonary hypertension. Eur Respir J 46:431–443. https://doi.org/10.1183/09031936.00009914

Quillard T, Araujo HA, Franck G, Shvartz E, Sukhova G, Libby P (2015) TLR2 and neutrophils potentiate endothelial stress, apoptosis and detachment: implications for superficial erosion. Eur Heart J 36:1394–1404. https://doi.org/10.1093/eurheartj/ehv044

Quillard T, Franck G, Mawson T, Folco E, Libby P (2017) Mechanisms of erosion of atherosclerotic plaques. Curr Opin Lipidol. https://doi.org/10.1097/mol.0000000000000440

Rainer TH, Wong LK, Lam W, Yuen E, Lam NY, Metreweli C, Lo YM (2003) Prognostic use of circulating plasma nucleic acid concentrations in patients with acute stroke. Clin Chem 49:562–569

Rao NV, Argyle B, Xu X, Reynolds PR, Walenga JM, Prechel M, Prestwich GD, MacArthur RB, Walters BB, Hoidal JR, Kennedy TP (2010) Low anticoagulant heparin targets multiple sites of inflammation, suppresses heparin-induced thrombocytopenia, and inhibits interaction of RAGE with its ligands. Am J Physiol Cell Physiol 299:C97–C110. https://doi.org/10.1152/ajpcell. 00009.2010

Rasmuson J, Kenne E, Wahlgren M, Soehnlein O, Lindbom L (2019) Heparinoid sevuparin inhibits streptococcus-induced vascular leak through neutralizing neutrophil-derived proteins. FASEB J:fj201900627R. https://doi.org/10.1096/fj.201900627R

Remijsen Q, Vanden Berghe T, Wirawan E, Asselbergh B, Parthoens E, De Rycke R, Noppen S, Delforge M, Willems J, Vandenabeele P (2011) Neutrophil extracellular trap cell death requires both autophagy and superoxide generation. Cell Res 21:290–304. https://doi.org/10.1038/cr. 2010.150

Rittersma SZ, van der Wal AC, Koch KT, Piek JJ, Henriques JP, Mulder KJ, Ploegmakers JP, Meesterman M, de Winter RJ (2005) Plaque instability frequently occurs days or weeks before occlusive coronary thrombosis: a pathological thrombectomy study in primary percutaneous coronary intervention. Circulation 111:1160–1165. https://doi.org/10.1161/01.cir.0000157141. 00778.ac

Rose F, Hattar K, Gakisch S, Grimminger F, Olschewski H, Seeger W, Tschuschner A, Schermuly RT, Weissmann N, Hanze J, Sibelius U, Ghofrani HA (2003) Increased neutrophil mediator release in patients with pulmonary hypertension--suppression by inhaled iloprost. Thromb Haemost 90:1141–1149. https://doi.org/10.1160/th03-03-0173

Rotzius P, Thams S, Soehnlein O, Kenne E, Tseng CN, Bjorkstrom NK, Malmberg KJ, Lindbom L, Eriksson EE (2010) Distinct infiltration of neutrophils in lesion shoulders in ApoE−/− mice. Am J Pathol 177:493–500 https://doi.org/10.2353/ajpath.2010.090480

Roumen-Klappe EM, den Heijer M, van Uum SH, van der Ven-Jongekrijg J, van der Graaf F, Wollersheim H (2002) Inflammatory response in the acute phase of deep vein thrombosis. J Vasc Surg 35:701–706

Roumen-Klappe EM, Janssen MC, Van Rossum J, Holewijn S, Van Bokhoven MM, Kaasjager K, Wollersheim H, Den Heijer M (2009) Inflammation in deep vein thrombosis and the development of post-thrombotic syndrome: a prospective study. J Thromb Haemost 7:582–587. https:// doi.org/10.1111/j.1538-7836.2009.03286.x

Sage AP, Tsiantoulas D, Binder CJ, Mallat Z (2019) The role of B cells in atherosclerosis. Nat Rev Cardiol 16:180–196. https://doi.org/10.1038/s41569-018-0106-9

Salas A, Sans M, Soriano A, Reverter JC, Anderson DC, Pique JM, Panes J (2000) Heparin attenuates TNF-alpha induced inflammatory response through a CD11b dependent mechanism. Gut 47:88–96. https://doi.org/10.1136/gut.47.1.88

Savchenko AS, Martinod K, Seidman MA, Wong SL, Borissoff JI, Piazza G, Libby P, Goldhaber SZ, Mitchell RN, Wagner DD (2014) Neutrophil extracellular traps form predominantly during the organizing stage of human venous thromboembolism development. J Thromb Haemost 12:860–870. https://doi.org/10.1111/jth.12571

Silvestre-Roig C, Braster Q, Wichapong K, Lee EY, Teulon JM, Berrebeh N, Winter J, Adrover JM, Santos GS, Froese A, Lemnitzer P, Ortega-Gomez A, Chevre R, Marschner J, Schumski A, Winter C, Perez-Olivares L, Pan C, Paulin N, Schoufour T, Hartwig H, Gonzalez-Ramos S, Kamp F, Megens RTA, Mowen KA, Gunzer M, Maegdefessel L, Hackeng T, Lutgens E, Daemen M, von Blume J, Anders HJ, Nikolaev VO, Pellequer JL, Weber C, Hidalgo A, Nicolaes GAF, Wong GCL, Soehnlein O (2019) Externalized histone H4 orchestrates chronic inflammation by inducing lytic cell death. Nature 569:236–240. https://doi.org/10.1038/s41586-019-1167-6

Stakos DA, Kambas K, Konstantinidis T, Mitroulis I, Apostolidou E, Arelaki S, Tsironidou V, Giatromanolaki A, Skendros P, Konstantinides S, Ritis K (2015) Expression of functional tissue factor by neutrophil extracellular traps in culprit artery of acute myocardial infarction. Eur Heart J 36:1405–1414. https://doi.org/10.1093/eurheartj/ehv007

Steffens S, Winter C, Schloss MJ, Hidalgo A, Weber C, Soehnlein O (2017) Circadian control of inflammatory processes in atherosclerosis and its complications. Arterioscler Thromb Vasc Biol 37:1022–1028. https://doi.org/10.1161/atvbaha.117.309374

Takei H, Araki A, Watanabe H, Ichinose A, Sendo F (1996) Rapid killing of human neutrophils by the potent activator phorbol 12-myristate 13-acetate (PMA) accompanied by changes different from typical apoptosis or necrosis. J Leukoc Biol 59:229–240

Tavora FR, Ripple M, Li L, Burke AP (2009) Monocytes and neutrophils expressing myeloperoxidase occur in fibrous caps and thrombi in unstable coronary plaques. BMC Cardiovasc Disord 9:27. https://doi.org/10.1186/1471-2261-9-27

Taylor AJ, Bobik A, Richards M, Kaye D, Raines G, Gould P, Jennings G (2004) Myocardial endothelin-1 release and indices of inflammation during angioplasty for acute myocardial infarction and stable coronary artery disease. Am Heart J 148:e10. https://doi.org/10.1016/j.ahj.2004.03.018

Tsai NW, Lin TK, Chen SD, Chang WN, Wang HC, Yang TM, Lin YJ, Jan CR, Huang CR, Liou CW, Lu CH (2011) The value of serial plasma nuclear and mitochondrial DNA levels in patients with acute ischemic stroke. Clin Chim Acta 412:476–479. https://doi.org/10.1016/j.cca.2010.11.036

Turunen S, Huhtakangas J, Nousiainen T, Valkealahti M, Melkko J, Risteli J, Lehenkari P (2016) Rheumatoid arthritis antigens homocitrulline and citrulline are generated by local myeloperoxidase and peptidyl arginine deiminases 2, 3 and 4 in rheumatoid nodule and synovial tissue. Arthritis Res Ther 18:239. https://doi.org/10.1186/s13075-016-1140-9

Valles J, Lago A, Santos MT, Latorre AM, Tembl JI, Salom JB, Nieves C, Moscardo A (2017) Neutrophil extracellular traps are increased in patients with acute ischemic stroke: prognostic significance. Thromb Haemost 117:1919–1929. https://doi.org/10.1160/th17-02-0130

van Leeuwen M, Gijbels MJ, Duijvestijn A, Smook M, van de Gaar MJ, Heeringa P, de Winther MP, Tervaert JW (2008) Accumulation of myeloperoxidase-positive neutrophils in atherosclerotic lesions in LDLR−/− mice. Arterioscler Thromb Vasc Biol 28:84–89. https://doi.org/10.1161/atvbaha.107.154807

van Montfoort ML, Stephan F, Lauw MN, Hutten BA, Van Mierlo GJ, Solati S, Middeldorp S, Meijers JC, Zeerleder S (2013) Circulating nucleosomes and neutrophil activation as risk factors for deep vein thrombosis. Arterioscler Thromb Vasc Biol 33:147–151. https://doi.org/10.1161/atvbaha.112.300498

Virmani R, Kolodgie FD, Burke AP, Farb A, Schwartz SM (2000) Lessons from sudden coronary death: a comprehensive morphological classification scheme for atherosclerotic lesions. Arterioscler Thromb Vasc Biol 20:1262–1275

Vogel B, Shinagawa H, Hofmann U, Ertl G, Frantz S (2015) Acute DNase1 treatment improves left ventricular remodeling after myocardial infarction by disruption of free chromatin. Basic Res Cardiol 110:15. https://doi.org/10.1007/s00395-015-0472-y

von Bruhl ML, Stark K, Steinhart A, Chandraratne S, Konrad I, Lorenz M, Khandoga A, Tirniceriu A, Coletti R, Kollnberger M, Byrne RA, Laitinen I, Walch A, Brill A, Pfeiler S, Manukyan D, Braun S, Lange P, Riegger J, Ware J, Eckart A, Haidari S, Rudelius M, Schulz C, Echtler K, Brinkmann V, Schwaiger M, Preissner KT, Wagner DD, Mackman N, Engelmann B, Massberg S (2012) Monocytes, neutrophils, and platelets cooperate to initiate and propagate venous thrombosis in mice in vivo. J Exp Med 209:819–835. https://doi.org/10.1084/jem.20112322

Wakefield TW, Strieter RM, Wilke CA, Kadell AM, Wrobleski SK, Burdick MD, Schmidt R, Kunkel SL, Greenfield LJ (1995) Venous thrombosis-associated inflammation and attenuation with neutralizing antibodies to cytokines and adhesion molecules. Arterioscler Thromb Vasc Biol 15:258–268

Wang J, Arase H (2014) Regulation of immune responses by neutrophils. Ann N Y Acad Sci 1319:66–81. https://doi.org/10.1111/nyas.12445

Wang J-G, Mu J-S, Zhu H-S, Geng J-G (2002) N-desulfated non-anticoagulant heparin inhibits leukocyte adhesion and transmigration in vitro and attenuates acute peritonitis and ischemia and reperfusion injury in vivo. Inflam Res 51:435–443. https://doi.org/10.1007/pl00012403

Wang Y, Wysocka J, Sayegh J, Lee YH, Perlin JR, Leonelli L, Sonbuchner LS, McDonald CH, Cook RG, Dou Y, Roeder RG, Clarke S, Stallcup MR, Allis CD, Coonrod SA (2004) Human PAD4 regulates histone arginine methylation levels via demethylimination. Science 306:279–283. https://doi.org/10.1126/science.1101400

Wang Y, Li M, Stadler S, Correll S, Li P, Wang D, Hayama R, Leonelli L, Han H, Grigoryev SA, Allis CD, Coonrod SA (2009) Histone hypercitrullination mediates chromatin decondensation and neutrophil extracellular trap formation. J Cell Biol 184:205–213. https://doi.org/10.1083/jcb.200806072

Warnatsch A, Ioannou M, Wang Q, Papayannopoulos V (2015) Inflammation. Neutrophil extracellular traps license macrophages for cytokine production in atherosclerosis. Science 349:316–320. https://doi.org/10.1126/science.aaa8064

Wildhagen KC, Garcia de Frutos P, Reutelingsperger CP, Schrijver R, Areste C, Ortega-Gomez A, Deckers NM, Hemker HC, Soehnlein O, Nicolaes GA (2014) Nonanticoagulant heparin prevents histone-mediated cytotoxicity in vitro and improves survival in sepsis. Blood 123:1098–1101. https://doi.org/10.1182/blood-2013-07-514984

Willis VC, Gizinski AM, Banda NK, Causey CP, Knuckley B, Cordova KN, Luo Y, Levitt B, Glogowska M, Chandra P, Kulik L, Robinson WH, Arend WP, Thompson PR, Holers VM (2011) N-alpha-benzoyl-N5-(2-chloro-1-iminoethyl)-L-ornithine amide, a protein arginine deiminase inhibitor, reduces the severity of murine collagen-induced arthritis. J Immunol 186:4396–4404. https://doi.org/10.4049/jimmunol.1001620

Witko-Sarsat V, Rieu P, Descamps-Latscha B, Lesavre P, Halbwachs-Mecarelli L (2000) Neutrophils: molecules, functions and pathophysiological aspects. Lab Investig 80:617–653

Zernecke A, Bot I, Djalali-Talab Y, Shagdarsuren E, Bidzhekov K, Meiler S, Krohn R, Schober A, Sperandio M, Soehnlein O, Bornemann J, Tacke F, Biessen EA, Weber C (2008) Protective role of CXC receptor 4/CXC ligand 12 unveils the importance of neutrophils in atherosclerosis. Circ Res 102:209–217. https://doi.org/10.1161/circresaha.107.160697

Zhang R, Brennan ML, Fu X, Aviles RJ, Pearce GL, Penn MS, Topol EJ, Sprecher DL, Hazen SL (2001) Association between myeloperoxidase levels and risk of coronary artery disease. JAMA 286:2136–2142

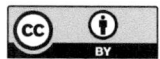

Part IV

Hypothesis-free Approaches to Unravel Novel Targets

Genomic Strategies Toward Identification of Novel Therapeutic Targets

Thorsten Kessler and Heribert Schunkert

Contents

1   Introduction 430
2   Methodological Aspects 430
    2.1   Techniques 431
    2.2   Selection of Individuals 431
    2.3   Statistical Analysis 433
    2.4   Mendelian Randomization Studies 433
3   Genetic Risk Factors Associated with Coronary Artery Disease 433
    3.1   Genome-Wide Association Studies 433
    3.2   Exome-Wide Association Studies 434
    3.3   Exome and Whole-Genome Sequencing 445
4   Genetic Overlap and Demarcation with Other Atherosclerotic Diseases 445
5   Pharmacological Targets Identified by Genomic Studies 447
    5.1   Lipid Metabolism 447
    5.2   Inflammation 450
    5.3   Platelet Function and Nitric Oxide Signaling 451
    5.4   Vascular Phenotypes 452
    5.5   Further Directions 453
6   Risk Scores and Risk Prediction 454
7   Summary 455
References 455

Abstract

Coronary artery disease, myocardial infarction, and secondary damages of the myocardium in the form of ischemic heart disease remain major causes of death in

T. Kessler (✉) · H. Schunkert
Deutsches Herzzentrum München, Klinik für Herz- und Kreislauferkrankungen, Technische Universität München, Munich, Germany

Deutsches Zentrum für Herz-Kreislauf-Forschung (DZHK) e.V., partner site Munich Heart Alliance, Munich, Germany
e-mail: thorsten.kessler@tum.de

© The Author(s) 2020
A. von Eckardstein, C. J. Binder (eds.), *Prevention and Treatment of Atherosclerosis*,
Handbook of Experimental Pharmacology 270, https://doi.org/10.1007/164_2020_360

429

Western countries. Beyond traditional risk factors such as smoking, hypertension, dyslipidemia, or diabetes, a positive family history is known to increase risk. The genetic factors underlying this observation remained unknown for decades until genetic studies were able to identify multiple genomic loci contributing to the heritability of the trait. Knowledge of the affected genes and the resulting molecular and cellular mechanisms leads to improved understanding of the pathophysiology leading to coronary atherosclerosis. Major goals are also to improve prevention and therapy of coronary artery disease and its sequelae via improved risk prediction tools and pharmacological targets. In this chapter, we recapitulate recent major findings. We focus on established novel targets and discuss possible further targets which are currently explored in translational studies.

Keywords

Coronary artery disease · Exome sequencing · Genomics · Genome-wide association studies · Myocardial infarction

1   Introduction

Coronary artery disease (CAD) and myocardial infarction (MI) are the main causes of morbidity and mortality. The identification of risk factors is a prerequisite to improve prevention and therapy of the disease via gaining knowledge about the underlying pathophysiological processes as well as the identification of therapeutic targets. Hyperlipidemia, hypertension, and diabetes mellitus are examples for risk factors which can be treated via pharmacological intervention, whereas smoking and obesity can be addressed by lifestyle interventions. Age and male gender, which are also major risk factors, cannot be addressed therapeutically. In the past, a positive family history has also been regarded as a non-modifiable risk factor. However, the underlying risk factors were not known for decades. In this chapter, we summarize the developments in the past years which led to the identification of a plethora of genomic loci which are associated with CAD with high statistical certainty.

2   Methodological Aspects

Over the past decades, the methodological spectrum has been vastly expanded to identify novel genetic risk factors of CAD and MI. Details on these methods have been discussed elsewhere (Kessler et al. 2016). In this section, we aim to briefly mention some important points.

2.1   Techniques

The development of arrays with hundred thousands of common single nucleotide polymorphisms (SNPs) distributed all over the genome of an individual enabled researchers to deeply genotype large numbers of individuals. An important prerequisite was knowledge of the human genome which has been mainly gained via projects as the human genome project (Lander et al. 2001; Sachidanandam et al. 2001). Subsequent projects as the *1000 Genomes Project* (1000 Genomes Project Consortium et al. 2012, 2015) raised further possibilities with the imputation of SNPs which had not been genotyped directly. As a consequence genome-wide association studies investigating millions of SNPs have been performed, and mostly common variants were found to be associated with the disease and lend support to the *common disease-common variant* hypothesis (Reich and Lander 2001). Thereby, since 2007, mostly genome-wide association studies and subsequent analyses led to the identification of genetic risk variants for various traits including CAD and traditional risk factors as blood pressure or lipids. Subsequently, large international consortia were formed that were responsible for the identification of most of the currently known CAD risk loci. Figure 1 illustrates the evolution of genome-wide association studies focusing on the CARDIoGRAMplusC4D consortium, a coalition of several individual studies to facilitate the identification of CAD risk factors (Schunkert et al. 2019) and further studies using data from UK Biobank (Littlejohns et al. 2019). The idea of exome-wide association studies is comparable to that of a genome-wide association study with the exception that the investigated SNPs are enriched for coding variants distributed over the genome (Myocardial Infarction Genetics and CARDIoGRAM Exome Consortia Investigators et al. 2016). Most of the currently known genetic CAD risk factors have been identified using these methods (Kessler et al. 2016; Khera and Kathiresan 2017a; Erdmann et al. 2018).

Apart from common variants, the association of rare variants and private mutations has also been extensively studied. To identify such genetic variation, mostly exome sequencing has been used in the past (Erdmann et al. 2013). As the name says, this next-generation sequencing method is able to determine the genomic sequence of an individual enriched for coding regions and thus renders the identification of missense variants co-segregating with a certain disease in, e.g., a family with high prevalence possible. Whole-genome sequencing is not restricted to coding sequences. However, due to costs and computational challenges of the different methods, whole-genome sequencing has not yet contributed to the current knowledge of genetic variation in CAD.

2.2   Selection of Individuals

Most large-scale genomic studies use a case-control design, i.e., a cohort of patients suffering from the trait of interest is compared to a group of healthy individuals free of the disease. Obviously, clear definitions of phenotypes are important to gain reliable results. Most GWAS on CAD/MI focused on cases suffering from the

Fig. 1 *Discovery of genomic variants associated with CAD/MI using genome-/exome-wide association studies* (modified after Kessler et al. 2016). (**a**) Over the past years, ongoing research led to the identification of increasing numbers of SNPs which are associated with CAD/MI at the genome-wide level of significance. Results from the CARDIoGRAMplusC4D-Million Hearts Initiative are awaited for 2019/2020. (**b**) The number of investigated individuals correlates with the number of identified risk variants which highlights the importance of international collaborations

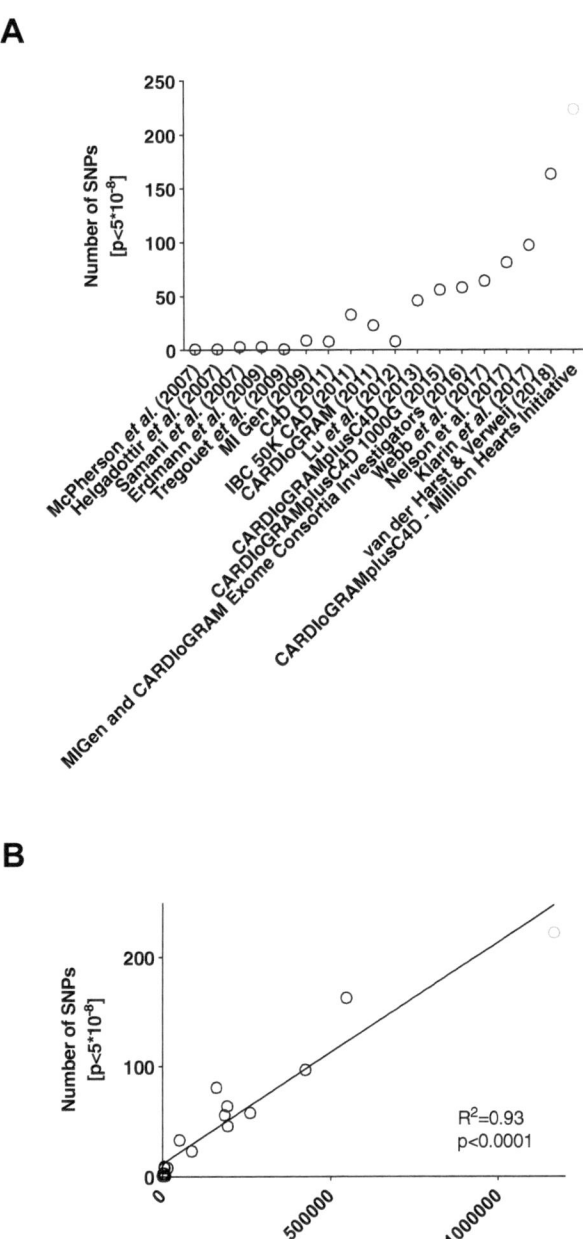

disease at an early age. This increased the possibility of identification of the genetic predisposition which, together with gender, still represents the strongest risk factor. For controls, population-based samples as well as individuals which have been diagnosed to not to suffer from CAD/MI have been included. An important resource that has increasingly been used in recent projects is the UK Biobank (https://www.ukbiobank.ac.uk/). It includes health information as well as genetic data for 500,000 individuals which can be accessed by researchers after approval of specific projects (Littlejohns et al. 2019). In the USA, the Million Veteran Project has formed and stated to provide likewise genome-wide data (Klarin et al. 2018).

2.3   Statistical Analysis

To reduce the possibility of a false-positive finding, rigorous statistical thresholds have been determined to identify a certain variant to be associated with a trait as CAD/MI. Currently, a p-value below 5×10^{-8} is commonly accepted as a genome-wide significant finding. The strict p-value is a result of the large number of statistical tests which are performed in parallel on one dataset in a genome-wide association study (Pe'er et al. 2008). However, it cannot be excluded that true positive signals are discarded because they do not reach the stringent p-value. Recent studies also reported loci below certain false discovery rate thresholds to address this issue.

2.4   Mendelian Randomization Studies

Mendelian randomization studies (for an overview see Jansen et al. 2014) enable to investigate whether a biomarker or a trait is causal in the development of a disease. In epidemiological research, associations between biomarkers and diseases are frequently observed. However, the association can be influenced by unknown factors. On the other hand, the investigated disease itself can influence a given biomarker. In Mendelian randomization studies, causality between a biomarker and development of a disease can be assumed if a genetic variant influences this biomarker in the same direction as the biomarker is associated with the disease. Important examples in CAD are biomarkers such as LDL-cholesterol or C-reactive protein as well as behavioral traits such as educational attainment (Zeng et al. 2019a) which are discussed in more detail below.

3   Genetic Risk Factors Associated with Coronary Artery Disease

3.1   Genome-Wide Association Studies

The discovery of genetic CAD/MI risk factors was launched in 2007 by three independent studies which reported the chromosome 9p21 locus as the first and, until today, strongest genetic risk locus (Helgadottir et al. 2007; McPherson et al. 2007; Samani et al. 2007). Since then, with the inclusion of more individuals and the possibility of analyzing a larger number of SNPs, more and more variants associated with CAD/MI have been reported (for an overview see Kessler et al. (2016), Khera and Kathiresan (2017b), and Erdmann et al. (2018)). The currently known loci are depicted in Table 1. Surprisingly, most of the SNPs tag genes which have not been studied in the pathophysiology of coronary atherosclerosis before. Another surprising finding was that only the minority of genes is also associated with traditional risk factors as hypertension or lipid metabolism rendering the involvement of other cellular mechanisms likely. Additionally, almost every lead SNP is located in a non-coding region of the genome. The most prominent example is again the chromosome 9p21 locus. Here, it is still unclear which gene might be responsible for the strong signal. Rather, there is much evidence that the effect might be mediated by the circular non-coding RNA *ANRIL* (Holdt et al. 2010, 2013, 2016). Overall, it has been estimated that the 163 so far known CAD risk loci explain between 30% and 40% of CAD heritability (Nelson et al. 2017). It has also been found that a large number of the reported loci also harbor multiple independent signals (van der Harst and Verweij 2018). Additionally, most of the loci show pleiotropy, i.e., a risk variant is associated with several phenotypes. About half of the currently known CAD risk loci have been reported to be associated with other traits (Webb et al. 2017).

The studies which led to the discovery of the currently known CAD/MI risk variants as well as studies which gave first insights into their involvement in CAD/MI are referenced in Table 1. Specific genes and pathways are further discussed below.

3.2   Exome-Wide Association Studies

As mentioned above, GWAS mainly led to the identification of non-coding variation associated with the disease. To specifically investigate the role of coding variants, dedicated arrays enriched for exonic variants were used. In an international effort, the Myocardial Infarction Genetics and CARDIoGRAM Exome Consortia Investigators performed the largest exome-wide association study so far (Myocardial Infarction Genetics and CARDIoGRAM Exome Consortia Investigators et al. 2016). The results are depicted in Table 2. In summary, only four variants were identified. First, it could be replicated that coding variation in the *LPA* and *PCSK9* genes is associated with CAD/MI. Second, two novel coding variants in *ANGPTL4* and *SVEP1* were found. Whereas *LPA*, *PCSK9*, and *ANGPTL4* are associated with lipid metabolism (see below), *SVEP1* only displayed association with blood pressure (Myocardial Infarction Genetics and CARDIoGRAM Exome Consortia Investigators et al. 2016). However, this effect cannot fully explain the association signal for CAD/MI.

Table 1 Loci associated with CAD/MI identified by GWAS (modified after Erdmann et al. (2018))

Chr.	Lead SNP	EA (EAF)	OR	Gene(s)	Association with traditional risk factors		Ref.
					HTN	Lipids	
1	rs36096196	T (0.15)	1.05	*MORN1*, **SKI**			Van der Harst and Verweij (2018)
	rs2493298	A (0.14)	1.06	**PRDM16**, *PEX10, PLCH2, RER1*			Van der Harst and Verweij (2018)
	rs61776719	A (0.53)	1.04	**FHL3**, *UTP11, SF3A3, MANEAL, INPP5B*			Van der Harst and Verweij (2018)
	rs11206510	T (0.82)	1.08	**PCSK9**		+	Abifadel et al. (2003), Cohen et al. (2006), Myocardial Infarction Genetics Consortium et al. (2009), and Teslovich et al. (2010)
	rs17114036	A (0.91)	1.17	**PPAP2B**			Teslovich et al. (2010), Schunkert et al. (2011)
	rs599839	A (0.78)	1.11	**SORT1**, *PSCR1, CELSR2*		+	Samani et al. (2007), Teslovich et al. (2010), and Schunkert et al. (2011)
	rs11806316	G (0.66)	1.04	**NGF, CASQ2**			Van der Harst and Verweij (2018)
	rs11810571	G (0.79)	1.07	**TDRKH**, *RP11-98D18.9*			Verweij et al. (2017), Nelson et al. (2017)
	rs4845625	T (0.47)	1.06	**IL6R**, *AQP10, ATP8B2, CHTOP, UBAP2L*			CARDIoGRAMplusC4D Consortium et al. (2013)
	rs1892094	C (0.50)	1.04	**ATP1B1**, *BLZF1, CCDC181, F5, NME7, SELP, SLC19A2*			Howson et al. (2017)
	rs6700559	C (0.53)	1.04	**DDX59, CAMSAP2**, *KIF14*			
	rs2820315	T (0.30)	1.05	**LMOD1**, *IPO9, NAV1, SHISA4, TIMM17A*			
	rs60154123	T (0.15)	1.05	**HHAT, SERTAD4, DIEXF**			Van der Harst and Verweij (2018)
	rs17465637	C (0.74)	1.14	**MIA3**, *AIDA, C1orf58*			Samani et al. (2007), Schunkert et al. (2011)
	rs699	G (0.42)	1.04	**AGT**, *CAPN9, GNPAT*			Van der Harst and Verweij (2018)

(continued)

Table 1 (continued)

Chr.	Lead SNP	EA (EAF)	OR	Gene(s)	Association with traditional risk factors		Ref.
					HTN	Lipids	
2	rs515135	G (0.83)	1.07	**APOB**		+	Teslovich et al. (2010), CARDIoGRAMplusC4D Consortium et al. (2013)
	rs6544713	T (0.30)	1.06	**ABCG5, ABCG8**		+	Teslovich et al. (2010), Schunkert et al. (2011), and IBC 50K CAD Consortium (2011)
	rs582384	A (0.53)	1.03	**PRKCE**, *TMEM247*			Van der Harst and Verweij (2018)
	rs1561198	A (0.45)	1.06	**VAMP5, VAMP8, GGCX**			CARDIoGRAMplusC4D Consortium et al. (2013)
	rs2252641	G (0.46)	1.06	**ZEB2, TEX41**			CARDIoGRAMplusC4D Consortium et al. (2013)
	rs12999907	A (0.82)	1.06	**FIGN**			Van der Harst and Verweij (2018)
	rs840616	C (0.65)	1.04	**CALCRL, TFPI**			Van der Harst and Verweij (2018)
	rs6725887	C (0.15)	1.14	**WDR12**, *CARF, FAM117B, ICA1L, NBEAL1*			Myocardial Infarction Genetics Consortium et al. (2009), Schunkert et al. (2011)
	rs1250229	T (0.26)	1.07	**FN1**, *ATIC, LOC102724849, ABCA12, LINC00607*		+	Klarin et al. (2017), Nelson et al. (2017)
	rs2571445	A (0.39)	1.04	**TNS1, CXCR2, RUFY4**			Howson et al. (2017)
	rs2972146	T (0.65)	1.07	*LOC646736*, **IRS1**, *MIR5702*	+	+	Klarin et al. (2017)
	rs1801251	A (0.35)	1.05	**KCNJ13**, *GIGYF2*			Webb et al. (2017)
	rs11677932	G (0.68)	1.03	**COL6A3**			Van der Harst and Verweij (2018)

	SNP	Allele (freq)		Gene(s)			Reference
3	rs748431	G (0.36)	1.04	**FGD5**			Klarin et al. (2017)
	rs7633770	A (0.41)	1.03	**ALS2CL, RTP3**	+		Van der Harst and Verweij (2018)
	rs7617773	T (0.67)	1.04	**CDC25A, SPINK8, MAP4, ZNF589**			Verweij et al. (2017), Klarin et al. (2017), Nelson et al. (2017), and Howson et al. (2017)
	rs7623687	A (0.86)	1.07	**RHOA**, *AMT, TCTA, CDHRA, KLHDC8B*, etc.			Verweij et al. (2017), Klarin et al. (2017), and Nelson et al. (2017)
	rs142695226	G (0.14)	1.08	**UMPS, ITGB5**			Verweij et al. (2017), Klarin et al. (2017), and Nelson et al. (2017)
	rs10512861	G (0.86)	1.04	**DNAJC13**, *NPHP3, ACAD11, UBA5*	+		Van der Harst and Verweij (2018)
	rs667920	T (0.78)	1.05	**STAG1, MSL2, NCK1, PPP2R3A**	+		Erdmann et al. (2009), Schunkert et al. (2011)
	rs2306374	C (0.18)	1.12	**MRAS**, *CEP70*			Verweij et al. (2017), Klarin et al. (2017), and Nelson et al. (2017)
	rs12493885	C (0.85)	1.07	**ARHGEF26**			Van der Harst and Verweij (2018)
	rs4266144	G (0.32)	1.03	*CCNL1, TIPARP*			
	rs12897	G (0.41)	1.04	**FNDC3B**			
4	rs16844401	A (0.07)	1.07	*HGFAC, RGS12, MSANTD1*	+		Nikpay et al. (2015)
	rs17087335	T (0.21)	1.06	**REST, NOA1**			Van der Harst and Verweij (2018)
	rs12500824	A (0.36)	1.04	*SHROOM3, SEPT11, FAM47E, STBD1*			
	rs10857147	T (0.27)	1.06	**PRDM8, FGF5**		+	Verweij et al. (2017), Klarin et al. (2017), and Nelson et al. (2017)
	rs11099493	A (0.69)	1.04	**HNRNPD**, *RASGEF1B*			Van der Harst and Verweij (2018)
	rs3775058	A (0.23)	1.04	**UNC5C**			
	rs11723436	G (0.31)	1.05	**MAD2L1, PDE5A**			Verweij et al. (2017), Klarin et al. (2017), and Nelson et al. (2017)
	rs35879803	C (0.70)	1.05	**ZNF827**			Verweij et al. (2017)
	rs1878406	T (0.15)	1.10	**EDNRA**			CARDIoGRAMplusC4D Consortium et al. (2013)
	rs7692387	G (0.81)	1.08	**GUCY1A1**		+	International Consortium for Blood Pressure Genome-Wide Association Studies et al. (2011), CARDIoGRAMplusC4D Consortium et al. (2013), and Erdmann et al. (2013)
	rs7696431	T (0.51)	1.04	**PALLD**, *DDX60L*			Van der Harst and Verweij (2018)

(continued)

Table 1 (continued)

Chr.	Lead SNP	EA (EAF)	OR	Gene(s)	Association with traditional risk factors		Ref.
					HTN	Lipids	
5	rs1508798	T (0.81)		**SEMA5A**, *TAS2R1*		+	Klarin et al. (2017)
	rs3936511	G (0.18)	1.04	**MAP3K1**, *MIER3*		+	
	rs1800449	T (0.17)	1.09	**LOX**			CARDIoGRAMplusC4D Consortium et al. (2013)
	rs273909	C (0.14)	1.07	**SLC22A4**			IBC 50K CAD Consortium (2011)
	rs2706399	G (0.51)	1.07	**IL5, RAD50**			Howson et al. (2017)
	rs246600	T (0.48)	1.05	**ARHGAP26**			Van der Harst and Verweij (2018)
6	rs9501744	C (0.87)	1.05	**FOXC1**			
	rs12526453	C (0.67)	1.10	**PHACTR1, EDN1**	+		Myocardial Infarction Genetics Consortium et al. (2009), Schunkert et al. (2011)
	rs35541991	C (0.31)	1.05	**HDGFL1**			Verweij et al. (2017), Nelson et al. (2017)
	rs3130683	T (0.86)	1.09	**C2**, *C4A*, etc.			Webb et al. (2017)
	rs17609940	G (0.75)	1.07	**ANKS1A**, *UHRF1BP1*			Schunkert et al. (2011)
	rs1321309	A (0.49)	1.03	*CDKN1A*, **PI16**		+	Van der Harst and Verweij (2018)
	rs10947789	T (0.76)	1.07	**KCNK5**			CARDIoGRAMplusC4D Consortium et al. (2013)
	rs6905288	A (0.57)	1.05	**VEGFA**, *MRPL14, TMEM63B*		+	Van der Harst and Verweij (2018)
	rs9367716	G (0.68)	1.04	*PRIM2*, **RAB23**, *DST, BEND6*			
	rs4613862	A (0.53)	1.03	**FAM46A**			
	rs1591805	A (0.49)	1.04	**CENPW**			
	rs12190287	C (0.62)	1.08	**TCF21**, *TARID (EYA4–AS1)*			Schunkert et al. (2011)
	rs17080091	C (0.92)	1.05	**PLEKHG1**, *IYD*		+	Van der Harst and Verweij (2018)
	rs3798220	C (0.02)	1.51	**LPA**, *SLC22A3, LPAL2*		+	Tregouet et al. (2009), Teslovich et al. (2010), and Schunkert et al. (2011)
	rs42252120	T (0.73)	1.07	**PLG**, *LPAL2*		+	CARDIoGRAMplusC4D Consortium et al. (2013)

7	rs10267593	G (0.8)	1.04		**MAD1L1**		Van der Harst and Verweij (2018)
	rs7797644	C (0.77)	1.04		**DAGLB, RAC1,** *FAM220A,* **KDELR2**		
	rs11509880	A (0.36)	1.04		**TMEM106B,** *THSD7A*		
	rs2023938	G (0.10)	1.08		**HDAC9**		CARDIoGRAMplusC4D Consortium et al. (2013)
	rs2107732	G (0.91)	1.06		**CCM2,** *MYO1G*	+	Van der Harst and Verweij (2018)
	rs10953541	C (0.80)	1.08		**BCAP29, GPR22**		Coronary Artery Disease C4D Genetics Consortium (2011a)
	rs975722	G (0.4)	1.03		*CTTNBP2,* **CFTR,** *ASZ1*		Van der Harst and Verweij (2018)
	rs11556924	C (0.62)	1.09		**ZC3HC1, KLHDC10**		Schunkert et al. (2011)
	rs10237377	G (0.65)	1.05		**PARP12, TBXAS1**		Howson et al. (2017)
	rs3918226	T (0.06)	1.14	+	**NOS3**		Nikpay et al. (2015)
8	rs6997340	T (0.31)	1.04		**NAT2**	+	Van der Harst and Verweij (2018)
	rs264	G (0.86)	1.11		**LPL**	+	Teslovich et al. (2010), CARDIoGRAMplusC4D Consortium et al. (2013), and Myocardial Infarction Genetics and CARDIoGRAM Exome Consortia Investigators et al. (2016)
	rs6984210	G (0.06)	1.08		**BMP1,** *SFTPC, DMTN, PHYHIP, DOK2, XPO7*		Van der Harst and Verweij (2018)
	rs10093110	G (0.58)	1.03		**ZFPM2**		
	rs2954029	A (0.55)	1.06		**TRIB1**	+	Teslovich et al. (2010), IBC 50K CAD Consortium (2011), and CARDIoGRAMplusC4D Consortium et al. (2013)
9	rs1333049	G (0.46)	1.29		**ANRIL,** *CDKN2B-AS*		Helgadottir et al. (2007), McPherson et al. (2007), Samani et al. (2007), Holdt et al. (2010), and Schunkert et al. (2011)
	rs944172	C (0.28)	1.04		**KLF4**		Van der Harst and Verweij (2018)
	rs885150	C (0.27)	1.03		**DAB2IP**		
	rs579459	C (0.21)	1.10		**ABO,** *SURF6, GBGT1*	+	Teslovich et al. (2010), Reilly et al. (2011), and Schunkert et al. (2011)

(continued)

Table 1 (continued)

Chr.	Lead SNP	EA (EAF)	OR	Gene(s)	Association with traditional risk factors		Ref.
					HTN	Lipids	
10	rs61848342	C (0.36)	1.04	**CDC123**, *NUDT5*, *OPTN*			Van der Harst and Verweij (2018)
	rs2505083	C (0.38)	1.07	**KIAA1462**			Coronary Artery Disease C4D Genetics Consortium (2011a), Erdmann et al. (2011)
	rs1746048	C (0.87)	1.09	**CXCL12**			Samani et al. (2007), Schunkert et al. (2011)
	rs17680741	T (0.72)	1.05	**TSPAN14**, *MAT1A*, **FAM213A**			Van der Harst and Verweij (2018)
	rs1412444	T (0.42)	1.09	**LIPA**			Coronary Artery Disease C4D Genetics Consortium (2011a)
	rs12413409	G (0.89)	1.12	**CYP17A1, CNNM2, NT5C2**	+		Levy et al. (2009), Newton-Cheh et al. (2009), and Schunkert et al. (2011)
	rs4918072	A (0.27)	1.04	*STN1*, **SH3PXD2A**			Van der Harst and Verweij (2018)
	rs4752700	G (0.45)	1.03	**HTRA1**, *PLEKHA1*			
11	rs11601507	A (0.07)	1.09	**TRIM5, TRIM22, TRIM6**, *OR52N1*, *OR52B6*			
	rs10840293	A (0.55)	1.06	**SWAP70**			Nikpay et al. (2015)
	rs11042937	T (0.49)	1.03	**MRVI1, CTR9**			Webb et al. (2017)
	rs1351525	T (0.67)	1.05	**ARNTL**			Verweij et al. (2017), Nelson et al. (2017)
	rs7116641	G (0.31)	1.03	**HSD17B12**			Van der Harst and Verweij (2018)
	rs12801636	G (0.77)	1.05	*PCNX3, POLA2, RELA*, **SIPA1**, etc.		+	Howson et al. (2017)
	rs590121	T (0.30)	1.05	**SERPINH1**			Howson et al. (2017)
	rs7947761	G (0.28)	1.04	**ARHGAP42**			Van der Harst and Verweij (2018)
	rs974819	T (0.32)	1.07	**PDGFD**			Coronary Artery Disease C4D Genetics Consortium (2011a)
	rs964184	G (0.13)	1.13	**APOA1-C3-A4-A5**		+	Schunkert et al. (2011), Do et al. (2015)
	rs11838267	T (0.87)	1.05	**C1S**			Van der Harst and Verweij (2018)

	SNP	Allele (Freq)	OR	Gene(s)			Reference
12	rs10841443	G (0.67)	1.06	RP11-664H17.1, PDE3A			Klarin et al. (2017)
	rs11170820	G (0.08)	1.10	HOXC4			Verweij et al. (2017)
	rs11172113	C (0.41)	1.06	LRP1, *STAT6*			Webb et al. (2017)
	rs7306455	G (0.9)	1.05	*NDUFA12, FGD6*			Van der Harst and Verweij (2018)
	rs3184504	T (0.44)	1.07	SH2B3, *FLJ21127, ATXN2*, etc.	+		Gudbjartsson et al. (2009), Levy et al. (2009), Newton-Cheh et al. (2009), Teslovich et al. (2010), and Schunkert et al. (2011)
	rs11830157	G (0.36)	1.12	KSR2			Nikpay et al. (2015)
	rs2244608	G (0.35)	1.06	HNF1A, *OASL, C12orf43, and others*		+	Verweij et al. (2017), Klarin et al. (2017), Nelson et al. (2017), and Howson et al. (2017)
	rs11057401	T (0.69)	1.08	CCDC92		+	Klarin et al. (2017)
	rs11057830	A (0.15)	1.07	SCARB1		+	Webb et al. (2017), Howson et al. (2017)
13	rs9319428	A (0.32)	1.06	FLT1			CARDIoGRAMplusC4D Consortium et al. (2013)
	rs9591012	G (0.66)	1.04	N4BP2L2, PDS5B			Van der Harst and Verweij (2018)
	rs4773144	G (0.44)	1.07	COL4A1, COL4A2			Schunkert et al. (2011)
	rs1317507	A (0.26)	1.04	MCF2L, *PCID2, CUL4A*			Van der Harst and Verweij (2018)
14	rs2145598	G (0.42)	1.03	ARID4A, PSMA3			Van der Harst and Verweij (2018)
	rs3832966	I (0.46)	1.05	TMED10, *ZC2HC1C, RPS6KL1, NEK9, EIF2B2e, ACYP1*			Verweij et al. (2017)
	rs112635299	G (0.92)	1.13	*SERPINA2,* SERPINA1			Van der Harst and Verweij (2018)
	rs2895811	C (0.43)	1.07	HHIPL1, YY1			Schunkert et al. (2011)
15	rs6494488	A (0.82)	1.05	*OAZ2, RBPMS2,* TRIP4, etc.			Howson et al. (2017)
	rs56062135	C (0.79)	1.07	SMAD3			Nikpay et al. (2015)
	rs3825807	A (0.57)	1.08	ADAMTS7			Reilly et al. (2011), Schunkert et al. (2011), and Coronary Artery Disease C4D Genetics Consortium (2011a)
	rs8042271	G (0.9)	1.10	MFGE8, *RP11-326A19.4, ABHD2*			Nikpay et al. (2015)
	rs17514846	A (0.44)	1.07	FURIN, FES	+		International Consortium for Blood Pressure Genome-Wide Association Studies et al. (2011), CARDIoGRAMplusC4D Consortium et al. (2013)
	rs17581137	A (0.75)	1.04	Gene desert			Van der Harst and Verweij (2018)

(continued)

Table 1 (continued)

Chr.	Lead SNP	EA (EAF)	OR	Gene(s)	Association with traditional risk factors		Ref.
					HTN	Lipids	
16	rs1800775	C (0.51)	1.03	**CETP**		+	Webb et al. (2017)
	rs1050362	A (0.38)	1.04	*DHX38*, **HP**, *DHODH*		+	Howson et al. (2017)
	rs3851738	C (0.60)	1.07	**CFDP1, BCAR1**			Verweij et al. (2017), Klarin et al. (2017)
	rs7199941	A (0.4)	1.04	**PLCG2**, *CENPN*			Van der Harst and Verweij (2018)
	rs7500448	A (0.77)	1.07	**CDH13**			Verweij et al. (2017), Klarin et al. (2017), and Nelson et al. (2017)
17	rs216172	C (0.37)	1.07	**SMG6**, *SRR*			Schunkert et al. (2011)
	rs12936587	G (0.56)	1.07	**Rai1, PEMT**, *RASD1, SMCR3, TOM1L2*			Schunkert et al. (2011)
	rs13723	G (0.49)	1.04	**CORO6, BLMH, ANKRD13B, GIT1, SSH2, EFCAB5**			Van der Harst and Verweij (2018)
	rs76954792	T (0.22)	1.04	**COPRS, RAB11FIP4**			
	rs2074158	C (0.18)	1.05	**DHX58, KAT2A, RAB5, NKIRAS2, DNAJC7, KCNH4, HCRT, GHDC**		+	
	rs17608766	C (0.14)	1.07	**GOSR2**, *MYL4, ARL17A*, etc.	+		Howson et al. (2017)
	rs46522	T (0.53)	1.06	**UBE2Z**, *GIP, ATP5G1*			Schunkert et al. (2011)
	rs7212798	C (0.15)	1.08	**BCAS3**			Nikpay et al. (2015)
	rs1867624	T (0.61)	1.04	**PECAM1, DDX5, TEX2**, etc.			Howson et al. (2017)
18	rs9964304	C (0.38)	1.04	**ACAA2, RPL17**		+	Van der Harst and Verweij (2018)
	rs663129	A (0.26)	1.06	**PMAIP1, MC4R**			Nikpay et al. (2015)

Chr	SNP	EA (EAF)	OR	Candidate gene		Ref
19	rs1122608	G (0.77)	1.14	**LDLR, SMARCA4**	+	Myocardial Infarction Genetics Consortium et al. (2009), Teslovich et al. (2010), Schunkert et al. (2011), and Do et al. (2015)
	rs73015714	G (0.2)	1.06	**FCHO1, COLGALT1**		Van der Harst and Verweij (2018)
	rs12976411	A (0.91)	1.33	**ZNF507**, *LOC400684*		Nikpay et al. (2015)
	rs8108632*	T (0.48)	1.05	**HNRNPUL1**, *CCDC97*, **TGFB1**, *B9D2*		Verweij et al. (2017), Klarin et al. (2017), and Nelson et al. (2017)
	rs2075650	G (0.14)	1.14	**APOE**, *APOC1*, *TOMM40*, **PVRL2**, **COTL1**	+	Teslovich et al. (2010), IBC 50K CAD Consortium (2011)
	rs1964272	G (0.51)	1.04	**SNRPD2**, *GIPR*		Nelson et al. (2017)
20	rs867186	A (0.89)	1.07	**PROCR**, *ASIP*, *NCOA6*, **ITGB4BP/EIF6**, etc.		Howson et al. (2017)
	rs6102343	A (0.25)	1.04	**ZHX3, PLCG1**, *TOP1*		Van der Harst and Verweij (2018)
	rs7270354	A (0.15)	1.06	*PCIF1*, *ZNF335*, *NEURL2*, **PLTP**, **MMP9**	+	Braenne et al. (2017)
	rs260020	T (0.13)	1.04	**ZNF831**		Van der Harst and Verweij (2018)
	rs2832227	G (0.18)	1.04	*MAP3K7CL*, **BACH1**		
21	rs9982601	T (0.15)	1.18	*MRPS6, SLC5A3*, **KCNE2**		Myocardial Infarction Genetics Consortium et al. (2009)
22	rs180803	G (0.97)	1.20	**ADORA2A**		Nikpay et al. (2015)

The most likely candidate gene at the locus is marked in bold (after McPherson and Tybjaerg-Hansen (2016)). *Chr* chromosome, *EA* effect allele, *EAF* effect allele frequency, *HTN* hypertension, *I/D* Indel/Deletion, *OR* odds ratio, *Ref* reference, *SNP* single nucleotide polymorphism

Table 2 Coding variants associated with CAD/MI risk identified by exome-wide association studies

Chr.	SNP (AA change)	EA (EAF)	OR	Gene(s)	Association with traditional risk factors		Ref.
					HTN	Lipids	
1	rs11591147 (p. R46L)	T (0.0152)	0.78	**PCSK9**		+	Myocardial Infarction Genetics and CARDIoGRAM Exome Consortia Investigators et al. (2016)
6	rs3798220 (p. I4399M)	C (0.019)	1.54	**LPA**		+	
9	rs111245230 (p. D2702G)	C (0.036)	1.14	**SVEP1**	+		
19	rs116843064 (p. E40K)	A (0.02)	0.86	**ANGPTL4**		+	

AA amino acid, *Chr* chromosome, *EA* effect allele, *EAF* effect allele frequency, *HTN* hypertension, *OR* odds ratio, *Ref* reference, *SNP* single nucleotide polymorphism

3.3   Exome and Whole-Genome Sequencing

As discussed above, due to still comparatively high costs, whole-genome sequencing has not yet significantly contributed to the knowledge of genetic CAD risk factors. In contrast, several studies made use of exome sequencing to identify variation in the coding sequence which is associated with CAD/MI. One scope of application the investigation of members of families with a high disease prevalence. Using this approach and subsequent co-segregation analyses genetic factors underlying the development of CAD/MI or its risk factors was possible. An important example is a mutation in the *GUCY1A3* gene, which has been – together with a coding mutation in the *CCT7* gene – shown to be responsible for the phenotype of premature CAD/MI in a family (Erdmann et al. 2013). As shown in Table 1, the *GUCY1A3* locus also harbors common, non-coding variants associated with CAD/MI. Thus, an allelic series has been shown at the locus with a mutation and common variants which lead to a strong or only moderate risk increase, respectively. Further loci have been identified by analyzing large cohorts of cases and controls comparable to the GWAS approach. Most of the genes that were thereby identified play a role in lipid metabolism. Some of the genes, e.g., *LDLR* or *PCSK9*, also demonstrate allelic series. A selection of genes which have been identified using exome sequencing is depicted in Table 3 and discussed below in more detail.

4   Genetic Overlap and Demarcation with Other Atherosclerotic Diseases

An increased prevalence of CAD risk alleles can be traced in a large number of cardiovascular conditions including heart failure, peripheral arterial disease, or atrial fibrillation (Ntalla et al. 2019). Large-scale genomic studies have also been published in particular for stroke (for a review see Dichgans et al. (2019)). Despite there is genetic overlap between CAD and atherosclerotic stroke (Dichgans et al. 2014; Kessler et al. 2015a), the genetic risk factors of CAD and stroke are not similar. The formation of large, international consortia has advanced the identification of risk genes in the fields of CAD and stroke genetics. In other atherosclerotic diseases as peripheral artery disease, genetic research will be facilitated by publicly available data from large-scale biobanks. Nevertheless, the identification of common genetic risk factors will be important to evaluate novel therapeutic strategies. Other genetic risk factors for CAD might also not play an important role in related diseases: as such, the strongest genetic risk factor reported so far, chromosome 9p21, is not associated with calcified aortic stenosis; in contrast, the *LPA* gene is associated with both diseases (Trenkwalder et al. 2018).

Table 3 Genes associated with CAD/MI which have been identified using exome sequencing

Chr.	Gene(s)	Mechanism	Ref.
1	ANGPTL3	• Angiopoietin-like 3 inhibits lipoprotein lipase • ANGPTL3 loss-of-function mutations are associated with reduced LDL-cholesterol and triglycerides as well as reduced CAD risk	Stitziel et al. (2017)
2	APOB	• Apolipoprotein B is a main component of LDL-cholesterol and triglyceride-rich lipoproteins • Truncating APOB mutations are associated with reduced LDL-cholesterol and reduced CAD risk	Peloso et al. (2019)
4/2	GUCY1A3/ CCT7	• Premature stop codon in GUCY1A3 leads to loss of α_1-subunit of the soluble guanylyl cyclase (sGC); missense mutation in CCT7 which encodes a chaperone protein stabilizing the sGC • Carriers of the GUCY1A3 +CCT7 mutation show reduced sGC-dependent cGMP formation in platelets • Coding variants in GUCY1A3 are overrepresented in young MI patients	CARDIoGRAMplusC4D Consortium et al. (2013), Erdmann et al. (2013), and Wobst et al. (2016)
7	NPC1L1	• Niemann-Pick C1-like protein 1 is responsible for the uptake of cholesterol from the intestine • NPC1L1 loss-of-function mutations are associated with reduced LDL-cholesterol and reduced risk of CAD/MI	Myocardial Infarction Genetics Consortium Investigators et al. (2014)
8	LPL	• Lipoprotein lipase reduced triglyceride levels • Loss-of-function variants are associated with increased triglyceride levels and CAD/MI	Myocardial Infarction Genetics and CARDIoGRAM Exome Consortia Investigators et al. (2016) and Khera et al. (2017)
11	APOA5	• Apolipoprotein A-V increases lipoprotein lipase activity • APOA5 loss-of-function mutations are associated with high triglyceride levels and CAD/MI	Do et al. (2015)
	APOC3	• Apolipoprotein C-III reduced lipoprotein lipase activity • APOC3 loss-of-function mutations are associated with	The TG and HDL Working Group of the Exome Sequencing Project, National Heart, Lung, and Blood Institute (2014)

(continued)

Table 3 (continued)

Chr.	Gene(s)	Mechanism	Ref.
		reduced triglyceride levels and CAD/MI risk	
16	*CETP*	• Cholesteryl ester transfer protein reduces HDL-cholesterol levels • Carriers of truncating CETP mutation displayed higher levels of HDL-cholesterol, lower levels of LDL-cholesterol, and a lower CAD risk	Nomura et al. (2017)
19	*LDLR*	• Loss of LDL-receptor function leads to reduced uptake of LDL-cholesterol and increased plasma LDL-cholesterol • High levels of LDL-cholesterol increase risk of CAD/MI	Do et al. (2015)

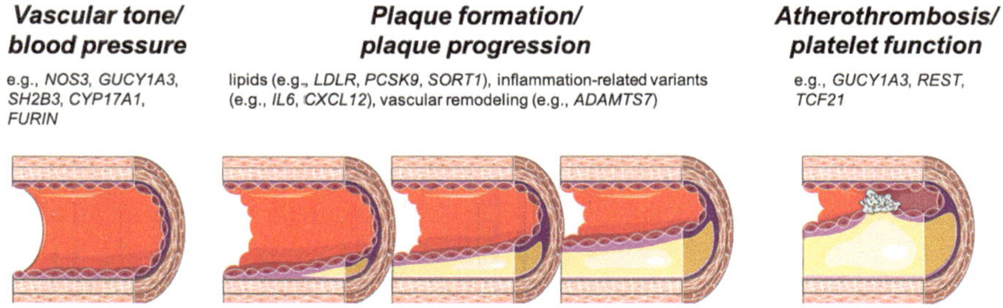

Vascular tone/ blood pressure	**Plaque formation/ plaque progression**	**Atherothrombosis/ platelet function**
e.g., *NOS3, GUCY1A3, SH2B3, CYP17A1, FURIN*	lipids (e.g., *LDLR, PCSK9, SORT1*), inflammation-related variants (e.g., *IL6, CXCL12*), vascular remodeling (e.g., *ADAMTS7*)	e.g., *GUCY1A3, REST, TCF21*

Fig. 2 *Examples of CAD risk genes involved in the sequence of atherosclerotic plaque formation and rupture.* Details see text. Contains modified image material available at Servier Medical Art under a Creative Commons Attribution 3.0 Unported License

5 Pharmacological Targets Identified by Genomic Studies

Genomic studies identified putative pharmacological targets at every stage of plaque formation, progression, and rupture (Fig. 2) which are discussed in this section.

5.1 Lipid Metabolism

While less than half of the identified variants tag genes which are associated with traditional risk factors, lipid metabolism represents a cluster of such variants.

LDL-Cholesterol Metabolism High levels of LDL-cholesterol are an established risk factors for CAD. Not surprisingly, the most prominent genes which are directly involved in LDL-cholesterol metabolism and have been tagged by GWAS are *LDLR*, *PCSK9*, and *SORT1*. In line, mutations in the *LDLR* gene leading to reduced hepatic uptake of LDL-cholesterol have been shown to underlie familial hypercholesterolemia which itself increases CAD risk (Tolleshaug et al. 1983; Brown and Goldstein 1986), and common variants at the LDLR locus have been associated with both phenotypes (Myocardial Infarction Genetics Consortium et al. 2009; Teslovich et al. 2010; Schunkert et al. 2011; Do et al. 2015). PCSK9 has been identified as an interaction partner of the LDL-receptor. If PCSK9 binds to the LDL-receptor, it is internalized and degraded resulting in reduced hepatic uptake and high plasma levels of LDL-cholesterol (Cameron et al. 2006). Gain-of-function mutations in *PCSK9* have been shown to increase LDL-cholesterol (Abifadel et al. 2003), whereas loss-of-function variants have been shown to reduce LDL-cholesterol and CAD risk (Cohen et al. 2006). PCSK9 has been targeted pharmacologically via different approaches. The inhibition of PCSK9 using, e.g., neutralizing antibodies resulted in a marked reduction of LDL-cholesterol and reduced risk of cardiovascular events in CAD patients (Sabatine et al. 2015, 2017). Sortilin 1 encoded by *SORT1* has also been shown to affect LDL-cholesterol (Samani et al. 2007; Musunuru et al. 2010; Teslovich et al. 2010; Schunkert et al. 2011). However, as it seems to also play a role in other processes and as the mechanism involving sortilin 1 in LDL-cholesterol metabolism has still not been fully understood, it might not represent an ideal drug target. NPC1L1, a membrane transporter leading to the uptake of cholesterol from the intestine encoded by the *NPC1L1* gene, also revealed a signal. Using exome sequencing, loss-of-function mutations were identified to be associated with reduced LDL-cholesterol and protection from CAD (Myocardial Infarction Genetics Consortium Investigators et al. 2014). In parallel, it has been shown that pharmacological targeting of NPC1L1 with ezetimibe also reduces the incidence of cardiovascular events in addition to a statin (Cannon et al. 2015). Figure 3 summarizes the multiple lines of evidence for an involvement of LDL-cholesterol metabolism in CAD/MI from a genetic point of view.

Triglyceride Metabolism Lipoprotein lipase has been identified as a central enzyme regulating triglyceride levels. In line, genetic variants in LPL have been associated with both triglyceride levels and CAD risk (Khera et al. 2017). Additionally, the genes encoding several modulators of lipoprotein lipase activity were found to be associated with CAD/MI risk: (1) apolipoprotein C-III reduces lipoprotein lipase activity, and mutations in *APOC3* are associated with both increased triglyceride levels and CAD risk (The TG and HDL Working Group of the Exome Sequencing Project, National Heart, Lung, and Blood Institute 2014; Klarin et al. 2018); (2) apolipoprotein A-V increases lipoprotein lipase activity, and mutations in *APOA5* increase triglyceride levels and CAD risk (Do et al. 2015); and (3) angiopoietin-like 4 inhibits lipoprotein lipase activity, and mutations in *ANGPTL4* reduce triglyceride levels and CAD risk (Myocardial Infarction Genetics and CARDIoGRAM Exome Consortia Investigators et al. 2016). Angiopoietin-like 3 seems to have comparable effects as deficiency was also associated with reduced triglycerides and CAD risk (Stitziel et al. 2017). Mainly apolipoprotein C-III but also

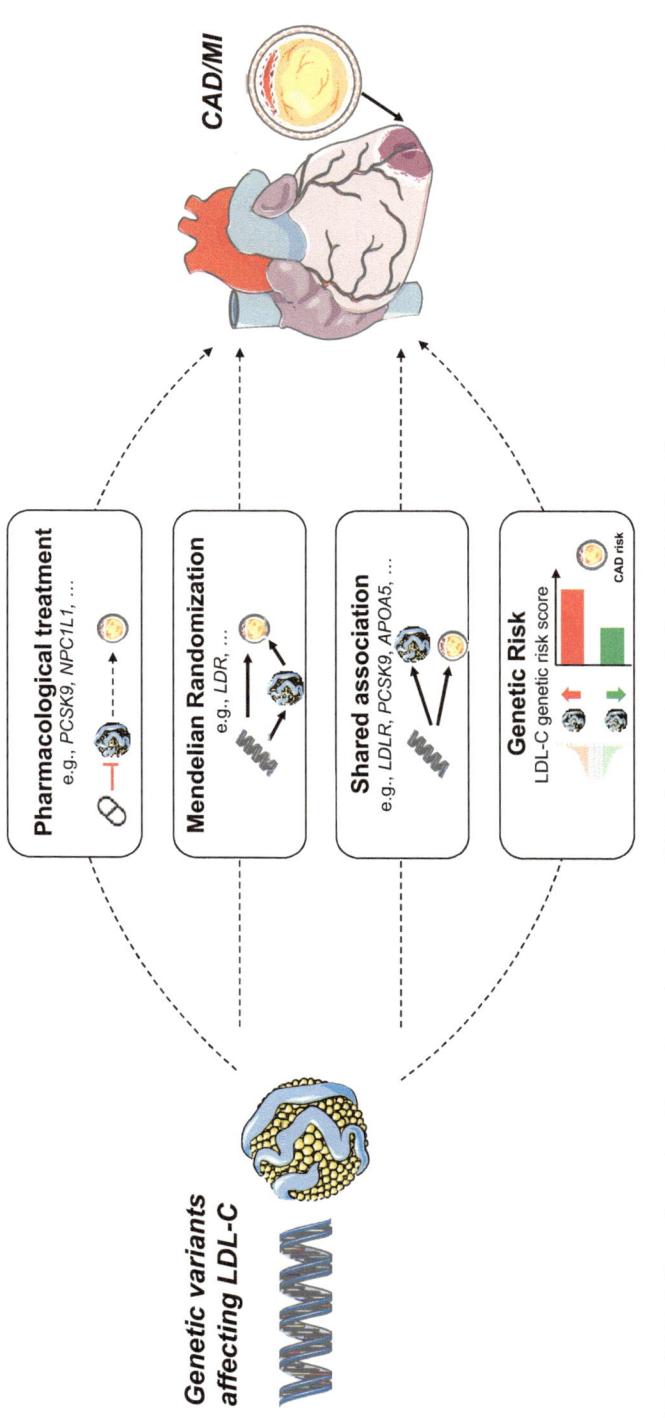

Fig. 3 *Multiple lines of genetic evidence for an involvement of LDL-cholesterol metabolism in CAD/MI. 1. Pharmacological treatments targeting genes which have been associated with LDL-cholesterol reduce risk of cardiovascular events. 2. Mendelian randomization studies have proven the causal influence of LDL-cholesterol metabolism in CAD/MI. 3. CAD/MI and LDL-cholesterol show shared genetic risk variants which are associated with both traits at the genome-wide level of statistical significance. 4. Genetic risk scores for LDL-cholesterol including genome-wide significant variants are also associated with CAD/MI risk, i.e., individuals with a high genetic LDL-cholesterol risk score are also at higher risk for CAD/MI and vice versa. Contains modified image material available at Servier Medical Art under a Creative Commons Attribution 3.0 Unported License*

angiopoietin-like 3 are subjects of research for novel strategies targeting lipoprotein lipase metabolism (Graham et al. 2013; Gaudet et al. 2015; Ahmad et al. 2019).

5.2 Inflammation

Vascular inflammation and the recruitment of leukocytes are the hallmarks of atherosclerosis (for reviews see Lusis (2000), Libby et al. (2011), and Swirski and Nahrendorf (2013)). Several clinical studies already in the past decades thus targeted inflammatory parameters. A prominent example is C-reactive protein (CRP), which has been regarded for a long time as a pathophysiological player. This was mainly due to the observation of elevated CRP levels in individuals suffering from CAD in epidemiological studies (Koenig et al. 1999; Danesh et al. 2004) making CRP a promising therapeutic target (Pepys et al. 2006). Indeed, clinical trials, e.g., the JUPITER trial which investigated the effect of rosuvastatin in individuals with elevated CRP levels, showed a benefit (Ridker et al. 2008). Genetic studies were, however, able to dissect this association and trial outcomes. As such, LDL-cholesterol could be clearly proven as a causal risk factor for CAD as a genetic risk score for LDL-cholesterol elevating variants was also associated with CAD risk (Kathiresan et al. 2008). In contrast, several variants found to increase CRP levels did not show an association with CAD risk (Lange et al. 2006; Zacho et al. 2008; Linsel-Nitschke et al. 2008; Schunkert and Samani 2008; C Reactive Protein Coronary Heart Disease Genetics Collaboration (CCGC) et al. 2011). While these studies on CRP remained disappointing, targeting inflammation has indeed lately been proven to be effective in CAD. In the CANTOS trial, the administration of an interleukin-1β neutralizing antibody was able to reduce the incidence of cardiovascular events ultimately proving the inflammation hypothesis (Ridker et al. 2017). This is in line with Mendelian randomization studies that revealed evidence for a causal role of interleukin-6/interleukin-6 receptor signaling, which is downstream of interleukin-1β, in CAD (Interleukin-6 Receptor Mendelian Randomisation Analysis Consortium et al. 2012).

GWAS led to the identification of a number of variants tagging genes which play a role in inflammatory processes to be associated with CAD/MI.

Autoimmune Processes CAD/MI and autoimmune disease share genetic risk factors. As such, the *SH2B3* locus has been identified to be associated with CAD/MI (Coronary Artery Disease C4D Genetics Consortium 2011b; Schunkert et al. 2011) but also, e.g., type 1 diabetes mellitus (Barrett et al. 2009) and celiac disease (Hunt et al. 2008). A role for the encoded protein, SH2B adaptor protein 3 (SH2B3), has been shown in post MI remodeling: lack of Sh2b3 in rats was associated with increased fibrosis, increased leukocyte infiltration, and decreased cardiac function (Flister et al. 2015). Additionally, it is involved in dendritic cell function leading to T-cell interferon signaling (Mori et al. 2014). Nevertheless, uncertainties remain as the locus was also found to be associated with blood pressure (Levy et al. 2009; Newton-Cheh et al. 2009) and hematologic parameters (Soranzo et al. 2009). The latter observation might be important as an involvement in megakaryopoiesis and stabilization of thrombi has also been shown experimentally (Tong and Lodish 2004; Takizawa et al. 2010). In a recent study, the *SH2B3* risk allele was found to be associated with decreased SH2B3 expression which, at least for the murine counterpart Sh2b3/Lnk, together with cholesterol loading promoted platelet production and activation (Wang et al. 2016).

Innate Immunity CXCL12 is a chemokine which is encoded by the CAD risk gene *CXCL12* (Myocardial Infarction Genetics Consortium et al. 2009; Coronary Artery Disease C4D Genetics Consortium 2011b) and has a function in various cellular processes. In atherosclerosis the CXCL12/CXCR4 axis has initially been described to have a rather protective role (Döring et al. 2014). Disruption of this axis led to increased plaque formation and proinflammatory plaque phenotypes in vivo (Zernecke et al. 2008). In line, CXCL12/CXCR4 signaling was shown to be important in endothelial cells and smooth muscle cells via maintaining barrier function and contractile responses, respectively (Döring et al. 2017). However, the interaction of CXCL12 and CXCR4 in atherosclerosis seems to be more complex. Whereas the atheroprotective findings were mainly derived from studies in which the interaction was inhibited by small molecules or genetic deletion of CXCR4, endothelial cell-derived CXCL12 was found to promote atherosclerosis (Döring et al. 2019). CXCR4 in contrast seems to be atheroprotective: in addition to the mentioned in vivo studies, the rs2322864 C-allele, which was found to be associated with CAD risk in a candidate gene study, was also associated with CXCR4 expression in plaques (Döring et al. 2017). The double-edged effects of CXCL12/CXCR4 signaling need to be considered to successfully target this pathway.

5.3 Platelet Function and Nitric Oxide Signaling

Genetic studies led to the identification of several genes which play a role in nitric oxide (NO) signaling leading to the formation or degradation of the second messenger cyclic guanosine monophosphate (cGMP), an endogenous inhibitor of platelet aggregation (Moro et al. 1996). Whereas several genes (e.g., *NOS3*, *PDE5A*, *MRVI1*, *PDE3A*) fulfill important functions in this pathway, most is known about *GUCY1A3* which encodes the α_1-subunit of the soluble guanylyl cyclase (α_1-sGC). As discussed above, a digenic mutation in *GUCY1A3* and the *CCT7* gene, which encodes the chaperone protein, was identified in a family by exome sequencing (Erdmann et al. 2013). At the same time, also a common non-coding variant (rs7678555) was identified in Europeans to be associated with CAD by GWAS (CARDIoGRAMplusC4D Consortium et al. 2013). Whereas the digenic mutation led to loss of α_1-sGC due to premature stop of translation (Erdmann et al. 2013), the common variant has been shown to influence *GUCY1A3* expression, i.e., the risk allele G was linked to reduced expression (Kessler et al. 2017). Both the digenic mutation and the common risk variant led to reduced cGMP formation in platelets (Erdmann et al. 2013; Kessler et al. 2017). As a consequence, platelets of carriers of the common risk variants showed impaired inhibition of platelet aggregation secondary to NO stimulation (Kessler et al. 2017). The sGC is a known pharmacological target. Specific stimulators and activators of the sGC are available (for an overview see Stasch et al. (2011)) and approved for other traits, e.g., pulmonary hypertension (Ghofrani et al. 2013a, b). First preclinical data also render a positive influence of sGC stimulators on atherosclerotic phenotypes possible (Tsou et al. 2014). Additionally, the impaired response to nitric oxide in carriers of the common risk allele G in platelets might also be targeted via unspecific inhibitors of platelet aggregation. Recently, we showed that homozygous risk allele carriers might benefit from aspirin treatment in the primary prevention of cardiovascular diseases, whereas homozygous or heterozygous carriers of the non-risk allele A seem to even display increased risk (Hall et al. 2019). Additionally, homozygous carriers of the risk allele G are at an increased risk of ischemic events after the implantation of coronary stents, at least in part via higher on-aspirin platelet reactivity (Kessler et al. 2019). While platelets, in addition to their well-known role in atherothrombosis, are also involved in atherosclerotic plaque formation (Gawaz et al. 2005) and despite the known influence of sGC function on inflammatory phenotypes (Ahluwalia et al. 2004), the exact mechanisms are still unknown. This is complicated by the fact that a complete knockout of the murine counterpart *Gucy1a3* led to the unexpected finding of reduced atherosclerotic plaque formation (Segura-Puimedon et al. 2016), whereas genetically determined reduced but not lacking expression of *Gucy1a3* was also associated with increased plaque formation (Kessler et al. 2017). The genetic findings at the further mentioned NO-cGMP-signaling loci associated with CAD/MI have been extensively discussed elsewhere (Wobst et al. 2018). A promising target in addition to sGC is phosphodiesterase 5A encoded by the *PDE5A* gene (Nelson et al. 2017) which leads to degradation of cGMP. However, there is currently no evidence for a beneficial effect of PDE5A inhibition in atherosclerosis.

5.4   Vascular Phenotypes

Several genes identified by GWAS have been linked to vascular phenotypes including the regulation of vascular tone and vascular remodeling.

Vascular Tone and Blood Pressure   Hypertension is a known risk factor for CAD (Yusuf et al. 2004). Some of the CAD risk genes also display genome-wide association with blood pressure. In particular, *NOS3*, encoding endothelial NO synthase (eNOS), and *GUCY1A3* (see above) have an established role also in smooth muscle cells leading to vasodilatation after production of cGMP (Moro et al. 1996). Both have been identified as blood pressure genes (International Consortium for Blood Pressure Genome-Wide Association Studies et al. 2011; Salvi et al. 2012). In line, a genetic risk score for *NOS3* and *GUCY1A3* was associated with increased CAD risk. However, the effect could only in part be explained by effects on blood pressure (Emdin et al. 2018). Further genes associated with both CAD and blood pressure include *SH2B3*, *CYP17A1*, *FURIN*, *AGT*, and *ARHGAP42*. Profound knowledge about the underlying mechanisms is still lacking. However, a genetic risk score for hypertension was strongly associated with CAD/MI and vice versa highlighting the importance of this risk factor which also has a strong heritability (Ntalla et al. 2019).

Vascular Remodeling A large number of genes have been linked to vascular remodeling (for an overview see Erdmann et al. (2018)). One example is the *REST* gene which has been identified as a CAD risk gene in 2017 (Nelson et al. 2017). *REST* encodes the RE-1 silencing transcription factor (REST) which has been mainly studied in neuronal diseases as Huntington disease (Zuccato et al. 2003) or seizures (McClelland et al. 2014). However, there is also evidence for a role in cardiac development where REST led to increased proliferation (Zhang et al. 2017). Additionally, REST has been described to inhibit microRNA-21 and to inhibit proliferation in vascular smooth muscle cells. As a consequence, REST might influence the formation of vulnerable atherosclerotic plaques (Jin et al. 2018). As it acts as a transcriptional regulator, several downstream transcripts might play important pathophysiological roles and represent novel targets. Another novel target is a disintegrin and metalloproteinase with thrombospondin motifs 7 (ADAMTS-7) which has been identified as a CAD risk gene (*ADAMTS7*) in 2011 (Reilly et al. 2011; Schunkert et al. 2011; Coronary Artery Disease C4D Genetics Consortium 2011a). It has been shown that *Adamts7* deficiency leads to reduced neointima formation after vascular injury (Bauer et al. 2015; Kessler et al. 2015b) as well as reduced atherosclerotic plaque formation under proatherogenic conditions (Bauer et al. 2015). Whereas the influence on vascular remodeling is influenced by ADAMTS-7-dependent degradation of cartilage oligomeric matrix protein (COMP) (Wang et al. 2009) and thrombospondin-1 (TSP-1) (Kessler et al. 2015b) with effects on vascular smooth muscle cells and endothelial cells, respectively, the mechanism underlying reduced atherosclerotic plaque formation in mice lacking *Adamts7* remains unknown so far. Of note, the *ADAMTS7* locus is the only locus that has been identified to exert a gene-environment interaction with smoking. In smokers, the protective effect of the *ADAMTS7* non-risk allele was outweighed in smokers, presumably via upregulation of *ADAMTS7* expression secondary to expo-sure to tobacco ingredients (Saleheen et al. 2017).

5.5   Further Directions

Other CAD risk genes have been clustered into similarly interesting pathways which could in principle be targets of therapeutic interventions. Genes have, for example, also been annotated to *transcriptional gene regulation*, *mitosis and proliferation*, or *neovascularization and angiogenesis* (Lempiäinen et al. 2018; Zeng et al. 2019b). The majority of variants and genes has nevertheless not yet been classified to such pathways (Erdmann et al. 2018). Also, the role of the first and strongest risk locus chromosome 9p21 is still not fully understood. Whereas studies initially focused on the role of the cyclin-dependent kinase inhibitors 2A/2B (CDKN2A/B) (Harismendy et al. 2011), the circular form of the non-coding RNA *ANRIL*, which is also located at the locus (Pasmant et al. 2011), was found to have an atheroprotective role through balanced regulation of vascular cells. In contrast, the linear form which is increased in carriers of the risk allele increases atherosclerosis risk (Holdt et al. 2016).

6   Risk Scores and Risk Prediction

Apart from identifying novel pharmacological targets, GWAS raised hope to identify patients at risk early on to improve prevention of CAD. Whereas initial studies including some of the identified variants only led to modest success in this regard (Hughes et al. 2012; for an overview see Kessler and Schunkert (2012)), recent studies using polygenic risk scores changed the scenario. A polygenic risk score for CSD including more than six millions of variants was able to identify individuals with a substantially elevated CAD risk. Strikingly, the score identified 20 times more individuals than familial hypercholesterolemia patients, while the carriers of a high genetic risk score were at even higher CAD risk (Khera et al. 2018). Even in a scenario in which high polygenic risk score and the presence of familial hypercholesterolemia lead to a same increase in CAD risk, the prevalence of a high polygenic risk score was ten times higher than that of familial hypercholesterolemia (Khera et al. 2019) illustrating the potential of including such scores in prevention programs.

Another field in which polygenic risk scores can be used is to investigate associations with other phenotypes. In particular, as discussed above it has been shown that CAD/MI and other cardiovascular phenotypes, e.g., peripheral arterial disease, stroke, or abdominal aneurysm, share genetic predisposition. In contrast, risk of migraine was reduced with increased genetic CAD/MI risk (Ntalla et al. 2019). Risk scores were also able to dissect an interrelationship between educational attainment, which is regarded as a determinant of lifestyle factors, and CAD/MI risk. Here, a genetic risk score including variants which are known to be associated with educational attainment was also associated with CAD risk. As the signal was lost after adjusting for body mass index and smoking, it can be hypothesized that a genetic predisposition to educational attainment might influence a healthier lifestyle and, subsequently, reduce CAD/MI risk (Zeng et al. 2019a).

Furthermore, there is hope that knowledge of particular genetic risk factors can be used to design individualized treatment strategies. *GUCY1A3* as an example has been discussed above. Here, knowledge of genotype could inform aspirin therapy in the setting of primary prevention (Hall et al. 2019) and ischemic risk in CAD patients after PCI (Kessler et al. 2019). Genetic risk scores have also been able to identify individuals who could have a larger benefit from statin treatment (Mega et al. 2015; Natarajan et al. 2017). In the future, polygenic risk scores might therefore also be used in the design of clinical trials. A recent post hoc study of the ODYSSEY trial which investigated the benefit from the PCSK9 inhibitor alirocumab in CAD (Schwartz et al. 2018) revealed that individuals with a higher polygenic risk score particularly benefited from treatment (Damask et al. 2020). Whereas this clearly indicated that polygenic risk scores might provide an excellent tool for risk stratification, a prospective benefit in the design of clinical trials needs to be demonstrated.

7 Summary

Genomic studies led to the identification of a large and still growing number of genes which play a role in the pathophysiology of CAD/MI. While only a few have been functionally investigated so far, novel therapeutic strategies have been developed in, e.g., LDL-cholesterol metabolism, and further promising targets might be identified. In addition, knowledge of genetic risk factors might facilitate prevention of the disease through early identification of individuals at risk and therapy via individualized treatment strategies.

References

1000 Genomes Project Consortium, Abecasis GR, Auton A et al (2012) An integrated map of genetic variation from 1,092 human genomes. Nature 491:56–65. https://doi.org/10.1038/nature11632

1000 Genomes Project Consortium, Auton A, Brooks LD et al (2015) A global reference for human genetic variation. Nature 526:68–74. https://doi.org/10.1038/nature15393

Abifadel M, Varret M, Rabès J-P et al (2003) Mutations in PCSK9 cause autosomal dominant hypercholesterolemia. Nat Genet 34:154–156. https://doi.org/10.1038/ng1161

Ahluwalia A, Foster P, Scotland RS et al (2004) Antiinflammatory activity of soluble guanylate cyclase: cGMP-dependent down-regulation of P-selectin expression and leukocyte recruitment. Proc Natl Acad Sci U S A 101:1386–1391. https://doi.org/10.1073/pnas.0304264101

Ahmad Z, Banerjee P, Hamon S et al (2019) Inhibition of Angiopoietin-Like Protein 3 with a Monoclonal antibody reduces triglycerides in hypertriglyceridemia. Circulation 140:470–486. https://doi.org/10.1161/CIRCULATIONAHA.118.039107

Barrett JC, Clayton DG, Concannon P et al (2009) Genome-wide association study and meta-analysis find that over 40 loci affect risk of type 1 diabetes. Nat Genet 41:703–707. https://doi.org/10.1038/ng.381

Bauer RC, Tohyama J, Cui J et al (2015) Knockout of Adamts7, a novel coronary artery disease locus in humans, reduces atherosclerosis in mice. Circulation 131:1202–1213. https://doi.org/10.1161/CIRCULATIONAHA.114.012669

Braenne I, Willenborg C, Tragante V et al (2017) A genomic exploration identifies mechanisms that may explain adverse cardiovascular effects of COX-2 inhibitors. Sci Rep 7:10252. https://doi.org/10.1038/s41598-017-10928-4

Brown MS, Goldstein JL (1986) A receptor-mediated pathway for cholesterol homeostasis. Science 232:34–47

C Reactive Protein Coronary Heart Disease Genetics Collaboration (CCGC), Wensley F, Gao P et al (2011) Association between C reactive protein and coronary heart disease: mendelian randomisation analysis based on individual participant data. BMJ 342:d548. https://doi.org/10.1136/bmj.d548

Cameron J, Holla ØL, Ranheim T et al (2006) Effect of mutations in the PCSK9 gene on the cell surface LDL receptors. Hum Mol Genet 15:1551–1558. https://doi.org/10.1093/hmg/ddl077

Cannon CP, Blazing MA, Giugliano RP et al (2015) Ezetimibe added to statin therapy after acute coronary syndromes. N Engl J Med 372:2387–2397. https://doi.org/10.1056/NEJMoa1410489

CARDIoGRAMplusC4D Consortium, Deloukas P, Kanoni S et al (2013) Large-scale association analysis identifies new risk loci for coronary artery disease. Nat Genet 45:25–33. https://doi.org/10.1038/ng.2480

Cohen JC, Boerwinkle E, Mosley TH, Hobbs HH (2006) Sequence variations in PCSK9, low LDL, and protection against coronary heart disease. N Engl J Med 354:1264–1272. https://doi.org/10.1056/NEJMoa054013

Coronary Artery Disease C4D Genetics Consortium (2011a) A genome-wide association study in Europeans and South Asians identifies five new loci for coronary artery disease. Nat Genet 43:339–344. https://doi.org/10.1038/ng.782

Coronary Artery Disease C4D Genetics Consortium (2011b) A genome-wide association study in Europeans and South Asians identifies five new loci for coronary artery disease. Nat Genet 43:339–344. https://doi.org/10.1038/ng.782

Damask A, Steg PG, Schwartz GG et al (2020) Patients with high genome-wide polygenic risk scores for coronary artery disease may receive greater clinical benefit from alirocumab treatment in the ODYSSEY OUTCOMES Trial. Circulation 141:624–636. https://doi.org/10.1161/CIRCULATIONAHA.119.044434

Danesh J, Wheeler JG, Hirschfield GM et al (2004) C-reactive protein and other circulating markers of inflammation in the prediction of coronary heart disease. N Engl J Med 350:1387–1397. https://doi.org/10.1056/NEJMoa032804

Dichgans M, Malik R, König IR et al (2014) Shared genetic susceptibility to ischemic stroke and coronary artery disease: a genome-wide analysis of common variants. Stroke 45:24–36. https://doi.org/10.1161/STROKEAHA.113.002707

Dichgans M, Pulit SL, Rosand J (2019) Stroke genetics: discovery, biology, and clinical applications. Lancet Neurol 18:587–599. https://doi.org/10.1016/S1474-4422(19)30043-2

Do R, Stitziel NO, Won H-H et al (2015) Exome sequencing identifies rare LDLR and APOA5 alleles conferring risk for myocardial infarction. Nature 518:102–106. https://doi.org/10.1038/nature13917

Döring Y, Pawig L, Weber C, Noels H (2014) The CXCL12/CXCR4 chemokine ligand/receptor axis in cardiovascular disease. Front Physiol 5:212. https://doi.org/10.3389/fphys.2014.00212

Döring Y, Noels H, van der Vorst EPC et al (2017) Vascular CXCR4 limits atherosclerosis by maintaining arterial integrity: evidence from mouse and human studies. Circulation 136:388–403. https://doi.org/10.1161/CIRCULATIONAHA.117.027646

Döring Y, van der Vorst EPC, Duchene J et al (2019) CXCL12 derived from endothelial cells promotes atherosclerosis to drive coronary artery disease. Circulation 139:1338–1340. https://doi.org/10.1161/CIRCULATIONAHA.118.037953

Emdin CA, Khera AV, Klarin D et al (2018) Phenotypic consequences of a genetic predisposition to enhanced nitric oxide signaling. Circulation 137:222–232. https://doi.org/10.1161/CIRCULATIONAHA.117.028021

Erdmann J, Grosshennig A, Braund PS et al (2009) New susceptibility locus for coronary artery disease on chromosome 3q22.3. Nat Genet 41:280–282. https://doi.org/10.1038/ng.307

Erdmann J, Willenborg C, Nahrstaedt J et al (2011) Genome-wide association study identifies a new locus for coronary artery disease on chromosome 10p11.23. Eur Heart J 32:158–168. https://doi.org/10.1093/eurheartj/ehq405

Erdmann J, Stark K, Esslinger UB et al (2013) Dysfunctional nitric oxide signalling increases risk of myocardial infarction. Nature 504:432–436. https://doi.org/10.1038/nature12722

Erdmann J, Kessler T, Munoz Venegas L, Schunkert H (2018) A decade of genome-wide association studies for coronary artery disease: the challenges ahead. Cardiovasc Res 114:1241–1257. https://doi.org/10.1093/cvr/cvy084

Flister MJ, Hoffman MJ, Lemke A et al (2015) SH2B3 is a genetic determinant of cardiac inflammation and fibrosis. Circ Cardiovasc Genet 8:294–304. https://doi.org/10.1161/CIRCGENETICS.114.000527

Gaudet D, Alexander VJ, Baker BF et al (2015) Antisense inhibition of apolipoprotein C-III in patients with hypertriglyceridemia. N Engl J Med 373:438–447. https://doi.org/10.1056/NEJMoa1400283

Gawaz M, Langer H, May AE (2005) Platelets in inflammation and atherogenesis. J Clin Invest 115:3378–3384. https://doi.org/10.1172/JCI27196

Ghofrani H-A, D'Armini AM, Grimminger F et al (2013a) Riociguat for the treatment of chronic thromboembolic pulmonary hypertension. N Engl J Med 369:319–329. https://doi.org/10.1056/NEJMoa1209657

Ghofrani H-A, Galiè N, Grimminger F et al (2013b) Riociguat for the treatment of pulmonary arterial hypertension. N Engl J Med 369:330–340. https://doi.org/10.1056/NEJMoa1209655

Graham MJ, Lee RG, Bell TA et al (2013) Antisense oligonucleotide inhibition of apolipoprotein C-III reduces plasma triglycerides in rodents, nonhuman primates, and humans. Circ Res 112:1479–1490. https://doi.org/10.1161/CIRCRESAHA.111.300367

Gudbjartsson DF, Bjornsdottir US, Halapi E et al (2009) Sequence variants affecting eosinophil numbers associate with asthma and myocardial infarction. Nat Genet 41:342–347. https://doi.org/10.1038/ng.323

Hall KT, Kessler T, Buring JE et al (2019) Genetic variation at the coronary artery disease risk locus GUCY1A3 modifies cardiovascular disease prevention effects of aspirin. Eur Heart J 40:3385–3392. https://doi.org/10.1093/eurheartj/ehz384

Harismendy O, Notani D, Song X et al (2011) 9p21 DNA variants associated with coronary artery disease impair interferon-γ signalling response. Nature 470:264–268. https://doi.org/10.1038/nature09753

Helgadottir A, Thorleifsson G, Manolescu A et al (2007) A common variant on chromosome 9p21 affects the risk of myocardial infarction. Science 316:1491–1493. https://doi.org/10.1126/science.1142842

Holdt LM, Beutner F, Scholz M et al (2010) ANRIL expression is associated with atherosclerosis risk at chromosome 9p21 Arterioscler Thromb Vasc Biol 30:620–627. https://doi.org/10.1161/ATVBAHA.109.196832

Holdt LM, Hoffmann S, Sass K et al (2013) ALU elements in ANRIL non-coding RNA at chromosome 9p21 modulate atherogenic cell functions through trans-regulation of gene networks. PLoS Genet 9:e1003588. https://doi.org/10.1371/journal.pgen.1003588

Holdt LM, Stahringer A, Sass K et al (2016) Circular non-coding RNA ANRIL modulates ribosomal RNA maturation and atherosclerosis in humans. Nat Commun 7:12429. https://doi.org/10.1038/ncomms12429

Howson JMM, Zhao W, Barnes DR et al (2017) Fifteen new risk loci for coronary artery disease highlight arterial-wall-specific mechanisms. Nat Genet 385:117–119. https://doi.org/10.1038/ng.3874

Hughes MF, Saarela O, Stritzke J et al (2012) Genetic markers enhance coronary risk prediction in men: the MORGAM prospective cohorts. PLoS One 7:e40922

Hunt KA, Zhernakova A, Turner G et al (2008) Newly identified genetic risk variants for celiac disease related to the immune response. Nat Genet 40:395–402. https://doi.org/10.1038/ng.102

IBC 50K CAD Consortium (2011) Large-scale gene-centric analysis identifies novel variants for coronary artery disease. PLoS Genet 7:e1002260. https://doi.org/10.1371/journal.pgen.1002260

Interleukin-6 Receptor Mendelian Randomisation Analysis (IL6R MR) Consortium, Swerdlow DI, Holmes MV et al (2012) The interleukin-6 receptor as a target for prevention of coronary heart disease: a mendelian randomisation analysis. 379:1214–1224. https://doi.org/10.1016/S0140-6736(12)60110-X

International Consortium for Blood Pressure Genome-Wide Association Studies, Ehret GB, Munroe PB et al (2011) Genetic variants in novel pathways influence blood pressure and cardiovascular disease risk. Nature 478:103–109. https://doi.org/10.1038/nature10405

Jansen H, Samani NJ, Schunkert H (2014) Mendelian randomization studies in coronary artery disease. Eur Heart J 35:1917–1924. https://doi.org/10.1093/eurheartj/ehu208

Jin H, Li DY, Chernogubova E et al (2018) Local delivery of miR-21 stabilizes fibrous caps in vulnerable atherosclerotic lesions. Mol Ther 26:1040–1055. https://doi.org/10.1016/j.ymthe. 2018.01.011

Kathiresan S, Melander O, Anevski D et al (2008) Polymorphisms associated with cholesterol and risk of cardiovascular events. N Engl J Med 358:1240–1249. https://doi.org/10.1056/ NEJMoa0706728

Kessler T, Schunkert H (2012) Clinical validation of genetic markers for improved risk estimation. Eur J Prev Cardiol 19:25–32. https://doi.org/10.1177/2047487312448993

Kessler T, Erdmann J, Dichgans M, Schunkert H (2015a) Shared genetic aetiology of coronary artery disease and atherosclerotic stroke-2015. Curr Atheroscler Rep 17:498. https://doi.org/10. 1007/s11883-015-0498-5

Kessler T, Zhang L, Liu Z et al (2015b) ADAMTS-7 inhibits re-endothelialization of injured arteries and promotes vascular remodeling through cleavage of Thrombospondin-1. Circulation 131:1191–1201. https://doi.org/10.1161/CIRCULATIONAHA.114.014072

Kessler T, Vilne B, Schunkert H (2016) The impact of genome-wide association studies on the pathophysiology and therapy of cardiovascular disease. EMBO Mol Med 8:688–701. https:// doi.org/10.15252/emmm.201506174

Kessler T, Wobst J, Wolf B et al (2017) Functional characterization of the GUCY1A3 coronary artery disease risk locus. Circulation 136:476–489. https://doi.org/10.1161/ CIRCULATIONAHA.116.024152

Kessler T, Wolf B, Eriksson N et al (2019) Association of the coronary artery disease risk gene GUCY1A3 with ischaemic events after coronary intervention. Cardiovasc Res 115:1512–1518. https://doi.org/10.1093/cvr/cvz015

Khera AV, Kathiresan S (2017a) Genetics of coronary artery disease: discovery, biology and clinical translation. Nat Rev Genet 18:331–344. https://doi.org/10.1038/nrg.2016.160

Khera AV, Kathiresan S (2017b) Genetics of coronary artery disease: discovery, biology and clinical translation. Nat Rev Genet 18:1–14. https://doi.org/10.1038/nrg.2016.160

Khera AV, Won H-H, Peloso GM et al (2017) Association of rare and common variation in the lipoprotein lipase gene with coronary artery disease. JAMA 317:937–946. https://doi.org/10. 1001/jama.2017.0972

Khera AV, Chaffin M, Aragam KG et al (2018) Genome-wide polygenic scores for common diseases identify individuals with risk equivalent to monogenic mutations. Nat Genet 50:1219–1224. https://doi.org/10.1038/s41588-018-0183-z

Khera AV, Chaffin M, Zekavat SM et al (2019) Whole-genome sequencing to characterize monogenic and polygenic contributions in patients hospitalized with early-onset myocardial infarction. Circulation 139:1593–1602. https://doi.org/10.1161/CIRCULATIONAHA.118. 035658

Klarin D, Zhu QM, Emdin CA et al (2017) Genetic analysis in UK Biobank links insulin resistance and transendothelial migration pathways to coronary artery disease. Nat Genet 49:1392–1397. https://doi.org/10.1038/ng.3914

Klarin D, Damrauer SM, Cho K et al (2018) Genetics of blood lipids among ~300,000 multi-ethnic participants of the Million Veteran Program. Nat Genet 50:1514–1523

Koenig W, Sund M, Fröhlich M et al (1999) C-Reactive protein, a sensitive marker of inflammation, predicts future risk of coronary heart disease in initially healthy middle-aged men: results from the MONICA (Monitoring Trends and Determinants in Cardiovascular Disease) Augsburg Cohort Study, 1984 to 1992. Circulation 99:237–242. https://doi.org/10.1161/01.cir.99.2.237

Lander ES, Linton LM, Birren B et al (2001) Initial sequencing and analysis of the human genome. Nature 409:860–921

Lange LA, Carlson CS, Hindorff LA et al (2006) Association of polymorphisms in the CRP gene with circulating C-reactive protein levels and cardiovascular events. JAMA 296:2703–2711. https://doi.org/10.1001/jama.296.22.2703

Lempiäinen H, Brænne I, Michoel T et al (2018) Network analysis of coronary artery disease risk genes elucidates disease mechanisms and druggable targets. Sci Rep 8:3434

Levy D, Ehret GB, Rice K et al (2009) Genome-wide association study of blood pressure and hypertension. Nat Genet 41:677–687. https://doi.org/10.1038/ng.384

Libby P, Ridker PM, Hansson GK (2011) Progress and challenges in translating the biology of atherosclerosis. Nature 473:317–325. https://doi.org/10.1038/nature10146

Linsel-Nitschke P, Götz A, Erdmann J et al (2008) Lifelong reduction of LDL-cholesterol related to a common variant in the LDL-receptor gene decreases the risk of coronary artery disease--a Mendelian Randomisation study. PLoS One 3:e2986. https://doi.org/10.1371/journal.pone.0002986

Littlejohns TJ, Sudlow C, Allen NE, Collins R (2019) UK Biobank: opportunities for cardiovascular research. Eur Heart J 40:1158–1166. https://doi.org/10.1093/eurheartj/ehx254

Lusis AJ (2000) Atherosclerosis. Nature 407:233–241. https://doi.org/10.1038/35025203

McClelland S, Brennan GP, Dubé C et al (2014) The transcription factor NRSF contributes to epileptogenesis by selective repression of a subset of target genes. Elife 3:e01267. https://doi.org/10.7554/eLife.01267

McPherson R, Tybjaerg-Hansen A (2016) Genetics of coronary artery disease. Circ Res 118:564–578. https://doi.org/10.1161/CIRCRESAHA.115.306566

McPherson R, Pertsemlidis A, Kavaslar N et al (2007) A common allele on chromosome 9 associated with coronary heart disease. Science 316:1488–1491. https://doi.org/10.1126/science.1142447

Mega JL, Stitziel NO, Smith JG et al (2015) Genetic risk, coronary heart disease events, and the clinical benefit of statin therapy: an analysis of primary and secondary prevention trials. Lancet 385:2264–2271. https://doi.org/10.1016/S0140-6736(14)61730-X

Mori T, Iwasaki Y, Seki Y et al (2014) Lnk/Sh2b3 controls the production and function of dendritic cells and regulates the induction of IFN-γ-producing T cells. J Immunol 193:1728–1736. https://doi.org/10.4049/jimmunol.1303243

Moro MA, Russel RJ, Cellek S et al (1996) cGMP mediates the vascular and platelet actions of nitric oxide: confirmation using an inhibitor of the soluble guanylyl cyclase. Proc Natl Acad Sci U S A 93:1480–1485

Musunuru K, Strong A, Frank-Kamenetsky M et al (2010) From noncoding variant to phenotype via SORT1 at the 1p13 cholesterol locus. Nature 466:714–719. https://doi.org/10.1038/nature09266

Myocardial Infarction Genetics and CARDIoGRAM Exome Consortia Investigators, Stitziel NO, Stirrups KE et al (2016) Coding variation in ANGPTL4, LPL, and SVEP1 and the risk of coronary disease. N Engl J Med 374:1134–1144. https://doi.org/10.1056/NEJMoa1507652

Myocardial Infarction Genetics Consortium Investigators, Stitziel NO, Won H-H et al (2014) Inactivating mutations in NPC1L1 and protection from coronary heart disease. N Engl J Med 371:2072–2082. https://doi.org/10.1056/NEJMoa1405386

Myocardial Infarction Genetics Consortium, Voight BF, Purcell S et al (2009) Genome-wide association of early-onset myocardial infarction with single nucleotide polymorphisms and copy number variants. Nat Genet 41:334–341. https://doi.org/10.1038/ng.327

Natarajan P, Young R, Stitziel NO et al (2017) Polygenic risk score identifies subgroup with higher burden of atherosclerosis and greater relative benefit from statin therapy in the primary prevention setting. Circulation 135:2091–2101. https://doi.org/10.1161/CIRCULATIONAHA.116.024436

Nelson CP, Goel A, Butterworth AS et al (2017) Association analyses based on false discovery rate implicate new loci for coronary artery disease. Nat Genet 49:1385–1391. https://doi.org/10.1038/ng.3913

Newton-Cheh C, Johnson T, Gateva V et al (2009) Genome-wide association study identifies eight loci associated with blood pressure. Nat Genet 41:666–676. https://doi.org/10.1038/ng.361

Nikpay M, Goel A, Won H-H et al (2015) A comprehensive 1,000 Genomes-based genome-wide association meta-analysis of coronary artery disease. Nat Genet 47:1121–1130. https://doi.org/10.1038/ng.3396

Nomura A, Won H-H, Khera AV et al (2017) Protein-truncating variants at the Cholesteryl Ester transfer protein gene and risk for coronary heart disease. Circ Res 121:81–88. https://doi.org/10. 1161/CIRCRESAHA.117.311145

Ntalla I, Kanoni S, Zeng L et al (2019) Genetic risk score for coronary disease identifies predispositions to cardiovascular and noncardiovascular diseases. J Am Coll Cardiol 73:2932–2942

Pasmant E, Sabbagh A, Vidaud M, Bièche I (2011) ANRIL, a long, noncoding RNA, is an unexpected major hotspot in GWAS. FASEB J 25:444–448. https://doi.org/10.1096/fj.10-172452

Pe'er I, Yelensky R, Altshuler D, Daly MJ (2008) Estimation of the multiple testing burden for genomewide association studies of nearly all common variants. Genet Epidemiol 32:381–385. https://doi.org/10.1002/gepi.20303

Peloso GM, Nomura A, Khera AV et al (2019) Rare protein-truncating variants in APOB, lower low-density lipoprotein cholesterol, and protection against coronary heart disease. Circ Genom Precis Med 12:e002376. https://doi.org/10.1161/CIRCGEN.118.002376

Pepys MB, Hirschfield GM, Tennent GA et al (2006) Targeting C-reactive protein for the treatment of cardiovascular disease. Nature 440:1217–1221. https://doi.org/10.1038/nature04672

Reich DE, Lander ES (2001) On the allelic spectrum of human disease. Trends Genet 17:502–510

Reilly MP, Li M, He J et al (2011) Identification of ADAMTS7 as a novel locus for coronary atherosclerosis and association of ABO with myocardial infarction in the presence of coronary atherosclerosis: two genome-wide association studies. Lancet 377:383–392. https://doi.org/10. 1016/S0140-6736(10)61996-4

Ridker PM, Danielson E, Fonseca FAH et al (2008) Rosuvastatin to prevent vascular events in men and women with elevated C-reactive protein. N Engl J Med 359:2195–2207. https://doi.org/10. 1056/NEJMoa0807646

Ridker PM, Everett BM, Thuren T et al (2017) Antiinflammatory therapy with Canakinumab for atherosclerotic disease. N Engl J Med 377:1119–1131. https://doi.org/10.1056/ NEJMoa1707914

Sabatine MS, Giugliano RP, Wiviott SD et al (2015) Efficacy and safety of evolocumab in reducing lipids and cardiovascular events. N Engl J Med 372:1500–1509. https://doi.org/10.1056/ NEJMoa1500858

Sabatine MS, Giugliano RP, Keech AC et al (2017) Evolocumab and clinical outcomes in patients with cardiovascular disease. N Engl J Med 376:1713–1722. https://doi.org/10.1056/ NEJMoa1615664

Sachidanandam R, Weissman D, Schmidt SC et al (2001) A map of human genome sequence variation containing 1.42 million single nucleotide polymorphisms. Nature 409:928–933. https://doi.org/10.1038/35057149

Saleheen D, Zhao W, Young R et al (2017) Loss of cardioprotective effects at the ADAMTS7 locus as a result of gene-smoking interactions. Circulation 135:2336–2353. https://doi.org/10.1161/ CIRCULATIONAHA.116.022069

Salvi E, Kutalik Z, Glorioso N et al (2012) Genomewide association study using a high-density single nucleotide polymorphism array and case-control design identifies a novel essential hypertension susceptibility locus in the promoter region of endothelial NO synthase. Hypertension 59:248–255. https://doi.org/10.1161/HYPERTENSIONAHA.111.181990

Samani NJ, Erdmann J, Hall AS et al (2007) Genomewide association analysis of coronary artery disease. N Engl J Med 357:443–453. https://doi.org/10.1056/NEJMoa072366

Schunkert H, Samani NJ (2008) Elevated C-reactive protein in atherosclerosis--chicken or egg? N Engl J Med 359:1953–1955

Schunkert H, König IR, Kathiresan S et al (2011) Large-scale association analysis identifies 13 new susceptibility loci for coronary artery disease. Nat Genet 43:333–338. https://doi.org/10.1038/ ng.784

Schunkert H, Erdmann J, Samani SNJ (2019) CARDIoGRAM celebrates its 10th Anniversary. Eur Heart J 40:1664–1666. https://doi.org/10.1093/eurheartj/ehz347

Schwartz GG, Steg PG, Szarek M et al (2018) Alirocumab and cardiovascular outcomes after acute coronary syndrome. N Engl J Med 379:2097–2107. https://doi.org/10.1056/NEJMoa1801174

Segura-Puimedon M, Mergia E, Al-Hasani J et al (2016) Proatherosclerotic effect of the α1-subunit of soluble Guanylyl Cyclase by promoting smooth muscle phenotypic switching. Am J Pathol 186:2220–2231. https://doi.org/10.1016/j.ajpath.2016.04.010

Soranzo N, Spector TD, Mangino M et al (2009) A genome-wide meta-analysis identifies 22 loci associated with eight hematological parameters in the HaemGen consortium. Nat Genet 41:1182–1190. https://doi.org/10.1038/ng.467

Stasch J-P, Pacher P, Evgenov OV (2011) Soluble guanylate cyclase as an emerging therapeutic target in cardiopulmonary disease. Circulation 123:2263–2273. https://doi.org/10.1161/CIRCULATIONAHA.110.981738

Stitziel NO, Khera AV, Wang X et al (2017) ANGPTL3 deficiency and protection against coronary artery disease. J Am Coll Cardiol 69:2054–2063. https://doi.org/10.1016/j.jacc.2017.02.030

Swirski FK, Nahrendorf M (2013) Leukocyte behavior in atherosclerosis, myocardial infarction, and heart failure. Science 339:161–166. https://doi.org/10.1126/science.1230719

Takizawa H, Nishimura S, Takayama N et al (2010) Lnk regulates integrin αIIbβ3 outside-in signaling in mouse platelets, leading to stabilization of thrombus development in vivo. J Clin Invest 120:179–190. https://doi.org/10.1172/JCI39503DS1

Teslovich TM, Musunuru K, Smith AV et al (2010) Biological, clinical and population relevance of 95 loci for blood lipids. Nature 466:707–713. https://doi.org/10.1038/nature09270

The TG and HDL Working Group of the Exome Sequencing Project, National Heart, Lung, and Blood Institute (2014) Loss-of-function mutations in APOC3, triglycerides, and coronary disease. N Engl J Med 371:22–31. https://doi.org/10.1056/NEJMoa1307095

Tolleshaug H, Hobgood KK, Brown MS, Goldstein JL (1983) The LDL receptor locus in familial hypercholesterolemia: multiple mutations disrupt transport and processing of a membrane receptor. Cell 32:941–951

Tong W, Lodish HF (2004) Lnk inhibits Tpo-mpl signaling and Tpo-mediated megakaryocytopoiesis. J Exp Med 200:569–580. https://doi.org/10.1084/jem.20040762

Tregouet D-A, König IR, Erdmann J et al (2009) Genome-wide haplotype association study identifies the SLC22A3-LPAL2-LPA gene cluster as a risk locus for coronary artery disease. Nat Genet 41:283–285. https://doi.org/10.1038/ng.314

Trenkwalder T, Nelson CP, Musameh MD et al (2018) Effects of the coronary artery disease associated LPA and 9p21 loci on risk of aortic valve stenosis. Int J Cardiol 276:212–217. https://doi.org/10.1016/j.ijcard.2018.11.094

Tsou C-Y, Chen C-Y, Zhao J-F et al (2014) Activation of soluble guanylyl cyclase prevents foam cell formation and atherosclerosis. Acta Physiol (Oxf) 210:799–810. https://doi.org/10.1111/apha.12210

van der Harst P, Verweij N (2018) Identification of 64 novel genetic loci provides an expanded view on the genetic architecture of coronary artery disease. Circ Res 122:433–443. https://doi.org/10.1161/CIRCRESAHA.117.312086

Verweij N, Eppinga RN, Hagemeijer Y, van der Harst P (2017) Identification of 15 novel risk loci for coronary artery disease and genetic risk of recurrent events, atrial fibrillation and heart failure. Sci Rep 7:2761. https://doi.org/10.1038/s41598-017-03062-8

Wang L, Zheng J, Bai X et al (2009) ADAMTS-7 mediates vascular smooth muscle cell migration and neointima formation in balloon-injured rat arteries. Circ Res 104:688–698. https://doi.org/10.1161/CIRCRESAHA.108.188425

Wang W, Tang Y, Wang Y et al (2016) LNK/SH2B3 loss of function promotes atherosclerosis and thrombosis. Circ Res 119:e91–e103. https://doi.org/10.1161/CIRCRESAHA.116.308955

Webb TR, Erdmann J, Stirrups KE et al (2017) Systematic evaluation of pleiotropy identifies 6 further loci associated with coronary artery disease. J Am Coll Cardiol 69:823–836. https://doi.org/10.1016/j.jacc.2016.11.056

Wobst J, Ameln Von S, Wolf B et al (2016) Stimulators of the soluble guanylyl cyclase: promising functional insights from rare coding atherosclerosis-related GUCY1A3 variants. Basic Res Cardiol 111:51. https://doi.org/10.1007/s00395-016-0570-5

Wobst J, Schunkert H, Kessler T (2018) Genetic alterations in the NO-cGMP pathway and cardiovascular risk. Nitric Oxide 76:105–112. https://doi.org/10.1016/j.niox.2018.03.019

Yusuf S, Hawken S, Ounpuu S et al (2004) Effect of potentially modifiable risk factors associated with myocardial infarction in 52 countries (the INTERHEART study): case-control study. Lancet 364:937–952. https://doi.org/10.1016/S0140-6736(04)17018-9

Zacho J, Tybjaerg-Hansen A, Jensen JS et al (2008) Genetically elevated C-reactive protein and ischemic vascular disease. N Engl J Med 359:1897–1908. https://doi.org/10.1056/NEJMoa0707402

Zeng L, Ntalla I, Kessler T et al (2019a) Genetically modulated educational attainment and coronary disease risk. Eur Heart J 40:2413–2420

Zeng L, Talukdar HA, Koplev S et al (2019b) Contribution of gene regulatory networks to heritability of coronary artery disease. J Am Coll Cardiol 73:2946–2957

Zernecke A, Bot I, Djalali-Talab Y et al (2008) Protective role of CXC receptor 4/CXC ligand 12 unveils the importance of neutrophils in atherosclerosis. Circ Res 102:209–217. https://doi.org/10.1161/CIRCRESAHA.107.160697

Zhang D, Wang Y, Lu P et al (2017) REST regulates the cell cycle for cardiac development and regeneration. Nat Commun 8:1979. https://doi.org/10.1038/s41467-017-02210-y

Zuccato C, Tartari M, Crotti A et al (2003) Huntingtin interacts with REST/NRSF to modulate the transcription of NRSE-controlled neuronal genes. Nat Genet 35:76–83. https://doi.org/10.1038/ng1219

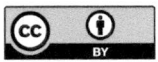

Regulatory Non-coding RNAs in Atherosclerosis

Andreas Schober, Saffiyeh Saboor Maleki, and
Maliheh Nazari-Jahantigh

Contents

1   Introduction 464
2   The Role of Non-coding RNAs in Arterial Endothelium 466
    2.1   miRNAs Drive Inflammatory Activation in Dysadapted Arterial ECs 467
    2.2   The miR-126 Strands in Apoptosis and Regeneration of Dysadapted ECs 470
    2.3   The miR-103–lncWDR59 Axis Limits Endothelial Regeneration and Promotes
          Aberrant Proliferation 471
3   Non-coding RNAs in Macrophage Function 472
    3.1   Regulatory RNAs in Macrophage Energy and Lipid Metabolism 473
    3.2   miR-155-5p and miR-146a/b: The LPS Mediators in Atherosclerosis 476
    3.3   Regulatory RNAs Control Macrophage Death and Efferocytosis in Necrotic Core
          Formation 480
4   MALAT1: The Master miRNA Sponge 481
5   The Simian lncRNA ANRIL and the Risk Locus for Atherosclerosis 482
6   Conclusions and Therapeutic Perspectives 483
References 484

Abstract

Regulatory RNAs like microRNAs (miRNAs) and long non-coding RNAs
(lncRNAs) control vascular and immune cells' phenotype and thus play a crucial
role in atherosclerosis. Moreover, the mutual interactions between miRNAs and
lncRNAs link both types of regulatory RNAs in a functional network that affects
lesion formation. In this review, we deduce novel concepts of atherosclerosis
from the analysis of the current data on regulatory RNAs' role in endothelial cells

A. Schober (✉) · S. S. Maleki · M. Nazari-Jahantigh
Institute for Cardiovascular Prevention, University Hospital, Ludwig-Maximilians-University,
Munich, Germany
e-mail: Andreas.Schober@med.uni-muenchen.de; saffiyeh.saboor@med.uni-muenchen.de;
mnazari@med.lmu.de

© The Author(s) 2020
A. von Eckardstein, C. J. Binder (eds.), *Prevention and Treatment of Atherosclerosis*,
Handbook of Experimental Pharmacology 270, https://doi.org/10.1007/164_2020_423

(ECs) and macrophages. In contrast to arterial ECs, which adopt a stable pheno-type by adaptation to high shear stress, macrophages are highly plastic and quickly change their activation status. At predilection sites of atherosclerosis, such as arterial bifurcations, ECs are exposed to disturbed laminar flow, which generates a dysadaptive stress response mediated by miRNAs. Whereas the highly abundant miR-126-5p promotes regenerative proliferation of dysadapted ECs, miR-103-3p stimulates inflammatory activation and impairs endothelial regeneration by aberrant proliferation and micronuclei formation. In macrophages, miRNAs are essential in regulating energy and lipid metabolism, which affects inflammatory activation and foam cell formation.

Moreover, lipopolysaccharide-induced miR-155 and miR-146 shape inflammatory macrophage activation through their oppositional effects on NF-kB. Most lncRNAs are not conserved between species, except a small group of very long lncRNAs, such as MALAT1, which blocks numerous miRNAs by providing non-functional binding sites. In summary, regulatory RNAs' roles are highly context-dependent, and therapeutic approaches that target specific functional interactions of miRNAs appear promising against cardiovascular diseases.

Keywords

Endothelial cell · Long non-coding RNA · Macrophage · MicroRNA

1   Introduction

RNA molecules have a great variety of functions in the cell, including the transfer of protein-coding information in the primary nucleotide sequence of the mRNA, reading the codons and matching them to amino acids by tRNA, catalysis of peptide bond formation by rRNA, and splicing of pre-mRNA by small nuclear RNAs in the spliceosome. Besides, regulatory non-coding RNAs, which have been grossly grouped into microRNAs (miRNAs) and long, non-coding RNAs (lncRNAs), play a critical role in the control of gene expression (Kopp and Mendell 2018). miRNAs have a comparatively confined length of 20–24 nucleotides and are processed from a primary transcript that contains a secondary hairpin structure with an imperfectly paired stem by endonucleases, such as Drosha and Dicer. By contrast, lncRNAs, linear and circular, are 200 to several thousand nucleotides long, which often adopt a complex secondary structure, and are generated in many different ways, such as RNaseP cleavage or back-splicing (Wu et al. 2017).

miRNAs play an essential role in nematodes, like miRNA let-7, the second described miRNA, which is critical in the development of *C. elegans* (Roush and Slack 2008). The nucleotides 2–7 at the 5′ end of the miRNA, also known as the "seed sequence," bind via Watson-Crick-based complementary base pairing to the recognition element mostly located in the 3′-UTR of mRNAs (Bartel 2018). However, also non-canonical interactions, including, e.g., G:U wobbles or bulges, can occur and mediate the effect of miRNAs (Chipman and Pasquinelli 2019). Thus, the seed sequence is essential for the function of miRNAs. Notably, some miRNAs share the same seed sequence but differ in one or two nucleotides outside the seed sequence, establishing a seed family of miRNAs. Moreover, multiple genomic loci may exist for a specific miRNA. For example, the human let-7 seed family, e.g., comprises 12 miRNAs, such as let-7a, let-7b, let-7c, etc., which share the same seed sequence (Lee et al. 2015). Moreover, three genomic loci encode the let-7a miRNA (let-7a-1, let-7a-2, and let-7a-3). Because of the same seed sequence, miRNA families may form a redundant system resistant to genetic losses and mutations.

Dicer cleaves the apical loop of the precursor hairpin and produces a miRNA duplex that contains the 5p (miRNA from the 5′ end of the precursor miRNA) and the 3p strand of the mature miRNA. Following cleavage of the precursor miRNA hairpin by Dicer in the cytoplasm, a miRNA duplex is loaded to Argonaute proteins constituting the RNA-induced silencing complex (RISC). The two miRNA strands are separated, and one of the two strands exits the RISC. Argonaute proteins present the seed sequence of the retained miRNA strand in the mature RISC, and thus greatly enhance the interaction with the mRNA target sequence. Following binding of the target, miRNAs mediate either translational inhibition or degradation of the target mRNA through GW182 proteins (Schober and Weber 2016). Many miRNAs target hundreds of mRNAs in a cell, but the level of suppression rarely exceeds 50%. An increase in miRNA genes parallels the development of vertebrates (Fromm et al. 2015). In humans, the number of miRNA genes expanded by 179 genes after the split from mouse, peaking at 585 miRNA genes with even many more mature miRNAs (Fromm et al. 2015). Therefore, miRNAs may play a role in the evolution of morphological complexity, probably by shaping specific cell phenotypes through buffering variations in gene expression due to environmental cues and internal noise (Kosik 2010; Siciliano et al. 2013). Thus, regulation by miRNAs confers robustness to differentiation processes during development (Ebert and Sharp 2012).

lncRNAs are not a homogenous class of molecules, but rather a mixture of different functional types with distinct biological mechanisms (Chen et al. 2016a). For example, a lncRNA can affect gene expression by the transcription of its genomic locus, by regulating chromatin states, influencing nuclear structure and organization, and interacting with and controlling proteins or other RNA molecules (Kopp and Mendell 2018; Yao et al. 2019). Many lncRNAs are biochemically identical to mRNAs, harboring a 5′ cap and a 3′ polyadenylated tail, and alternative splicing can produce numerous lncRNA transcripts. Whereas many miRNAs are highly conserved between species, most lncRNAs are evolutionary "novel" (< 50 Million years), and conservation even between humans and mice is rare (Ulitsky 2016). In humans, around 50–90,000 genomic lncRNA loci are annotated (Ulitsky 2016; Uszczynska-Ratajczak et al. 2018), the majority is expressed at a very low level and may not play a functional role. However, a small group of very long, highly expressed, and evolutionarily conserved lncRNAs exists, including, e.g., metastasis-associated lung adenocarcinoma transcript (MALAT)1 and myocardial infarction associated transcript (MIAT). Notably, these lncRNAs contain binding sites for a large number of miRNAs and interact with those in the RISC, the so-called sponge effect. Numerous reports have shown that the functional effect of sponging lncRNAs is due to the inhibition and suppression of the bound miRNAs. Thus, sponging miRNAs appears to be an evolutionarily conserved function of this group of lncRNAs, which closely links the miRNA and the lncRNA world in a complex interaction network.

2   The Role of Non-coding RNAs in Arterial Endothelium

The arterial system is inherently vulnerable to chronic, low-grade endothelial injury at branching sites and curvatures due to disturbed laminar blood flow (Chen et al. 1997). Considering the specifications of ECs in different vascular regions and organs, the response of arterial ECs to non-laminar blood flow appears as if they are maladapted to this physiologic condition at branching arteries. Whereas the low shear stress generated by non-laminar blood flow is stable, the direction of the shear stress and blood flow near the arterial wall in these regions changes randomly, indicating complex vortices. Accordingly, ECs do not align to the direction of the blood flow at branching sites like at arterial areas exposed to laminar blood flow (Gau et al. 1980).

Interestingly, the multidirectionality of near-wall shear stress better predicts the effect of non-laminar blood flow on the localization of atherosclerotic lesions than low shear stress (Peiffer et al. 2013; Mohamied et al. 2015, 2017). Because cellular adaptation to chaotic conditions is impossible, the unpredictable changes of the shear stress direction prevent the adaptation of arterial ECs to non-laminar blood flow and trigger a heterogeneous stress response (Fig. 1). Although at a low frequency, the non-laminar blood flow induces apoptosis of ECs by activating the endoplasmatic reticulum stress response and SUMOylation of p53 (Kim and Woo 2018; Bjorkerud and Bondjers 1972; Zeng et al. 2009; Pan et al. 2017; Hansson et al. 1985; Heo et al. 2011, 2013). Apoptotic ECs are rapidly replaced by the migration and proliferation of adjacent ECs. The endothelial dysadaptation to disturbed laminar blood flow also triggers inflammatory activation and increased adhesiveness to leukocytes, which may play a role in endothelial repair (Tsao et al. 1995). Stress-induced transcription factors, such as NF-κb and hypoxia-inducible factor (HIF)-1α, shape the inflammatory phenotype of dysadapted arterial ECs (Akhtar et al. 2015).

Moreover, chronic endothelial healing in arterial regions exposed to disturbed laminar blood flow impairs endothelial barrier function and increases the permeability to macromolecules, such as lipoproteins (Mundi et al. 2018). Low-density lipoproteins (LDL) are trapped in the subendothelial space and become oxidized by ECs (van Hinsbergh et al. 1986). Oxidized LDL constitutes the second cause of endothelial death (Salvayre et al. 2002) and drives the accumulation of monocyte-derived macrophages in the vessel wall. In arterial regions exposed to laminar blood flow, which stimulates the expression of the transcription factors Krüppel-like factor (KLF) 2 and KLF4, endothelial turnover and vascular permeability are low (Gerrity et al. 1977). KLF2 and KLF4 contribute to a quiescent endothelial phenotype by regulating up to 15% of the flow-regulated genes in a partially redundant manner resulting in the reduction of vascular permeability, inflammatory gene expression, and thrombogenicity (Schober et al. 2015). Moreover, high shear stress-exposed

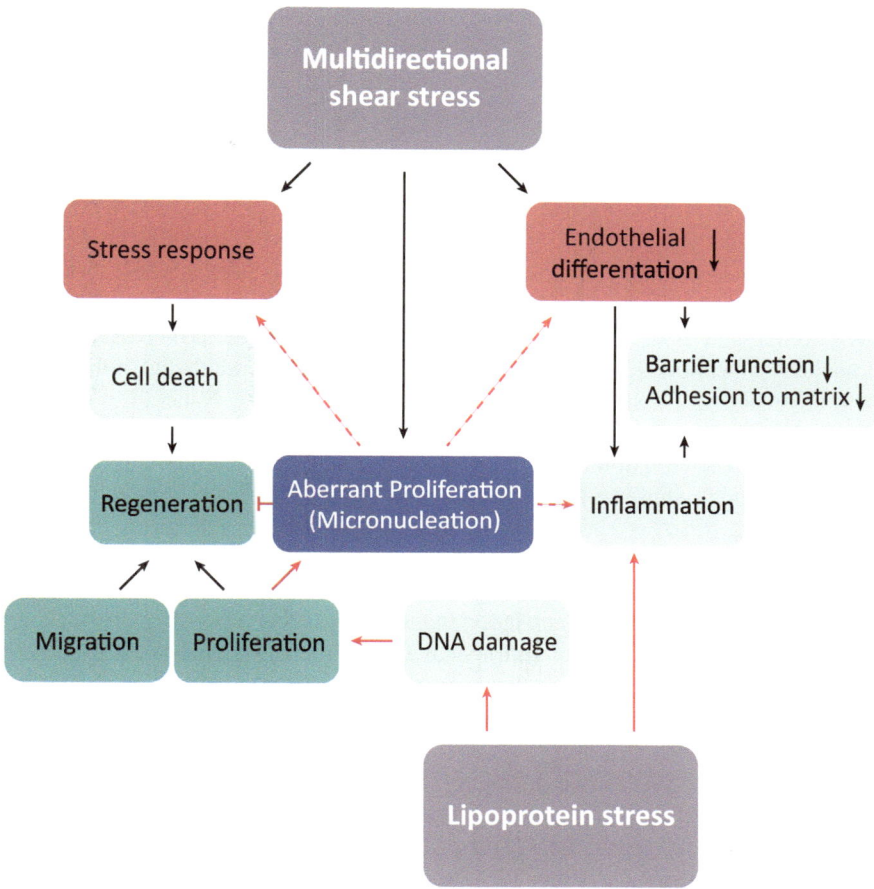

Fig. 1 Dysadaptation of arterial ECs sensitizes to lipoprotein stress. The unpredictable changes in the direction of near-wall shear stress and blood flow at arterial bifurcations make the adaptation of arterial ECs impossible. The dysadaptation induces a stress response characterized by EC death and a lack of endothelial differentiation. The damaged endothelium is regenerated by migrating and proliferating ECs; however, the chronic endothelial wound healing poses a risk for aberrant proliferation due to DNA damage of mitotic ECs by oxidative lipoprotein stress. Dashed lines indicate hypothetical effects

ECs can rapidly proliferate and regenerate the endothelium in response to acute injury (Hansson et al. 1985).

2.1 miRNAs Drive Inflammatory Activation in Dysadapted Arterial ECs

ECs express 164 to 315 miRNAs, and the miRNA expression profile differs significantly between ECs from different vascular regions (McCall et al. 2011; Voellenkle et al. 2012). miR-21-5p (32% of all endothelial miRNAs) is by far the most abundant miRNA in human umbilical vein ECs, followed by miR-126-3p (7%) (Voellenkle et al. 2012). Surprisingly, *Mir21* knockout mice do not have any gross phenotypic changes and develop normally (Patrick et al. 2010). By contrast, 50% of all *Mir126* knockout mice die during development due to vascular leakage, but the surviving mice develop normally (Kuhnert et al. 2008). Notably, specific miRNA families and clusters are primarily expressed in ECs, such as the miR-221/222 cluster, the let-7 miRNA family, and the miR-17-92 cluster. Endothelial Dicer is not essential in embryonic development, and, surprisingly, Dicer suppresses endothelial differentiation in vitro by downregulating KLF2 and by upregulating inflammatory genes, such as CXCL1 and IL-8 (Suarez et al. 2007, 2008; Wu et al. 2011). Accordingly, knockout of endothelial Dicer in $Apoe^{-/-}$ mice limits endothelial inflammation and atherosclerotic lesion formation (Hartmann et al. 2016; Natarelli et al. 2018), indicating that the whole miRNA system counter regulates high shear stress-induced endothelial differentiation. This effect was associated with the downregulation of a relatively small subset of miRNAs, including miR-103-3p, miR-652-3p, and miR-433-3p, whereas miR-126-3p was not reduced, indicating substantial differences in the turnover rates of these miRNAs. In general, the stability of miRNAs is more than ten times higher than that of mRNAs; however, turnover rates significantly differ between individual miRNAs (Hartmann et al. 2016; Gantier et al. 2011). Thus, the role of endothelial Dicer in atherosclerosis and endothelial differentiation may depend on the generation of miRNAs with a short half-life. Similar to the in vitro results, endothelial Dicer increases inflammatory gene expression, such as Cxcl1 and Ccl2, and reduces the expression of endothelial genes such as cadherin 5 and SRY-box transcription factor (Sox) 17, in murine atherosclerotic arteries. Also, Dicer significantly regulates KLF4, Notch, and β-catenin signaling pathways in atherosclerotic ECs (Hartmann et al. 2016).

miR-103-3p mediates many of the inflammatory effects of Dicer in ECs (Hartmann et al. 2016). The *Mir103* gene is expressed from two different genomic loci located in the intronic sequences of the pantothenate kinase (Pank) 2 and Pank3 genes. These genomic loci and the sequence of the mature miR-103-3p are highly conserved within deuterostomes (Finnerty et al. 2010). Notably, miR-103-3p is abundant in ECs at branching sites of arteries, probably due to disturbed flow-induced NF-κB activation (Hartmann et al. 2016; Tzima et al. 2005). Hyperlipidemia and mildly oxidized LDL also upregulate miR-103-3p expression in arterial ECs (Hartmann et al. 2016). miR-103-3p promotes dedifferentiation by targeting KLF4 and increases Cxcl1-dependent monocyte recruitment to atherosclerotic arteries. Accordingly, inhibiting the interaction between miR-103-3p and KLF4 with a sequence-specific oligonucleotide ameliorates atherosclerosis (Hartmann et al. 2016). Moreover, inhibition of miR-103-3p also reduces atherosclerosis, endothelial inflammation, and endoplasmic reticulum stress in $Apoe^{-/-}$ mice (Jiang et al. 2020). In human aortic ECs, miR-103-3p targets phosphatase and tensin homolog (PTEN) through a canonical binding site, which is not conserved in mouse (Jiang et al. 2020).

In addition to miR-103-3p, the expression of miR-652-3p in ECs promotes atherosclerosis (Huang et al. 2019). The development of atherosclerosis is reduced in $Mir652^{-/-}/Apoe^{-/-}$ mice, probably due to increased endothelial regeneration, because miR-652-3p inhibits endothelial proliferation and repair following mechanical injury (Huang et al. 2019). miR-652-3p suppresses endothelial proliferation by targeting the G1 cyclin, cyclin D2 (Ccnd2) in human and mouse via different non-canonical sites, indicating functional conservation of this interaction (Huang et al. 2019). Ccnd2 is targeted by two other miRNAs, miR-494, and the let-7 family member miR-98, in ECs, which thereby inhibit endothelial proliferation (Li et al. 2016; Wu et al. 2016). Besides, the expression of miR-652-3p inversely correlates with the endothelial expression of CCND2 and EC proliferation in human atherosclerosis, suggesting that miR-652-3p plays a vital role in endothelial dysadaptation (Huang et al. 2019).

miR-92a-3p is another important miRNA in endothelial dysadaptation and inflammation, which is, like miR-103-3p, upregulated in ECs by low shear stress, oxidized LDL, and oxidative stress (Chen et al. 2015; Fang and Davies 2012). miR-92a-3p cooperates with miR-103-3p in suppressing KLF4 and enhancing inflammatory gene expression through activation of NF-κB. Moreover, miR-92a-3p targets several other transcripts in ECs, like KLF2, SOCS5, and SIRT1 (Chen et al. 2015), which also contributes to the inflammatory phenotype of dysadapted ECs. Accordingly, inhibition of miR-92a-3p by antisense oligonucleotides in $Apoe^{-/-}$ and $Ldlr^{-/-}$ mice reduced atherosclerosis and endothelial inflammation (Chen et al. 2015; Loyer et al. 2014). However, after subtotal nephrectomy in $Apoe^{-/-}$ mice on a regular diet, as a model of atherosclerosis triggered by chronic renal failure, locked nucleic acid-based inhibitors of miR-92a-3p applied together with HDL did not reduce lesion formation, despite a strong decrease in endothelial miR-92a-3p expression (Wiese et al. 2019). This result indicates that the role of endothelial miR-92a-3p in atherosclerosis may be model dependent. ECs also release miR-92a-3p in microvesicles, which increases the level of miR-92a-3p in the circulation of patients with coronary atherosclerosis (Liu et al. 2019). miR-92a-3p is processed from the 7-kb long lncRNA MIR17HG together with five other miRNAs, including miR-17-5p, miR-18a-5p, miR-20a-5p, miR-19a-3p, and miR-19b-3p (Mogilyansky and Rigoutsos 2013). Whereas miR-92a and miR-19b are additionally processed from the miR-106a-363 cluster transcript, miR-19a is only expressed from the miR-17-92a locus. Activation of HIF-1α in arterial ECs by turbulent flow and lipoprotein-derived lysophosphatidic acid selectively upregulates miR-19a-3p (Akhtar et al. 2015). Because HIF-1α-mediated miR-19a-3p expression in ECs increases monocyte adhesion by activating NF-κB, this mechanism may mediate the atherogenic effect of endothelial HIF-1α activation (Akhtar et al. 2015). Accordingly, blocking miR-19a-3p by systemic injection of antisense oligonucleotides decreases atherosclerosis in $Apoe^{-/-}$ mice (Chen et al. 2017).

The miR-106b-25 cluster contains three miRNAs, including miR-106b, miR-93, and miR-25, and closely relates to the miRNAs of the miR-17-92a locus. Whereas miR-106b and miR-25 belong to the miR-17 family of miRNAs, miR-25 shares the same seed sequence with miR-92a (Mogilyansky and Rigoutsos 2013). Knockout of the miR-106b-25 cluster in $Apoe^{-/-}$ mice decreases atherosclerosis, reduces the cholesterol content in VLDL and LDL in the blood, and increases VLDL and LDL receptor expression in splenocytes (Semo et al. 2019). These findings indicate that the miRNAs of the miR-106b-25 cluster elevate plasma lipid levels by suppressing lipoprotein clearance by the spleen (Semo et al. 2019).

2.2 The miR-126 Strands in Apoptosis and Regeneration of Dysadapted ECs

MiR-126-3p is one of the most highly expressed miRNAs in ECs. Apoptosis triggers the packaging of miR-126-3p into apoptotic bodies, which are released to the extracellular space, and adjacent ECs take up the apoptotic vesicles. The paracrine transfer of miR-126-3p from apoptotic ECs upregulates the chemokine CXCL12 in the recipient ECs and reduces atherosclerosis (Zernecke et al. 2009). However, the role of CXCL12 and its receptor CXCR4 in atherosclerosis is ambiguous. Whereas endothelial knockout of CXCL12 decreases lesion formation, deletion of its receptor CXCR4 in ECs promotes atherosclerosis (Döring et al. 2017, 2019). These findings suggest that the absence of endothelial CXCL12 expression, which reduces circulating CXCL12 levels, limits lipid deposition in the arterial wall, probably due to its inhibitory effect on cholesterol efflux from macrophages (Gao et al. 2019a). By contrast, local delivery of miR-126-3p in apoptotic vesicles to ECs may support endothelial function by CXCR4-mediated activation of the AKT pathway (Döring et al. 2017). Interestingly, miR-126-3p increases AKT signaling in ECs (Chen et al. 2016b; Fish et al. 2008), reduces endothelial apoptosis, and supports endothelial barrier function (Döring et al. 2017; Cheng et al. 2017a). Several miR-126-3p targets, such as RGS16, phosphatidylinositol 3-kinase regulatory subunit beta, and transforming growth factor-β may play a role in the protection of ECs from apoptosis.

Processing of the precursor miR-126 by Dicer also produces a mature miRNA from its 5p end. Although the miR-126-5p expression level is lower than that of miR-126-3p, it is still one of the most highly expressed miRNAs in ECs. Disturbed laminar flow suppresses miR-126-5p expression in dysadapted ECs and limits, thereby their capacity to compensate additional hyperlipidemia-induced injury by increased proliferation (Schober and Weber 2016). Conversely, higher miR-126-5p levels in ECs exposed to laminar flow increase their proliferative reserve compared with dysadapted ECs (Schober et al. 2014). miR-126-5p generates an endothelial proliferative reserve by suppressing delta like non-canonical notch ligand (DLK) 1, an inhibitor of the Notch1 signaling pathway (Schober et al. 2014). Derepression of DLK1 in dysadapted ECs limits endothelial regeneration in response to hyperlipidemic stress (Fig. 2). Thus, inhibition of miR-126-5p expression in ECs by disturbed flow promotes atherosclerosis (Schober et al. 2014). The inhibition of Notch1 may at least partially mediate the effects of DLK1. Accordingly, disturbed flow reduces endothelial Notch1 activation, and knockout of Notch1 in ECs increases lesion formation (Mack et al. 2017). Moreover, high shear stress reduces endothelial apoptosis by miR-126-5p-mediated inhibition of caspase 3 in the nucleus (Santovito et al. 2020). These results indicate a dual role of miR-126-5p in ECs; in

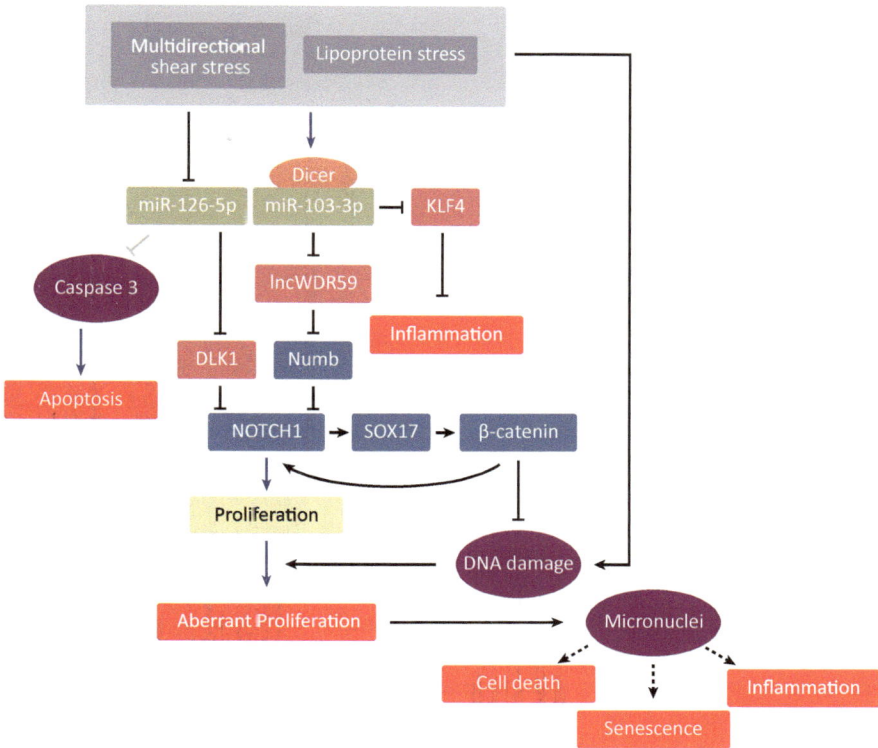

Fig. 2 miRNAs modulate endothelial dysadaptation. The protective miR-126-5p is downregulated in dysadapted ECs, which limits NOTCH1-mediated endothelial regeneration and increases EC apoptosis through a non-canonical mechanism. By contrast, Dicer produces increased levels of miR-103 in dysadapted ECs, which promotes inflammation by targeting KLF4. Moreover, miR-103 inhibits EC proliferation and promotes DNA damage, thus impairing the chronic wound healing response of dysadapted ECs

the cytoplasm, it facilitates Notch1 signaling and thus promotes endothelial regeneration; in the nucleus, it limits apoptosis through a non-canonical mechanism.

2.3 The miR-103–lncWDR59 Axis Limits Endothelial Regeneration and Promotes Aberrant Proliferation

In arteries, endothelial repair by proliferation is a delicate process because blood flow can detach mitotic ECs and increase vascular permeability (Wechezak et al. 1994). Moreover, mitotic cells are incredibly vulnerable to DNA damage because double-strand breaks cannot be repaired and may lead to errors in chromosomal segregation and the formation of micronuclei consisting of chromatin surrounded by its nuclear membrane (Blackford and Stucki 2020). Chromosomes in micronuclei accumulate DNA damage and replicate imperfectly, leading to genomic instability, which can induce growth arrest, senescence, apoptosis, and inflammation (Blackford and Stucki 2020; Zhang et al. 2015; Shah and Bennett 2017). Atherogenic LDL triggers DNA damage in aortic ECs in a LOX-1-dependent manner, probably by increasing mitochondrial ROS production (Wang et al. 2018). Moreover, chronic inflammation may enhance DNA damage due to environmental exposures in tissues that are continuously regenerating (Kiraly et al. 2015). Thus, aberrant proliferation characterized by DNA damage and micronuclei formation may impair chronic regeneration of dysadapted arterial ECs and promote atherosclerosis. Accordingly, high-fat diet (HFD) feeding enhances micronuclei formation and DNA damage in ECs, primarily at predilection sites of atherosclerosis (Natarelli et al. 2018; Thum and Borlak 2008). This finding indicates that disturbed laminar blood flow and oxidized LDL synergistically promote genomic instability (Fig. 1).

In addition to inflammation, Dicer increases DNA damage and micronuclei formation in ECs and inhibits endothelial proliferation at predilection sites of atherosclerosis (Natarelli et al. 2018). These effects are due to the suppression of the lncRNA lncWDR59 by miR-103-3p. lncWDR59 promotes Notch1 activation and endothelial proliferation by competitive binding to the Notch1 inhibitor Numb (Natarelli et al. 2018). Moreover, Notch1 induces SOX17 expression and thus increases β-catenin activity, which inhibits oxLDL-mediated DNA damage and micronuclei formation in ECs. Therefore, the interaction between miR-103-3p and lncWDR59 promotes aberrant EC proliferation by abolishing β-catenin-mediated protection against DNA damage. Accordingly, blocking the targeting of lncWDR59 by miR-103-3p in Apoe$^{-/-}$ mice reduces atherosclerosis and endothelial DNA damage and increases endothelial proliferation (Fig. 2). Notably, a human lncWDR59 homolog with a conserved genomic location exists. In human lesions, ECs express lncWDR59, and its expression level correlates with endothelial proliferation, indicating that the targeting of lncWDR59 by miR-103-3p also plays a role in humans (Natarelli et al. 2018).

3   Non-coding RNAs in Macrophage Function

Macrophages drive the progression of atherosclerosis from a clinically silent condition to advanced lesions with a thrombogenic core. Uncontrolled uptake of modified lipoproteins from the extracellular space by macrophages promotes their transformation into foam cells characterized by the accumulation of cholesterol esters and triglycerides in lipid droplets, similar as in adipocytes. Whereas cholesterol is removed from foam cells by ATP binding cassette subfamily A member (ABCA) 1 and ATP binding cassette subfamily G member (ABCG) 1 transporters, triglycerides and fatty acids can be degraded by foam cells and fuel mitochondrial energy production. However, the ongoing influx of lipoproteins exceeds the capacity of macrophages to store cholesterol intracellularly or transfer it to HDL, which causes cell death and the formation of cholesterol crystals. Accordingly, macrophages death by apoptosis or necroptosis increases during the progression of atherosclerosis (Lin et al. 2013). Besides, the phagocytic removal of dying foam cells is impaired or insufficient in advanced atherosclerosis resulting in the formation of a lipid-rich, necrotic core with cholesterol crystals encapsulated by macrophages.

In contrast to arterial ECs, which have a more stable phenotype, macrophages undergo considerable phenotypic changes during inflammatory activation. Bacterial products such as lipopolysaccharide (LPS) and the T_h1 cell cytokine IFNγ activate the NF-κB and HIF-1α pathway and thus shift mitochondrial function from energy production to the generation of reactive oxygen species (ROS) and reactive nitrogen species (RNS) to combat microbes (Cameron et al. 2019). In turn, energy production is shifted to aerobic glycolysis, which reduces ATP supply. By contrast, stimulation with IL-4 evokes a different response characterized by signal transducer and activator of transcription (STAT) 6 and peroxisome proliferator-activated receptor (PPAR) activation, which reduces nitric oxide (NO) and promotes mitochondrial ATP production by oxidative phosphorylation (OXPHOS) of fatty acids. The latter effect may support phagocytosing macrophages, which need more energy and are challenged by the influx of lipids.

3.1 Regulatory RNAs in Macrophage Energy and Lipid Metabolism

miR-10a-5p, miR-146a-5p, and let-7 family members, and miR-21a-5p are among the most abundant miRNAs in murine macrophages (Canfran-Duque et al. 2017). Dicer knockout reduces the expression of a great majority of miRNAs in macrophages, including miR-21a-5p, miR-342-5p, miR-10a-5p, and miR-503-5p (Wei et al. 2018). In contrast to ECs, knockout of Dicer in macrophages increases the development of atherosclerosis, macrophage apoptosis, and the expression of NOS2 and inflammatory cytokines, such as IL-1β (Wei et al. 2018). Moreover, Dicer knockout impairs OXPHOS in IL-4 stimulated but not in unstimulated or LPS/IFN-γ-stimulated macrophages, suggesting a central role of miRNAs in the energy metabolism of IL-4-stimulated, anti-inflammatory macrophages (Wei et al. 2018). Notably, Dicer also increases oxygen consumption and mitochondrial oxidation in macrophage-derived foam cells, and thus limits the accumulation of lipids probably by the oxidation of fatty acids (Wei et al. 2018). Ligand-dependent corepressor (LCOR) is a crucial target of miRNAs in macrophages and contains numerous highly conserved miRNA-binding sites in its 3′-UTR. LCOR inhibits retinoid X receptor alpha (RXRA), which promotes the expression of OXPHOS-related genes and increases mitochondrial function through interaction with peroxisome proliferator-activated receptor-gamma coactivator (PGC)-1 (Chae et al. 2013). Among the miRNAs predicted to target LCOR, miR-10a-5p most strongly promoted OXPHOS in IL-4-stimulated macrophages and foam cells through targeting LCOR (Wei et al. 2018). Moreover, miR-10a-5p increases OXPHOS also by interacting with another corepressor of nuclear receptors, nuclear receptor corepressor 2 (NCOR2), which inhibits the activity of the PPARα (Wei et al. 2018). Blocking the interaction between miR-10a-5p and LCOR in macrophages by target site-specific antisense oligonucleotides increases atherosclerosis in mice, suggesting

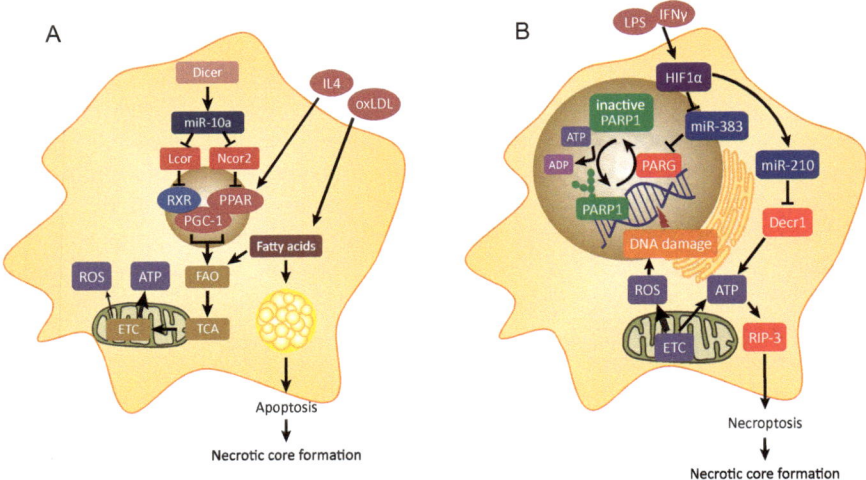

Fig. 3 Effects of miRNAs in macrophages on energy metabolism and cell death. (**a**) In anti-inflammatory macrophages, Dicer promotes mitochondrial energy production by generating miR-10a, which targets the corepressors of nuclear receptors, such as LCOR and NCOR2. miR-10a improves fatty acid oxidation (FAO) and reduces foam cell formation, thus enhancing cell survival. (**b**) In inflammatory macrophages, HIF-1α activation switches the mitochondrial metabolism from ATP to ROS production, thus generating a pseudo-hypoxic state. This effect of HIF-1α is mediated by the suppression of Decr1 by miR-210, which reduces ATP synthesis and necroptotic cell death. Moreover, HIF-1α activation lowers cellular ATP levels by hyper activating PARP-1 due to the derepression of the miR-383 target PARG. ETC, electron transport chain; TCA, tri-carboxyl acid

that miRNA-mediated OXPHOS in macrophages protects from atherosclerosis (Wei et al. 2018). Notably, RXRα agonists upregulate miR-10a-5p in ECs, indicating a positive forward loop in which RXRα increases its activity by miR-10a-5p-meditated suppression of LCOR (Lee et al. 2018). Moreover, treatment of $Apoe^{-/-}$ mice with miR-10a-5p mimics reduces atherosclerosis (Lee et al. 2018). Besides let-7b-5p, but not other members of the let-7 family increases mitochondrial function, indicating that the functional role between the members of a miRNA family can differ despite having the same seed sequence (Fig. 3).

Hypoxia-inducible factor 1α (HIF-1α) is an essential transcription factor in the regulation of mitochondrial energy metabolism in inflammatory macrophages. Stimulation of macrophages with LPS and IFNγ activates HIF-1α, which generates a pseudo-hypoxic state by shutting down OXPHOS and increasing ROS and RNS production. Although this metabolic switch aids to fight off infections, the concomitantly reduced energy supply and enhanced exposure to oxidizing agents can lead to macrophage necroptosis (Pajuelo et al. 2018; He et al. 2011). In atherosclerotic lesions, HIF-1α activation increases receptor-interacting serine/threonine kinase 3 (RIP3)-mediated macrophage necroptosis and necrotic core formation (Lin et al. 2013; Karshovska et al. 2020). This effect is probably mediated by HIF-1α-induced upregulation of miR-210, which lowers ATP levels by suppressing OXPHOS and increasing ROS through targeting 2,4-dienoyl-CoA reductase1 (Decr1) (Karshovska et al. 2020). Decr1 is an essential enzyme in the β-oxidation of unsaturated fatty acids and in the adaptation to metabolic stress during fasting (Miinalainen et al. 2009). Thus, β-oxidation of unsaturated fatty acids may be critical for the survival of energy-depleted inflammatory macrophages by maintaining a basal level of oxidative ATP production. miR-210 is highly abundant in human atherosclerosis, and HIF-1α activation in macrophages increases lesional miR-210 expression in $Apoe^{-/-}$ mice (Karshovska et al. 2020; Raitoharju et al. 2011). However, the functional role of miR-210 in atherosclerosis has not yet been studied.

Similar to LCOR, the 3'-UTR of the ABCA1 transcript contains numerous conserved binding sites for miRNAs, indicating a significant role of miRNAs in foam cell formation, efferocytosis, and inflammatory activation by regulating ABCA1 expression (Zannis et al. 2006; Wei and Schober 2016). In addition to the transcriptional regulation by the nuclear sterol-activated liver-X-receptors (LXRs), post-transcriptional targeting of the ABCA1 transcript by at least 15 miRNAs, such as miR-33-5p, miR-302a-3p, and miR-23a-3p, has been experimentally confirmed (Yang et al. 2018; Rayner et al. 2010; Meiler et al. 2015).

miR-33a-5p (only miR-33-5p in mice) is co-transcribed from an intronic region of the transcription factor sterol regulatory element-binding protein-2, and both synergistically promote cellular cholesterol accumulation in macrophages (Schober and Weber 2016). miR-33-5p is one of the most extensively studied miRNA in atherosclerosis, initially because blocking miR-33-5p raised HDL levels, an effect that is likely due to the targeting of ABCA1 in the liver. The role of miR-33-5p in atherosclerosis has been controversially discussed. Studies in genetically modified mice show conflicting results. In $Apoe^{-/-}$ mice, the whole-body knockout of the $Mir33$ gene reduces atherosclerosis, whereas the absence of miR-33-5p expression in bone marrow cells does not alter lesion formation (Horie et al. 2012). However, in $Ldlr^{-/-}$ mice, only deletion of $Mir33$ in bone marrow cells slightly reduces lesion formation, whereas the whole-body knockout of $Mir33$ surprisingly does not affect atherosclerosis (Price et al. 2017). These results indicate that the expression of miR-33-5p in bone marrow cells promotes atherosclerosis in $Ldlr^{-/-}$ mice, whereas its expression in non-bone-marrow cells is athero-protective. Interestingly, $Ldlr^{-/-}$ mice with bone marrow cells that harbor a mutation of the miR-33-5p binding site in the ABCA1 3'-UTR develop less atherosclerosis, similar to the effect of the $Mir33$ knockout in bone marrow cells (Price et al. 2019). Although this mechanism can explain not all impacts of miR-33-5p, targeting of ABCA1 in macrophages appears to play a crucial role in atherogenesis in $Ldlr^{-/-}$ mice.

miR-34a-5p is highly abundant in atherosclerotic lesions and targets ABCA1 and ABCG1 in macrophages (Xu et al. 2020). Interestingly, the ABCA1 and ABCG1 binding sites of miR-34a-5p are not conserved between human and mouse, and only the site in the human ABCA1 3'-UTR is canonical (Xu et al. 2020). This finding suggests that non-canonical sites are functional and that miRNA sites can have the same effect in mouse and human despite the lack of a conserved binding site. Consistently, the conditional knockout of $Mir34a$ in myeloid cells and the knockout of *Mir34a* in bone marrow cells reduces atherosclerosis in *Apoe*$^{-/-}$ and *Ldlr*$^{-/-}$ mice, respectively (Xu et al. 2020). This effect has been attributed to improved cholesterol efflux from macrophages due to increased expression of ABCA1, ABCG1, and LXRα.

Notably, several ABCA1-targeting miRNAs promote lesion formation in athero-sclerotic mouse models, such as miR-302a-3p (Meiler et al. 2015), miR-23a-5p (Yang et al. 2018), miR-17-5p (Tan et al. 2019), miR-20a/b-5p (Liang et al. 2017), and miR-19b-5p (Lv et al. 2014). However, it is unclear whether the effects of these miRNAs on lesion formation are due to ABCA1 suppression.

LXR activation induces not only ABCA1 expression but also upregulates several lncRNAs, which further increase ABCA1 levels. For example, the primate-specific lncRNA cholesterol homeostasis regulator of miRNA expression (*CHROME*) is upregulated in atherosclerotic lesions and derepresses ABCA1 expression by inactivating several ABCA1-targeting miRNAs, such as miR-27b, miR-33a/b, and miR-128 (Hennessy et al. 2019). Another LXR-induced lncRNA is macrophage-expressed LXR-induced sequence (MeXis), which is transcribed from a gene located near the ABCA1 gene (Sallam et al. 2018). MeXis acts as a nuclear RNA that influences chromatin architecture and facilitates the accessibility of the nuclear receptor coactivator DDX17 at the ABCA1 locus, thus enhancing LXR-mediated ABCA1 expression in response to cholesterol loading in macrophages (Sallam et al. 2018). Knockout of MeXis in bone marrow cells reduces atherosclerosis and increases ABCA1 expression in *Ldlr*$^{-/-}$ mice (Sallam et al. 2018). Notably, a genomic region surrounding the MeXis/ABCA1 locus revealed some degree of conservation between species. In humans, a non-coding RNA transcript in this region was identified as TCONS00016111 with some sequence conservation with MeXis (Sallam et al. 2018). However, its role in lipid metabolism in human lesional macrophages is not fully understood.

3.2   miR-155-5p and miR-146a/b: The LPS Mediators in Atherosclerosis

miR-155-5p is a highly conserved miRNA and predominantly expressed in hematopoietic cells, such as lymphocytes and macrophages. The precursor miR-155 hairpin is encoded in the third exon of a lncRNA called MIR155HG. The expression of MIR155HG is driven by a promoter that is strongly activated by NF-κB (Schober and Weber 2016; Thompson et al. 2013). Thereby, LPS selectively induces miR-155-5p in macrophages together with a small number of other miRNAs, such as miR-147-5p and miR-210-5p (Androulidaki et al. 2009; Nazari-Jahantigh et al. 2012; Dueck et al. 2014), and miR-155-5p mediates many pro-inflammatory effects of LPS by targeting inhibitors of NF-κB signaling, such as suppressor of cytokine signaling 1 and brain and muscle ARNTL-like 1 (Curtis et al. 2015; Wang et al. 2016). Interestingly, low amounts of LPS continuously leak from the intestine to the blood, enhanced by an HFD, where LPS is inactivated by binding to lipoproteins, such as LDL and VLDL. However, chemical modification of LDL leads to reactivation of LPS (Zhu et al. 2017) and upregulation of miR-155-5p in macrophages via toll-like receptor 4 (TLR4) (Du et al. 2014). Accordingly, LPS is detectable in human atherosclerotic lesions, and patients with carotid stenosis have higher blood levels of LPS (Carnevale et al. 2018). Moreover, miR-342-5p, which is abundantly expressed in atherosclerotic lesions, promotes LPS-induced inflammatory macrophage activation by targeting Akt1 and thus upregulates miR-155-5p expression (Wei et al. 2013) (Fig. 4). Blocking miR-342-5p in $Apoe^{-/-}$ mice reduces atherosclerosis and miR-155-5p expression in atherosclerotic vessels (Wei et al.

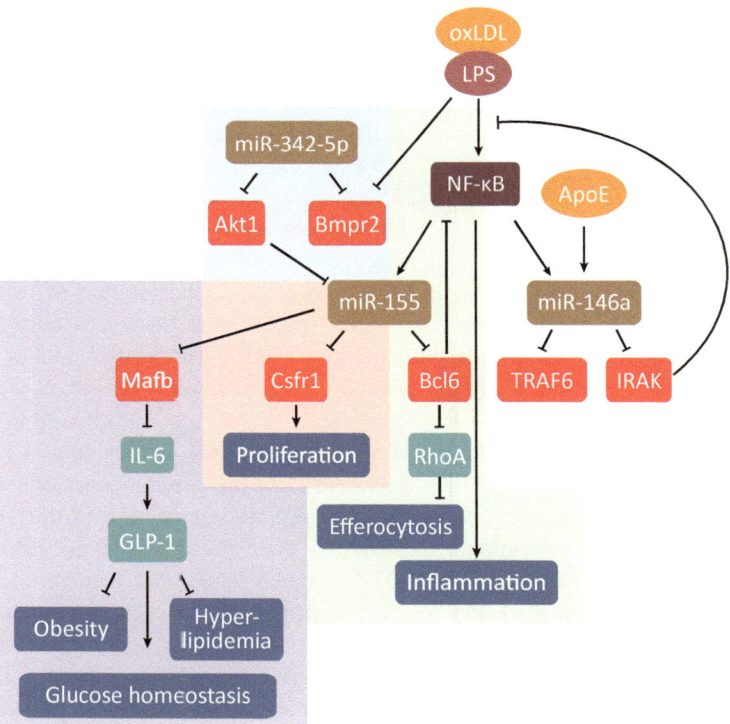

Fig. 4 The complex roles of the LPS mediators miR-155 and miR-146a in atherosclerosis. The stimulation of macrophages with LPS upregulates miR-155 and miR-146a via NF-κB activation. Whereas miR-155 promotes the NF-κB-mediated inflammatory response in macrophages by targeting Bcl6, miR-146a suppresses mediators of LPS signaling and NF-κB activation. MiR-155 increases advanced atherosclerosis by targeting Bcl6, which drives inflammation and inhibits efferocytosis, thus resulting in necrotic core formation in $Apoe^{-/-}$ mice (green). In early atherosclerosis, however, miR-155 decreases lesion growth by blocking macrophage proliferation (pink). Moreover, miR-155 improves glucose homeostasis and reduces atherosclerosis in obese $Ldlr^{-/-}$ mice by targeting Mafb in pancreatic β-cells (violet). The effect of miR-146a in macrophages on atherosclerosis is less clear. Although treatment with miR-146a mimics reduces atherosclerosis and macrophage activation, the anti-inflammatory role of miR-146a in ECs may also protect from lesion formation

2013). The expression level of miR-342-5p and inflammatory cytokines is increased in peripheral leukocytes from patients with coronary artery disease (Ahmadi et al. 2018). However, the effect of miR-155-5p on macrophages during lesion formations differs considerably between early and advanced lesions (Nazari-Jahantigh et al. 2012; Wei et al. 2015). Whereas miR-155-5p expression in early atherosclerosis limits lesion formation by reducing macrophage proliferation, the formation of advanced lesions is promoted by miR-155-5p through inflammation-induced impairment of efferocytosis (Wei et al. 2015). The latter effect is mediated by the targeting of *B cell leukemia/lymphoma 6*(BCL6), a transcriptional repressor of NF-κB-induced genes, which improves efferocytosis through inhibition of *Ras homolog family member A* (RhoA) (Fig. 4) (Wei et al. 2015).

In contrast to its role in *Apoe*$^{-/-}$ mice, miR-155-5p limits advanced atherosclerosis in *Ldlr*$^{-/-}$ mice (Zhu et al. 2017). This effect is due to the upregulation of miR-155-5p in pancreatic β-cells, which promotes insulin secretion by targeting v-maf musculoaponeurotic fibrosarcoma oncogene family, protein B (MafB). The suppression of MafB by miR-155-5p increases IL-6 secretion from β-cells, which stimulates glucagon-like peptide (GLP)-1 expression in α-cells (Fig. 4). In hyperlipidemic *Ldlr*$^{-/-}$ mice, *Mir155* knockout increases obesity, adipose tissue inflammation, blood lipid levels, and blood glucose levels (Zhu et al. 2017). GLP-1 inhibits glucagon production and increases insulin secretion, which may explain how miR-155-5p in β-cells improves the metabolic status of obese and hyperlipidemic mice. Moreover, miR-155-5p expression increases GLP-1 plasma levels, which may limit vascular inflammation and atherosclerosis (Zhu et al. 2017; Rakipovski et al. 2018). Hyperlipidemia stimulates miR-155-5p expression in β-cells probably due to HFD-induced endotoxemia because LPS bound to oxidized LDL is deposited in pancreatic islets and oxidation of LDL reactivates LPS (Zhu et al. 2017). *Apoe*$^{-/-}$ mice are more sensitive to the pro-inflammatory effects of LPS than *Ldlr*$^{-/-}$ mice (Ali et al. 2005). Thus, the pro-atherogenic role of miR-155-5p in macrophages may predominate in *Apoe*$^{-/-}$ mice (Schreyer et al. 2002, 2003), whereas metabolic effects of miR-155-5p related to glucose hemostasis, obesity, and adipose tissue inflammation are more critical for the development of atherosclerosis in *Ldlr*$^{-/-}$ mice. Thus, hyperlipidemia improves glucose metabolism and adipose tissue inflammation by LPS-mediated upregulation of miR-155-5p in β-cells. This mechanism may explain why patients with familial hypercholesterolemia have a reduced risk for type 2 diabetes (Besseling et al. 2015).

Besides, exosomes transfer miR-155-5p from hematopoietic cells, such as dendritic cells and neutrophils, and smooth muscle cells to other cell types like ECs (Gomez et al. 2020; Zheng et al. 2017). The uptake of exosomal miR-155-5p sensitizes the recipient cells to LPS-induced inflammatory activation by suppressing its target genes (Alexander et al. 2015). In neutrophils, HFD increases the packaging of miR-155-5p into microvesicles and stimulates their release into the circulation, where they are preferentially taken up by ECs exposed to disturbed blood flow (Gomez et al. 2020). The uptake of the neutrophil-derived microvesicles by ECs promotes their inflammatory activation by miR-155-5p-mediated suppression of BCL6 and increases atherosclerosis (Gomez et al. 2020). Thus, the exosomal transfer of miR-155-5p from neutrophils is essential for the pro-atherogenic role of this miRNA in ECs (Gomez et al. 2020) because the endogenous level of miR-155-5p in ECs is not high enough to drive lesion formation in $Apoe^{-/-}$ mice (Wei et al. 2015).

In macrophages, NF-κB activation by LPS also induces the expression of miR-146a-5p, which antagonizes the pro-inflammatory effects of miR-155-5p by targeting components of the TLR4 signaling pathway, such as *interleukin 1 receptor-associated kinase* (IRAK) and *TNF receptor-associated factor 6* (TRAF6) (Fig. 4) (Mann et al. 2017; Su et al. 2020). Moreover, constitutive NF-κB activation in *Mir146a* knockout mice drives the development of myeloid malignancies (Zhao et al. 2011). Notably, increased levels of miR-155-5p in macrophages mediate the chronic inflammatory response in $Mir146a^{-/-}$ mice by hyper activating NF-κB (Mann et al. 2017). Treatment of $Ldlr^{-/-}$ mice with miR-146a mimics reduces atherosclerosis and inflammatory macrophage accumulation (Li et al. 2015). Notably, the anti-inflammatory effects of ApoE are partially mediated by the upregulation of miR-146a (Li et al. 2015). However, the atherosclerosis phenotype of HFD-fed $Mir146a^{-/-}/Ldlr^{-/-}$ mice, which develop bone marrow failure and splenomegaly, is unexpected. Although *Mir146a* knockout increases inflammatory cytokine levels in the blood, it decreases lipid levels and the progression of advanced atherosclerosis (Cheng et al. 2017b). This effect was due to the lack of miR-146a expression in bone marrow cells, probably because it leads to bone marrow failure and reduced production of pro-atherogenic hematopoietic cells (Cheng et al. 2017b). By contrast, *Mir146a* knockout in $Ldlr^{-/-}$ mice harboring *Mir146a* wildtype bone marrow cells develop increased atherosclerotic lesions. These mice are also more sensitive to arterial inflammation, which may be due to increased NF-κB activation in ECs (Cheng et al. 2013, 2017b). Although another study using the same mouse model also found lower blood lipid levels, it did not detect an effect of *Mir146a* knockout in bone marrow cells on the development of atherosclerosis (Del Monte et al. 2018).

miR-146b is the second member of the miR-146 seed family and differs from miR-146a in two nucleotides at the 3′ end. Similar to miR-146a, miR-146b inhibits NF-κB activation and the TLR4 pathway (Taganov et al. 2006). $Mir146b^{-/-}$ knockout mice also develop hematologic malignancies and splenomegaly, although less frequently than $Mir146a^{-/-}$ mice (Mitsumura et al. 2018). It remains unclear whether miR-146b expression, which is not affected by *Mir146a* knockout because it is transcribed from a different genomic locus, can compensate for the lack of miR-146a expression. Notably, murine macrophages stimulated with IL-4 release exosomes that contain preferentially miR-146b together with miR-99a and miR-378a (Bouchareychas et al. 2020). The transfer of each of these miRNAs to LPS-stimulated macrophages reduces NF-κB activation. Moreover, treatment with exosomes from IL-4-treated macrophages reduces inflammation in atherosclerotic lesions but not lesion size (Bouchareychas et al. 2020).

3.3 Regulatory RNAs Control Macrophage Death and Efferocytosis in Necrotic Core Formation

Necrotic core formation results from the disbalance between cell death and efferocytosis. As reported in the previous chapter, miR-155-5p establishes an essential link between inflammatory activation and impaired efferocytosis during the progression of atherosclerosis, which promotes the formation of a necrotic core (Wei et al. 2015). Besides miR-155-5p, miR-21a-5p, one of the most abundant miRNAs in atherosclerotic lesions, has been implicated in necrotic core formation. miR-21 is an oncomiR that inhibits apoptosis by targeting, e.g., programmed cell death protein 4 (Krichevsky and Gabriely 2009; Hatley et al. 2010). Accordingly, knockout of *Mir21a* in bone marrow cells promotes lesional apoptosis, necrotic core formation, and atherosclerosis in HFD-fed $Ldlr^{-/-}$ mice, but it reduces lesions in the aortic sinus in $Apoe^{-/-}$ mice fed a regular diet (Canfran-Duque et al. 2017; Chipont et al. 2019). Whole-body *Mir21a* knockout also reduces atherosclerotic lesions, although not in every arterial region studied, in $Apoe^{-/-}$ mice fed an HFD and in aged $Apoe^{-/-}$ mice fed a regular diet (Chipont et al. 2019; Gao et al. 2019b). Chipont et al. reported the conflicting finding that the inhibition of lesion formation by *Mir21a* knockout is associated with increased apoptosis of lesional macrophages and impaired efferocytosis in the peritoneum (Chipont et al. 2019). Another puzzling finding in this regard is that Jin et al. described increased lesion size by *Mir21a* knockout in $Apoe^{-/-}$ mice fed a regular diet (Jin et al. 2018). Unfortunately, the mechanisms of these *Mir21a* effects are incompletely understood.

As discussed in the section "Regulatory RNAs in macrophage energy and lipid metabolism," HIF-1α activation in macrophages drives necrotic core formation in part by inducing miR-210, which inhibits OXPHOS and promotes necroptosis. Besides, HIF-1α activation lowers ATP levels in macrophages by suppressing miR-383-5p expression (Karshovska et al. 2020). miR-383-5p limits ATP consumption by targeting poly(ADP-ribose) glycohydrolase (PARG) (Karshovska et al. 2020), which removes poly(ADP-)ribose polymers from DNA strand breaks and thus antagonizes the ATP-dependent role of poly(ADP-ribose) polymerase (PARP)-1 in response to RNS-induced DNA damage (Ying et al. 2001). The increased activity of PARG following HIF-1α-mediated suppression of miR-383-5p leads to hyperactivation of PARP-1, and thus to ATP depletion and RIP3-mediated necroptosis (Karshovska et al. 2020). Blocking the interaction between miR-383-5p and PARG in mice reversed the protective effect of *Hif1a* knockout in myeloid cells on the lesion and necrotic core formation, demonstrating the critical role of miR-383-5p in HIF-1α-mediated lesional macrophage necroptosis (Karshovska et al. 2020).

A genome-wide screen for SNPs associated with myocardial infarction discovered the lncRNA MIAT. Six SNPs in the MIAT gene are strongly associated with myocardial infarction, indicating that they contribute to the genetic risk of cardiovascular disease (Ishii et al. 2006). MIAT expression is upregulated in atherosclerotic lesions, and adenoviral knockdown of MIAT in $Apoe^{-/-}$ mice reduced advanced atherosclerosis, necrotic core formation, and efferocytosis (Ye et al.

2019). Notably, MIAT impairs the phagocytic activity of macrophages by binding to miR-149-5p in the RISC, thus upregulating the anti-phagocytic receptor CD47, a target of miR-149-5p (Ye et al. 2019; Kojima et al. 2016).

4   MALAT1: The Master miRNA Sponge

The evolutionary conserved lncRNA MALAT1 (Johnsson et al. 2014) is transcribed from a single exon into a 7-kb long RNA molecule, which adopts a complex secondary structure, including a triple helix and a t-RNA-like cloverleaf at the 3′ end (McCown et al. 2019). The triple helix structure is conserved and increases the stability of the poly(A) tail-lacking MALAT1 lncRNA. Cleavage by RNase P releases the cloverleaf structure from the 3′ end, which is called *Malat1-associated small cytoplasmic RNA* (mascRNA). In contrast to the processed MALAT1, which is predominantly retained in the nuclear speckles, mascRNA is transferred into the cytoplasm.

The term "miRNA sponge" fits no other lncRNA better than to MALAT1, which contains an extensively high number of canonical miRNA binding sites (Plotnikova et al. 2019). Several studies have shown that MALAT1 is associated with Ago2 in the RISC, where miRNAs, such as miR-22-3p and miR-155-5p, target MALAT1 (Cao et al. 2016; Tang et al. 2015). Surprisingly, the interaction with MALAT1 also reduces the expression of the targeting miRNA (Tang et al. 2015). The functional interaction with more than 50 miRNAs has been established experimentally in various cell types. In ECs, several MALAT1-binding miRNAs have been described, such as miR-19b-3p, miR-216-5p, miR-181b, and miR-155 (Liu et al. 2020; Wang et al. 2019a; Li et al. 2018).

In macrophages, LPS stimulation increases MALAT1 expression in an NF-κB-dependent manner, whereas IL-4 downregulates MALAT1 (Cui et al. 2019; Zhao et al. 2016). In mice, MALAT1 promotes LPS-induced inflammatory activation of macrophages by upregulating C-type lectin domain family 16, member A, indicating a pro-inflammatory role of MALAT1 (Cui et al. 2019). Moreover, MALAT1 inhibits IL-4-induced anti-inflammatory and pro-fibrotic macrophage polarization by glucose-dependent OXPHOS (Cui et al. 2019). LPS also induces MALAT1 via activating NF-κB in human THP-1 macrophages. However, in contrast to murine macrophages, MALAT1 reduces inflammatory cytokine expression in THP-1 cells by binding NF-κB in the nucleus (Zhao et al. 2016).

In patients with atherosclerosis, MALAT1 expression is reduced in lesions (Cremer et al. 2019; Arslan et al. 2017) and increased in the circulation (Wang et al. 2019a; Zhu et al. 2019). By contrast, lesional *Malat1* expression is upregulated in *Apoe*$^{-/-}$ mice (Li et al. 2019). Treatment with an antagomir against *Malat1* for 4 weeks reduces lesion size by almost 50% in *Apoe*$^{-/-}$ mice fed an HFD for 12 weeks (Zhu et al. 2019). This study indicates that *Malat1* promotes atherosclerosis in mice. However, the effect of *Malat1* knockout on atherosclerosis is quite different. Notably, none of the three existing strains of *Malat1*$^{-/-}$ mice has an obvious phenotype (Eissmann et al. 2012; Nakagawa et al. 2012; Zhang et al.

2012). Unexpectedly, crossing *Malat1(LacZ)*$^{-/-}$ mice, generated by insertion of the LacZ gene into the promoter region of *Malat1*, with *Apoe*$^{-/-}$ mice resulted in intrauterine death, whereas *Apoe*$^{-/-}$ mice heterozygous for *Malat1(LacZ)* develop normally (Gast et al. 2019). Interestingly, severe atherosclerosis develops in 8-week-old *Malat1(LacZ)*$^{+/-}$/*Apoe*$^{-/-}$ mice even without feeding them an HFD (Gast et al. 2019), which is probably related to the hyperinflammatory state of these mice (Gast et al. 2019). Whether this effect is due to lower mascRNA levels, which promotes inflammatory cytokine expression in THP-1 cells (Gast et al. 2019), remains unclear. By contrast, *Malat1*$^{-/-}$ mice produced by Cre-mediated excision of the whole *Malat1* gene could be crossed with *Apoe*$^{-/-}$ mice without having a spontaneous phenotype (Cremer et al. 2019). Moreover, feeding these mice an HFD with only a comparably small amount of cholesterol for 12 weeks did not change lesion size, but slightly increased lesional leukocyte accumulation (Cremer et al. 2019). Besides, *Malat1* knockout in bone marrow cells slightly increased lesion size, and the production of inflammatory leukocytes in *Apoe*$^{-/-}$ after 16 weeks of HFD feeding, probably due to the loss of miR-503-5p sponging by *Malat1* in macrophages (Cremer et al. 2019; Yan et al. 2017). Unfortunately, it is not clear whether also non-irradiated *Malat1*$^{-/-}$/*Apoe*$^{-/-}$ mice show the same changes in the production of inflammatory leukocytes as irradiated mice. The expression of numerous miRNAs is increased in *Malat1(LacZ)*$^{+/-}$/*Apoe*$^{-/-}$ mice; however, not that of miR-503-5p (Gast et al. 2019). Taken together, studies in mice with a deletion of the *Malat1* gene indicate a protective role of *Malat1* in macrophages, although the extent of its effect differs considerably between the models. A significant difference between the two *Malat1*$^{-/-}$ mouse strains consists in the regulation of NEAT1, a lncRNA transcribed from a neighboring gene of MALAT1. In *Malat1*$^{-/-}$/*Apoe*$^{-/-}$ mice, NEAT1 is upregulated in lung tissue (Cremer et al. 2019), whereas *Malat1(LacZ)*$^{+/-}$/*Apoe*$^{-/-}$ mice express lower levels of NEAT1 in splenocytes than *Malat1* wildtype mice (Gast et al. 2019). NEAT1 enhances oxidized LDL-induced inflammatory activation and foam cell formation in human and mouse macrophage cell lines by the sponging of miRNAs, such as miR-342-3p and miR-128, and by the formation of paraspeckles (Chen et al. 2018; Huang-Fu et al. 2018; Wang et al. 2019b).

5   The Simian lncRNA ANRIL and the Risk Locus for Atherosclerosis

The chromosome 9p21.3 in humans represents a risk locus for many different diseases, including atherosclerosis and coronary artery disease (CAD) (Chen et al. 2014). The 58 kb-long CAD risk region includes 59 single nucleotide polymorphisms and is devoid of protein-coding genes, but encodes the 3′ end of the lncRNA ANRIL. Therefore, changes in one of the various ANRIL transcripts by the risk haplotype have been linked to atherosclerosis (Lo Sardo et al. 2018). During rodent evolution, ANRIL was gradually lost and is absent in mouse and rat (He et al. 2013). However, mice have a syntenic region on chromosome 4 ortholog to the 9p21.3 locus, which encodes a lncRNA that is different from ANRIL (Visel et al.

2010). Knockout of the murine 9p21.3 ortholog in $Apoe^{-/-}$ mice increases atherosclerosis and lesion calcification but not lesion vulnerability (Kojima et al. 2020). Remarkably, the histological changes in mice were matched with those determined in human lesions from patients carrying the 9p21 risk allele, indicating that it promotes atherosclerosis by lesion calcification independent of ANRIL (Kojima et al. 2020).

6 Conclusions and Therapeutic Perspectives

The world of regulatory RNAs in atherosclerosis has expanded considerably by the combined effects of miRNAs and lncRNAs. Especially the small number of conserved lncRNAs plays an essential role in regulating miRNA activities in atherosclerosis. However, more details about the mechanisms of miRNA sponging and the mutual regulation of miRNAs and lncRNAs are needed. Besides, the fact that the great majority of lncRNAs is species-specific raises the possibility that the often-claimed lack of transferability of mouse data into humans is, at least partly, related to lncRNAs. Whether the conservation of lncRNAs goes beyond pure sequence similarities and could be related to structural conservation or conservation of the genomic locus is unclear. Besides, we think it is also essential to reconsider the conservation of miRNA functions against this background because it might not always be possible to predict that a miRNA in mice and humans only from the sequence conservation of its binding site.

Beyond the species-specific differences of regulatory RNA functions, the chronic course of atherosclerosis passing through various, considerably different stages, which may all be present in one patient simultaneously, is a significant obstacle for any kind of drug therapy of this disease. Therefore, it is essential to identify the stage(s) of atherosclerosis that is/are most suitable for therapeutic interventions and ideally develop a transient treatment with long-term beneficial effects avoiding continuous drug application. According to the regulatory RNA functions described in this article, miRNAs tightly control two critical processes in the pathogenesis of atherosclerosis, which can be targeted by miRNA-based therapies: endothelial dysadaptation and necrotic core formation. In a preventive approach, miRNA-based drugs could reprogram dysadapted ECs to develop an arterial endothelial phenotype without the correct hemodynamic stimulus. By contrast, limiting necrotic core formation and plaque rupture by miRNA-based drugs would make it necessary to define and identify lesions where cell apoptosis begins to exceed the lesional efferocytosis capacity. Although different strategies of miRNA-based therapies are currently tested (Roberts et al. 2020; Herrera et al. 2018), it remains unclear how promising the application of drugs comprising miRNA duplexes and oligonucleotide-based competitive miRNA inhibitors is. One miRNA, such as miR-155, may have opposing effects in different atherosclerosis stages through distinct targets. Thus, tailored miRNA inhibitors, such as target site blockers, which specifically block the interaction of a miRNA with only one of its targets, maybe an alternative approach to reduce unwanted effects. Moreover, more specific targeting of individual miRNA interactions may enhance efficacy and require lower doses of therapeutic oligonucleotides, thus improving safety.

References

Ahmadi R, Heidarian E, Fadaei R, Moradi N, Malek M, Fallah S (2018) miR-342-5p expression levels in coronary artery disease patients and its association with inflammatory cytokines. Clin Lab 64(4):603–609

Akhtar S, Hartmann P, Karshovska E, Rinderknecht FA, Subramanian P, Gremse F et al (2015) Endothelial hypoxia-inducible factor-1α promotes atherosclerosis and monocyte recruitment by upregulating microRNA-19a. Hypertension 66(6):1220–1226

Alexander M, Hu R, Runtsch MC, Kagele DA, Mosbruger TL, Tolmachova T et al (2015) Exosome-delivered microRNAs modulate the inflammatory response to endotoxin. Nat Commun 6:7321

Ali K, Middleton M, Pure E, Rader DJ (2005) Apolipoprotein E suppresses the type I inflammatory response in vivo. Circ Res 97(9):922–927

Androulidaki A, Iliopoulos D, Arranz A, Doxaki C, Schworer S, Zacharioudaki V et al (2009) The kinase Akt1 controls macrophage response to lipopolysaccharide by regulating microRNAs. Immunity 31(2):220–231

Arslan S, Berkan O, Lalem T, Ozbilum N, Goksel S, Korkmaz O et al (2017) Long non-coding RNAs in the atherosclerotic plaque. Atherosclerosis 266:176–181

Bartel DP (2018) Metazoan microRNAs. Cell 173(1):20–51

Besseling J, Kastelein JJ, Defesche JC, Hutten BA, Hovingh GK (2015) Association between familial hypercholesterolemia and prevalence of type 2 diabetes mellitus. JAMA 313 (10):1029–1036

Bjorkerud S, Bondjers G (1972) Endothelial integrity and viability in the aorta of the normal rabbit and rat as evaluated with dye exclusion tests and interference contrast microscopy. Atherosclerosis 15(3):285–300

Blackford AN, Stucki M (2020) How cells respond to DNA breaks in mitosis. Trends Biochem Sci 45(4):321–331

Bouchareychas L, Duong P, Covarrubias S, Alsop E, Phu TA, Chung A et al (2020) Macrophage exosomes resolve atherosclerosis by regulating hematopoiesis and inflammation via microRNA cargo. Cell Rep 32(2):107881

Cameron AM, Castoldi A, Sanin DE, Flachsmann LJ, Field CS, Puleston DJ et al (2019) Inflammatory macrophage dependence on NAD(+) salvage is a consequence of reactive oxygen species-mediated DNA damage. Nat Immunol 20(4):420–432

Canfran-Duque A, Rotllan N, Zhang X, Fernandez-Fuertes M, Ramirez-Hidalgo C, Araldi E et al (2017) Macrophage deficiency of miR-21 promotes apoptosis, plaque necrosis, and vascular inflammation during atherogenesis. EMBO Mol Med 9(9):1244–1262

Cao S, Wang Y, Li J, Lv M, Niu H, Tian Y (2016) Tumor-suppressive function of long noncoding RNA MALAT1 in glioma cells by suppressing miR-155 expression and activating FBXW7 function. Am J Cancer Res 6(11):2561–2574

Carnevale R, Nocella C, Petrozza V, Cammisotto V, Pacini L, Sorrentino V et al (2018) Localization of lipopolysaccharide from *Escherichia Coli* into human atherosclerotic plaque. Sci Rep 8 (1):3598

Chae S, Ahn BY, Byun K, Cho YM, Yu MH, Lee B et al (2013) A systems approach for decoding mitochondrial retrograde signaling pathways. Sci Signal 6(264):rs4

Chen YL, Jan KM, Lin HS, Chien S (1997) Relationship between endothelial cell turnover and permeability to horseradish peroxidase. Atherosclerosis 133(1):7–14

Chen HH, Almontashiri NA, Antoine D, Stewart AF (2014) Functional genomics of the 9p21.3 locus for atherosclerosis: clarity or confusion? Curr Cardiol Rep 16(7):502

Chen Z, Wen L, Martin M, Hsu CY, Fang L, Lin FM et al (2015) Oxidative stress activates endothelial innate immunity via sterol regulatory element binding protein 2 (SREBP2) transactivation of microRNA-92a. Circulation 131(9):805–814

Chen J, Shishkin AA, Zhu X, Kadri S, Maza I, Guttman M et al (2016a) Evolutionary analysis across mammals reveals distinct classes of long non-coding RNAs. Genome Biol 17:19

Chen L, Wang J, Wang B, Yang J, Gong Z, Zhao X et al (2016b) MiR-126 inhibits vascular endothelial cell apoptosis through targeting PI3K/Akt signaling. Ann Hematol 95(3):365–374

Chen H, Li X, Liu S, Gu L, Zhou X (2017) MircroRNA-19a promotes vascular inflammation and foam cell formation by targeting HBP-1 in atherogenesis. Sci Rep 7(1):12089

Chen DD, Hui LL, Zhang XC, Chang Q (2018) NEAT1 contributes to ox-LDL-induced inflammation and oxidative stress in macrophages through inhibiting miR-128. J Cell Biochem 120 (2):2493–2501

Cheng HS, Sivachandran N, Lau A, Boudreau E, Zhao JL, Baltimore D et al (2013) MicroRNA-146 represses endothelial activation by inhibiting pro-inflammatory pathways. EMBO Mol Med 5 (7):949–966

Cheng XW, Wan YF, Zhou Q, Wang Y, Zhu HQ (2017a) MicroRNA126 inhibits endothelial permeability and apoptosis in apolipoprotein E-knockout mice fed a high-fat diet. Mol Med Rep 16(3):3061–3068

Cheng HS, Besla R, Li A, Chen Z, Shikatani EA, Nazari-Jahantigh M et al (2017b) Paradoxical suppression of therosclerosis in the absence of microRNA-146a. Circ Res 121(4):354–367

Chipman LB, Pasquinelli AE (2019) miRNA targeting: growing beyond the seed. Trends Genet 35 (3):215–222

Chipont A, Esposito B, Challier I, Montabord M, Tedgui A, Mallat Z et al (2019) MicroRNA-21 deficiency alters the survival of Ly-6C(lo) monocytes in ApoE(−/−) mice and reduces early-stage atherosclerosis-brief report. Arterioscler Thromb Vasc Biol 39(2):170–177

Cremer S, Michalik KM, Fischer A, Pfisterer L, Jae N, Winter C et al (2019) Hematopoietic deficiency of the long noncoding RNA MALAT1 promotes atherosclerosis and plaque inflammation. Circulation 139(10):1320–1334

Cui H, Banerjee S, Guo S, Xie N, Ge J, Jiang D et al (2019) Long noncoding RNA Malat1 regulates differential activation of macrophages and response to lung injury. JCI Insight 4(4):e124522

Curtis AM, Fagundes CT, Yang G, Palsson-McDermott EM, Wochal P, McGettrick AF et al (2015) Circadian control of innate immunity in macrophages by miR-155 targeting Bmal1. Proc Natl Acad Sci U S A 112(23):7231–7236

Del Monte A, Arroyo AB, Andres-Manzano MJ, Garcia-Barbera N, Caleprico MS, Vicente V et al (2018) miR-146a deficiency in hematopoietic cells is not involved in the development of atherosclerosis. PLoS One 13(6):e0198932

Döring Y, Noels H, van der Vorst EPC, Neideck C, Egea V, Drechsler M et al (2017) Vascular CXCR4 limits atherosclerosis by maintaining arterial integrity: evidence from mouse and human studies. Circulation 136(4):388–403

Doring Y, van der Vorst EPC, Duchene J, Jansen Y, Gencer S, Bidzhekov K et al (2019) CXCL12 derived from endothelial cells promotes atherosclerosis to drive coronary artery disease. Circulation 139(10):1338–1340

Du F, Yu F, Wang Y, Hui Y, Carnevale K, Fu M et al (2014) MicroRNA-155 deficiency results in decreased macrophage inflammation and attenuated atherogenesis in apolipoprotein E-deficient mice. Arterioscler Thromb Vasc Biol 34(4):759–767

Dueck A, Eichner A, Sixt M, Meister G (2014) A miR-155-dependent microRNA hierarchy in dendritic cell maturation and macrophage activation. FEBS Lett 588(4):632–640

Ebert MS, Sharp PA (2012) Roles for MicroRNAs in conferring robustness to biological processes. Cell 149(3):515–524

Eissmann M, Gutschner T, Hammerle M, Gunther S, Caudron-Herger M, Gross M et al (2012) Loss of the abundant nuclear non-coding RNA MALAT1 is compatible with life and development. RNA Biol 9(8):1076–1087

Fang Y, Davies PF (2012) Site-specific microRNA-92a regulation of Kruppel-like factors 4 and 2 in atherosusceptible endothelium. Arterioscler Thromb Vasc Biol 32(4):979–987

Finnerty JR, Wang WX, Hebert SS, Wilfred BR, Mao G, Nelson PT (2010) The miR-15/107 group of microRNA genes: evolutionary biology, cellular functions, and roles in human diseases. J Mol Biol 402(3):491–509

Fish JE, Santoro MM, Morton SU, Yu S, Yeh RF, Wythe JD et al (2008) miR-126 regulates angiogenic signaling and vascular integrity. Dev Cell 15(2):272–284

Fromm B, Billipp T, Peck LE, Johansen M, Tarver JE, King BL et al (2015) A uniform system for the annotation of vertebrate microRNA genes and the evolution of the human microRNAome. Annu Rev Genet 49:213–242

Gantier MP, McCoy CE, Rusinova I, Saulep D, Wang D, Xu D et al (2011) Analysis of microRNA turnover in mammalian cells following Dicer1 ablation. Nucleic Acids Res 39(13):5692–5703

Gao JH, He LH, Yu XH, Zhao ZW, Wang G, Zou J et al (2019a) CXCL12 promotes atherosclerosis by downregulating ABCA1 expression via the CXCR4/GSK3beta/beta-catenin(T120)/TCF21 pathway. J Lipid Res 60(12):2020–2033

Gao L, Zeng H, Zhang T, Mao C, Wang Y, Han Z et al (2019b) MicroRNA-21 deficiency attenuated atherogenesis and decreased macrophage infiltration by targeting Dusp-8. Atherosclerosis 291:78–86

Gast M, Rauch BH, Nakagawa S, Haghikia A, Jasina A, Haas J et al (2019) Immune system-mediated atherosclerosis caused by deficiency of long non-coding RNA MALAT1 in ApoE−/− mice. Cardiovasc Res 115(2):302–314

Gau GS, Ryder TA, Mackenzie ML (1980) The effect of blood flow on the surface morphology of the human endothelium. J Pathol 131(1):55–64

Gerrity RG, Richardson M, Somer JB, Bell FP, Schwartz CJ (1977) Endothelial cell morphology in areas of in vivo Evans blue uptake in the aorta of young pigs. II. Ultrastructure of the intima in areas of differing permeability to proteins. Am J Pathol 89(2):313–334

Gomez I, Ward B, Souilhol C, Recarti C, Ariaans M, Johnston J et al (2020) Neutrophil microvesicles drive atherosclerosis by delivering miR-155 to atheroprone endothelium. Nat Commun 11(1):214

Hansson GK, Chao S, Schwartz SM, Reidy MA (1985) Aortic endothelial cell death and replication in normal and lipopolysaccharide-treated rats. Am J Pathol 121(1):123–127

Hartmann P, Zhou Z, Natarelli L, Wei Y, Nazari-Jahantigh M, Zhu M et al (2016) Endothelial dicer promotes atherosclerosis and vascular inflammation by miRNA-103-mediated suppression of KLF4. Nat Commun 7:10521

Hatley ME, Patrick DM, Garcia MR, Richardson JA, Bassel-Duby R, van Rooij E et al (2010) Modulation of K-Ras-dependent lung tumorigenesis by MicroRNA-21. Cancer Cell 18 (3):282–293

He S, Liang Y, Shao F, Wang X (2011) Toll-like receptors activate programmed necrosis in macrophages through a receptor-interacting kinase-3-mediated pathway. Proc Natl Acad Sci U S A 108(50):20054–20059

He S, Gu W, Li Y, Zhu H (2013) ANRIL/CDKN2B-AS shows two-stage clade-specific evolution and becomes conserved after transposon insertions in simians. BMC Evol Biol 13(1):247

Hennessy EJ, van Solingen C, Scacalossi KR, Ouimet M, Afonso MS, Prins J et al (2019) The long noncoding RNA CHROME regulates cholesterol homeostasis in primate. Nat Metab 1 (1):98–110

Heo KS, Lee H, Nigro P, Thomas T, Le NT, Chang E et al (2011) PKCzeta mediates disturbed flow-induced endothelial apoptosis via p53 SUMOylation. J Cell Biol 193(5):867–884

Heo KS, Chang E, Le NT, Cushman H, Yeh ET, Fujiwara K et al (2013) De-SUMOylation enzyme of sentrin/SUMO-specific protease 2 regulates disturbed flow-induced SUMOylation of ERK5 and p53 that leads to endothelial dysfunction and atherosclerosis. Circ Res 112(6):911–923

Herrera VL, Colby AH, Ruiz-Opazo N, Coleman DG, Grinstaff MW (2018) Nucleic acid nanomedicines in phase II/III clinical trials: translation of nucleic acid therapies for reprogramming cells. Nanomedicine (Lond) 13(16):2083–2098

Horie T, Baba O, Kuwabara Y, Chujo Y, Watanabe S, Kinoshita M et al (2012) MicroRNA-33 deficiency reduces the progression of atherosclerotic plaque in ApoE−/− mice. J Am Heart Assoc 1(6):e003376

Huang R, Hu Z, Cao Y, Li H, Zhang H, Su W et al (2019) MiR-652-3p inhibition enhances endothelial repair and reduces atherosclerosis by promoting cyclin D2 expression. EBioMedicine 40:685–694

Huang-Fu N, Cheng JS, Wang Y, Li ZW, Wang SH (2018) Neat1 regulates oxidized low-density lipoprotein-induced inflammation and lipid uptake in macrophages via paraspeckle formation. Mol Med Rep 17(2):3092–3098

Ishii N, Ozaki K, Sato H, Mizuno H, Saito S, Takahashi A et al (2006) Identification of a novel non-coding RNA, MIAT, that confers risk of myocardial infarction. J Hum Genet 51 (12):1087–1099

Jiang L, Qiao Y, Wang Z, Ma X, Wang H, Li J (2020) Inhibition of microRNA-103 attenuates inflammation and endoplasmic reticulum stress in atherosclerosis through disrupting the PTEN-mediated MAPK signaling. J Cell Physiol 235(1):380–393

Jin H, Li DY, Chernogubova E, Sun C, Busch A, Eken SM et al (2018) Local delivery of miR-21 stabilizes fibrous caps in vulnerable atherosclerotic lesions. Mol Ther 26(4):1040–1055

Johnsson P, Lipovich L, Grander D, Morris KV (2014) Evolutionary conservation of long non-coding RNAs; sequence, structure, function. Biochim Biophys Acta 1840(3):1063–1071

Karshovska E, Wei Y, Subramanian P, Mohibullah R, Geissler C, Baatsch I et al (2020) HIF-1alpha (Hypoxia-inducible factor-1alpha) promotes macrophage necroptosis by regulating miR-210 and miR-383. Arterioscler Thromb Vasc Biol 40(3):583–596

Kim S, Woo CH (2018) Laminar flow inhibits ER stress-induced endothelial apoptosis through PI3K/Akt-dependent signaling pathway. Mol Cells 41(11):964–970

Kiraly O, Gong G, Olipitz W, Muthupalani S, Engelward BP (2015) Inflammation-induced cell proliferation potentiates DNA damage-induced mutations in vivo. PLoS Genet 11(2):e1004901

Kojima Y, Volkmer JP, McKenna K, Civelek M, Lusis AJ, Miller CL et al (2016) CD47-blocking antibodies restore phagocytosis and prevent atherosclerosis. Nature 536(7614):86–90

Kojima Y, Ye J, Nanda V, Wang Y, Flores AM, Jarr KU et al (2020) Knockout of the murine ortholog to the human 9p21 coronary artery disease locus leads to smooth muscle cell proliferation, vascular calcification, and advanced atherosclerosis. Circulation 141(15):1274–1276

Kopp F, Mendell JT (2018) Functional classification and experimental dissection of long noncoding RNAs. Cell 172(3):393–407

Kosik KS (2010) MicroRNAs and cellular phenotypy. Cell 143(1):21–26

Krichevsky AM, Gabriely G (2009) miR-21: a small multi-faceted RNA. J Cell Mol Med 13 (1):39–53

Kuhnert F, Mancuso MR, Hampton J, Stankunas K, Asano T, Chen CZ et al (2008) Attribution of vascular phenotypes of the murine Egfl7 locus to the microRNA miR-126. Development 135 (24):3989–3993

Lee H, Han S, Kwon CS, Lee D (2015) Biogenesis and regulation of the let-7 miRNAs and their functional implications. Protein Cell 7(2):100–113

Lee DY, Yang TL, Huang YF, Lee CI, Chen LJ, Shih YT et al (2018) Induction of microRNA-10a using retinoic acid receptor-alpha and retinoid x receptor-alpha agonists inhibits atherosclerotic lesion formation. Atherosclerosis 271:36–44

Li K, Ching D, Luk FS, Raffai RL (2015) Apolipoprotein E enhances microRNA-146a in monocytes and macrophages to suppress nuclear factor-kappaB-driven inflammation and atherosclerosis. Circ Res 117(1):e1–e11

Li XX, Liu YM, Li YJ, Xie N, Yan YF, Chi YL et al (2016) High glucose concentration induces endothelial cell proliferation by regulating cyclin-D2-related miR-98. J Cell Mol Med 20 (6):1159–1169

Li S, Sun Y, Zhong L, Xiao Z, Yang M, Chen M et al (2018) The suppression of ox-LDL-induced inflammatory cytokine release and apoptosis of HCAECs by long non-coding RNA-MALAT1 via regulating microRNA-155/SOCS1 pathway. Nutr Metab Cardiovasc Dis 28(11):1175–1187

Li H, Zhao Q, Chang L, Wei C, Bei H, Yin Y et al (2019) LncRNA MALAT1 modulates ox-LDL induced EndMT through the Wnt/beta-catenin signaling pathway. Lipids Health Dis 18(1):62

Liang B, Wang X, Song X, Bai R, Yang H, Yang Z et al (2017) MicroRNA-20a/b regulates cholesterol efflux through post-transcriptional repression of ATP-binding cassette transporter A1. Biochim Biophys Acta Mol Cell Biol Lipids 1862(9):929–938

Lin J, Li H, Yang M, Ren J, Huang Z, Han F et al (2013) A role of RIP3-mediated macrophage necrosis in atherosclerosis development. Cell Rep 3(1):200–210

Liu Y, Li Q, Hosen MR, Zietzer A, Flender A, Levermann P et al (2019) Atherosclerotic conditions promote the packaging of functional microRNA-92a-3p into endothelial microvesicles. Circ Res 124(4):575–587

Liu H, Shi C, Deng Y (2020) MALAT1 affects hypoxia-induced vascular endothelial cell injury and autophagy by regulating miR-19b-3p/HIF-1alpha axis. Mol Cell Biochem 466(1–2):25–34

Lo Sardo V, Chubukov P, Ferguson W, Kumar A, Teng EL, Duran M et al (2018) Unveiling the role of the most impactful cardiovascular risk locus through haplotype editing. Cell 175 (7):1796–810.e20

Loyer X, Potteaux S, Vion AC, Guerin CL, Boulkroun S, Rautou PE et al (2014) Inhibition of microRNA-92a prevents endothelial dysfunction and atherosclerosis in mice. Circ Res 114 (3):434–443

Lv YC, Tang YY, Peng J, Zhao GJ, Yang J, Yao F et al (2014) MicroRNA-19b promotes macrophage cholesterol accumulation and aortic atherosclerosis by targeting ATP-binding cassette transporter A1. Atherosclerosis 236(1):215–226

Mack JJ, Mosqueiro TS, Archer BJ, Jones WM, Sunshine H, Faas GC et al (2017) NOTCH1 is a mechanosensor in adult arteries. Nat Commun 8(1):1620

Mann M, Mehta A, Zhao JL, Lee K, Marinov GK, Garcia-Flores Y et al (2017) An NF-kappaB-microRNA regulatory network tunes macrophage inflammatory responses. Nat Commun 8 (1):851

McCall MN, Kent OA, Yu J, Fox-Talbot K, Zaiman AL, Halushka MK (2011) MicroRNA profiling of diverse endothelial cell types. BMC Med Genet 4:78

McCown PJ, Wang MC, Jaeger L, Brown JA (2019) Secondary structural model of human MALAT1 reveals multiple structure-function relationships. Int J Mol Sci 20(22):5610

Meiler S, Baumer Y, Toulmin E, Seng K, Boisvert WA (2015) MicroRNA 302a is a novel modulator of cholesterol homeostasis and atherosclerosis. Arterioscler Thromb Vasc Biol 35 (2):323–331

Miinalainen IJ, Schmitz W, Huotari A, Autio KJ, Soininen R, Ver Loren van Themaat E et al (2009) Mitochondrial 2,4-dienoyl-CoA reductase deficiency in mice results in severe hypoglycemia with stress intolerance and unimpaired ketogenesis. PLoS Genet 5(7):e1000543

Mitsumura T, Ito Y, Chiba T, Matsushima T, Kurimoto R, Tanaka Y et al (2018) Ablation of miR-146b in mice causes hematopoietic malignancy. Blood Adv 2(23):3483–3491

Mogilyansky E, Rigoutsos I (2013) The miR-17/92 cluster: a comprehensive update on its genomics, genetics, functions and increasingly important and numerous roles in health and disease. Cell Death Differ 20(12):1603–1614

Mohamied Y, Rowland EM, Bailey EL, Sherwin SJ, Schwartz MA, Weinberg PD (2015) Change of direction in the biomechanics of atherosclerosis. Ann Biomed Eng 43(1):16–25

Mohamied Y, Sherwin SJ, Weinberg PD (2017) Understanding the fluid mechanics behind transverse wall shear stress. J Biomech 50:102–109

Mundi S, Massaro M, Scoditti E, Carluccio MA, van Hinsbergh VWM, Iruela-Arispe ML et al (2018) Endothelial permeability, LDL deposition, and cardiovascular risk factors-a review. Cardiovasc Res 114(1):35–52

Nakagawa S, Ip JY, Shioi G, Tripathi V, Zong X, Hirose T et al (2012) Malat1 is not an essential component of nuclear speckles in mice. RNA 18(8):1487–1499

Natarelli L, Geissler C, Csaba G, Wei Y, Zhu M, di Francesco A et al (2018) miR-103 promotes endothelial maladaptation by targeting lncWDR59. Nat Commun 9(1):2645

Nazari-Jahantigh M, Wei Y, Noels H, Akhtar S, Zhou Z, Koenen RR et al (2012) MicroRNA-155 promotes atherosclerosis by repressing Bcl6 in macrophages. J Clin Investig 122 (11):4190–4202

Pajuelo D, Gonzalez-Juarbe N, Tak U, Sun J, Orihuela CJ, Niederweis M (2018) NAD(+) depletion triggers macrophage necroptosis, a cell death pathway exploited by *Mycobacterium tuberculosis*. Cell Rep 24(2):429–440

Pan L, Hong Z, Yu L, Gao Y, Zhang R, Feng H et al (2017) Shear stress induces human aortic endothelial cell apoptosis via interleukin-1 receptor-associated kinase 2-induced endoplasmic reticulum stress. Mol Med Rep 16(5):7205–7212

Patrick DM, Montgomery RL, Qi X, Obad S, Kauppinen S, Hill JA et al (2010) Stress-dependent cardiac remodeling occurs in the absence of microRNA-21 in mice. J Clin Investig 120 (11):3912–3916

Peiffer V, Sherwin SJ, Weinberg PD (2013) Computation in the rabbit aorta of a new metric - the transverse wall shear stress - to quantify the multidirectional character of disturbed blood flow. J Biomech 46(15):2651–2658

Plotnikova O, Baranova A, Skoblov M (2019) Comprehensive analysis of human microRNA-mRNA interactome. Front Genet 10:933

Price NL, Rotllan N, Canfran-Duque A, Zhang X, Pati P, Arias N et al (2017) Genetic dissection of the impact of miR-33a and miR-33b during the progression of atherosclerosis. Cell Rep 21 (5):1317–1330

Price NL, Rotllan N, Zhang X, Canfran-Duque A, Nottoli T, Suarez Y et al (2019) Specific disruption of Abca1 targeting largely mimics the effects of miR-33 knockout on macrophage cholesterol efflux and atherosclerotic plaque development. Circ Res 124(6):874–880

Raitoharju E, Lyytikainen LP, Levula M, Oksala N, Mennander A, Tarkka M et al (2011) miR-21, miR-210, miR-34a, and miR-146a/b are up-regulated in human atherosclerotic plaques in the Tampere vascular study. Atherosclerosis 219(1):211–217

Rakipovski G, Rolin B, Nøhr J, Klewe I, Frederiksen KS, Augustin R et al (2018) The GLP-1 analogs liraglutide and semaglutide reduce atherosclerosis in ApoE(−/−) and LDLr(−/−) mice by a mechanism that includes inflammatory pathways. JACC Basic Transl Sci 3(6):844–857

Rayner KJ, Suarez Y, Davalos A, Parathath S, Fitzgerald ML, Tamehiro N et al (2010) MiR-33 contributes to the regulation of cholesterol homeostasis. Science 328(5985):1570–1573

Roberts TC, Langer R, Wood MJA (2020) Advances in oligonucleotide drug delivery. Nat Rev Drug Discov 19(10):673–694

Roush S, Slack FJ (2008) The let-7 family of microRNAs. Trends Cell Biol 18(10):505–516

Sallam T, Jones M, Thomas BJ, Wu X, Gilliland T, Qian K et al (2018) Transcriptional regulation of macrophage cholesterol efflux and atherogenesis by a long noncoding RNA. Nat Med 24 (3):304–312

Salvayre R, Auge N, Benoist H, Negre-Salvayre A (2002) Oxidized low-density lipoprotein-induced apoptosis. Biochim Biophys Acta 1585(2–3):213–221

Santovito D, Egea V, Bidzhekov K, Natarelli L, Mourão A, Blanchet X et al (2020) Noncanonical inhibition of caspase-3 by a nuclear microRNA confers endothelial protection by autophagy in atherosclerosis. Sci Transl Med 12(546):eaaz2294

Schober A, Weber C (2016) Mechanisms of microRNAs in atherosclerosis. Annu Rev Pathol 11:583–616

Schober A, Nazari-Jahantigh M, Wei Y, Bidzhekov K, Gremse F, Grommes J et al (2014) MicroRNA-126-5p promotes endothelial proliferation and limits atherosclerosis by suppressing Dlk1. Nat Med 20(4):368–376

Schober A, Nazari-Jahantigh M, Weber C (2015) MicroRNA-mediated mechanisms of the cellular stress response in atherosclerosis. Nat Rev Cardiol 12(6):361–374

Schreyer SA, Vick C, Lystig TC, Mystkowski P, LeBoeuf RC (2002) LDL receptor but not apolipoprotein E deficiency increases diet-induced obesity and diabetes in mice. Am J Physiol Endocrinol Metab 282(1):E207–E214

Schreyer SA, Lystig TC, Vick CM, LeBoeuf RC (2003) Mice deficient in apolipoprotein E but not LDL receptors are resistant to accelerated atherosclerosis associated with obesity. Atherosclerosis 171(1):49–55

Semo J, Chernin G, Jonas M, Shimoni S, George J (2019) Deletion of the Mir-106b~ 25 MicroRNA cluster attenuates atherosclerosis in apolipoprotein E knockout mice. Lipids Health Dis 18 (1):208

Shah AV, Bennett MR (2017) DNA damage-dependent mechanisms of ageing and disease in the macro- and microvasculature. Eur J Pharmacol 816:116–128

Siciliano V, Garzilli I, Fracassi C, Criscuolo S, Ventre S, di Bernardo D (2013) MiRNAs confer phenotypic robustness to gene networks by suppressing biological noise. Nat Commun 4:2364

Su YL, Wang X, Mann M, Adamus TP, Wang D, Moreira DF et al (2020) Myeloid cell-targeted miR-146a mimic inhibits NF-kappaB-driven inflammation and leukemia progression in vivo. Blood 135(3):167–180

Suarez Y, Fernandez-Hernando C, Pober JS, Sessa WC (2007) Dicer dependent microRNAs regulate gene expression and functions in human endothelial cells. Circ Res 100(8):1164–1173

Suarez Y, Fernandez-Hernando C, Yu J, Gerber SA, Harrison KD, Pober JS et al (2008) Dicer-dependent endothelial microRNAs are necessary for postnatal angiogenesis. Proc Natl Acad Sci U S A 105(37):14082–14087

Taganov KD, Boldin MP, Chang KJ, Baltimore D (2006) NF-kappaB-dependent induction of microRNA miR-146, an inhibitor targeted to signaling proteins of innate immune responses. Proc Natl Acad Sci U S A 103(33):12481–12486

Tan L, Liu L, Jiang Z, Hao X (2019) Inhibition of microRNA-17-5p reduces the inflammation and lipid accumulation, and up-regulates ATP-binding cassette transporterA1 in atherosclerosis. J Pharmacol Sci 139(4):280–288

Tang Y, Jin X, Xiang Y, Chen Y, Shen CX, Zhang YC et al (2015) The lncRNA MALAT1 protects the endothelium against ox-LDL-induced dysfunction via upregulating the expression of the miR-22-3p target genes CXCR2 and AKT. FEBS Lett 589(20 Pt B):3189–3196

Thompson RC, Vardinogiannis I, Gilmore TD (2013) Identification of an NF-kappaB p50/p65-responsive site in the human MIR155HG promoter. BMC Mol Biol 14:24

Thum T, Borlak J (2008) LOX-1 receptor blockade abrogates oxLDL-induced oxidative DNA damage and prevents activation of the transcriptional repressor Oct-1 in human coronary arterial endothelium. J Biol Chem 283(28):19456–19464

Tsao PS, Lewis NP, Alpert S, Cooke JP (1995) Exposure to shear stress alters endothelial adhesiveness. Role of nitric oxide. Circulation 92(12):3513–3519

Tzima E, Irani-Tehrani M, Kiosses WB, Dejana E, Schultz DA, Engelhardt B et al (2005) A mechanosensory complex that mediates the endothelial cell response to fluid shear stress. Nature 437(7057):426–431

Ulitsky I (2016) Evolution to the rescue: using comparative genomics to understand long non-coding RNAs. Nat Rev Genet 17(10):601–614

Uszczynska-Ratajczak B, Lagarde J, Frankish A, Guigo R, Johnson R (2018) Towards a complete map of the human long non-coding RNA transcriptome. Nat Rev Genet 19(9):535–548

van Hinsbergh VW, Scheffer M, Havekes L, Kempen HJ (1986) Role of endothelial cells and their products in the modification of low-density lipoproteins. Biochim Biophys Acta 878(1):49–64

Visel A, Zhu Y, May D, Afzal V, Gong E, Attanasio C et al (2010) Targeted deletion of the 9p21 non-coding coronary artery disease risk interval in mice. Nature 464(7287):409–412

Voellenkle C, Rooij J, Guffanti A, Brini E, Fasanaro P, Isaia E et al (2012) Deep-sequencing of endothelial cells exposed to hypoxia reveals the complexity of known and novel microRNAs. RNA 18(3):472–484

Wang W, Liu Z, Su J, Chen WS, Wang XW, Bai SX et al (2016) Macrophage micro-RNA-155 promotes lipopolysaccharide-induced acute lung injury in mice and rats. Am J Physiol Lung Cell Mol Physiol 311(2):L494–L506

Wang Y-C, Lee A-S, Lu L-S, Ke L-Y, Chen W-Y, Dong J-W et al (2018) Human electronegative LDL induces mitochondrial dysfunction and premature senescence of vascular cells in vivo. Aging Cell 17(4):e12792-e

Wang K, Yang C, Shi J, Gao T (2019a) Ox-LDL-induced lncRNA MALAT1 promotes autophagy in human umbilical vein endothelial cells by sponging miR-216a-5p and regulating Beclin-1 expression. Eur J Pharmacol 858:172338

Wang L, Xia JW, Ke ZP, Zhang BH (2019b) Blockade of NEAT1 represses inflammation response and lipid uptake via modulating miR-342-3p in human macrophages THP-1 cells. J Cell Physiol 234(4):5319–5326

Wechezak AR, Viggers RF, Coan DE, Sauvage LR (1994) Mitosis and cytokinesis in subconfluent endothelial cells exposed to increasing levels of shear stress. J Cell Physiol 159(1):83–91

Wei Y, Schober A (2016) MicroRNA regulation of macrophages in human pathologies. Cell Mol Life Sci 73(18):3473–3495

Wei Y, Nazari-Jahantigh M, Chan L, Zhu M, Heyll K, Corbalan-Campos J et al (2013) The microRNA-342-5p fosters inflammatory macrophage activation through an Akt1- and microRNA-155-dependent pathway during atherosclerosis. Circulation 127(15):1609–1619

Wei Y, Zhu M, Corbalan-Campos J, Heyll K, Weber C, Schober A (2015) Regulation of Csf1r and Bcl6 in macrophages mediates the stage-specific effects of microRNA-155 on atherosclerosis. Arterioscler Thromb Vasc Biol 35(4):796–803

Wei Y, Corbalan-Campos J, Gurung R, Natarelli L, Zhu M, Exner N et al (2018) Dicer in macrophages prevents atherosclerosis by promoting mitochondrial oxidative metabolism. Circulation 138(18):2007–2020

Wiese CB, Zhong J, Xu ZQ, Zhang Y, Ramirez Solano MA, Zhu W et al (2019) Dual inhibition of endothelial miR-92a-3p and miR-489-3p reduces renal injury-associated atherosclerosis. Atherosclerosis 282:121–131

Wu W, Xiao H, Laguna-Fernandez A, Villarreal G Jr, Wang KC, Geary GG et al (2011) Flow-dependent regulation of kruppel-like factor 2 is mediated by MicroRNA-92a. Circulation 124 (5):633–641

Wu R, Tang S, Wang M, Xu X, Yao C, Wang S (2016) MicroRNA-497 induces apoptosis and suppresses proliferation via the Bcl-2/Bax-Caspase9-Caspase3 pathway and cyclin D2 protein in HUVECs. PLoS One 11(12):e0167052

Wu H, Yang L, Chen L-L (2017) The diversity of long noncoding RNAs and their generation. Trends Genet 33(8):540–552

Xu Y, Xu Y, Zhu Y, Sun H, Juguilon C, Li F et al (2020) Macrophage miR-34a is a key regulator of cholesterol efflux and atherosclerosis. Mol Ther 28(1):202–216

Yan W, Wu Q, Yao W, Li Y, Liu Y, Yuan J et al (2017) MiR-503 modulates epithelial-mesenchymal transition in silica-induced pulmonary fibrosis by targeting PI3K p85 and is sponged by lncRNA MALAT1. Sci Rep 7(1):11313

Yang S, Ye ZM, Chen S, Luo XY, Chen SL, Mao L et al (2018) MicroRNA-23a-5p promotes atherosclerotic plaque progression and vulnerability by repressing ATP-binding cassette transporter A1/G1 in macrophages. J Mol Cell Cardiol 123:139–149

Yao RW, Wang Y, Chen LL (2019) Cellular functions of long noncoding RNAs. Nat Cell Biol 21 (5):542–551

Ye ZM, Yang S, Xia YP, Hu RT, Chen S, Li BW et al (2019) LncRNA MIAT sponges miR-149-5p to inhibit efferocytosis in advanced atherosclerosis through CD47 upregulation. Cell Death Dis 10(2):138

Ying W, Sevigny MB, Chen Y, Swanson RA (2001) Poly(ADP-ribose) glycohydrolase mediates oxidative and excitotoxic neuronal death. Proc Natl Acad Sci U S A 98(21):12227–12232

Zannis VI, Chroni A, Krieger M (2006) Role of apoA-I, ABCA1, LCAT, and SR-BI in the biogenesis of HDL. J Mol Med (Berl) 84(4):276–294

Zeng L, Zampetaki A, Margariti A, Pepe AE, Alam S, Martin D et al (2009) Sustained activation of XBP1 splicing leads to endothelial apoptosis and atherosclerosis development in response to disturbed flow. Proc Natl Acad Sci U S A 106(20):8326–8331

Zernecke A, Bidzhekov K, Noels H, Shagdarsuren E, Gan L, Denecke B et al (2009) Delivery of microRNA-126 by apoptotic bodies induces CXCL12-dependent vascular protection. Sci Signal 2(100):ra81

Zhang B, Arun G, Mao YS, Lazar Z, Hung G, Bhattacharjee G et al (2012) The lncRNA Malat1 is dispensable for mouse development but its transcription plays a cis-regulatory role in the adult. Cell Rep 2(1):111–123

Zhang CZ, Spektor A, Cornils H, Francis JM, Jackson EK, Liu S et al (2015) Chromothripsis from DNA damage in micronuclei. Nature 522(7555):179–184

Zhao JL, Rao DS, Boldin MP, Taganov KD, O'Connell RM, Baltimore D (2011) NF-{kappa}B dysregulation in microRNA-146a-deficient mice drives the development of myeloid malignancies. Proc Natl Acad Sci U S A 108(22):9184–9189

Zhao G, Su Z, Song D, Mao Y, Mao X (2016) The long noncoding RNA MALAT1 regulates the lipopolysaccharide-induced inflammatory response through its interaction with NF-kappaB. FEBS Lett 590(17):2884–2895

Zheng B, Yin WN, Suzuki T, Zhang XH, Zhang Y, Song LL et al (2017) Exosome-mediated miR-155 transfer from smooth muscle cells to endothelial cells induces endothelial injury and promotes atherosclerosis. Mol Ther 25(6):1279–1294

Zhu M, Wei Y, Geissler C, Abschlag K, Corbalan Campos J, Hristov M et al (2017) Hyperlipidemia-induced microRNA-155-5p improves beta-cell function by targeting Mafb. Diabetes 66(12):3072–3084

Zhu Y, Yang T, Duan J, Mu N, Zhang T (2019) MALAT1/miR-15b-5p/MAPK1 mediates endothelial progenitor cells autophagy and affects coronary atherosclerotic heart disease via mTOR signaling pathway. Aging 11(4):1089–1109

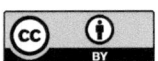

Lipidomics in Biomarker Research

Thorsten Hornemann

Contents

1 Introduction 494
2 Biochemistry of Lipids 494
3 Lipidomics 496
   3.1 Mass Spectrometry and Chromatography 497
   3.2 Pre-analytical Considerations 500
   3.3 Lipid Extraction 501
   3.4 Targeted vs. Untargeted Lipidomics 502
   3.5 Annotation 502
   3.6 Biostatistics 503
4 Application of Lipidomics in Clinical and Epidemiological Studies 503
References 505

Abstract

Lipids are natural substances found in all living organisms and involved in many biological functions. Imbalances in the lipid metabolism are linked to various diseases such as obesity, diabetes, or cardiovascular disease. Lipids comprise thousands of chemically distinct species making them a challenge to analyze because of their great structural diversity.

Thanks to the technological improvements in the fields of chromatography, high-resolution mass spectrometry, and bioinformatics over the last years, it is now possible to perform global lipidomics analyses, allowing the concomitant detection, identification, and relative quantification of hundreds of lipid species. This review shall provide an insight into a general lipidomics workflow and its application in metabolic biomarker research.

T. Hornemann (✉)
University Zurich and University Hospital Zurich, Zurich, Switzerland
e-mail: thorsten.hornemann@usz.ch

© The Author(s) 2021
A. von Eckardstein, C. J. Binder (eds.), *Prevention and Treatment of Atherosclerosis*,
Handbook of Experimental Pharmacology 270, https://doi.org/10.1007/164_2021_517

Keywords

Biomarkers · Data analysis · Dyslipidemia · LC/MS · Lipids · Metabolic disease ·
Metabolites

1   Introduction

Metabolic diseases can present long before becoming clinically apparent. Early
predictors of metabolic disease are of particular importance since a delay or prevention of morbidity is possible via pharmacological and behavioral interventions.
Thus, biomarkers are essential tools to select patients for appropriate treatment
schemes, optimally providing the right treatment to the right patient at the right time.
     Cardiovascular diseases (CVDs) and associated mortality have a high prevalence
in western societies. For coronary artery disease (CAD), the average annual mortality ranges between 1 and 3% (for fatal and non-fatal myocardial infarctions) and
remains a clinical challenge (Morrow 2010). In patients who survived an acute event
of a coronary syndrome (ACS), the rate of myocardial infarction and death is
markedly increased (Hamm et al. 2012). However, at the individual patient level,
the risk may vary considerably and therefore risk estimation tools are needed to
better manage such patients. A better risk stratification would also help to identify
individuals at risk who require interventions that are more intensive. Conversely, it is
equally important to identify patients with a good prognosis, to avoid unnecessary
procedures   or   aggressive   drug   treatments   with   associated   side   effects.
Concentrations of cholesterol in total plasma (TC), low density lipoproteins
(LDL-C), and high density lipoproteins (HDL-C) as well as triglycerides
(TG) have been used for risk prediction. LDL-C has become the main therapeutic
target in the management of patients with CAD. However, a number of studies have
failed to show any association between LDL-C and outcomes in large series of CAD
patients (Puri et al. 2013). There is a clinical need for additional risk markers in CVD
as well as a better understanding on how lipids relate with established metabolic risk
factors to evaluate their potential as clinical biomarkers.

2   Biochemistry of Lipids

Biological systems are comprised of thousands of chemically distinct lipids. The
structural diversity of lipids confers a broad spectrum of functionality. For most
lipids, their functions depend on their molecular structure and can be very different
for the different lipid classes as well as for different lipid species within the same
lipid class (Stahlman et al. 2012). Lipids are found in all living organisms. They are
involved in many critical cellular functions such as energy storage, structural plasma
membrane integrity, and cell signaling. Imbalances of lipid metabolism are linked to
the pathology of various diseases such as diabetes, Alzheimer's, obesity, cancer, and
atherosclerosis (Cavojsky et al. 2016; Jung and Choi 2014; Steinberg 2006; Tan
et al. 2017; Watson 2006; Wenk 2005). While routine plasma lipid analysis precedes

prescription of lipid-lowering drugs (Quehenberger et al. 2010), the abundance of particular lipid species may be indicative of a specific disease (Quehenberger and Dennis 2011). Abnormal concentrations of lipids are observed in various metabolic disorders.

Moreover, many inborn errors of metabolism are related to alterations in the metabolism of lipids, and particularly that of sphingolipids. Sphingolipidoses are monogenic inherited diseases caused by defects in the sphingolipid degradation pathways (Kolter and Sandhoff 2006; Sandhoff and Harzer 2013), leading to a massive storage of undegraded sphingolipid species in the lysosomes, causing neuroinflammation and neurodegeneration. Sphingolipids also emerged over the last years as significant factors in the pathogenesis of cardiometabolic diseases (Cowart 2009; Summers 2006; Deevska and Nikolova-Karakashian 2011).

Lipids show a large structural diversity that is comprised in the term "lipidome." According to the comprehensive classification system proposed by the LIPID MAPS consortium (http://www.lipidmaps.org), lipids can be classified into eight different classes (Fig. 1): glycerophospholipids (GP), sphingolipids (SL), glycerolipids, sterol lipids, free fatty acids, prenol lipids, saccharolipids, and polyketides (Fahy et al. 2005; Fahy et al. 2009).

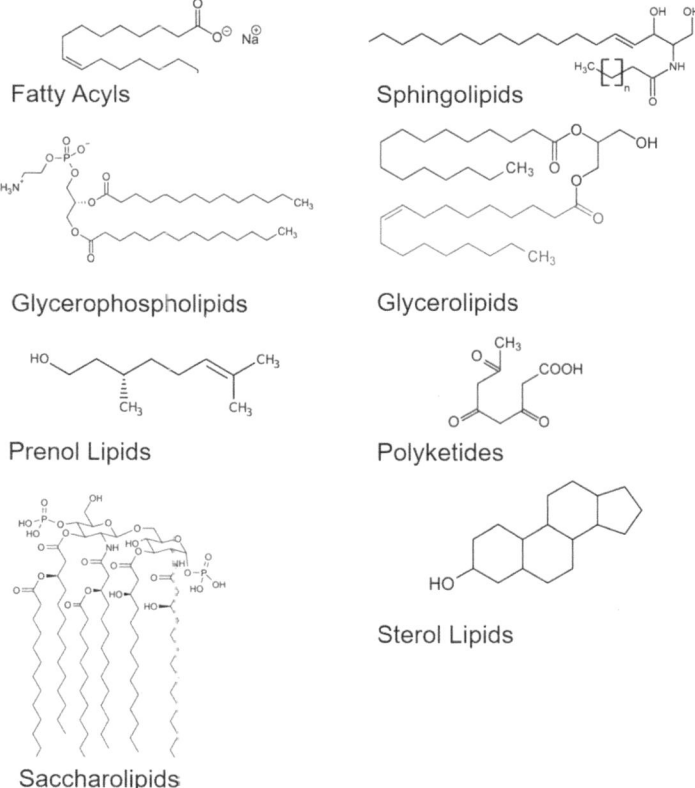

Fig. 1 Structures of the most abundant lipid families

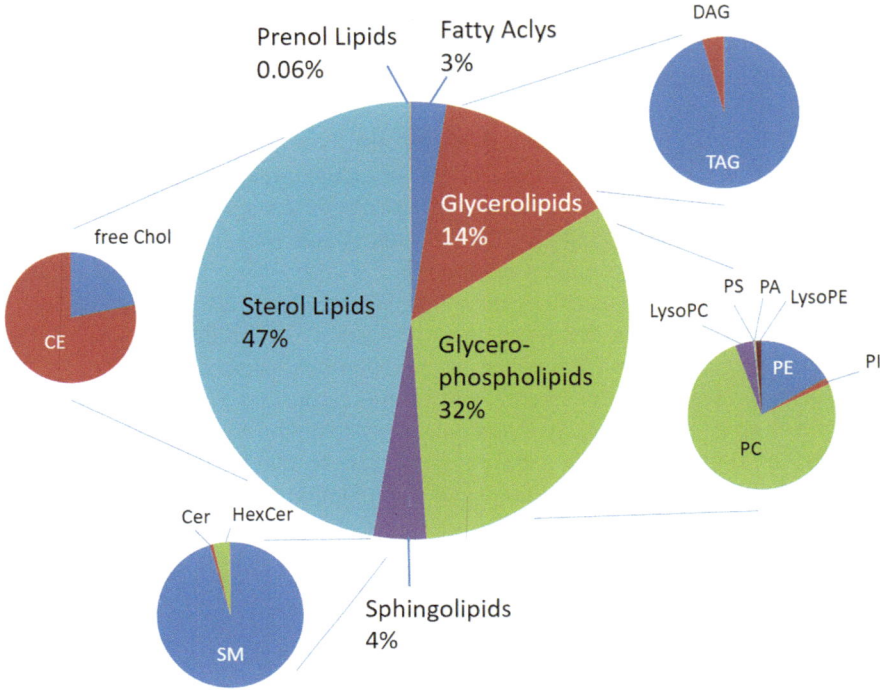

Fig. 2 Distribution of the individual lipid classes in human plasma (reproduced from Quehenberger et al. (2010))

GP constitute the largest lipid class and are derived from sn-glycero-3-phosphoric acid. Nearly 200 GP species were identified in human plasma (Fig. 2). Among them glycerophosphocholines and glycerophosphoethanolamines are most abundant and glycerophosphoserines least abundant (Quehenberger et al. 2010; Quehenberger and Dennis 2011). Lyso-GPs only bear one fatty acid that is esterified to a hydroxyl group either at sn-1 or sn-2 position.

Human plasma contains more than 200 different SL species. The largest SL fraction in human plasma is sphingomyelin, while ceramides are least abundant.

Among sterols cholesterol is most abundant in plasma followed by lathosterol and desmosterol. The largest part of cholesterol in plasma is esterified (Fig. 2). Among the cholesteryl esters (CE) of human plasma, CE(18:2) and CE(20:4) contribute the major fraction (Quehenberger et al. 2010).

Prenol lipids are built from five carbon isoprene units. The two main prenol lipids in plasma are dolichol and ubiquinone (Shiota et al. 2008).

3   Lipidomics

Lipidomics is a relatively young field of science, which aims to identify and quantify all individual lipid species and their functions within a biological system (Han and Gross 2003). Lipidomics technologies are increasingly applied to biomarker discovery. They offer great promise for new-generation biomarkers in common and complex phenotypes such as dyslipidemia and cardiovascular diseases (CVDs).

3.1   Mass Spectrometry and Chromatography

A lipidomics analysis provides an overall picture of the lipids in a sample, thanks to the combined use of analytical chemistry and data mining tools. However, the comprehensive characterization of a lipidome in biological samples is still challenging. The huge structural diversity of lipids that primarily arises from the combination of various fatty acids and functional head groups makes a complete molecular profiling of the lipidome difficult. In particular, the presence of multiple isobaric lipid species increases the complexity. Also the detection of quantitatively minor lipid species remains a challenge.

The development of mass spectrometry (MS) based technologies over the last decade has rapidly expanded research in the field of lipidomics. In lipidomics, the mass spectrometer can be used without prior separation ("shot-gun lipidomics") or connected to chromatographic systems in order to provide an additional dimension of separation.

In the shot-gun strategy, the crude lipid extract is directly introduced into the MS system (Han and Gross 1994), which is a fast and simple method to obtain a quantitative lipid profile from biological matrices. However, as the trade-off, the technology suffers from a limited dynamic range and the risk of ion suppression, making the detection of isobaric and low concentrated lipid species difficult. Therefore, recent methodologies are often based on the progress in high-resolution (HR) MS, such as Orbitrap (Ejsing et al. 2009; Schwudke et al. 2011) or Q-TOF detectors (Guo et al. 2012; Li et al. 2013). Using HR-MS, individual lipid species are identified and quantified according to their exact chemical mass. Nevertheless, the major limitation of shot-gun MS is the lack of discrimination between isobaric species. Because of the building block-like nature of many lipid families, isobaric species are frequently found in the lipidome. This is in particular the case for certain glycero- and sphingolipids, which have a very similar accurate mass (Schwudke et al. 2011).

Thin layer chromatography (TLC) was one of the earliest chromatographic methods applied in lipid analysis. However, it is time-consuming and lacks resolution power and reproducibility. Nevertheless, TLC is still widely used, because of its simplicity and low cost. Also, with gas chromatography (GC), it is possible to obtain information on individual lipid species. Volatile lipid classes, in particular triacylglycerols, can be separated directly and without any chemical modification, whereas the analysis of more polar compounds such as fatty acids, phospholipids, and sphingolipids requires initial derivatization or hydrolysis. Also capillary electrophoresis has been applied for the separation of phospholipids at high data acquisition speed (Jang et al. 2011). However, (ultra) high-performance liquid chromatography ((U)HPLC) is the most versatile method and the majority of lipid classes including glycerophospholipids, glycerolipids, sphingolipids, sterols, and fatty acids can be separated directly by (U)HPLC (Wenk 2005).

In lipidomics studies, either normal-phase (NPLC) or reversed-phase (RPLC) liquid chromatography is used. In NPLC, lipid species are primarily separated by the polarity of their head groups, while RPLC separates the lipids based on their lipophilicity which is primarily determined by the acyl chain length, the number of double bonds, and hydroxylations (Merrill Jr. et al. 2005). In RPLC, lipids with shorter acyl chains and/or a higher degree of unsaturation elute earlier. Furthermore, RPLC can separate isomeric species based on the type of double bond (*cis* or *trans*) or whether a fatty acid is in sn-1 or sn-2 position (Bird et al. 2012). Other HPLC based separation techniques have been developed recently and show a great potential for lipidomics. In particular, supercritical fluid chromatography-mass spectrometry (SFC-MS) has been used for the separation of lipids over a wide range of polarities depending on the choice of the chromatographic columns (Bamba et al. 2012). In lipidomics, MS instruments are mostly combined with LC systems. This strategy drastically decreases ion suppression and improved the separation of isobaric and low-abundance species (Taguchi and Ishikawa 2010). In addition, ion mobility (IM) separation offers an additional dimension for the separation of isobaric lipid species which can even be combined with LC based separation methods (Kliman et al. 2011). Also, HR-MS is often combined with high- or ultra-performance liquid chromatography (Bird et al. 2011a, b) or ion mobility spectroscopy (Kliman et al. 2011).

In addition to chromatography, technological advancements in MS, particularly in the field of ionization methods, have played a critical role in advancing the lipid analysis from complex matrices. Electrospray ionization (ESI) and atmospheric pressure ion (API) sources, including atmospheric pressure chemical ionization (APCI) and atmospheric pressure photoionization (APPI) are most widely used. Other methods such as matrix-assisted laser desorption ionization (MALDI) are also applied but are not the most established methods for lipid profiling. In contrast to ESI or atmospheric pressure ion sources, MALDI cannot be easily coupled to chromatographic systems. However, MALDI-MS is used in mass spectrometry imaging (MSI) (Aichler and Walch 2015) to analyze individual lipid species directly in tissue sections. Also, the combination of MALDI-MS with TLC provides direct information about the molecular species and the molecular weight (Guittard et al. 1999) as by TLC, lipids are normally separated according to their classes.

The first analysis of a complex lipid mixture using an ESI source was reported by Han and Gross (Han and Gross 1994). Today, ESI is the most widely used method for lipidomic studies, although some important classes, such as cholesteryl esters and glycerolipids (mono-, di- and tri-acylglycerols) are not well ionized with ESI and therefore require the addition of ammonium, lithium, or copper ions to increase signal strength (Murphy and Axelsen 2011; Murphy and Gaskell 2011).

With the advent of high-resolution MS and the capability to perform simultaneous HR-MS and MS/MS analysis, the major challenge for LC-MS based lipidomics is to deal with the vast amount of information generated during data acquisitions. Therefore, bioinformatics tools (Table 1) have been developed to

Table 1 Publically available software tools for the processing and annotation of MS data

	Application	URL
Databases		
LIPID MAPS	Lipid database and classification	http://www.lipidmaps.org
LipidBank	Official database of Japanese Conference on the Biochemistry of lipids	http://www.lipidbank.jp
LMSD	Structure and annotation of lipid species	http://www.lipidmaps.org/data/structure/index.html
Massbank	High resolution mass spectral database	http://www.massbank.jp
IUPAC	IUPAC lipid nomenclature	http://www.chem.qmul.ac.uk/iupac/lipid
LIPIDAT	Thermodynamic data of lipids	http://www.lipidat.tcd.ie
Cyberlipids	Dedicated site for lipid analysis	http://www.cyberlipid.org
Lipid Library	Dedicated site for lipid analysis	http://lipidlibrary.aocs.org
SphingoMAP	Sphingolipid metabolism	http://www.sphingomap.org
KEGG	Fatty acid, sterol, and phospholipid metabolism	http://www.genome.jp/kegg/pathway.html
METACYC	Lipid metabolism	http://metacyc.org
HMDB	Metabolome database (MS and MS/MS spectra)	http://www.hmdb.ca
METLIN	Metabolome database (MS and MS/MS spectra)	http://metlin.scripps.edu/index.php
mzCloud	High resolution mass spectral database	http://www.mzcloud.org
Free software		
Mzmine 2	Open source software for LC-MS data processing	http://mzmine.github.io/
XCMS	Framework for processing and visualization of LC-MS data	https://bioconductor.org/packages/release/bioc/html/xcms.html
metAlign	Pre-processing and comparison of full scan LC-MS and GC-MS data	https://www.wur.nl/en/show/MetAlign-1.htm
LipidBlast	Tandem mass spectrometry database for lipid identification	https://fiehnlab.ucdavis.edu/projects/LipidBlast
LipidXplorer	Molecular fragmentation query language (MFQL) in shot-gun lipidomics	https://wiki.mpi-cbg.de/lipidx/Main_Page
Lipid Data Analyzer (LDA)	Identifying novel lipid molecular species from mass spectrometry data	http://genome.tugraz.at/lda/lda_description.shtml
LipidIMMS Analyzer	Integrates multidimensional LC-MS/MS spectra and ion mobility data for lipid identification	http://imms.zhulab.cn/LipidIMMS/
Skyline	Powerful open source application for the analysis of proteomics and lipidomics data	https://skyline.ms/project/home/software/Skyline/begin.view
Lipidcreator	Skyline plugin for targeted LC-MS/MS-based lipidomics	https://lifs.isas.de/lipidcreator.html
LIQUID	Open source software for identifying lipids in LC-MS/MS-based data	https://github.com/PNNL-Comp-Mass-Spec/LIQUID

(continued)

Table 1 (continued)

	Application	URL
LIMSA	Integrates and matches MS peaks with a user list of expected lipids, corrects for isotopic patterns, and quantifies the identified lipid species	https://omictools.com/limsa-tool
LipiDex	Unifies LC-MS/MS-based lipid identification using intelligent data filtering	https://github.com/coongroup/LipiDex
LipidHunter	de novo identification of native phospholipids	https://home.uni-leipzig.de/fedorova/software/lipidhunter/
LipidMatch	Rule-based lipid identification using untargeted high-resolution MS/MS data	https://omictools.com/lipidmatch-tool
LipidMS	Lipid annotation in untargeted lipidomics based on fragmentation and intensity rules	https://rdrr.io/cran/LipidMS/
Commercial software		*Manufacturer*
LipidView	LC-MS data processing	AB/Sciex
Marketlynx	LC-MS, LC-MS/MS, GC/MS, and GC-MS/MS data processing	Waters
Metabolic Profiler	NMR and MS data processing	Bruker
Lipid Search	LC-MS/MS data processing	ThermoScientific

handle, process, and interpret large amounts of data generated during lipidomics analysis. Typically, a lipidomics workflow includes four steps.

I. Sample preparation, II. LC-MS/MS analysis, III. Automatic data processing for peak detection and alignment based on commercial or freely available software algorithms, and IV. Feature identification using public or proprietary databases (Fig. 3).

3.2 Pre-analytical Considerations

A key factor for the quality of a lipid profiling study is the integrity of the samples (Ellervik and Vaught 2015). Errors during the pre-analytical phase including sample collection, processing, and storage may severely affect subsequent downstream analyses and resulting data (Ellervik and Vaught 2015). Anticoagulants are commonly used in plasma preparation and the most common anticoagulants such as EDTA and heparin plasma as well as serum are compatible with lipidomics studies. Nonetheless, the peak responses of a number of lipid species can be influenced by the material (Hammad et al. 2010). Therefore, the same anticoagulant should be used throughout a study. In addition, the correct storage of the samples is of importance. Particularly in large clinical cohorts, batches of samples may be stored for a long period of time. Samples are commonly stored at $-80\ °C$ or lower before they undergo a lipidomics profiling. However, certain lipids such as sphingomyelins were lost from plasma samples over 5 years of storage (Haid et al. 2018). Plasma

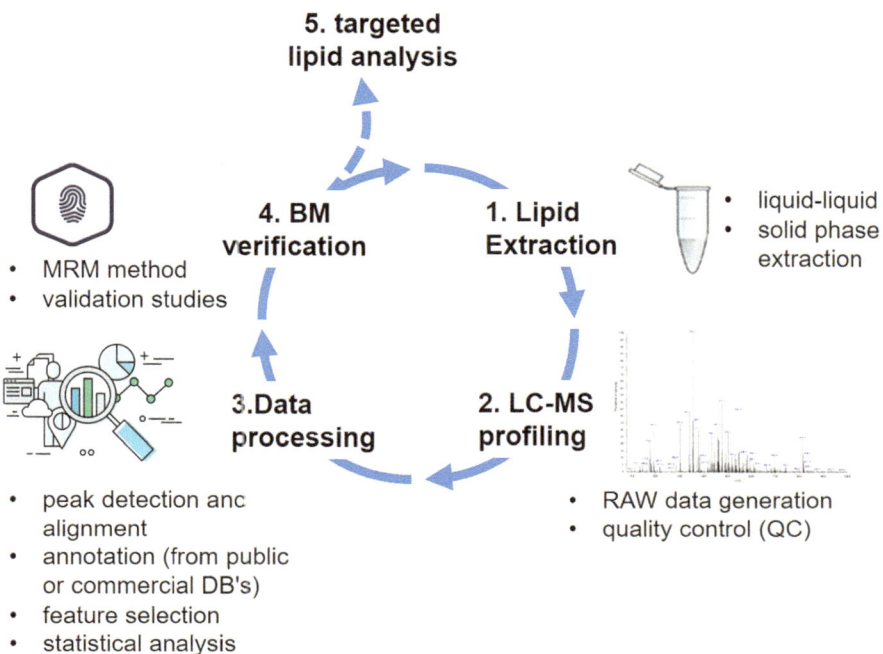

Fig. 3 Typical workflow for lipid biomarker identification

concentrations of cholesterol and triglycerides were shown to decrease in serum samples stored over 7 and 5 years, respectively (Shih et al. 2000) even at −80 °C. This should be considered as the time-dependent degradation of certain lipids may lead to biased results. Consequently, the time between sampling and analysis should be kept as short as possible.

3.3   Lipid Extraction

Usually, lipids are extracted from biological sources using liquid–liquid extractions. Lipid extraction is a crucial step in obtaining global coverage of the lipidome. The two most commonly applied methods are using either a 2/1 mixture of chloroform and methanol according to Folch (Folch et al. 1957) or a 1/1 mixture of chloroform and methanol according to Bligh and Dyer (Bligh and Dyer 1959). Based on these traditional protocols, new methods have been developed, although most of them are adaptations of either the one or the other. Chloroform and methanol can be replaced by either dichloromethane (Hu et al. 2008), methyl *tert*-butyl ether (MTBE) or by heptane and ethyl acetate (Lofgren et al. 2012). Comparing the yeast lipidome prepared by three extraction methods (chloroform/methanol 17/1 (v/v), chloroform/methanol 2/1 (v/v). or chloroform/methanol/H2O 1/1/0.9 (v/v/v) showed a large heterogeneity in the extraction yield which was also dependent on the respective lipid classes (Ejsing et al. 2009). Therefore, the appropriate extraction protocol depends on the underlying analytical question and the lipid class of interest (Danne-Rasche et al. 2018).

3.4   Targeted vs. Untargeted Lipidomics

LC-MS is typically applied in two distinct operational modes – targeted or untargeted. A targeted approach is normally chosen for a limited, predefined number of lipid species. It is typically more sensitive and specific than untargeted approaches. In a targeted approach, often low-resolution MS systems are used, such as triple quadrupole or quadrupole linear ion trap instruments, because of their speed, sensitivity, and quantification capabilities (Bielawski et al. 2009). However, the development of HR-MS instruments such as Orbitrap and quadrupole time-of-flight MS also allows untargeted lipidomic approaches, which is independent of a predefined compound list (Junot et al. 2014). HR-MS enables the concomitant analysis of multiple lipid families without the need for extensive fragmentation. Improvements in the duty cycle allow the combination of high-resolution MS and higher energy collisional dissociation (HCD) scans, which provides further information about the accurate mass of precursor and fragment ions of the detected lipids (Bird et al. 2013, 2015). Depending on the model and MS manufacturer, also combined approaches of HR-MS together with ion fragmentation are possible. Many instrument manufacturers offer the possibility to generate HR-MS fragment data using either a data dependent (DDA) or data independent (DIA) acquisition mode.

3.5   Annotation

Lipid species detected by MS-based approaches are typically annotated with the help of dedicated databases. Numerous lipid databases have been developed in the field of lipidomics (see Table 1). The LIPID MAPS consortium has developed the structure database LIPID MAPS (Schmelzer et al. 2007), wherein lipid species are classified by families, class, and subclasses according to their accurate mass and structure. This database is openly available and can be downloaded allowing an automatic annotation. This database consists of compiled databases such as LipidBank, LIPIDAT, or LipidBlast (Cajka and Fiehn 2017). Also databases commonly used in the field of metabolomics, such as HMDB, METLIN, and KEGG, contain data on lipid species as well as other sources such as Cyberlipids and Lipid Library.

However, before the individual lipid species can be annotated, the raw data obtained from an MS analyzer must be pre-processed. Typically, raw MS data are first converted into either a proprietary data format of the respective MS manufacturer or an open data container such as NetCDF, mzXML, or mzData (i.e., XCMS or MZmine). In parallel with advances in instrumentation technology (particularly for high-resolution mass spectrometers), manufacturers have developed commercial software packages for direct interpretation of the raw data obtained. In contrast to manufacturer specific data formats, which normally can only be read in combination with branded software packages, open data formats are commonly used in freely available software programs such as MZmine (Katajamaa et al. 2006) or XCMS (Smith et al. 2006) (Table 1). Data processing in MZmine is based on algorithms for spectral filtering, alignments according to the retention time, peak picking detection, normalization, and visualization. XCMS in contrast uses non-linear retention time peak alignment, matching by a filter process and peak matching.

Many of these data processing tools allow to perform univariate or multi-variate statistical analysis to identify discriminant variables (potential biomarker lipid species, for example). However, in case of unclear structural definitions, often further MS/MS experiments are needed to identify the lipid metabolite of interest unambiguously.

3.6 Biostatistics

Finally, advanced biostatistical tools are needed to process, analyze, and interpret high-dimensional lipidomics data in the context of clinical information. Based on the typically large and comprehensive dataset, supervised and unsupervised statistical methods are applied. This includes but is not limited to partial least squares discriminant analysis (PLS-DA), orthogonal projection-potential structure analysis (OPLS-DA), principal component analysis (PCA), clustering analysis, linear discriminant analysis, or other stoichiometric methods (Liland et al. 2010). Tools such as MetaboAnalyst can help to identify relevant markers and lipid signatures (Xia and Wishart 2016).

4 Application of Lipidomics in Clinical and Epidemiological Studies

In plasma, lipids are mostly transported and distributed by lipoproteins (e.g., HDL, LDL, VLDL). Several studies have examined the lipid components of lipoproteins among healthy participants (Quehenberger et al. 2010; Christinat and Masoodi 2017; Kontush et al. 2013). However, the lipid composition of lipoproteins varies (Cardner et al. 2020). Triacylglycerols (TAGs) are the predominant core lipid in VLDL, while CEs predominate in the core of LDL and HDL. Compared to LDL, HDL contains a higher amount of phospholipids, particularly PC and LPC. The fatty acid composition of phospholipids, TAGs, and CE is similar in HDL, LDL, and VLDL.

CVD is mostly associated with increased blood levels for one or more lipid classes. These hyperlipicemias (HL) can be linked to familial or non-familial reasons. Familial HL are caused by genetic alterations in lipoprotein metabolism but the penetrance can vary considerably depending on the condition (De Castro-Oros et al. 2010). Non-familial HL occur due to adverse lifestyle behavior such as physical inactivity, intake of lipid-rich diet, smoking, and alcohol consumption or due to underlying diseases such as obesity, liver diseases, and diabetes. Urban diets, stress, and unhealthy eating pattern have made non-familial HL highly prevalent and a focal topic in health prevention. HL affects a large proportion of the human lipidome, resulting in changes in plasma levels of saturated diacylglycerols (DAGs), TAGs, SM, and phospholipids in obese individuals (Graessler et al. 2009; Hanamatsu et al. 2014; Kim et al. 2010). Plasma levels of PC, phosphatidyl-ethanolamine, ether-linked lipids, phosphatidylinositol (PI), LPC, and CE (Barber et al. 2012; Donovan et al. 2013; Eisinger et al. 2014; Graessler et al. 2009; Hanamatsu et al. 2014; Kim et al. 2010; Samad et al. 2006) were also altered while LPCs showed a mixed behavior. At present, hyperlipidemic conditions are monitored routinely by the measurement of cholesterol and TAG in total plasma, LDL, and HDL. However, lipidomics demonstrated that besides cholesterol also other lipid classes and lipid species of the plasma lipidome are associated with the risk for CVD (Razquin et al. 2018). In particular plasma levels of ceramides show a positive association with the risk of CVD (Laaksonen et al. 2016). Ceramides are primarily present in LDL and may influence the function and atherogenicity of LDL. In fact, LDL extracted from human atherosclerosis lesions are highly enriched in ceramides (Schissel et al. 1996), and animal studies showed a decrease in athero-sclerotic lesion size when ceramide synthesis was inhibited (Hojjati et al. 2005).

Relatively few studies have compared the lipidomics profile of lipoproteins in relation to CVD outcomes. Higher TAGs, lower PUFAs, lower phospholipids, and lower sphingomyelin (SM) in HDL may be associated with higher risks of CVD and type 2 diabetes (T2D), although it is currently unknown whether these associations are confounded by HDL-C. In two studies, a low HDL-C has been associated with higher TAGs, lower PUFAs, lower LPC, and lower SM levels (Kontush et al. 2013). Another study found that, compared to participants without CVD or at early stages of CVD, participants with severe CVD had higher levels of short chain FAs in both HDL and non-HDL particles. PC and SM levels were lower in HDL, and PUFAs reduced in non-HDL particles. Additionally, two studies showed that lower levels of PC-plasmalogens were associated with a higher risk of CVD, particularly pf acute CVD (Meikle et al. 2019; Sutter et al. 2015).

Obesity also leads to increased lipolysis in adipose tissues and thus increases plasma level of FFAs (Haus et al. 2009). There is a direct relationship between increased intake of saturated fatty acids (e.g., lauric, myristic, or palmitic acid) and an increase in TAGs (Fernandez and West 2005; Steinberg 2005). Increased FFAs and MAGs in plasma can be attributed to an increased lipolysis of TAGs obtained from high fat diet (Ho and Storch 2001). Dietary saturated fatty acids have a tendency to increase TAG while polyunsaturated fatty acids have the ability to lower TAG and LDL-C (Siri-Tarino et al. 2010; Williams and Salter 2016). On the other hand, diets rich in SM were shown to specifically increase HDL-C without affecting other lipids (Ramprasath et al. 2013).

Mouse models of diet-induced obesity showed elevation in plasma ceramide level and alterations in PCs, LPCs, and SMs (Barber et al. 2012; Samad et al. 2006). Perturbation in lipid levels is also associated with both type 1 (T1D) (Fox et al. 2011; Sorensen et al. 2010) and type 2 diabetes (T2D) (Graessler et al. 2009; Barber et al.

2012; Samad et al. 2006). In diabetes, plasma levels of most LPC decrease, while PCs showed a mixed behavior. An important hallmark of T2D is an increase in plasma concentration of FFA (Barber et al. 2012; Samad et al. 2006), ceramides (Samad et al. 2006; Haus et al. 2009; Kang et al. 2013), and TAGs enriched with short chain saturated fatty acids (Rhee et al. 2011). Moreover, atypical 1-deoxy-Spingolipids (1-deoxySL) were found to be elevated in T2DM and showed a similar or even closer association with T2DM or metabolic syndrome than established markers such as waist circumference, glucose, triglycerides, HDL cholesterol, and blood pressure (Bertea et al. 2010; Othman et al. 2012; Othman et al. 2015a). Further studies showed that elevated plasma 1-deoxySL levels are strong and independent risk predictors of future T2DM, especially for non-obese individuals in the general population (Mwinyi et al. 2017). Plasma C20-Sphingolipids were also shown to indicate cardiovascular events independently from conventional cardiovascular risk factors in patients undergoing coronary angiography (Othman et al. 2015b).

High-throughput lipidomics analyses were recently applied to plasma samples of 10,339 participants from the Australian Diabetes, Obesity and Lifestyle Study (AusDiab) (Huynh et al. 2019; Beyene and Olshansky 2020). The data were validated in a second cohort with 4,207 participants (the Busselton Health Study) (Beyene and Olshansky 2020). The studies showed differences in the plasma lipidome related to metabolic disease and gender. A class of specific ether-phospholipids and lysophospholipids were inversely associated with age in men. The comparison of post- and premenopausal women showed higher TAG and lower lysoPC species in the postmenopausal group. Lysophospholipids were negatively associated with BMI in both sexes (with a larger effect size in men). Based on specific lipid ratios the authors identified the lipid metabolizing enzymes stearoyl CoA desaturase (SCD-1), fatty acid desaturase 3 (FADS3), and plasmanylethanolamine Δ1-desaturase, as well as the sphingolipid metabolic pathway as relevant factors associated with cardiometabolic phenotypes.

In conclusion, MS-based lipid analysis combined with bioinformatics tools have revolutionized the field of lipidomics. Thanks to commercial and freely available software packages that allow automatic peak detection, alignment, and feature annotation using public or proprietary databases to study large cohorts of patients and identify novel biomarkers which are getting increasingly important particularly in the growing field of precision and personalized medicine.

Acknowledgments This work was supported by the Swiss Science Foundation (#31003A), the Herzog-Egli Stiftung, and the Swiss Life foundation. I also would like to thank Dr. A. Hülsmeier for his corrections and comments on this manuscript.

References

Aichler M, Walch A (2015) MALDI imaging mass spectrometry: current frontiers and perspectives in pathology research and practice. Lab Investig 95:422–431

Bamba T, Lee JW, Matsubara A, Fukusaki E (2012) Metabolic profiling of lipids by supercritical fluid chromatography/mass spectrometry. J Chromatogr A 1250:212–219

Barber MN, Risis S, Yang C, Meikle PJ, Staples M, Febbraio MA, Bruce CR (2012) Plasma lysophosphatidylcholine levels are reduced in obesity and type 2 diabetes. PLoS One 7:e41456

Bertea M, Rutti MF, Othman A, Marti-Jaun J, Hersberger M, von Eckardstein A, Hornemann T (2010) Deoxysphingoid bases as plasma markers in diabetes mellitus. Lipids Health Dis 9:84

Beyene HB, Olshansky G, Adam Alexander TS, Giles C, Huynh K, Cinel M, Mellett NA, Cadby G, Hung J, Hui J et al (2020) High-coverage plasma lipidomics reveals novel sex-specific lipidomic fingerprints of age and BMI: evidence from two large population cohort studies. PLoS Biol 18: e3000870

Bielawski J, Pierce JS, Snider J, Rembiesa B, Szulc ZM, Bielawska A (2009) Comprehensive quantitative analysis of bioactive sphingolipids by high-performance liquid chromatography-tandem mass spectrometry. Methods Mol Biol 579:443–467

Bird SS, Marur VR, Sniatynski MJ, Greenberg HK, Kristal BS (2011a) Serum lipidomics profiling using LC-MS and high-energy collisional dissociation fragmentation: focus on triglyceride detection and characterization. Anal Chem 83:6648–6657

Bird SS, Marur VR, Sniatynski MJ, Greenberg HK, Kristal BS (2011b) Lipidomics profiling by high-resolution LC-MS and high-energy collisional dissociation fragmentation: focus on characterization of mitochondrial cardiolipins and monolysocardiolipins. Anal Chem 83:940–949

Bird SS, Marur VR, Stavrovskaya IG, Kristal BS (2012) Separation of cis-trans phospholipid isomers using reversed phase LC with high resolution MS detection. Anal Chem 84:5509–5517

Bird SS, Marur VR, Stavrovskaya IG, Kristal BS (2013) Qualitative characterization of the rat liver mitochondrial lipidome using LC-MS profiling and high energy collisional dissociation (HCD) all ion fragmentation. Metabolomics 9:67–83

Bird SS, Stavrovskaya IG, Gathungu RM, Tousi F, Kristal BS (2015) Qualitative characterization of the rat liver mitochondrial lipidome using all ion fragmentation on an Exactive benchtop Orbitrap MS. Methods Mol Biol 1264:441–452

Bligh EG, Dyer WJ (1959) A rapid method of total lipid extraction and purification. Can J Biochem Physiol 37:911–917

Cajka T, Fiehn O (2017) LC-MS-based lipidomics and automated identification of lipids using the LipidBlast in-silico MS/MS library. Methods Mol Biol 1609:149–170

Cardner M, Yalcinkaya M, Goetze S, Luca E, Balaz M, Hunjadi M, Hartung J, Shemet A, Krankel N, Radosavljevic S et al (2020) Structure-function relationships of HDL in diabetes and coronary heart disease. JCI Insight 5:e131491

Cavojsky T, Bilka F, Paulikova I (2016) The relationship of lipid imbalance and chronic inflammation mediated by PPAR. Ceska Slov Farm 65:3–9

Christinat N, Masoodi M (2017) Comprehensive lipoprotein characterization using lipidomics analysis of human plasma. J Proteome Res 16:2947–2953

Cowart LA (2009) Sphingolipids: players in the pathology of metabolic disease. Trends Endocrinol Metab 20:34–42

Danne-Rasche N, Coman C, Ahrends R (2018) Nano-LC/NSI MS refines lipidomics by enhancing lipid coverage, measurement sensitivity, and linear dynamic range. Anal Chem 90:8093–8101

De Castro-Oros I, Pocovi M, Civeira F (2010) The genetic basis of familial hypercholesterolemia: inheritance, linkage, and mutations. Appl Clin Genet 3:53–64

Deevska GM, Nikolova-Karakashian MN (2011) The twists and turns of sphingolipid pathway in glucose regulation. Biochimie 93(1):32–38

Donovan EL, Pettine SM, Hickey MS, Hamilton KL, Miller BF (2013) Lipidomic analysis of human plasma reveals ether-linked lipids that are elevated in morbidly obese humans compared to lean. Diabetol Metab Syndr 5:24

Eisinger K, Liebisch G, Schmitz G, Aslanidis C, Krautbauer S, Buechler C (2014) Lipidomic analysis of serum from high fat diet induced obese mice. Int J Mol Sci 15:2991–3002

Ejsing CS, Sampaio JL, Surendranath V, Duchoslav E, Ekroos K, Klemm RW, Simons K, Shevchenko A (2009) Global analysis of the yeast lipidome by quantitative shotgun mass spectrometry. Proc Natl Acad Sci U S A 106:2136–2141

Ellervik C, Vaught J (2015) Preanalytical variables affecting the integrity of human biospecimens in biobanking. Clin Chem 61:914–934

Fahy E, Subramaniam S, Brown HA, Glass CK, Merrill AH Jr, Murphy RC, Raetz CR, Russell DW, Seyama Y, Shaw W et al (2005) A comprehensive classification system for lipids. J Lipid Res 46:839–861

Fahy E, Subramaniam S, Murphy RC, Nishijima M, Raetz CR, Shimizu T, Spener F, van Meer G, Wakelam MJ, Dennis EA (2009) Update of the LIPID MAPS comprehensive classification system for lipids. J Lipid Res 50(Suppl):S9–S14

Fernandez ML, West KL (2005) Mechanisms by which dietary fatty acids modulate plasma lipids. J Nutr 135:2075–2078

Folch J, Lees M, Sloane Stanley GH (1957) A simple method for the isolation and purification of total lipides from animal tissues. J Biol Chem 226:497–509

Fox TE, Bewley MC, Unrath KA, Pedersen MM, Anderson RE, Jung DY, Jefferson LS, Kim JK, Bronson SK, Flanagan JM, Kester M (2011) Circulating sphingolipid biomarkers in models of type 1 diabetes. J Lipid Res 52:509–517

Graessler J, Schwudke D, Schwarz PE, Herzog R, Shevchenko A, Bornstein SR (2009) Top-down lipidomics reveals ether lipid deficiency in blood plasma of hypertensive patients. PLoS One 4: e6261

Guittard J, Hronowski XL, Costello CE (1999) Direct matrix-assisted laser desorption/ionization mass spectrometric analysis of glycosphingolipids on thin layer chromatographic plates and transfer membranes. Rapid Commun Mass Spectrom 13:1838–1849

Guo Y, Wang X, Qiu L, Qin X, Liu H, Wang Y, Li F, Wang X, Chen G, Song G et al (2012) Probing gender-specific lipid metabolites and diagnostic biomarkers for lung cancer using Fourier transform ion cyclotron resonance mass spectrometry. Clin Chim Acta 414:135–141

Haid M, Muschet C, Wahl S, Romisch-Margl W, Prehn C, Moller G, Adamski J (2018) Long-term stability of human plasma metabolites during storage at −80 degrees C. J Proteome Res 17:203–211

Hamm CW, Bassand JP, Agewall S, Bax J, Boersma E, Bueno H, Caso P, Dudek D, Gielen S, Huber K et al (2012) ESC guidelines for the management of acute coronary syndromes in patients presenting without persistent ST-segment elevation. The task force for the management of acute coronary syndromes (ACS) in patients presenting without persistent ST-segment elevation of the European Society of Cardiology (ESC). G Ital Cardiol (Rome) 13:171–228

Hammad SM, Pierce JS, Soodavar F, Smith KJ, Al Gadban MM, Rembiesa B, Klein RL, Hannun YA, Bielawski J, Bielawska A (2010) Blood sphingolipidomics in healthy humans: impact of sample collection methodology. J Lipid Res 51:3074–3087

Han X, Gross RW (1994) Electrospray ionization mass spectroscopic analysis of human erythrocyte plasma membrane phospholipids. Proc Natl Acad Sci U S A 91:10635–10639

Han X, Gross RW (2003) Global analyses of cellular lipidomes directly from crude extracts of biological samples by ESI mass spectrometry: a bridge to lipidomics. J Lipid Res 44:1071–1079

Hanamatsu H, Ohnishi S, Sakai S, Yuyama K, Mitsutake S, Takeda H, Hashino S, Igarashi Y (2014) Altered levels of serum sphingomyelin and ceramide containing distinct acyl chains in young obese adults. Nutr Diabetes 4:e141

Haus JM, Kashyap SR, Kasumov T, Zhang R, Kelly KR, Defronzo RA, Kirwan JP (2009) Plasma ceramides are elevated in obese subjects with type 2 diabetes and correlate with the severity of insulin resistance. Diabetes 58:337–343

Ho SY, Storch J (2001) Common mechanisms of monoacylglycerol and fatty acid uptake by human intestinal Caco-2 cells. Am J Physiol Cell Physiol 281:C1106–C1117

Hojjati MR, Li Z, Zhou H, Tang S, Huan C, Ooi E, Lu S, Jiang XC (2005) Effect of myriocin on plasma sphingolipid metabolism and atherosclerosis in apoE-deficient mice. J Biol Chem 280:10284–10289

Hu C, van Dommelen J, van der Heijden R, Spijksma G, Reijmers TH, Wang M, Slee E, Lu X, Xu G, van der Greef J, Hankemeier T (2008) RPLC-ion-trap-FTMS method for lipid profiling of plasma: method validation and application to p53 mutant mouse model. J Proteome Res 7:4982–4991

Huynh K, Barlow CK, Jayawardana KS, Weir JM, Mellett NA, Cinel M, Magliano DJ, Shaw JE, Drew BG, Meikle PJ (2019) High-throughput plasma lipidomics: detailed mapping of the associations with cardiometabolic risk factors. Cell Chem Biol 26:71–84.e74

Jang R, Kim KH, Zaidi SA, Cheong WJ, Moon MH (2011) Analysis of phospholipids using an open-tubular capillary column with a monolithic layer of molecularly imprinted polymer in capillary electrochromatography-electrospray ionization-tandem mass spectrometry. Electrophoresis 32:2167–2173

Jung UJ, Choi MS (2014) Obesity and its metabolic complications: the role of adipokines and the relationship between obesity, inflammation, insulin resistance, dyslipidemia and nonalcoholic fatty liver disease. Int J Mol Sci 15:6184–6223

Junot C, Fenaille F, Colsch B, Becher F (2014) High resolution mass spectrometry based techniques at the crossroads of metabolic pathways. Mass Spectrom Rev 33:471–500

Kang SC, Kim BR, Lee SY, Park TS (2013) Sphingolipid metabolism and obesity-induced inflammation. Front Endocrinol (Lausanne) 4:67

Katajamaa M, Miettinen J, Oresic M (2006) MZmine: toolbox for processing and visualization of mass spectrometry based molecular profile data. Bioinformatics 22:634–636

Kim JY, Park JY, Kim OY, Ham BM, Kim HJ, Kwon DY, Jang Y, Lee JH (2010) Metabolic profiling of plasma in overweight/obese and lean men using ultra performance liquid chromatography and Q-TOF mass spectrometry (UPLC-Q-TOF MS). J Proteome Res 9:4368–4375

Kliman M, May JC, McLean JA (2011) Lipid analysis and lipidomics by structurally selective ion mobility-mass spectrometry. Biochim Biophys Acta 1811:935–945

Kolter T, Sandhoff K (2006) Sphingolipid metabolism diseases. Biochim Biophys Acta 1758:2057–2079

Kontush A, Lhomme M, Chapman MJ (2013) Unraveling the complexities of the HDL lipidome. J Lipid Res 54:2950–2963

Laaksonen R, Ekroos K, Sysi-Aho M, Hilvo M, Vihervaara T, Kauhanen D, Suoniemi M, Hurme R, Marz W, Scharnagl H et al (2016) Plasma ceramides predict cardiovascular death in patients with stable coronary artery disease and acute coronary syndromes beyond LDL-cholesterol. Eur Heart J 37:1967–1976

Li F, Qin X, Chen H, Qiu L, Guo Y, Liu H, Chen G, Song G, Wang X, Li F et al (2013) Lipid profiling for early diagnosis and progression of colorectal cancer using direct-infusion electrospray ionization Fourier transform ion cyclotron resonance mass spectrometry. Rapid Commun Mass Spectrom 27:24–34

Liland KH, Almoy T, Mevik BH (2010) Optimal choice of baseline correction for multivariate calibration of spectra. Appl Spectrosc 64:1007–1016

Lofgren L, Stahlman M, Forsberg GB, Saarinen S, Nilsson R, Hansson GI (2012) The BUME method: a novel automated chloroform-free 96-well total lipid extraction method for blood plasma. J Lipid Res 53:1690–1700

Meikle PJ, Formosa MF, Mellett NA, Jayawardana KS, Giles C, Bertovic DA, Jennings GL, Childs W, Reddy M, Carey AL et al (2019) HDL phospholipids, but not cholesterol distinguish acute coronary syndrome from stable coronary artery disease. J Am Heart Assoc 8:e011792

Merrill AH Jr, Sullards MC, Allegood JC, Kelly S, Wang E (2005) Sphingolipidomics: high-throughput, structure-specific, and quantitative analysis of sphingolipids by liquid chromatography tandem mass spectrometry. Methods 36:207–224

Morrow DA (2010) Cardiovascular risk prediction in patients with stable and unstable coronary heart disease. Circulation 121:2681–2691

Murphy RC, Axelsen PH (2011) Mass spectrometric analysis of long-chain lipids. Mass Spectrom Rev 30:579–599

Murphy RC, Gaskell SJ (2011) New applications of mass spectrometry in lipid analysis. J Biol Chem 286:25427–25433

Mwinyi J, Bostrom A, Fehrer I, Othman A, Waeber G, Marti-Soler H, Vollenweider P, Marques-Vidal P, Schioth HB, von Eckardstein A, Hornemann T (2017) Plasma 1-deoxysphingolipids are early predictors of incident type 2 diabetes mellitus. PLoS One 12:e0175776

Othman A, Rutti MF, Ernst D, Saely CH, Rein P, Drexel H, Porretta-Serapiglia C, Lauria G, Bianchi R, von Eckardstein A, Hornemann T (2012) Plasma deoxysphingolipids: a novel class of biomarkers for the metabolic syndrome? Diabetologia 55:421–431

Othman A, Saely CH, Muendlein A, Vonbank A, Drexel H, von Eckardstein A, Hornemann T (2015a) Plasma 1-deoxysphingolipids are predictive biomarkers for type 2 diabetes mellitus. BMJ Open Diabetes Res Care 3:e000073

Othman A, Saely CH, Muendlein A, Vonbank A, Drexel H, von Eckardstein A, Hornemann T (2015b) Plasma C20-sphingolipids predict cardiovascular events independently from conventional cardiovascular risk factors in patients undergoing coronary angiography. Atherosclerosis 240:216–221

Puri R, Nissen SE, Libby P, Shao M, Ballantyne CM, Barter PJ, Chapman MJ, Erbel R, Raichlen JS, Uno K et al (2013) C-reactive protein, but not low-density lipoprotein cholesterol levels, associate with coronary atheroma regression and cardiovascular events after maximally intensive statin therapy. Circulation 128:2395–2403

Quehenberger O, Dennis EA (2011) The human plasma lipidome. N Engl J Med 365:1812–1823

Quehenberger O, Armando AM, Brown AH, Milne SB, Myers DS, Merrill AH, Bandyopadhyay S, Jones KN, Kelly S, Shaner RL et al (2010) Lipidomics reveals a remarkable diversity of lipids in human plasma. J Lipid Res 51:3299–3305

Ramprasath VR, Jones PJ, Buckley DD, Woollett LA, Heubi JE (2013) Effect of dietary sphingomyelin on absorption and fractional synthetic rate of cholesterol and serum lipid profile in humans. Lipids Health Dis 12:125

Razquin C, Liang L, Toledo E, Clish CB, Ruiz-Canela M, Zheng Y, Wang DD, Corella D, Castaner O, Ros E et al (2018) Plasma lipidome patterns associated with cardiovascular risk in the PREDIMED trial: a case-cohort study. Int J Cardiol 253:126–132

Rhee EP, Cheng S, Larson MG, Walford GA, Lewis GD, McCabe E, Yang E, Farrell L, Fox CS, O'Donnell CJ et al (2011) Lipid profiling identifies a triacylglycerol signature of insulin resistance and improves diabetes prediction in humans. J Clin Invest 121:1402–1411

Samad F, Hester KD, Yang G, Hannun YA, Bielawski J (2006) Altered adipose and plasma sphingolipid metabolism in obesity: a potential mechanism for cardiovascular and metabolic risk. Diabetes 55:2579–2587

Sandhoff K, Harzer K (2013) Gangliosides and gangliosidoses: principles of molecular and metabolic pathogenesis. J Neurosci 33:10195–10208

Schissel SL, Tweedie-Hardman J, Rapp JH, Graham G, Williams KJ, Tabas I (1996) Rabbit aorta and human atherosclerotic lesions hydrolyze the sphingomyelin of retained low-density lipoprotein. Proposed role for arterial-wall sphingomyelinase in subendothelial retention and aggregation of atherogenic lipoproteins. J Clin Invest 98:1455–1464

Schmelzer K, Fahy E, Subramaniam S, Dennis EA (2007) The lipid maps initiative in lipidomics. Methods Enzymol 432:171–183

Schwudke D, Schuhmann K, Herzog R, Bornstein SR, Shevchenko A (2011) Shotgun lipidomics on high resolution mass spectrometers. Cold Spring Harb Perspect Biol 3:a004614

Shih WJ, Bachorik PS, Haga JA, Myers GL, Stein EA (2000) Estimating the long-term effects of storage at −70 degrees C on cholesterol, triglyceride, and HDL-cholesterol measurements in stored sera. Clin Chem 46:351–364

Shiota Y, Kiyota K, Kobayashi T, Kano S, Kawamura M, Matsushima T, Miyazaki S, Uchino K, Hashimoto F, Hayashi E (2008) Distribution of dolichol in the serum and relationships between serum dolichol levels and various laboratory test values. Biol Pharm Bull 31:340–347

Siri-Tarino PW, Sun Q, Hu FB, Krauss RM (2010) Saturated fatty acids and risk of coronary heart disease: modulation by replacement nutrients. Curr Atheroscler Rep 12:384–390

Smith CA, Want EJ, O'Maille G, Abagyan R, Siuzdak G (2006) XCMS: processing mass spectrometry data for metabolite profiling using nonlinear peak alignment, matching, and identification. Anal Chem 78:779–787

Sorensen CM, Ding J, Zhang Q, Alquier T, Zhao R, Mueller PW, Smith RD, Metz TO (2010) Perturbations in the lipid profile of individuals with newly diagnosed type 1 diabetes mellitus: lipidomics analysis of a diabetes antibody standardization program sample subset. Clin Biochem 43:948–956

Stahlman M, Boren L, Ekross K (2012) High-throughput molecular lipidomics. In: Ekross K (ed) Lipidomics. Wiley-VCH Verlag GmbH & Co. KGaA, Weinheim, pp 35–51

Steinberg D (2005) Thematic review series: the pathogenesis of atherosclerosis. An interpretive history of the cholesterol controversy: part II: the early evidence linking hypercholesterolemia to coronary disease in humans. J Lipid Res 46:179–190

Steinberg D (2006) Thematic review series: the pathogenesis of atherosclerosis. An interpretive history of the cholesterol controversy, part V: the discovery of the statins and the end of the controversy. J Lipid Res 47:1339–1351

Summers SA (2006) Ceramides in insulin resistance and lipotoxicity. Prog Lipid Res 45:42–72

Sutter I, Velagapudi S, Othman A, Riwanto M, Manz J, Rohrer L, Rentsch K, Hornemann T, Landmesser U, von Eckardstein A (2015) Plasmalogens of high-density lipoproteins (HDL) are associated with coronary artery disease and anti-apoptotic activity of HDL. Atherosclerosis 241:539–546

Taguchi R, Ishikawa M (2010) Precise and global identification of phospholipid molecular species by an Orbitrap mass spectrometer and automated search engine lipid search. J Chromatogr A 1217:4229–4239

Tan L, Xing A, Zhao DL, Sun FR, Tan MS, Wan Y, Tan CC, Zhang W, Miao D, Yu JT, Tan L (2017) Strong association of lipid metabolism related microRNA binding sites polymorphisms with the risk of late onset Alzheimer's disease. Curr Neurovasc Res 14:3–10

Watson AD (2006) Thematic review series: systems biology approaches to metabolic and cardiovascular disorders. Lipidomics: a global approach to lipid analysis in biological systems. J Lipid Res 47:2101–2111

Wenk MR (2005) The emerging field of lipidomics. Nat Rev Drug Discov 4:594–610

Williams CM, Salter A (2016) Saturated fatty acids and coronary heart disease risk: the debate goes on. Curr Opin Clin Nutr Metab Care 19:97–102

Xia J, Wishart DS (2016) Using MetaboAnalyst 3.0 for comprehensive metabolomics data analysis. Curr Protoc Bioinformatics 55:14 10 11–14 10 91

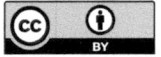

The Epigenome in Atherosclerosis

Sarah Costantino and Francesco Paneni

Contents

1   Discovery and Impact of Epigenetics 512
2   Classification of Epigenetic Modifications 513
    2.1   DNA Methylation 513
    2.2   Histone Posttranslational Modifications 516
3   Epigenetic Inheritance and Vascular Disease 517
4   Epigenetic Processing in Atherosclerotic Vascular Disease 519
    4.1   DNA Methylation 519
    4.2   Histone Posttranslational Modifications 522
5   Chromatin Signatures as Epigenetic Biomarkers in Atherosclerosis 524
6   Epigenetic Drugs 525
7   Conclusions 528
References 529

Abstract

Emerging evidence suggests the growing importance of "nongenetic factors" in the pathogenesis of atherosclerotic vascular disease. Indeed, the inherited genome determines only part of the risk profile as genomic approaches do not take into account additional layers of biological regulation by "epi"-genetic changes. Epigenetic modifications are defined as plastic chemical changes of DNA/histone complexes which critically affect gene activity without altering the DNA

S. Costantino
Center for Molecular Cardiology, University of Zürich, Zürich, Switzerland

F. Paneni (✉)
Center for Molecular Cardiology, University of Zürich, Zürich, Switzerland

University Heart Center, Cardiology, University Hospital Zürich, Zürich, Switzerland

Department of Research and Education, University Hospital Zürich, Zürich, Switzerland
e-mail: francesco.paneni@uzh.ch

© The Author(s) 2020   511
A. von Eckardstein, C. J. Binder (eds.), *Prevention and Treatment of Atherosclerosis*,
Handbook of Experimental Pharmacology 270, https://doi.org/10.1007/164_2020_422

sequence. These modifications include DNA methylation, histone posttranslational modifications, and non-coding RNAs and have the ability to modulate gene expression at both transcriptional and posttranscriptional level. Notably, epigenetic signals are mainly induced by environmental factors (i.e., pollution, smoking, noise) and, once acquired, may be transmitted to the offspring. The inheritance of adverse epigenetic changes may lead to premature deregulation of pathways involved in vascular damage and endothelial dysfunction. Here, we describe the emerging role of epigenetic modifications as fine-tuners of gene transcription in atherosclerosis. Specifically, the following aspects are described in detail: (1) discovery and impact of the epigenome in cardiovascular disease, (2) the epigenetic landscape in atherosclerosis; (3) inheritance of epigenetic signals and premature vascular disease; (4) epigenetic control of lipid metabolism, vascular oxidative stress, inflammation, autophagy, and apoptosis; (5) epigenetic biomarkers in patients with atherosclerosis; (6) novel therapeutic strategies to modulate epigenetic marks. Understanding the individual epigenetic profile may pave the way for new approaches to determine cardiovascular risk and to develop personalized therapies to treat atherosclerosis and its complications.

Keywords

Atherosclerotic plaque · Epigenetic therapies · Epigenome · Inflammation · Vascular disease

1   Discovery and Impact of Epigenetics

Although inborn genetic variation can influence disease susceptibility, accumulating evidence supports the notion that cardiovascular diseases (CVD) are heavily affected by non-genetic factors. Indeed, the inherited genome determines only part of the risk profile as genomic approaches do not take into account additional layers of biological regulation by "epi"-genetic changes – defined as acquired modifications to the genome subject to influence by the environment (Handy et al. 2011). The discovery of epigenetic modifications dates back to 1956, when the British developmental biologist Conrad Waddington demonstrated for the first time the inheritance of a characteristic acquired in a population in response to an environmental stimulus (Slack 2002). Waddington's experimental work showed that embryo fruit flies carrying an identical genetic background displayed different thorax and wing structures when exposed to different temperature or chemical stimuli (Noble 2015). While the term "epigenetics" initially embraced the process by which a fertilized zygote develops into a complex organism, the concept was refined over the next years by the observations that cells sharing the same genetic information can exhibit clear differences in gene expression. Waddington's work has contributed to understand that heritable traits can associate not only with changes in nucleotide sequence, but also with chemical modifications of DNA or proteins interacting with DNA. Later experiments in 1975 showed that epigenetic changes could be transmitted to daughter cells, thus regulating gene expression across multiple generations (Gonzalez-Recio et al. 2015). There are several examples outlining the importance of epigenetic processing in health and disease. First, epigenetic regulation of gene expression is a major determinant of cell fate. Epigenetic signals occurring at the levels of DNA and histones have the ability to license regions of the genome while shutting down others, thus favoring specific transcriptional programs which enable the differentiation of genetically identical pluripotent stem cells toward different cell types (i.e. myocytes, endothelial cells, adipocytes) (Brunet and Berger 2014). Along the same line, monozygotic twins who share an identical genetic make-up may display different physical and behavioral traits when raised under different environmental conditions (Fraga et al. 2005). Chronic exposure to different stimuli (i.e., pollution, noise) will enable the induction of specific epigenetic programs eventually leading to different gene expression profiles over the lifetime (Baccarelli and Ghosh 2012). Of note, epigenetic-induced deregulation of longevity genes was shown to accelerate cellular senescence and vascular aging (Sen et al. 2016). On the other hand, specific interventions such as caloric restriction have shown to delay age-dependent onset of diseases mostly via an epigenetic reprogramming. Taken together, epigenetic regulation of gene transcription represents a pivotal mechanism of adaptation to different environmental conditions and is among the most important mechanisms underlying cardiovascular diseases. A deep understanding of the epigenetic machinery may enable the characterization of cell-specific transcriptional programs in patients with atherosclerosis and could offer the tools for personalized therapeutic approaches to prevent cardiovascular diseases. The availability of new technologies for the study of our genome has indeed allowed a deep characterization of chromatin structure and function thus unveiling an array of epigenetic changes at the level of DNA and histones. This important information has enabled to understand inter-individual diversity and has prompted us to strive for an ever greater level of personalization in cardiovascular medicine.

2 Classification of Epigenetic Modifications

Epigenetic modifications fall into three main categories: (1) chemical modifications of DNA (i.e., methylation); (2) posttranslational modifications of histone tails; (3) regulation of gene expression by non-coding RNAs [i.e., microRNAs, PIWI-interacting RNAs, endogenous short interfering RNAs, long non-coding RNAs (lncRNAs)] (Fig. 1). The present chapter will focus on the role of chromatin modifications in atherosclerosis. The function of ncRNAs in this setting is described extensively in a different chapter.

2.1 DNA Methylation

Nuclear DNA is tightly wrapped around a core of eight histone proteins (two copies each of H2A, H2B, H3, and H4), generating repetitive units known as nucleosomes.

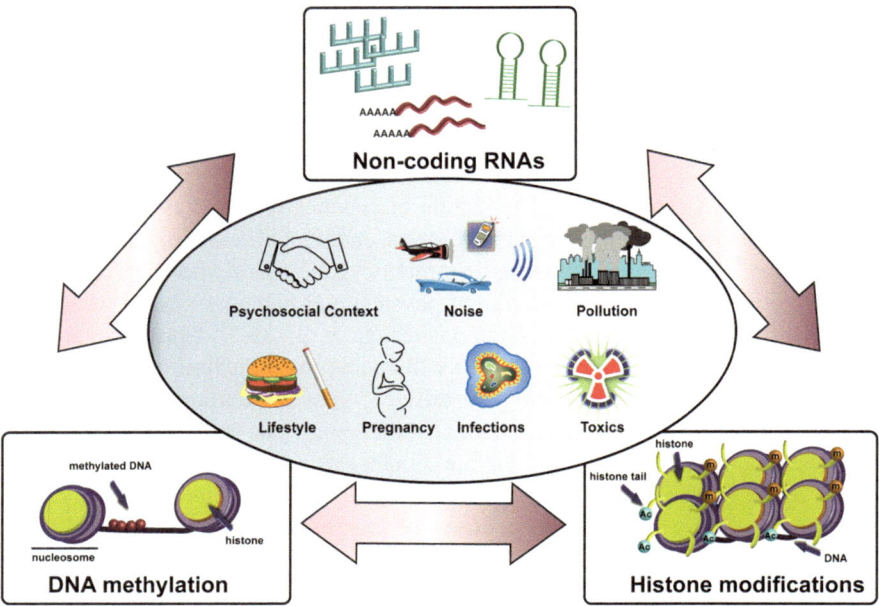

Fig. 1 Role of epigenetic inheritance in vascular disease. Environmental factors induce epigenetic changes which are transmitted to the offspring, thus leading to maladaptive transcriptional programs responsible for early vascular damage

These structures enable a very efficient packaging of DNA within the cell nucleus, through the formation of chromatin. Despite its complex three-dimensional structure, chromatin is a very dynamic entity where DNA and histones can be chemically modified. This alters the accessibility of transcriptional factors to genes and, thus, modulates transcription (Goldberg et al. 2007).

DNA methylation plays an important role in the regulation of chromatin structure and gene expression, and therefore, participates in a variety of biological processes (Hamidi et al. 2015), including tissue-specific regulation of gene expression, genomic imprinting, X chromosome inactivation, silencing of transposable elements, and defense against viral sequences (Prasher et al. 2019). This epigenetic modification is relatively stable, it is tissue-specific and can be transmitted to the offspring (Izquierdo and Crujeiras 2019). Methylation of DNA mainly occurs through attachment of methyl group (CH3) from S-adenosyl methionine (SAM) to the C5 position in the cytosine-paired-with-guanine (CpG) dinucleotide sequences thus forming 5-methylcytosine (5mC) (Davis and Gallagher 2019). Furthermore, non-CpG methylation (i.e., CHG or CHH region) may also occur and this signature is usually observed in embryonic stem cells (Bernstein et al. 2007).

CpG sequences are generally located into promoter regions of genes, however, they can also be located within gene bodies (Costantino et al. 2015). Promoter methylation is generally associated with transcriptional repression, while gene body methylation is associated with enhanced transcription (Maunakea et al. 2010). Although both transcriptional repression and activation have been reported, DNA methylation leads – in >95% of cases – to gene silencing (Xiao et al. 2019). Specifically, methylated cytosines are recognized by DNA methyl-binding proteins (MBPs) that prevent the binding of transcription factors to DNA (Prasher et al. 2019). Alternatively, DNA methylation may recruit specific proteins, such as the methyl-CpG binding protein 2 (MeCP2), that specifically bind to methylated regions to foster transcriptional repression (Jones et al. 1998). Besides methylation, other chemical modifications of cytosine have been identified, such as hydroxymethylation, formylation, and carboxylation, but their interrelation with methylation is not completely understood yet (Elia and Condorelli 2019).

DNA methylation is catalyzed by the DNA methyltransferase 1 (DNMT1), 3a (DNMT3a), and 3b (DNMT3b) and is reversed by Tet methylcytosine dioxygenases (TET1, 2, and 3) (Xu et al. 2018). Among these enzymes, Dnmt1 is responsible for the maintenance of methylation patterns in the genome by replicating the hemi-methylated CpG sites (Vilkaitis et al. 2005), whereas Dnmt3a/b are considered de novo methyltransferases (Okano et al. 1999). The activity of DNMT1 has been demonstrated to be dependent on a co-factor that recognizes hemi-methylated DNA. The Ubiquitin-like with PHD and Ring Finger Domains 1 (UHRF1), were shown to be essential for maintenance of the methylation status of DNA by directing the recruitment of DNMT1 to the replication forks (Bostick et al. 2007). DNMT3 can also methylate non-CpG sites (at CpA and CHG) and the presence of methylated non-CpG sites in the human genome indicates that there is ongoing de novo DNA methylation at each round of genome replication (Aavik et al. 2019).

DNA demethylation can be achieved by either passive or active mechanisms (Costantino et al. 2015). Passive demethylation can be the result of Dnmt1 inhibition during cell replication (Wolffe et al. 1999) while active demethylation is modulated by DNA demethylases. DNA demethylation may follow two main pathways: the first is dependent on cytosine deamination (AID, APOBEC3G, FTO) while the second is dependent on the oxidation of methylated cytosines (Aavik et al. 2019). The latter reaction is catalyzed by members of the Ten-eleven translocation (TET) proteins family (TET1-3) which convert 5-methylcytosine (5mC) into 5-hydroxymethylcytosine (5hmC) (Wu and Zhang 2010). TET1 is mostly found in embryonic stem cells, whereas TET2 and TET3 are ubiquitously expressed (Costantino et al. 2015). TET1 is low in normal tissues, whereas TET2 is an abundant protein in most tissues/cell types and TET3 expression is overlapping with TET2 in many tissues (Kohli and Zhang 2013). The observed abundance of TET2 and TET3 enzymes in various tissues indicates that DNA demethylation must have an important role in cellular homeostasis (Aavik et al. 2019). The TET family enzymes represent promising therapeutic targets given their ability to oxidize 5mC thus leading to the reversal of gene repression by DNA methylation (Greco et al. 2016).

2.2   Histone Posttranslational Modifications

DNA is packaged into repeating units called nucleosomes by wrapping around multimeric histone proteins. When nucleosomes are organized into tightly packed bundles (heterochromatin), the transcriptional machinery is hampered by a reduction of chromatin accessibility. Conversely, when chromatin is relaxed (euchromatin), DNA is more accessible to transcription factors and gene transcription may occur. Each histone (H) protein is an octamer comprised of 2 sets of H2A, H2B, H3, and H4 proteins with a single histone H1 linker protein between nucleosomes. Each histone subunit has an N-terminal tail containing a lysine (K) residue that protrudes away from the surface of the histone octamer creating an exposed surface (Davis and Gallagher 2019). Histones are amenable to many posttranslational modifications (PTMs), which include methylation, acetylation, ubiquitination, phosphorylation, SUMOylation, GlcNAcylation, carbonylation, and ADP-ribosylation (Zhang et al. 2018). Histone modifications are induced by specific enzymes that act predominantly at histone N-terminal tails primarily involving the amino acids lysine (K) and arginine (R). These modifications can be present on multiple (but specific) sites on histones (Kouzarides 2007).

In addition to DNA modifications, PTMs of histone tails may serve as a repressive or activating signal depending on the specific histone tail, the number of groups added, and the region of chromatin where the modification occurs (Bauer and Martin 2017). Although the biological significance of many PTMs remains to be elucidated, considerable advances have been made in the understanding of lysine acetylation and methylation (Bernstein et al. 2007). The first PTM reported is histone acetylation, an epigenetic signature characterized by the addition of positively charged acetyl groups to amino acid residues on the histones, which neutralizes the negative charges of DNA. This modification reduces the affinity of the histone for DNA and consequently results in the formation of a more relaxed chromatin structure, eventually increasing chromatin accessibility (Nicorescu et al. 2019). Acetylation occurs mainly on lysine residues on histones H3 and H4; this mark mainly associates with activation of transcription by enhancing chromatin accessibility (Gillette and Hill 2015). In this context, bromodomain and extra-terminal proteins recognize histone acetylation marks and initiate the assembly of the transcriptional machinery (Filippakopoulos and Knapp 2014). Acetylation is modulated by histone acetyltransferases (HATs) and histone deacetylases (HDACs) which are involved in the addition or removal of an acetyl group, respectively (Baccarelli and Ghosh 2012). This modification is driven by recognition and binding of transcription factors able to recruit one of a growing family of HATs, namely CBP/p300, MYST, and GNAT (Kouzarides 2007). Under physiological conditions, lysine residues on histone tails are positively charged and can bind DNA which is a negatively charged molecule due to its phosphate components. The interaction between histone and DNA favors a compact chromatin structure, with scarce accessibility to transcription factors. Conversely, when lysine residues are acetylated they lose their positive charge, thus favoring an open chromatin and, hence, enhanced gene expression (Costantino et al. 2015). HATs catalyze the addition of two-carbon acetyl groups to lysine residues from acetyl-CoA (Carrozza et al. 2003). On the other hand, removal of acetyl groups from histone residues by HDACs represses gene transcription (Stratton et al. 2019). Specifically, HDACs catalyze removal of acetyl groups from lysine residues and are distributed among four classes (Class I, IIa, IIb, III, and IV) (Haberland et al. 2009).

In contrast to lysine acetylation, a process known to enhance gene expression, histone methylation is a more complex modification which may result in different chromatin states according to the methylated residue and the number of added methyl groups (Cooper and El-Osta 2010). For instance, the lysine residues at positions 4, 9, and 27 on histone H3 can be methylated to different levels (mono-, bi-, and tri-methylation), resulting in different states of chromatin accessibility (Elia and Condorelli 2019). Histone methylation is defined as the transfer of methyl group from S-adenosyl-L-methionine to lysine or arginine residues of histone proteins by histone methyltransferases (HMTs). While lysines may be mono-, di-, or tri-methylated, arginines may be monomethylated or demethylated (symmetrically or asymmetrically) (Bannister and Kouzarides 2011). Histone methyltransferases (HMTs) include the EZH, SETD, PRDM, PRMT, METTL, and MLL enzyme families (Stratton et al. 2019).

Over the last few years, a well-established theory was that histone turnover was the only mechanism regulating histone methylation. More recently, histone demethylases (HDMs) have been reported as a novel mechanism capable of demethylating lysine residues on histone tails (Handy et al. 2011). Indeed, histone methylation is a very dynamic process regulated by histone demethylases, which remove the methyl groups from lysine residues with a high gene specificity (Tsukada et al. 2006). HDMs include members of UTX/Y, JARID1, JMJD, LSD, PHF, and FBXL enzyme families (Stratton et al. 2019).

Two important studies have identified the first HDM, lysine demethylase 1 (LSD1) which is able to remove methyl group from H3K4 and H3K9, suggesting that lysine demethylation is subjected to dynamic modulation (Metzger et al. 2005). Several lysine demethylases specific for diverse histone lysine residues have been identified (Costantino et al. 2015). A better comprehension of how such demethylases are regulated during disease states is of paramount importance.

Interestingly, studies have shown that DNA methylase (DNMTs), histone methyltransferase (HMTs), and histone acetyltransferase (HATs) are closely interconnected to regulate chromatin remodelling under specific stimuli (Li et al. 2007). For example, H3K9 methylation induces DNA methylation while CpG methylation favors H3K9m (Cedar and Bergman 2009). Therefore, chromatin modifications may influence each other and can propagate.

3 Epigenetic Inheritance and Vascular Disease

An important aspect to consider when dealing with epigenetics is that epigenetic modifications are heritable. Epigenetic signals acquired during the lifetime are transmitted to the offspring, where they participate to determine substantial changes

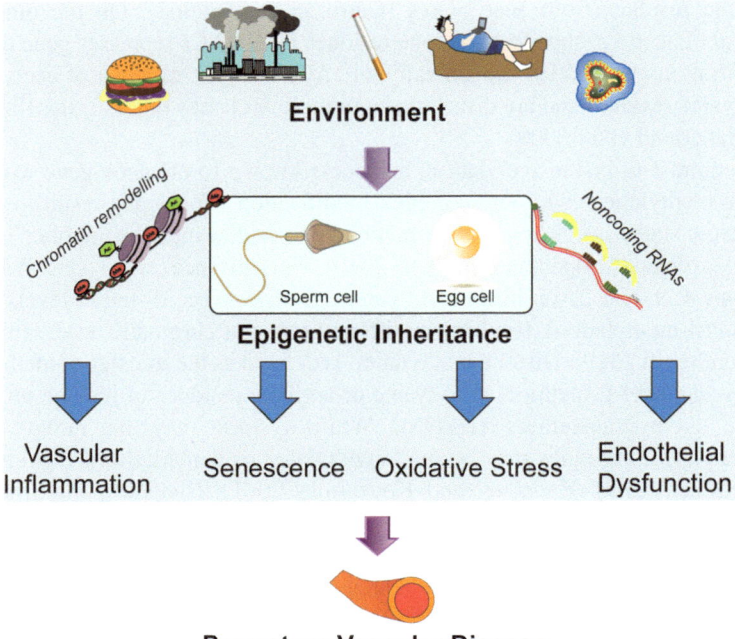

Fig. 2 Epigenetic changes and environmental factors. Exposure to different environmental factors induces several epigenetic modifications. These entail changes of DNA methylation, posttranslational histone modifications, and altered expression of non-coding RNAs. Reproduced with permission from Costantino et al. Eur Heart J. 2018;39:4150–4158

in phenotype (Fig. 2) (Heard and Martienssen 2014). In the Överkalix study, conducted in northern Sweden to investigate the physiological effects of various environmental factors on transgenerational epigenetic inheritance, three cohorts born in 1890, 1905, and 1920 were studied until death. The study showed that overeating during a child's slow growth period (SGP), before their prepubertal peak in growth velocity, influences descendants' risk of death from cardiovascular disease and diabetes (Pembrey et al. 2006). If food was not readily available during the father's slow growth period, then cardiovascular disease mortality of the proband was low. By contrast, diabetes mortality increased if the paternal grandfather was exposed to a surfeit of food during his slow growth period (Odds Ratio 4.1, 95% confidence interval 1.33–12.93, $P = 0.01$) (Pembrey et al. 2006). This study was one of the first to demonstrate that a nutrition-linked mechanism through the male line seems to have influenced the risk of developing cardiovascular and metabolic diseases. Periconceptional diet was shown to influence DNA methylation levels with phenotypic consequences. A genome-scale analysis of differential DNA methylation in whole blood after periconceptional exposure to the Dutch Hunger Winter famine revealed changes of differentially methylated regions (Tobi et al. 2014). These changes were preferentially observed at regulatory regions of genes relevant for metabolic homeostasis, inflammation and longevity, key processes underlying the pathogenesis of atherosclerosis. Specifically, individuals conceived during the Dutch famine showed, six decades later, reduced methylation levels at the promoter of insulin-like growth factor type 2 (IGF-2), a gene regulating of glucose homeostasis, cardiovascular function, and lipid metabolism (Heijmans et al. 2008). Overall, these data suggest that epigenetic modulation of pathways by prenatal malnutrition may promote adverse cardiometabolic phenotypes during childhood. Inheritance of specific epigenetic patterns may contribute to explain the alarming increase in childhood obesity from 32 million in 1990 to around 42 million in 2016 (Brown et al. 2015). Notably, early metabolic alterations in obese children are associated with low-grade inflammation, high oxidative stress levels, impaired nitric oxide bioavailability, endothelial dysfunction, and arterial stiffness (Suglia et al. 2018). Macrophage polarization and adipose tissue inflammation are also important features commonly found in obese children (Singer and Lumeng 2017). Epigenetic modulation of inflammation is supported by the notion that promoter methylation of *TNF-α*, pyruvate dehydrogenase kinase 4 (*PDK4*), and leptin (*LEP*) are all reduced in obese as compared to lean children, while methylation of peroxisome proliferator-activated receptor gamma coactivator 1-alpha (*PGC-1α*) and proopiomelanocortin (*POMC)* genes are increased (Garcia-Cardona et al. 2014). As a consequence of these alterations, risk of diabetes, dyslipidemia, and silent heart disease are significantly higher in obese as compared to non-obese children (Juonala et al. 2011). Despite emerging evidence indicates the existence of a transgenerational epigenetic inheritance in humans, data still remain inconclusive due to relevant confounders represented by genetic, ecological, and cultural inheritance. Parents and offspring may share the same epigenomic features, but it is challenging to understand whether these features are being transmitted through the germline or are newly established in each generation by the action of shared genes and shared environments (Horsthemke 2018). The most difficult aspect in humans is the demonstration that a specific epigenetic factor in the germ cells is responsible for the phenotypic effect in the next generation. While this phenomenon was clearly described in plants, nematodes, and fruit flies, its occurrence in humans remains controversial. This important aspect of epigenetic regulation is the object of intense investigation and future studies will contribute to clarify the contribution of inheritable epigenetic traits to global vascular risk in humans.

4 Epigenetic Processing in Atherosclerotic Vascular Disease

4.1 DNA Methylation

Reduced DNA methylation is an important signature of atherosclerotic lesions both in humans and in experimental models, such as apolipoprotein E knockout mice (*Apoe*$^{-/-}$) and neointima of balloon-denuded New Zealand White (NZW) rabbit aortas (Napoli et al. 2012). Several studies have shown profound changes of atherosclerosis-specific methylated CpGs in human atherosclerotic plaques

EPIGENETIC LANDSCAPE IN ATHEROSCLEROSIS

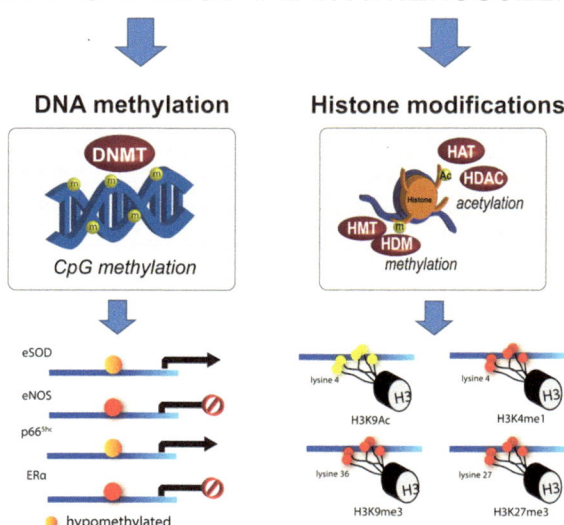

Fig. 3 Alterations of the chromatin landscape in atherosclerosis. *HAT* histone methyltransferase, *HDAC* histone deacetylase, *HMT* histone methyltransferase, *HDM* histone demethylase, *H3* histone 3, *K* lysine residue

(hypomethylation of 3,997 promoter sites = 84%) with a progressive increase in gene methylation as the lesions matured (Aavik et al. 2015). Global hypomethylation of DNA in human aortic lesions was the result of a near-complete demethylation of the subset of CpG islands that were hypermethylated in control aortas (Aavik et al. 2019). Beside global variations in methylation status, alterations in the methylation pattern of specific genes have been causally implicated in the pathogenesis of atherosclerosis. Methylation of genes regulating cellular proliferation, namely genes encoding for estrogen receptor-α (ERα) was found in atherosclerotic plaques from human subjects (Fig. 3). Moreover, ERα gene was also shown to be methylated in vascular smooth muscle cells (SMCs) in vitro during their phenotypic switch (Aavik et al. 2019). Methylation-dependent increase in proliferation of SMCs may represent an important epigenetic mechanism underpinning atherogenesis. Indeed – under physiological conditions – arterial SMCs are terminally differentiated and replication does not occur. This associates with a low activity of the epigenetic machinery. By contrast, during lesion development, changes in DNA methylation affect transcriptional programs fostering SMCs proliferation. The effects of DNA methylation may be the direct result of gene hypomethylation or can be due to methylation-induced alterations of DNA integrity and function. DNA hypomethylation of 15-lipoxygenase and extracellular superoxide dismutase (eSOD) genes were found during SMCs replications (Napoli et al. 2012). Epigenetic remodelling of growth regulatory genes such as platelet-derived growth factor and c-*myc* might also contribute to SMCs proliferation (Hiltunen and Yla-Herttuala

2003). De novo methylation of genes is the most plausible mechanism to explain the dynamic effects of epigenetic processing in atherosclerosis. Intervention studies in cellular models have clearly shown that treatment with the methylation inhibitor 5-azadeoxycytidine heavily affects gene expression in vitro and in vivo (Yang et al. 2010). The importance of de novo methylation is supported by the notion that overexpression of Dnmt, an enzyme which lacks de novo methylation activity, does not reverse genomic hypomethylation in cancer (Zhang and Xu 2017).

The accumulation of reactive oxygen species (ROS) is a key promoter of epigenetic signatures. It has been shown that ROS may foster changes in DNA methylation, and in turn, methylation chances may induce the upregulation of pro-oxidant genes. Reduced methylation of CpG islands at the promoter of the *shc1* gene, encoding for the mitochondrial adaptor p66^{Shc}, has been associated with high oxidative stress levels, mitochondrial insufficiency, apoptosis, and endothelial dysfunction (Paneni et al. 2012). Both diabetic mice and humans display reduced DNA methylation of *shc1* promoter in the vasculature and the heart, and this epigenetic signature persists despite intensive glycemic control (Paneni et al. 2012; Costantino et al. 2017). Interestingly, epigenetic reprogramming by selective targeting of dnmt3b restores promoter methylation thus repressing p66^{Shc} transcription (Costantino et al. 2018a). Other genes implicated in oxidative stress and vascular disease, namely the AP-1 transcription factor JunD and the prolyil-isomerase-1 (Pin1) were also shown to be modulated by specific changes of CpG methylation (Paneni et al. 2013, 2015a). DNA methylation was also reported to affect the expression of inflammatory genes including TNF-α, COX-2, and IL-1β (Stylianou 2019). Genetic deletion of Tet methylcytosine dioxygenase 2 (TET2) in macrophages leads to increased expression of inflammatory cytokines and chemokines in response to native LDL (Peng et al. 2016). A similar increase in plasma interleukin-8 was observed in people with TET2 mutations but not in those without the mutations suggesting that control of DNA methylation by TET2 regulates inflammation in atherosclerosis (Fuster et al. 2017).

Atherosclerosis and ageing are highly interconnected, and age-dependent epigenetic modifications may significantly contribute to vascular disease (Paneni et al. 2017). Aging is generally associated with a progressive decline in global DNA methylation (Hannum et al. 2013). Indeed, DNA methylation content assessed by whole-genome bisulfite is heavily reduced in centenarians as compared with newborns (Heyn et al. 2012). Reduced DNA methylation at the promoter of genes associated with self-renewal was also found in stem cells isolated from aged versus young subjects and associated with functional defects and reduced ability to differentiate (Sun et al. 2014). DNMT3A, TET2, and ASXL1 are key regulators of DNA methylation status and their deregulation is associated with clonal expansion in hematopoiesis and functional defects, a phenomenon known as clonal hematopoiesis of indeterminate potential (CHIP). CHIP was found to be associated with an increased risk of CVD, stroke, coronary calcification, malignancies, and all-cause mortality (Jaiswal et al. 2017). Dnmt3a gene was the most recurrently mutated in individuals with CHIP. Hematopoietic tissue-specific conditional Dnmt3a deletion in mouse models led to a progressive expansion of long-term HSC with impaired differentiation by incomplete epigenetic repression of HSC-specific genes (Challen et al. 2011). Hematopoietic tissue-specific Tet2 loss leads to decreased levels of 5hmC, increased stem cell self-renewal, delayed HSC differentiation, and skewed development toward the monocyte/macrophage lineage (Moran-Crusio et al. 2011). Thus, hematopoietic stressors can induce stable epigenetic reprogramming of bone marrow HSCs contributing to clonal hematopoiesis and myeloid skewing. Albeit DNMT3A and TET2 exert opposite functions in terms of DNA methylation, a recent study showed that these chromatin modifiers both repress the erythroid regulator *Klf1* suggesting a model of cooperative inhibition resulting in HSCs transformation (Zhang et al. 2016). Methylation changes at the promoter of eNOS, GATA-2, and GATA-3 during aging were also associated with functional defects and reduced differentiation potential of endothelial progenitor cells (EPCs), whereas reprogramming approaches aimed at restoring promoter methylation of these genes contributed to cell rejuvenation and longevity (Chan et al. 2004). Beside modulating EPCs functionality, DNA methylation directly regulates endothelial cell function mainly via TET2 signaling. TET2 promotes endothelial autophagy and downregulates inflammatory factors such as VCAM1, ICAM1, MCP1, and IL-1β in lesions of high fat fed $ApoE^{-/-}$ mice (Peng et al. 2016). Moreover, TET2 overexpression decreased the methylation levels of Beclin-1 promoter, thus leading to increased endothelial cell autophagy and decreased inflammatory factors in endothelial cells exposed to oxidized LDL (Li et al. 2015). Epigenetic changes of p66^{Shc} and eNOS have also shown to affect endothelial function in vivo as well as in patients with obesity and type 2 diabetes (Costantino et al. 2017, 2019).

4.2 Histone Posttranslational Modifications

Growing evidence indicates that posttranslational modifications of histones, mainly at lysine and arginine residues, significantly affect chromatin accessibility thus enabling cell-specific transcriptional programs implicated in the pathophysiology of atherosclerotic vascular disease (Jiang et al. 2018) (Fig. 3). Chromatin modifications play a pivotal role in regulating vascular inflammation by epigenetic modulation of nuclear factor kappa-B (NF-kB) signaling. Several cardiovascular risk factors have shown to modulate histone marks and gene expression. In primary human aortic endothelial cells, hyperglycemia induces a specific mono-methylation of histone 3 at lysine 4 (H3K4m1) thus enabling chromatin accessibility at the level of NF-kB p65 promoter (El-Osta et al. 2008). Hyperglycemia-related H3K4m1 is induced by the mammalian methyltransferase SETD7, which is emerging as a key player in the regulation of vascular inflammation and oxidative stress (Okabe et al. 2012). Several stimuli, including reactive oxygen species are able to increase SETD7 activity. Indeed, overexpression of scavenger enzymes (e.g., uncoupling protein-1) blunted SETD7-dependent H3K4m1 and subsequent activation of NF-kB p65 and downstream inflammatory genes, namely MCP-1, VCAM-1, and ICAM-1 (El-Osta et al. 2008). Of note, SETD7 expression is increased in peripheral blood monocytes from patients with type 2 diabetes, and correlated with endothelial function and oxidative stress levels, as assessed by flow-mediated dilation (FMD) of the brachial artery and urinary levels of isoPGF$_{2\alpha}$, respectively (Paneni et al. 2015b). Moreover, SETD7 induction positively correlated with the expression of proatherosclerotic genes including COX-2, iNOS, and VCAM-1 (Paneni et al. 2015b). Chromatin immunoprecipitation experiments revealed that SETD7 specifically binds a specific region of the human NF-kB p65 promoter thus fostering the expression of inflammatory genes. Beside SETD7, other chromatin modifiers such as the methyltransferase Suv39h1 and LSD1 have shown their ability to modulate NF-kB-dependent inflammatory genes (IL-6 and MCP-1) by reducing the levels of dimethylation (H3K9m2) and trimethylation of H3 at lysine 9 (H3K9m3) in SMCs (Brasacchio et al. 2009). Suv39h1 gain- and loss-of-function approaches in experimental models of type 2 diabetes showed that H3K9m2 and H3K9m3 can be dynamically modulated thus reverting the SMCs phenotype. Histone acetyltransferases, such as CBP/p300 and p/CAF, were found to be critically involved in the NF-kB signaling and upregulation of TNF-α and COX-2, master regulators of the atherosclerotic process (Deng et al. 2004). Mechanistically, p300 interacts with the p65 (RELA) subunit of NF-kB in the nucleus to displace repressive p50– HDAC1 interactions (Ashburner et al. 2001). This results in increased acetylation of both p65 itself and histones in proximity of NF-kB promoter. The p65–p300 interaction has been found to be critical for the inflammatory activation of both macrophages and endothelial cells (Jiang et al. 2018). The relevance of this epigenetic route is supported by the notion that inhibition of p300 by curcumin enhances macrophage cholesterol efflux in human and mouse macrophages in vitro, and exerts an anti-inflammatory effect by suppressing NF-kB activity (Khyzha et al. 2017). Deregulation of histone deacetylases, namely sirtuins, also represents a major underpinning of vascular disease and atherosclerosis via modulation of oxidative stress, endothelial function, inflammation, mitochondrial bioenergetics, and cellular metabolism (Winnik et al. 2015). SIRT1 activity is reduced in patients with obesity and significantly contributes to endothelial dysfunction (Masi et al. 2020). By contrast, pharmacological activation of SIRT1 by resveratrol restores endothelial function and NO availability and attenuates dyslipidemia and obesity-induced metabolic alterations in human subjects (Carrizzo et al. 2013). Overexpression of SIRT1 in endothelial cells increases their sprouting and migration, whereas SIRT1 depletion impairs angiogenic response, mainly via FLT1 and CXCR4 (Potente et al. 2007). SIRT1 was also found to regulate the transcription of the mitochondrial adaptor p66[Shc], thus leading to oxidative stress and endothelial dysfunction (Zhou et al. 2011; Mohammed et al. 2020). Furthermore, pharmacological activation of SIRT1 by visfatin has shown to attenuate oxLDL-induced senescence of EPCs through the PI3K/Akt/ERK pathway (Ming et al. 2016). SIRT3 and SIRT6 have also recently emerged as an essential regulator of endothelial cell senescence and angiogenesis, key alterations commonly observed in atherosclerosis (Costantino et al. 2018b). Deregulation of chromatin modifying enzymes SUV39H1, JMJD2C, and SRC-1 in visceral fat arteries from obese patients was associated with increased di-(H3K9me2) and trimethylation (H3K9me3) as well as acetylation (H3K9ac) of histone 3 lysine 9 (H3K9) (Costantino et al. 2019). This epigenetic pattern was found to promote transcriptional signatures involved in endothelial ROS generation and vascular dysfunction. Interestingly, in vivo editing of SUV39H1, JMJD2C, and SRC-1 blunted obesity-related endothelial dysfunction in obese mice (Costantino et al. 2019). Other histone deacetylases have shown to affect the atherosclerotic phenotype, although often with conflicting results. HDAC3, HDAC5, and HDAC7 were shown to repress KLF2 expression in human endothelial cells, while their overexpression fostered a proatherogenic phenotype (Kwon et al. 2014). In mice, HDAC3 and HDAC9 deletion in macrophages favors the upregulation of pro-inflammatory signatures eventually leading to a proatherosclerotic phenotype (Stratton et al. 2019). Consistently, $Apoe^{-/-}$ mice with endothelial specific deletion of HDAC3 displayed increased neointimal formation, suggesting an atheroprotective role of endothelial HDAC3 (Zampetaki et al. 2010). Along the same line, $Ldlr^{-/-}$ mice treated with the HDAC inhibitor Trichostatin A exhibited increased plaque size and enhanced macrophage infiltration (Choi et al. 2005). In rats, HDACs are upregulated in aortic SMCs under mitogenic stimulation and their inhibition alters the expression of cell cycle genes, resulting in diminished SMC proliferation, which might be expected to be atheroprotective (Findeisen et al. 2011).

Specific chromatin modifications occurring in macrophages, namely increased activity of the demethylase JMJD3, were also found to act as pivotal regulator of pro-inflammatory cytokines (i.e., TNFα), by erasing the H3K27me3 mark (Yan et al. 2014). Further work is needed to test whether chemical inhibition of JMJD3 has a protective effect in atherosclerotic mouse models. Technologies to probe H3K27me3 and other histone PTMs genome-wide in small samples will be vital to fully understand the cause and consequence of epigenetic changes that occur during atherogenesis.

5   Chromatin Signatures as Epigenetic Biomarkers in Atherosclerosis

Epigenetic signals acquired during the life course can be employed as potential biomarkers of cardiovascular disease. Indeed, modifications of the epigenetic landscape may reflect dynamic changes in expression of genes relevant to vascular homeostasis. A global reduction of DNA methylation was reported in patients with coronary atherosclerosis. The evaluation of the methylation status of LINE-1 due to its high representation in the human genome (55%) and its high methylation levels can be used to evaluate global methylation changes (Aavik et al. 2019). Hypomethylation of the IL-6 promoter, leading to its upregulation and systemic inflammation, was also associated with a higher risk of coronary heart disease (Zuo et al. 2016). The promoter of two atheroprotective genes, namely the estrogen receptor α (ESR1) and estrogen receptor β (ESR2), was hypermethylated in atherosclerotic vascular tissues as well as in cultured vascular SMCs (Napoli et al. 2012). Age-related mutations of key epigenetic regulators including DNMT3A, TET2, and ASXL1 in hematopoietic stem cells (HSCs) is emerging as a major mechanism underlying clonal expansion of HSCs, a phenomenon known as clonal hematopoiesis of indeterminate potential (CHIP) (Li et al. 2018). Notably, the presence of CHIP was associated with an increased risk of CVD and all-cause mortality (Jaiswal et al. 2017). In the northern Sweden population health study, individuals with a history of MI showed differential DNA methylation at 211 CpG-sites representing genes related to CVD, cardiac function, cardiogenesis and recovery after ischemic injury (Rask-Andersen et al. 2016). Hence, epigenetic information may explain the alterations in cardiovascular gene expression trajectories and offer biomarkers for the follow-up of these patients. Overall, available evidence suggests that the epigenome represents a fundamental biological layer in the regulation of gene expression, and epigenetic information may contribute to advance CV risk stratification. The "epigenetic landscape" may provide a real post-genomic snapshot offering the tools to build individual maps of CV risk (Costantino et al. 2018c). Hence, epigenetic changes accumulated during the lifetime may be employed to customize diagnostic and therapeutic approaches in primary and secondary prevention of CVD. Individual epigenetic maps will be invaluable to define new risk scores predicting beyond traditional calculators. This innovative approach will be invaluable for the development of personalized therapies in patients with atherosclerosis (Fig. 4).

6   Epigenetic Drugs

Targeting epigenetic modifications is a highly promising approach to restore gene expression and to rescue or prevent alterations of vascular phenotype (Masi et al. 2020; Landmesser et al. 2020). There are several examples of how specific interventions can be employed to modify the landscape of DNA/histone modifications (Table 1). Emerging evidence indicates that circulating angiogenic cells (CACs), endothelial progenitor cells (EPCs) and, more in general, bone marrow-derived stem cells are critically involved in vascular repair and maintenance of vascular homeostasis via different mechanisms which include local engraftment and paracrine actions. Epigenetic mechanisms substantially contribute to the functional decline of these cells during life (Costantino et al. 2018b). Indeed, DNA methylation is decreased at the promoter of genes associated with self-renewal, whereas promoters of genes regulating differentiation are generally hypermethylated (Sun et al. 2014). Pharmacological blockade of the DNA methyltransferase by RG108 has shown to rejuvenate BM-derived stem cells by resetting the expression of senescence-related genes (Oh et al. 2015). These findings may open perspectives for the ex vivo epigenetic reprogramming of BM-derived cells for the treatment of atherosclerosis and ischemic heart failure. However, pharmacological editing of global DNA methylation lacks specificity and may be associated with undesirable effects, such as autoimmune diseases (lupus erythematosus was reported in 25–30% of patients) (Chen et al. 2017). The relevance of epigenetic drugs is outlined by the notion that several of these compounds are being tested in clinical trials for the treatment of cancer, neurological and cardiovascular diseases (Costantino et al. 2015). More than 20 years ago, Decitabine (5-aza-2′-deoxycytidine) was found to

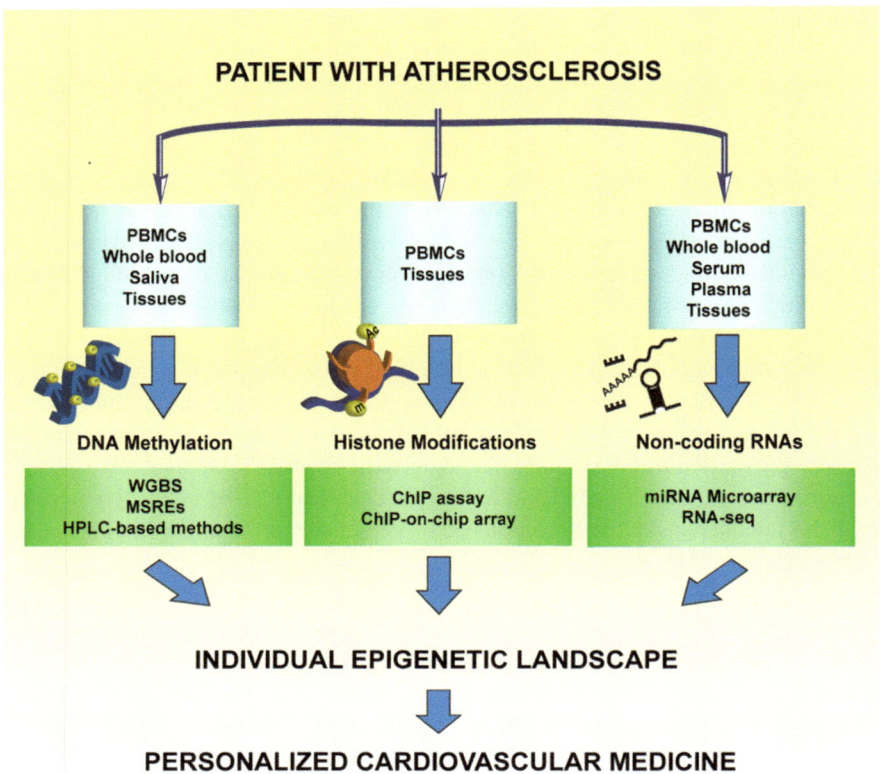

Fig. 4 Approaches to detect epigenetic biomarkers in patients with atherosclerosis. *PBMCs* peripheral blood mononuclear cells, *WGBS* whole-genome bisulfite sequencing, *MSREs* methylation sensitive restriction enzymes, *HPLC* high-performance liquid chromatography, *ChIP* chromatin immunoprecipitation, *miRNAs* microRNAs, *RNA-seq* RNA sequencing. Modified from Costantino et al. Eur Heart J. 2018;39:4150-4158

reactivate ESR1 and ESR2 expression in cancer cells and used to treat myelodysplastic syndromes. However almost 20 years later this drug was reported to blunt inflammation in endothelial cells in a mouse model of atherosclerosis (Dunn et al. 2014). The FDA-approved drug Vorinostat (suberoylanilide hydroxamic acid), a histone deacetylase inhibitor, has shown to prevent eNOS uncoupling, NF-kB signaling, and oxidative stress in experimental diabetes (Advani et al. 2011). Vorinostat also promotes the autophagic flux, a process which is defective in atherosclerosis (Xie et al. 2014). In experimental models of atherosclerosis, the HDAC inhibitor sodium butyrate was shown to blunt NF-kB signaling and inflammatory molecules, namely TNF-α, IL-6, VCAM-1, and ICAM-1 (Hu et al. 2014). Chronic treatment with the SIRT1 activator resveratrol improves endothelial function and insulin sensitivity in patients with obesity and T2D (Pollack and Crandall 2013). Metformin and glucagon-like peptide 1 (GLP-1), widely-used anti-diabetic

Table 1 Epigenetic drugs with potential application for the prevention and treatment of atherosclerosis

Drug	Epigenetic mechanism	Main finding
RG108	DNMT inhibitor	RG108 resets the expression of senescence-related genes in BM-derived stem cells
Azaticidine (5-AZA)	DNMT inhibitor	Blunts the upregulation of inflammatory genes in endothelial cells
(SAHA)/ Vorinostat	HDAC inhibitor	Prevents eNOS uncoupling and activation of NF-kB signalling in the setting of diabetes. Reactivates autophagy
Sodium butyrate	HDAC inhibitor	Suppresses NF-kB signaling and transcription of NF-kB-dependent inflammatory molecules
Resveratrol	HDAC activator	Improves endothelial function in obese and diabetic patients by activating SIRT1
Metformin	HDAC activator	Preserves the expression of genes implicated in beta cell function and insulin signaling via activation of SIRT1
GLP-1	HDAC activator	Modulates SIRT1 activity thus preserving insulin signaling
Curcumin	HAT inhibitor	Reduces the expression of proatherogenic cytokines and attenuates atherosclerotic lesion size in ApoE and LDLR double knockout mice. Curcumin supplementation in diabetic patients ameliorates proteinuria, reduces pro-fibrotic cytokines and improves microangiopathy.
Apabetalone	BET inhibitor	Stimulates reverse cholesterol transport by inducing ApoAI expression and increasing HDL levels. It has also shown to decrease systemic inflammation in humans, as assessed by C-reactive protein as well as to act as an anti-thrombotic agent.

DNMT DNA methyltransferase, *HAT* histone acetyltransferase, *HDAC* histone deacetylase, *HMT* histone methyltransferase

medications, have also shown to modulate SIRT1 activity, thus affecting histone acetylation and transcription of genes implicated in beta cell function and preservation of insulin signaling (Costantino et al. 2015). The histone acetyltransferase p300 inhibitor curcumin has shown to reduce lipopolysaccharide-induced expression of key proatherogenic cytokines such as MCP-1, IL-1β, and TNF-α in primary human monocytes as well as to reduce macrophage polarization (Moss and Ramji 2016). Chronic treatment (4 months) with curcumin reduced atherosclerotic lesion size in ApoE and LDLr double knockout mice (Hasan et al. 2014). Moreover, a randomized double-blind trial involving 240 individuals with T2D reported a decrease in CVD risk with 6 months of curcumin dietary supplementation, exemplified through a lower pulse wave velocity and improved metabolic profile (Chuengsamarn et al. 2014). In T2D patients, chronic supplementation with curcumin (1–2 months) ameliorated proteinuria, reduced pro-fibrotic cytokines (i.e., TGF-β and IL-8), and improved microangiopathy (Khajehdehi et al. 2011). Current limitations in the use of curcumin include its poor bioavailability due to a very rapid excretion from the body (Lopresti 2018). The use of liposomal curcumin, nanoparticles, and a curcumin phospholipid complex represents current strategies to boost the clinical applicability of this compound. Several other compounds including folates, apicidin, PPARγ agonists, and valproic acid have shown the ability to revert chromatin modifications in cardiometabolic states (Napoli et al. 2012). Recent evidence indicates that apabetalone (RVX-208) – an epigenetic regulator targeting bromodomain and extra-terminal (BET) proteins – stimulates reverse cholesterol transport by inducing ApoAI expression and increasing HDL levels (Ghosh et al. 2017). This drug has also shown to decrease systemic inflammation in humans, as assessed by C-reactive protein as well as to act as an anti-thrombotic agent (Schooling and Zhao 2019). Pooled analysis of short-term non-randomized studies showed fewer cardiovascular events among patients treated with apabetalone as compared to placebo (Nicholls et al. 2018). The recent phase III BETonMACE trial, designed to investigate the impact of apabetalone on cardiovascular outcomes in 2425 patients with diabetes after an ACS, failed to meet the primary endpoint (cardiovascular death, non-fatal myocardial infarction, or stroke) (Ray et al. 2020). However, the drug showed to significantly impact on secondary endpoints. Undoubtedly, larger clinical trials are needed to better explore the safety and efficacy of apabetalone for the treatment of cardiovascular disease.

7   Conclusions

Evidence discussed here suggests that epigenetic processing plays a central role in the pathogenesis of atherosclerosis. Specific epigenetic patterns, characterized by modifications of DNA/histone complexes as well as by ncRNAs, have shown to promote transcriptional programs involved in inflammation, oxidative stress, and endothelial dysfunction. Plastic changes may also contribute to the phenotypic switch of SMCs, a key factor involved in the pathophysiology of atherosclerosis. A careful analysis of the individual epigenetic landscape may furnish novel biomarkers of atherosclerotic vascular disease. An important challenge is the demonstration that epigenetic signals are causally linked to vascular disease phenotypes. The causality of presumed epigenetic events and atherosclerotic phenotypes can be assessed by using different strategies. One possibility would be using longitudinal studies whereby the epigenome can be profiled before the onset of the disease and during follow-up. Alternatively, specific tools, such as the framework of Mendelian randomization which explores the causal link between exposure, epigenetic marks and outcome, can be employed to discriminate between epigenetic phenomena and epi-phenomena. Ongoing epigenomic studies will help to unveil the complex relationship among genetics, epigenetics, and CVD, and will contribute to characterize the incremental value of epigenetic information over established clinical and genetic scores. Epigenetic information can also be used to develop new mechanism-based therapies. The growing understanding of chromatin architecture and metabolism has led to the design of specific molecules able to modulate chromatin accessibility by enhancing or repressing epigenetic marks on DNA/histone complexes. Noteworthy, some of these drugs have been already approved for the treatment of several conditions including cancer, neurological and cardiovascular disease. Taken together, epigenetic information could advance individualized risk assessment and personalized therapeutic approaches in patients with cardiometabolic disturbances.

Acknowledgments F.P. is the recipient of a H.H. Sheikh Khalifa bin Hamad Al Thani Foundation Assistant Professorship at the Faculty of Medicine, University of Zurich. The present work is supported by the Zürich Heart House, the Swiss Heart Foundation, Swiss Life Foundation, Kurt und Senta-Hermann Stiftung, the EMDO Stiftung, the Olga Mayenfisch Stiftung and the Schweizerische Diabetes-Stiftung to F.P; the Holcim Foundation and the Swiss Heart Foundation to S.C

References

Aavik E, Lumivuori H, Leppanen O, Wirth T, Hakkinen SK, Brasen JH, Beschorner U, Zeller T, Braspenning M, van Criekinge W, Makinen K, Yla-Herttuala S (2015) Global DNA methylation analysis of human atherosclerotic plaques reveals extensive genomic hypomethylation and reactivation at imprinted locus 14q32 involving induction of a miRNA cluster. Eur Heart J 36 (16):993–1000

Aavik E, Babu M, Yla-Herttuala S (2019) DNA methylation processes in atheosclerotic plaque. Atherosclerosis 281:168–179

Advani A, Huang Q, Thai K, Advani SL, White KE, Kelly DJ, Yuen DA, Connelly KA, Marsden PA, Gilbert RE (2011) Long-term administration of the histone deacetylase inhibitor vorinostat attenuates renal injury in experimental diabetes through an endothelial nitric oxide synthase-dependent mechanism. Am J Pathol 178(5):2205–2214

Ashburner BP, Westerheide SD, Baldwin AS Jr (2001) The p65 (RelA) subunit of NF-kappaB interacts with the histone deacetylase (HDAC) corepressors HDAC1 and HDAC2 to negatively regulate gene expression. Mol Cell Biol 21(20):7065–7077

Baccarelli A, Ghosh S (2012) Environmental exposures, epigenetics and cardiovascular disease. Curr Opin Clin Nutr Metab Care 15(4):323–329

Bannister AJ, Kouzarides T (2011) Regulation of chromatin by histone modifications. Cell Res 21 (3):381–395

Bauer AJ, Martin KA (2017) Coordinating regulation of gene expression in cardiovascular disease: interactions between chromatin modifiers and transcription factors. Front Cardiovasc Med 4:19

Bernstein BE, Meissner A. Lander ES (2007) The mammalian epigenome. Cell 128(4):669–681

Bostick M, Kim JK, Esteve PO, Clark A, Pradhan S, Jacobsen SE (2007) UHRF1 plays a role in maintaining DNA methylation in mammalian cells. Science 317(5845):1760–1764

Brasacchio D, Okabe J, Tikellis C, Balcerczyk A, George P, Baker EK, Calkin AC, Brownlee M, Cooper ME, El-Osta A (2009) Hyperglycemia induces a dynamic cooperativity of histone methylase and demethylase enzymes associated with gene-activating epigenetic marks that coexist on the lysine tail. Diabetes 58(5):1229–1236

Brown CL, Halvorson EE, Cohen GM, Lazorick S, Skelton JA (2015) Addressing childhood obesity: opportunities for prevention. Pediatr Clin North Am 62(5):1241–1261

Brunet A, Berger SL (2014) Epigenetics of aging and aging-related disease. J Gerontol A Biol Sci Med Sci 69(Suppl 1):S17–S20

Carrizzo A, Puca A, Damato A, Marino M, Franco E, Pompeo F, Traficante A, Civitillo F, Santini L, Trimarco V, Vecchione C (2013) Resveratrol improves vascular function in patients with hypertension and dyslipidemia by modulating NO metabolism. Hypertension 62 (2):359–366

Carrozza MJ, Utley RT, Workman JL, Cote J (2003) The diverse functions of histone acetyltransferase complexes. Trends Genet 19(6):321–329

Cedar H, Bergman Y (2009) Linking DNA methylation and histone modification: patterns and paradigms. Nat Rev Genet 10(5):295–304

Challen GA, Sun D, Jeong M, Luo M, Jelinek J, Berg JS, Bock C, Vasanthakumar A, Gu H, Xi Y, Liang S, Lu Y, Darlington GJ, Meissner A, Issa JP, Godley LA, Li W, Goodell MA (2011) Dnmt3a is essential for hematopoietic stem cell differentiation. Nat Genet 44(1):23–31

Chan Y, Fish JE, D'Abreo C, Lin S, Robb GB, Teichert AM, Karantzoulis-Fegaras F, Keightley A, Steer BM, Marsden PA (2004) The cell-specific expression of endothelial nitric-oxide synthase: a role for DNA methylation. J Biol Chem 279(33):35087–35100

Chen SH, Lv QL, Hu L, Peng MJ, Wang GH, Sun B (2017) DNA methylation alterations in the pathogenesis of lupus. Clin Exp Immunol 187(2):185–192

Choi JH, Nam KH, Kim J, Baek MW, Park JE, Park HY, Kwon HJ, Kwon OS, Kim DY, Oh GT (2005) Trichostatin A exacerbates atherosclerosis in low density lipoprotein receptor-deficient mice. Arterioscler Thromb Vasc Biol 25(11):2404–2409

Chuengsamarn S, Rattanamongkolgul S, Phonrat B, Tungtrongchitr R, Jirawatnotai S (2014) Reduction of atherogenic risk in patients with type 2 diabetes by curcuminoid extract: a randomized controlled trial. J Nutr Biochem 25(2):144–150

Cooper ME, El-Osta A (2010) Epigenetics: mechanisms and implications for diabetic complications. Circ Res 107(12):1403–1413

Costantino S, Paneni F, Cosentino F (2015) Targeting chromatin remodeling to prevent cardiovascular disease in diabetes. Curr Pharm Biotechnol 16(6):531–543

Costantino S, Paneni F, Battista R, Castello L, Capretti G, Chiandotto S, Tanese L, Russo G, Pitocco D, Lanza GA, Volpe M, Luscher TF, Cosentino F (2017) Impact of glycemic variability on chromatin remodeling, oxidative stress, and endothelial dysfunction in patients with type 2 diabetes and with target HbA1c levels. Diabetes 66(9):2472–2482

Costantino S, Paneni F, Mitchell K, Mohammed SA, Hussain S, Gkolfos C, Berrino L, Volpe M, Schwarzwald C, Luscher TF, Cosentino F (2018a) Hyperglycaemia-induced epigenetic changes drive persistent cardiac dysfunction via the adaptor p66(Shc). Int J Cardiol 268:179–186

Costantino S, Camici GG, Mohammed SA, Volpe M, Luscher TF, Paneni F (2018b) Epigenetics and cardiovascular regenerative medicine in the elderly. Int J Cardiol 250:207–214

Costantino S, Libby P, Kishore R, Tardif JC, El-Osta A, Paneni F (2018c) Epigenetics and precision medicine in cardiovascular patients: from basic concepts to the clinical arena. Eur Heart J 39 (47):4150–4158

Costantino S, Paneni F, Virdis A, Hussain S, Mohammed SA, Capretti G, Akhmedov A, Dalgaard K, Chiandotto S, Pospisilik JA, Jenuwein T, Giorgio M, Volpe M, Taddei S, Luscher TF, Cosentino F (2019) Interplay among H3K9-editing enzymes SUV39H1, JMJD2C and SRC-1 drives p66Shc transcription and vascular oxidative stress in obesity. Eur Heart J 40 (4):383–391

Davis FM, Gallagher KA (2019) Epigenetic mechanisms in monocytes/macrophages regulate inflammation in cardiometabolic and vascular disease. Arterioscler Thromb Vasc Biol 39 (4):623–634

Deng WG, Zhu Y, Wu KK (2004) Role of p300 and PCAF in regulating cyclooxygenase-2-promoter activation by inflammatory mediators. Blood 103(6):2135–2142

Dunn J, Qiu H, Kim S, Jjingo D, Hoffman R, Kim CW, Jang I, Son DJ, Kim D, Pan C, Fan Y, Jordan IK, Jo H (2014) Flow-dependent epigenetic DNA methylation regulates endothelial gene expression and atherosclerosis. J Clin Invest 124(7):3187–3199

Elia L, Condorelli G (2019) The involvement of epigenetics in vascular disease development. Int J Biochem Cell Biol 107:27–31

El-Osta A, Brasacchio D, Yao D, Pocai A, Jones PL, Roeder RG, Cooper ME, Brownlee M (2008) Transient high glucose causes persistent epigenetic changes and altered gene expression during subsequent normoglycemia. J Exp Med 205(10):2409–2417

Filippakopoulos P, Knapp S (2014) Targeting bromodomains: epigenetic readers of lysine acetylation. Nat Rev Drug Discov 13(5):337–356

Findeisen HM, Gizard F, Zhao Y, Qing H, Heywood EB, Jones KL, Cohn D, Bruemmer D (2011) Epigenetic regulation of vascular smooth muscle cell proliferation and neointima formation by histone deacetylase inhibition. Arterioscler Thromb Vasc Biol 31(4):851–860

Fraga MF, Ballestar E, Paz MF, Ropero S, Setien F, Ballestar ML, Heine-Suner D, Cigudosa JC, Urioste M, Benitez J, Boix-Chornet M, Sanchez-Aguilera A, Ling C, Carlsson E, Poulsen P, Vaag A, Stephan Z, Spector TD, Wu YZ, Plass C, Esteller M (2005) Epigenetic differences arise during the lifetime of monozygotic twins. Proc Natl Acad Sci U S A 102(30):10604–10609

Fuster JJ, MacLauchlan S, Zuriaga MA, Polackal MN, Ostriker AC, Chakraborty R, Wu CL, Sano S, Muralidharan S, Rius C, Vuong J, Jacob S, Muralidhar V, Robertson AA, Cooper MA, Andres V, Hirschi KK, Martin KA, Walsh K (2017) Clonal hematopoiesis associated with TET2 deficiency accelerates atherosclerosis development in mice. Science 355(6327):842–847

Garcia-Cardona MC, Huang F, Garcia-Vivas JM, Lopez-Camarillo C, Del Rio Navarro BE, Navarro Olivos E, Hong-Chong E, Bolanos-Jimenez F, Marchat LA (2014) DNA methylation of leptin and adiponectin promoters in children is reduced by the combined presence of obesity and insulin resistance. Int J Obes 38(11):1457–1465

Ghosh GC, Bhadra R, Ghosh RK, Banerjee K, Gupta A (2017) RVX 208: a novel BET protein inhibitor, role as an inducer of apo A-I/HDL and beyond. Cardiovasc Ther 35(4):e12265

Gillette TG, Hill JA (2015) Readers, writers, and erasers: chromatin as the whiteboard of heart disease. Circ Res 116(7):1245–1253

Goldberg AD, Allis CD, Bernstein E (2007) Epigenetics: a landscape takes shape. Cell 128 (4):635–638

Gonzalez-Recio O, Toro MA, Bach A (2015) Past, present, and future of epigenetics applied to livestock breeding. Front Genet 6:305

Greco CM, Kunderfranco P, Rubino M, Larcher V, Carullo P, Anselmo A, Kurz K, Carell T, Angius A, Latronico MV, Papait R, Condorelli G (2016) DNA hydroxymethylation controls cardiomyocyte gene expression in development and hypertrophy. Nat Commun 7:12418

Haberland M, Montgomery RL, Olson EN (2009) The many roles of histone deacetylases in development and physiology: implications for disease and therapy. Nat Rev Genet 10(1):32–42

Hamidi T, Singh AK, Chen T (2015) Genetic alterations of DNA methylation machinery in human diseases. Epigenomics 7(2):247–265

Handy DE, Castro R, Loscalzo J (2011) Epigenetic modifications: basic mechanisms and role in cardiovascular disease. Circulation 123(19):2145–2156

Hannum G, Guinney J, Zhao L, Zhang L, Hughes G, Sadda S, Klotzle B, Bibikova M, Fan JB, Gao Y, Deconde R, Chen M, Rajapakse I, Friend S, Ideker T, Zhang K (2013) Genome-wide methylation profiles reveal quantitative views of human aging rates. Mol Cell 49(2):359–367

Hasan ST, Zingg JM, Kwan P, Noble T, Smith D, Meydani M (2014) Curcumin modulation of high fat diet-induced atherosclerosis and steatohepatosis in LDL receptor deficient mice. Atherosclerosis 232(1):40–51

Heard E, Martienssen RA (2014) Transgenerational epigenetic inheritance: myths and mechanisms. Cell 157(1):95–109

Heijmans BT, Tobi EW, Stein AD, Putter H, Blauw GJ, Susser ES, Slagboom PE, Lumey LH (2008) Persistent epigenetic differences associated with prenatal exposure to famine in humans. Proc Natl Acad Sci U S A 105(44):17046–17049

Heyn H, Li N, Ferreira HJ, Moran S, Pisano DG, Gomez A, Diez J, Sanchez-Mut JV, Setien F, Carmona FJ, Puca AA, Sayols S, Pujana MA, Serra-Musach J, Iglesias-Platas I, Formiga F, Fernandez AF, Fraga MF, Heath SC, Valencia A, Gut IG, Wang J, Esteller M (2012) Distinct DNA methylomes of newborns and centenarians. Proc Natl Acad Sci U S A 109 (26):10522–10527

Hiltunen MO, Yla-Herttuala S (2003) DNA methylation, smooth muscle cells, and atherogenesis. Arterioscler Thromb Vasc Biol 23(10):1750–1753

Horsthemke B (2018) A critical view on transgenerational epigenetic inheritance in humans. Nat Commun 9(1):2973

Hu X, Zhang K, Xu C, Chen Z, Jiang H (2014) Anti-inflammatory effect of sodium butyrate preconditioning during myocardial ischemia/reperfusion. Exp Ther Med 8(1):229–232

Izquierdo AG, Crujeiras AB (2019) Role of epigenomic mechanisms in the onset and management of insulin resistance. Rev Endocr Metab Disord 20(1):89–102

Jaiswal S, Natarajan P, Silver AJ, Gibson CJ, Bick AG, Shvartz E, McConkey M, Gupta N, Gabriel S, Ardissino D, Baber U, Mehran R, Fuster V, Danesh J, Frossard P, Saleheen D, Melander O, Sukhova GK, Neuberg D, Libby P, Kathiresan S, Ebert BL (2017) Clonal hematopoiesis and risk of atherosclerotic cardiovascular disease. N Engl J Med 377(2):111–121

Jiang W, Agrawal DK, Boosani CS (2018) Cellspecific histone modifications in atherosclerosis (review). Mol Med Rep 18(2):1215–1224

Jones PL, Veenstra GJ, Wade PA, Vermaak D, Kass SU, Landsberger N, Strouboulis J, Wolffe AP (1998) Methylated DNA and MeCP2 recruit histone deacetylase to repress transcription. Nat Genet 19(2):187–191

Juonala M, Magnussen CG, Berenson GS, Venn A, Burns TL, Sabin MA, Srinivasan SR, Daniels SR, Davis PH, Chen W, Sun C, Cheung M, Viikari JS, Dwyer T, Raitakari OT (2011) Childhood adiposity, adult adiposity, and cardiovascular risk factors. N Engl J Med 365 (20):1876–1885

Khajehdehi P, Pakfetrat M, Javidnia K, Azad F, Malekmakan L, Nasab MH, Dehghanzadeh G (2011) Oral supplementation of turmeric attenuates proteinuria, transforming growth factor-beta and interleukin-8 levels in patients with overt type 2 diabetic nephropathy: a randomized, double-blind and placebo-controlled study. Scand J Urol Nephrol 45(5):365–370

Khyzha N, Alizada A, Wilson MD, Fish JE (2017) Epigenetics of atherosclerosis: emerging mechanisms and methods. Trends Mol Med 23(4):332–347

Kohli RM, Zhang Y (2013) TET enzymes, TDG and the dynamics of DNA demethylation. Nature 502(7472):472–479

Kouzarides T (2007) Chromatin modifications and their function. Cell 128(4):693–705

Kwon IS, Wang W, Xu S, Jin ZG (2014) Histone deacetylase 5 interacts with Kruppel-like factor 2 and inhibits its transcriptional activity in endothelium. Cardiovasc Res 104(1):127–137

Landmesser U, Poller W, Tsimikas S, Most P, Paneni F, Luscher TF (2020) From traditional pharmacological towards nucleic acid-based therapies for cardiovascular diseases. Eur Heart J. https://doi.org/10.1093/eurheartj/ehaa229

Li B, Carey M, Workman JL (2007) The role of chromatin during transcription. Cell 128 (4):707–719

Li G, Peng J, Liu Y, Li X, Yang Q, Li Y, Tang Z, Wang Z, Jiang Z, Wei D (2015) Oxidized low-density lipoprotein inhibits THP-1-derived macrophage autophagy via TET2 down-regulation. Lipids 50(2):177–183

Li F, Wu X, Zhou Q, Zhu DW (2018) Clonal hematopoiesis of indeterminate potential (CHIP): a potential contributor to atherlosclerotic cardio/cerebro-vascular diseases? Genes Dis 5(2):75–76

Lopresti AL (2018) The problem of curcumin and its bioavailability: could its gastrointestinal influence contribute to its overall health-enhancing effects? Adv Nutr 9(1):41–50

Masi S, Ambrosini S, Mohammed SA, Sciarretta S, Luscher TF, Paneni F, Costantino S (2020) Epigenetic remodeling in obesity-related vascular disease. Antioxid Redox Signal. https://doi.org/10.1089/ars.2020.8040

Maunakea AK, Nagarajan RP, Bilenky M, Ballinger TJ, D'Souza C, Fouse SD, Johnson BE, Hong C, Nielsen C, Zhao Y, Turecki G, Delaney A, Varhol R, Thiessen N, Shchors K, Heine VM, Rowitch DH, Xing X, Fiore C, Schillebeeckx M, Jones SJ, Haussler D, Marra MA, Hirst M, Wang T, Costello JF (2010) Conserved role of intragenic DNA methylation in regulating alternative promoters. Nature 466(7303):253–257

Metzger E, Wissmann M, Yin N, Muller JM, Schneider R, Peters AH, Gunther T, Buettner R, Schule R (2005) LSD1 demethylates repressive histone marks to promote androgen-receptor-dependent transcription. Nature 437(7057):436–439

Ming GF, Tang YJ, Hu K, Chen Y, Huang WH, Xiao J (2016) Visfatin attenuates the ox-LDL-induced senescence of endothelial progenitor cells by upregulating SIRT1 expression through the PI3K/Akt/ERK pathway. Int J Mol Med 38(2):643–649

Mohammed SA, Ambrosini S, Luscher T, Paneni F, Costantino S (2020) Epigenetic control of mitochondrial function in the vasculature. Front Cardiovasc Med 7:28

Moran-Crusio K, Reavie L, Shih A, Abdel-Wahab O, Ndiaye-Lobry D, Lobry C, Figueroa ME, Vasanthakumar A, Patel J, Zhao X, Perna F, Pandey S, Madzo J, Song C, Dai Q, He C, Ibrahim S, Beran M, Zavadil J, Nimer SD, Melnick A, Godley LA, Aifantis I, Levine RL (2011) Tet2 loss leads to increased hematopoietic stem cell self-renewal and myeloid transformation. Cancer Cell 20(1):11–24

Moss JW, Ramji DP (2016) Nutraceutical therapies for atherosclerosis. Nat Rev Cardiol 13 (9):513–532

Napoli C, Crudele V, Soricelli A, Al-Omran M, Vitale N, Infante T, Mancini FP (2012) Primary prevention of atherosclerosis: a clinical challenge for the reversal of epigenetic mechanisms? Circulation 125(19):2363–2373

Nicholls SJ, Ray KK, Johansson JO, Gordon A, Sweeney M, Halliday C, Kulikowski E, Wong N, Kim SW, Schwartz GG (2018) Selective BET protein inhibition with apabetalone and cardiovascular events: a pooled analysis of trials in patients with coronary artery disease. Am J Cardiovasc Drugs 18(2):109–115

Nicorescu I, Dallinga GM, de Winther MPJ, Stroes ESG, Bahjat M (2019) Potential epigenetic therapeutics for atherosclerosis treatment. Atherosclerosis 281:189–197

Noble D (2015) Conrad Waddington and the origin of epigenetics. J Exp Biol 218(Pt 6):816–818

Oh YS, Jeong SG, Cho GW (2015) Anti-senescence effects of DNA methyltransferase inhibitor RG108 in human bone marrow mesenchymal stromal cells. Biotechnol Appl Biochem 62 (5):583–590

Okabe J, Orlowski C, Balcerczyk A, Tikellis C, Thomas MC, Cooper ME, El-Osta A (2012) Distinguishing hyperglycemic changes by Set7 in vascular endothelial cells. Circ Res 110 (8):1067–1076

Okano M, Bell DW, Haber DA, Li E (1999) DNA methyltransferases Dnmt3a and Dnmt3b are essential for de novo methylation and mammalian development. Cell 99(3):247–257

Paneni F, Mocharla P, Akhmedov A, Costantino S, Osto E, Volpe M, Luscher TF, Cosentino F (2012) Gene silencing of the mitochondrial adaptor p66(Shc) suppresses vascular hyperglycemic memory in diabetes. Circ Res 111(3):278–289

Paneni F, Osto E, Costantino S, Mateescu B, Briand S, Coppolino G, Perna E, Mocharla P, Akhmedov A, Kubant R, Rohrer L, Malinski T, Camici GG, Matter CM, Mechta-Grigoriou F, Volpe M, Luscher TF, Cosentino F (2013) Deletion of the activated protein-1 transcription factor JunD induces oxidative stress and accelerates age-related endothelial dysfunction. Circulation 127(11):1229–1240. e1221-1221

Paneni F, Costantino S, Castello L, Battista R, Capretti G, Chiandotto S, D'Amario D, Scavone G, Villano A, Rustighi A, Crea F, Pitocco D, Lanza G, Volpe M, Del Sal G, Luscher TF, Cosentino F (2015a) Targeting prolyl-isomerase Pin1 prevents mitochondrial oxidative stress and vascular dysfunction: insights in patients with diabetes. Eur Heart J 36(13):817–828

Paneni F, Costantino S, Battista R, Castello L, Capretti G, Chiandotto S, Scavone G, Villano A, Pitocco D, Lanza G, Volpe M, Luscher TF, Cosentino F (2015b) Adverse epigenetic signatures by histone methyltransferase Set7 contribute to vascular dysfunction in patients with type 2 diabetes mellitus. Circ Cardiovasc Genet 8(1):150–158

Paneni F, Diaz Canestro C, Libby P, Luscher TF, Camici GG (2017) The aging cardiovascular system: understanding it at the cellular and clinical levels. J Am Coll Cardiol 69(15):1952–1967

Pembrey ME, Bygren LO, Kaati G, Edvinsson S, Northstone K, Sjostrom M, Golding J, Team AS (2006) Sex-specific, male-line transgenerational responses in humans. Eur J Hum Genet 14 (2):159–166

Peng J, Yang Q, Li AF, Li RQ, Wang Z, Liu LS, Ren Z, Zheng XL, Tang XQ, Li GH, Tang ZH, Jiang ZS, Wei DH (2016) Tet methylcytosine dioxygenase 2 inhibits atherosclerosis via upregulation of autophagy in ApoE−/− mice. Oncotarget 7(47):76423–76436

Pollack RM, Crandall JP (2013) Resveratrol: therapeutic potential for improving cardiometabolic health. Am J Hypertens 26(11):1260–1268

Potente M, Ghaeni L, Baldessari D, Mostoslavsky R, Rossig L, Dequiedt F, Haendeler J, Mione M, Dejana E, Alt FW, Zeiher AM, Dimmeler S (2007) SIRT1 controls endothelial angiogenic functions during vascular growth. Genes Dev 21(20):2644–2658

Prasher D, Greenway SC, Singh RB (2019) The impact of epigenetics on cardiovascular disease. Biochem Cell Biol 98(1):12–22. https://doi.org/10.1139/bcb-2019-0045

Rask-Andersen M, Martinsson D, Ahsan M, Enroth S, Ek WE, Gyllensten U, Johansson A (2016) Epigenome-wide association study reveals differential DNA methylation in individuals with a history of myocardial infarction. Hum Mol Genet 25(21):4739–4748

Ray KK, Nicholls SJ, Buhr KA, Ginsberg HN, Johansson JO, Kalantar-Zadeh K, Kulikowski E, Toth PP, Wong N, Sweeney M, Schwartz GG, Investigators BE Committees (2020) Effect of apabetalone added to standard therapy on major adverse cardiovascular events in patients with recent acute coronary syndrome and type 2 diabetes: a randomized clinical trial. JAMA 323 (16):1565–1573. https://doi.org/10.1001/jama.2020.3308

Schooling CM, Zhao JV (2019) How might bromodomain and extra-terminal (BET) inhibitors operate in cardiovascular disease? Am J Cardiovasc Drugs 19(2):107–111

Sen P, Shah PP, Nativio R, Berger SL (2016) Epigenetic mechanisms of longevity and aging. Cell 166(4):822–839

Singer K, Lumeng CN (2017) The initiation of metabolic inflammation in childhood obesity. J Clin Invest 127(1):65–73

Slack JM (2002) Conrad Hal Waddington: the last renaissance biologist? Nat Rev Genet 3 (11):889–895

Stratton MS, Farina FM, Elia L (2019) Epigenetics and vascular diseases. J Mol Cell Cardiol 133:148–163

Stylianou E (2019) Epigenetics of chronic inflammatory diseases. J Inflamm Res 12:1–14

Suglia SF, Koenen KC, Boynton-Jarrett R, Chan PS, Clark CJ, Danese A, Faith MS, Goldstein BI, Hayman LL, Isasi CR, Pratt CA, Slopen N, Sumner JA, Turer A, Turer CB, Zachariah JP, American Heart Association Council on E, Prevention, Council on Cardiovascular Disease in the Y, Council on Functional G, Translational B, Council on C, Stroke N, Council on Quality of C, Outcomes R (2018) Childhood and adolescent adversity and cardiometabolic outcomes: a scientific statement from the American Heart Association. Circulation 137(5):e15–e28

Sun D, Luo M, Jeong M, Rodriguez B, Xia Z, Hannah R, Wang H, Le T, Faull KF, Chen R, Gu H, Bock C, Meissner A, Gottgens B, Darlington GJ, Li W, Goodell MA (2014) Epigenomic profiling of young and aged HSCs reveals concerted changes during aging that reinforce self-renewal. Cell Stem Cell 14(5):673–688

Tobi EW, Goeman JJ, Monajemi R, Gu H, Putter H, Zhang Y, Slieker RC, Stok AP, Thijssen PE, Muller F, van Zwet EW, Bock C, Meissner A, Lumey LH, Eline Slagboom P, Heijmans BT (2014) DNA methylation signatures link prenatal famine exposure to growth and metabolism. Nat Commun 5:5592

Tsukada Y, Fang J, Erdjument-Bromage H, Warren ME, Borchers CH, Tempst P, Zhang Y (2006) Histone demethylation by a family of JmjC domain-containing proteins. Nature 439 (7078):811–816

Vilkaitis G, Suetake I, Klimasauskas S, Tajima S (2005) Processive methylation of hemimethylated CpG sites by mouse Dnmt1 DNA methyltransferase. J Biol Chem 280(1):64–72

Winnik S, Auwerx J, Sinclair DA, Matter CM (2015) Protective effects of sirtuins in cardiovascular diseases: from bench to bedside. Eur Heart J 36(48):3404–3412

Wolffe AP, Jones PL, Wade PA (1999) DNA demethylation. Proc Natl Acad Sci U S A 96 (11):5894–5896

Wu SC, Zhang Y (2010) Active DNA demethylation: many roads lead to Rome. Nat Rev Mol Cell Biol 11(9):607–620

Xiao FH, Wang HT, Kong QP (2019) Dynamic DNA methylation during aging: a "prophet" of age-related outcomes. Front Genet 10:107

Xie M, Kong Y, Tan W, May H, Battiprolu PK, Pedrozo Z, Wang ZV, Morales C, Luo X, Cho G, Jiang N, Jessen ME, Warner JJ, Lavandero S, Gillette TG, Turer AT, Hill JA (2014) Histone deacetylase inhibition blunts ischemia/reperfusion injury by inducing cardiomyocyte autophagy. Circulation 129(10):1139–1151

Xu S, Pelisek J, Jin ZG (2018) Atherosclerosis is an epigenetic disease. Trends Endocrinol Metab 29(11):739–742

Yan Q, Sun L, Zhu Z, Wang L, Li S, Ye RD (2014) Jmjd3-mediated epigenetic regulation of inflammatory cytokine gene expression in serum amyloid A-stimulated macrophages. Cell Signal 26(9):1783–1791

Yang X, Lay F, Han H, Jones PA (2010) Targeting DNA methylation for epigenetic therapy. Trends Pharmacol Sci 31(11):536–546

Zampetaki A, Zeng L, Margariti A, Xiao Q, Li H, Zhang Z, Pepe AE, Wang G, Habi O, deFalco E, Cockerill G, Mason JC, Hu Y, Xu Q (2010) Histone deacetylase 3 is critical in endothelial survival and atherosclerosis development in response to disturbed flow. Circulation 121 (1):132–142

Zhang W, Xu J (2017) DNA methyltransferases and their roles in tumorigenesis. Biomark Res 5:1

Zhang X, Su J, Jeong M, Ko M, Huang Y, Park HJ, Guzman A, Lei Y, Huang YH, Rao A, Li W, Goodell MA (2016) DNMT3A and TET2 compete and cooperate to repress lineage-specific transcription factors in hematopoietic stem cells. Nat Genet 48(9):1014–1023

Zhang W, Song M, Qu J, Liu GH (2018) Epigenetic modifications in cardiovascular aging and diseases. Circ Res 123(7):773–786

Zhou S, Chen HZ, Wan YZ, Zhang QJ, Wei YS, Huang S, Liu JJ, Lu YB, Zhang ZQ, Yang RF, Zhang R, Cai H, Liu DP, Liang CC (2011) Repression of P66Shc expression by SIRT1 contributes to the prevention of hyperglycemia-induced endothelial dysfunction. Circ Res 109 (6):639–648

Zuo HP, Guo YY, Che L, Wu XZ (2016) Hypomethylation of interleukin-6 promoter is associated with the risk of coronary heart disease. Arq Bras Cardiol 107(2):131–136

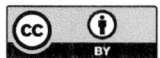

Correction to: Blood Pressure-Lowering Therapy

Isabella Sudano ⓘ, Elena Osto ⓘ, and Frank Ruschitzka ⓘ

Correction to:
Chapter "Blood Pressure-Lowering Therapy" in:
Isabella Sudano et al., Handbook of Experimental
Pharmacology,
https://doi.org/10.1007/164_2020_372

The Open Access chapter 'Blood Pressure-Lowering Therapy' was published online unfortunately without the Conflict of Interest statement. The COI statement should appear as:

FR reports grant support for the ESC-HFA Postgraduate Course in Heart Failure from Novartis, Servier, Bayer, Abbott and Astra Zeneca and the VASCEND trial from Novartis (all payments directly to the University of Zurich).

FR has been paid for the time spent as a committee member for clinical trials, advisory boards, other forms of consulting and lectures or presentations. These payments were made directly to the University of Zurich and no personal payments were received in relation to these trials or other activities since January 2018.

The updated online version of this chapter can be found at
https://doi.org/10.1007/164_2020_372

I. Sudano · F. Ruschitzka (✉)
Department of Cardiology, University Heart Center Zurich, Zürich, Switzerland
e-mail: frank.ruschitzka@usz.ch

E. Osto
Department of Cardiology, University Heart Center Zurich, Zürich, Switzerland

Institute of Clinical Chemistry, University of Zurich, University Hospital Zurich, Zürich, Switzerland

© The Author(s) 2020
A. von Eckardstein, C. J. Binder (eds.), *Prevention and Treatment of Atherosclerosis*,
Handbook of Experimental Pharmacology 270, https://doi.org/10.1007/164_2020_410

Before 2018, FR reports grants and personal fees from SJM/Abbott, Servier, Novartis and Bayer, personal fees from Zoll, Astra Zeneca, Sanofi, Amgen, BMS, Pfizer, Fresenius, Vifor, Roche, Cardiorentis and Boehringer Ingelheim, other from Heartware and grants from Mars, outside the submitted work.

These corrections have been updated in the original chapter.